# The *Physician Manager's* Handbook

## *Essential Business Skills for Succeeding in Health Care*

### Second Edition

**Robert J. Solomon, PhD**
*Professor of Business Administration*
*Mason School of Business*
*The College of William and Mary*
*Williamsburg, Virginia*

**JONES AND BARTLETT PUBLISHERS**
*Sudbury, Massachusetts*
BOSTON   TORONTO   LONDON   SINGAPORE

*World Headquarters*

Jones and Bartlett Publishers
40 Tall Pine Drive
Sudbury, MA 01776
978-443-5000
info@jbpub.com
www.jbpub.com

Jones and Bartlett Publishers
Canada
6339 Ormindale Way
Mississauga, Ontario L5V 1J2
CANADA

Jones and Bartlett Publishers
International
Barb House, Barb Mews
London W6 7PA
United Kingdom

Jones and Bartlett's books and products are available through most bookstores and online booksellers. To contact Jones and Bartlett Publishers directly, call 800-832-0034, fax 978-443-8000, or visit our website www.jbpub.com.

Substantial discounts on bulk quantities of Jones and Bartlett's publications are available to corporations, professional associations, and other qualified organizations. For details and specific discount information, contact the special sales department at Jones and Bartlett via the above contact information or send an email to specialsales@jbpub.com.

This publication is designed to provide accurate and authoritative information in regard to the subject matter covered. It is sold with the understanding that the publisher is not engaged in rendering legal, accounting, or other professional service. If legal advice or other expert assistance is required, the service of a competent professional person should be sought.

**Production Credits**
Executive Editor: David Cella
Editorial Assistant: Lisa Gordon
Production Director: Amy Rose
Production Editor: Renée Sekerak
Production Assistant: Julia Waugaman
Associate Marketing Manager: Jennifer Bengtson
Manufacturing and Inventory Control Supervisor: Amy Bacus
Composition: Auburn Associates, Inc.
Cover Design: Kate Ternullo
Printing and Binding: Malloy Incorporated
Cover Printing: Malloy Incorporated

**Library of Congress Cataloging-in-Publication Data**
Solomon, Robert J., 1947-
   The physician manager's handbook : essential business skills for succeeding in health care / by Robert Solomon. — 2nd ed.
      p. ; cm.
   Includes bibliographical references and index.
   ISBN 978-0-7637-4603-2
   1. Health services administration—United States—Handbooks, manuals, etc. 2. Health facilities—United States—Business management—Handbooks, manuals, etc. 3. Physician executives—United States—Handbooks, manuals, etc.
I. Title.
   [DNLM: 1. Practice Management, Medical—organization & administration—United States. 2. Financial Management—organization & administration—United States. 3. Personnel Management—methods—United States.
   W 80 S689p 2008]
   RA971.S677 2008
   610.68—dc22
                                                                                    2007032483
6048

Printed in the United States of America
11 10 09 08 07   10 9 8 7 6 5 4 3 2 1

# Contents

Acknowledgments . . . . . . . . . . . . . . . . . . . . . . . . . . . . . . . . . . . . . . . . . vii
Introduction . . . . . . . . . . . . . . . . . . . . . . . . . . . . . . . . . . . . . . . . . . . . . . viii

**Chapter 1**  **Financial Management** . . . . . . . . . . . . . . . . . . . . . . . . . . . . . . . 1
                CVP Analysis . . . . . . . . . . . . . . . . . . . . . . . . . . . . . . . . . . . 2
                Capital Asset Planning . . . . . . . . . . . . . . . . . . . . . . . . . . . . 11
                Lease Versus Purchase Decisions . . . . . . . . . . . . . . . . . . . . . 21
                Financial Statements, Reports, and Accounting Systems . . . . . . . 22
                Uses for Ratios . . . . . . . . . . . . . . . . . . . . . . . . . . . . . . . . . 36
                Control and Budgeting . . . . . . . . . . . . . . . . . . . . . . . . . . . . 36
                Activity-Based Costing . . . . . . . . . . . . . . . . . . . . . . . . . . . . 46
                Conclusion . . . . . . . . . . . . . . . . . . . . . . . . . . . . . . . . . . . . 57

**Chapter 2**  **Cash Management and Collection in Private Practices** . . . . . . . 61
                Cash Management . . . . . . . . . . . . . . . . . . . . . . . . . . . . . . . 62
                Revenue and Procedure Database . . . . . . . . . . . . . . . . . . . . . 65
                Cash Receipts and Disbursements . . . . . . . . . . . . . . . . . . . . . 66
                Applied Cash Management Procedures . . . . . . . . . . . . . . . . . . 70
                Case Illustrations . . . . . . . . . . . . . . . . . . . . . . . . . . . . . . . . 72
                The Small Practice Physician Manager's Role in Cash Control . . . . 72
                Collection Management . . . . . . . . . . . . . . . . . . . . . . . . . . . . 74
                Collection Roles and Responsibilities . . . . . . . . . . . . . . . . . . . 74
                Case Analysis: Rewards and Behaviors . . . . . . . . . . . . . . . . . . 82
                Collecting from Patients . . . . . . . . . . . . . . . . . . . . . . . . . . . 83
                The Patient Intake Process . . . . . . . . . . . . . . . . . . . . . . . . . . 86
                Patient Education . . . . . . . . . . . . . . . . . . . . . . . . . . . . . . . . 87
                Billing Strategies . . . . . . . . . . . . . . . . . . . . . . . . . . . . . . . . 90
                Collecting Overdue Patient Balances . . . . . . . . . . . . . . . . . . . 92
                Placing an Account in Collection . . . . . . . . . . . . . . . . . . . . . . 96
                Collecting from Insurance Companies . . . . . . . . . . . . . . . . . . 98
                Problem Account Detection and Timing . . . . . . . . . . . . . . . . . 102
                Collection Database . . . . . . . . . . . . . . . . . . . . . . . . . . . . . . 103
                The Collection Plan . . . . . . . . . . . . . . . . . . . . . . . . . . . . . . 104
                What to Do if Your Accounts Are Out of Control . . . . . . . . . . . 104
                Conclusion . . . . . . . . . . . . . . . . . . . . . . . . . . . . . . . . . . . . 106

Appendix 2A   Sample Collection Plan (Partial)............................107
              Patient Intake Process.....................................107
              Patient Education Process..................................107
              Verification and Preauthorizations.........................107
              Copayment Collection Procedures............................108
              Insurance Billing Procedures...............................108
              Problem Account Detection..................................108
              Collection Steps and Sequencing............................108

**Chapter 3    Evaluating Performance................................109**
              Performance Appraisal: Context.............................109
              Performance Appraisal: The Short Course....................111
              Conducting the Annual Appraisal............................121
              Performance Evaluation Data................................128
              Performance Standards......................................129
              Rating Forms...............................................130
              Improving Performance......................................132
              Evaluating Physician Performance...........................132
              Performance-Appraisal Summary..............................136

**Chapter 4    Employment Methods....................................137**
              Introduction...............................................137
              Using the Job Description: Identifying Selection Factors....139
              Recruiting.................................................141
              Developing Selection Procedures: The Big Picture...........143
              Selection Procedures.......................................147
              Who Should Design and Conduct Your Testing?................155
              The Résumé.................................................156
              The Application Form.......................................157
              Additional Testing.........................................158
              Work Samples...............................................163
              References and Recommendations.............................165
              Selection Strategy.........................................165
              Selecting Physicians and Other Professional Employees......168
              Equal Employment Opportunity...............................170
              Case Application: Hiring a Business Manager.................172
              Case Application: A Selection Failure—A Personal Perspective..179
              Conclusion.................................................179

**Chapter 5    Compensating Employees................................183**
              Who Should Construct Your Compensation Plan?...............184
              Equity: A Theory and Strategy for Determining Compensation...184
              Using Equity to Construct a Compensation Plan..............186

Job Evaluation Methods for Achieving Internal and
    External Equity . . . . . . . . . . . . . . . . . . . . . . . . . . . . . . . 190
Ranking Job Evaluation Method. . . . . . . . . . . . . . . . . . . . . . . 191
Going Beyond a Ranking Method . . . . . . . . . . . . . . . . . . . . . 197
Pay Ranges . . . . . . . . . . . . . . . . . . . . . . . . . . . . . . . . . . . . . . 200
Inflation. . . . . . . . . . . . . . . . . . . . . . . . . . . . . . . . . . . . . . . . . 202
Compensation Plan Coverage . . . . . . . . . . . . . . . . . . . . . . . . 202
Practical Considerations . . . . . . . . . . . . . . . . . . . . . . . . . . . . 202
Incentive Plans . . . . . . . . . . . . . . . . . . . . . . . . . . . . . . . . . . . 203
Benefits. . . . . . . . . . . . . . . . . . . . . . . . . . . . . . . . . . . . . . . . . 206
Case Application: Mrs. Wilson's Equity . . . . . . . . . . . . . . . . 209
Physician Compensation. . . . . . . . . . . . . . . . . . . . . . . . . . . . 210
Conclusion . . . . . . . . . . . . . . . . . . . . . . . . . . . . . . . . . . . . . . 215
Appendix 5A  Point System of Job Evaluation . . . . . . . . . . . . . . . . . . . . . 217
Knowledge (Table 5A–1) . . . . . . . . . . . . . . . . . . . . . . . . . . . 217
Nonsupervisory Responsibility (Table 5A–2) . . . . . . . . . . . . 217
Ingenuity (Table 5A–3). . . . . . . . . . . . . . . . . . . . . . . . . . . . . 217
Personnel Management Responsibility (Table 5A–4) . . . . . . . 221
Outside Relationships (Table 5A–5). . . . . . . . . . . . . . . . . . . . 223

**Chapter 6**   **Leading Your Employees and Colleagues** . . . . . . . . . . . . . . . . . **225**
Introduction. . . . . . . . . . . . . . . . . . . . . . . . . . . . . . . . . . . . . . 225
Leadership. . . . . . . . . . . . . . . . . . . . . . . . . . . . . . . . . . . . . . . 226
Leading the Change Process. . . . . . . . . . . . . . . . . . . . . . . . . . 237
Motivation. . . . . . . . . . . . . . . . . . . . . . . . . . . . . . . . . . . . . . . 245
Conclusion . . . . . . . . . . . . . . . . . . . . . . . . . . . . . . . . . . . . . . 250
Appendix 6A  United Family Practices, Ltd. . . . . . . . . . . . . . . . . . . . . . . . . 253

**Chapter 7**   **Marketing** . . . . . . . . . . . . . . . . . . . . . . . . . . . . . . . . . . . . . . . **257**
Introduction. . . . . . . . . . . . . . . . . . . . . . . . . . . . . . . . . . . . . . 257
Developing a Marketing Plan . . . . . . . . . . . . . . . . . . . . . . . . 259
Generic Marketing Strategies . . . . . . . . . . . . . . . . . . . . . . . . 266
Outcome: The Marketing Plan . . . . . . . . . . . . . . . . . . . . . . . 271
Focusing on Promotion. . . . . . . . . . . . . . . . . . . . . . . . . . . . . 273
Market Segmentation . . . . . . . . . . . . . . . . . . . . . . . . . . . . . . 286
The Internet. . . . . . . . . . . . . . . . . . . . . . . . . . . . . . . . . . . . . . 291
Other Considerations . . . . . . . . . . . . . . . . . . . . . . . . . . . . . . 298
The Internet—Your Role. . . . . . . . . . . . . . . . . . . . . . . . . . . . 300
Conclusions. . . . . . . . . . . . . . . . . . . . . . . . . . . . . . . . . . . . . . 300

**Chapter 8**   **Negotiation.** . . . . . . . . . . . . . . . . . . . . . . . . . . . . . . . . . . . . . **303**
The Art of Negotiation: Key Concepts . . . . . . . . . . . . . . . . . 304
Integrative and Distributive Negotiating. . . . . . . . . . . . . . . . 309

The Prisoners' Dilemma: A Metaphor for
    Many Negotiation Issues...................................318
Case Analysis: The Black Book ..........................321
Conclusion ...........................................326
Appendix 8A  The Black Book Proposal..............................328
Proposal for Lease Modification .........................328

**Chapter 9    Organizational Integration...........................331**
Introduction..........................................331
Structure ............................................333
Factors Inhibiting Integration ...........................342
Integration Mechanisms ................................343
Small Practice Structures ...............................347
Conclusion ...........................................350
Northeast HealthCare Case Analysis .....................351
Appendix 9A  Northeast HealthCare .................................353

**Chapter 10   Business Law .......................................355**
General Torts.........................................357
Classification ........................................358
Intentional Torts .....................................358
Negligence Torts .....................................361
Malpractice ..........................................362
Contracts............................................367
Employment Issues....................................370
Antikickbacks and Antireferral Legislation .................385
Selecting an Attorney ..................................390
Conclusion ...........................................391

**Chapter 11   Quality Improvement ...............................393**
Total Quality Management (TQM) Concepts................394
Teamwork: The Core of TQM and Organization Integration .....402
Six Sigma ...........................................404
Case Analysis: Higher Quality and Lower Costs in Dialysis .....405
Conclusion ...........................................408

**Chapter 12   Final Thoughts.....................................411**
The Physician Manager's Personal Challenge ...............411
Expectations of Others and Self .........................412
Business Expectations..................................414

**Index .......................................................417**

# Acknowledgments

William T. Geary, PhD, CPA, wrote and co-authored many of the financial cases and exhibits in this book for the physician leadership programs that we have been conducting for healthcare systems. His permission to use these materials is greatly appreciated. Irving M. Pike, MD, has provided many insightful observations about practice management over the years, which contributed to the content and direction of this manuscript. Finally, I want to thank my wife, Bernadette, who has tolerated yet another book writing endeavor.

# Introduction

## SUCCEEDING AS A PHYSICIAN MANAGER: ESSENTIAL BUSINESS SKILLS

Many physicians think of physician managers as having developed an alternative employment path to traditional clinical practice. Generally, this path is seen as one that emphasizes management responsibility instead of clinical practice—in some cases to the total exclusion of clinical practice. The focus of this book is at odds with this limited view of who is the physician manager. It is my contention that management skills should now be an essential part of *every* physician's repertoire, and that physicians who do not possess these skills are less able to provide their patients with the highest levels of clinical care, as well as to personally survive and prosper in the current healthcare environment.

Many physician managers are employed by large healthcare organizations, including hospitals, healthcare systems, HMOs, insurers, and large single-specialty or multispecialty private practices. There is another physician manager, however, who often is overlooked and who needs to be as much the physician manager as his or her colleagues working in large organizations. This physician manager works in, and probably owns part of, a small group or solo practice. Historically, private-practice physicians have always had to manage their practices' business affairs. Often, one physician undertakes these responsibilities, perhaps reluctantly, through default, rotation, or self-interest. All too often, important management responsibilities are delegated to a practice business manager, without retaining sufficient physician involvement or control. This can be a formula for disaster because there are many situations in which a business manager's self-interest does not coincide with those who own the practice. Other physicians, realizing the importance of their participation in management decision making, actively manage their practices, although many do so without adequate management skills.

All of these physicians are in situations that call for physician management skills and can benefit from this book. The core knowledge areas that physician managers need are the same irrespective of whether they manage in a large healthcare system, a solo private practice, or anything in between. What varies, as one progresses from a solo practice to a large healthcare system, is the complexity of the situation, the amount of data available, and the degree to which and the immediacy with which decisions will directly affect the physician. All physician managers must become proficient in the *same* body of knowledge. *How* a physician uses this knowledge, and the extent to which it will be the central focus of his or her work, will vary depending on the specific nature of the physician manager's responsibilities.

Medical practices, hospitals, and healthcare systems *are* businesses. Health care currently constitutes about 16 percent of the U.S. gross domestic product.[1] Unfortunately, the recognition of this fact by physicians and those who train them is only now beginning to occur.

Medicine has been slow to acquire management skills for two reasons. First, for most of the 20th century, medicine was very profitable. When times are good, patients are plentiful, and an industry is growing, many don't feel the need to operate efficiently. A thick salve of cash will cover many business mistakes and inefficiencies. Second, medical academicians, who are often unfamiliar with and uninterested in the nonmedical aspects of health care, design medical school and residency curricula. As such, they generally have little appreciation of the need for their students and their profession to acquire business and management skills. As a result, these skills are generally not adequately represented in their curricula.

## THE PHYSICIAN MANAGER'S ROLE DEFINITION

In working and consulting with medical practices, I have seen two fundamental errors as physician managers try to determine their appropriate role. Some physician managers make the mistake of being a micromanager. Micromanagers look over everyone's shoulder. They routinely second guess subordinates' and perhaps colleagues' daily operational decisions, and in general become very intrusive in everyone's lives. This reduces employee discretion and initiative, and in some cases employees become fearful and resentful of not being trusted to do their work. In addition, practice-based micromanaging physician managers are doing less of what arguably is the *most* critical function in their job description, and what only they can do: generate revenue! Time devoted to micromanaging is time taken away from clinical work.

The other role definition error that physician managers make is to be the absentee physician manager. These physician managers often say, "I hired a business manager and staff to take care of all that stuff," or "The hospital has numerous administrators to take care of all those business issues," and in both cases the physician concludes, "so I'm not going to get involved in any of it—I'm going to focus on my patients." Going to this other extreme also creates problems. If the physician manager is uninvolved in important decisions, then choices will be made without physician perspective and input. It's not necessarily that the others who will be making decisions are trying to be malevolent. It's just that business managers, employees, nurses, administrators, and other stakeholders have different perspectives and self-interests, and as a result the physician's point of view will not be adequately represented when important decisions are being made.

To help you define the appropriate level of physician manager involvement, I propose the following criteria. Physician managers should know enough and be involved enough in business decision making to:

- Know when you are getting a good job from employees and others, and lead change when needed. For example, you are not satisfied with the quality of your practice's clinical support staff. You need to know enough about employment methods, so when you inquire about how applicants are evaluated, you know that the unstructured anecdotal interviews and references currently used are not the best selection methods. You then can lead your business manager or human resources director toward more effective methods (Chapter 4). You personally will not be involved in utilizing these more effective methods. That would be getting too far down in the trenches, because it is not the best use of valuable physician time.[2]

Your role in this case is to make certain that the *employment system* is functioning appropriately by identifying the problem and leading the change process.

• Ask questions and obtain critical information for decision making. For example, if you are on a hospital committee considering purchasing new laparoscopic surgery equipment, then this means knowing enough to ask for the necessary financial information to make a *financially,* as well as medically, informed decision. You need to know, for example, that you want to see a breakeven analysis sensitized to several critical success factors, such as volume and fees (Chapter 1). You also want to see the investment characteristics of the project, such as the project's internal rate of return (IRR) and net present value (NPV), once again sensitized to critical success factors. You will *not* be collecting the data yourself to do these analysis, nor will you be assembling them into spreadsheets, because if you did you would be too far down in the trenches. But, you know enough about these issues to be certain to utilize this information, and if necessary cause it to be generated, and then make an informed decision that is sensitive to both clinical and business considerations.

• Have the management skills necessary to achieve outcomes that meet *physicians'* needs. For example, your health care system is in the process of selecting an electronic medical record (EMR). You have seen several of the proposed systems, and note that from a physician's perspective they are all deficient in important ways, such as easy access to appropriate fields, intrusive data entry, decision support, security, etc. First, you need to have a vision of the physician manager's *appropriate* role in the EMR system design and selection process to effectively negotiate with administration, IT, pharmacy, and other physicians, in order to get a system that works better for physicians. Second, this means that you need the business skills described below in order to have the ammunition to make changes consistent with physicians' needs. Third, this means having negotiation (Chapter 8) and change management skills (Chapter 6) necessary to successfully execute the change.

## PHYSICIAN MANAGER SKILLS

Physician managers must develop skills in several business disciplines in order to achieve the three goals listed here. These skill areas form the chapters of this book. The following is a brief description of some of the major subject areas.

### Management

Management is the glue that holds all organizations together. It is the process of obtaining, organizing, and directing all the human resources associated with a healthcare organization. Whether the physician manages in a solo practice with one secretary, in a group practice with many physicians and diverse job descriptions, or in a large multihospital healthcare system, the quality of management will determine whether personnel operate as an effective team. In some organizations, employees and groups are constantly fighting border disputes; in others, they work together synergistically to achieve a common vision of what needs to be achieved.

There are many aspects of managing a healthcare organization's human resources. They include the following:

- *Leadership*: guiding and inspiring physician and nonphysician employees to work toward a common goal. Leadership skills can range from being directive, to consulting with others, to delegating tasks to others. It also can involve empowering others, such as giving subordinates decision-making responsibilities that might normally be reserved for more senior managers. Often, in larger healthcare organizations, physician managers are working with groups of employees where there is no clear manager–subordinate relationship. Physician leaders also must learn, therefore, to lead when they do not have line control. Leadership is not only leading through inspiration, but knowing how to involve others, such as when to be directive and when to hand off a decision.
- *Performance Appraisal*: evaluating the job performance of employees, and using this information to make personnel decisions, such as training needed, compensation, discipline, termination, promotion, etc. Appraisal of physician performance is becoming increasingly important. Medical outcomes, patient satisfaction, and cost are increasingly being used to evaluate physician performance. The physician manager's role is to ensure that performance appraisal systems are in place to motivate appropriate employee, peer, and partner behavior.
- *Employment Methods*: knowing how to hire both professional and clerical employees. Knowledge of this function fits the classic physician manager role definition. The physician manager will not be doing the hiring personally, but as a physician he or she clearly has to live with the *consequences* of good or poor employment decisions.
- *Motivation*: understanding what drives employees to act in specific ways when given a task to perform or a goal to achieve. By understanding what motivates employees, the physician leader can structure the work–reward relationship to best achieve his or her objectives. Similarly, he or she can influence his or her organization to structure rewards to better meet employees' needs.
- *Compensation*: determining equitable pay and benefits for employees, including physicians.
- *Organizational Integration*: getting the parts of the healthcare organization to work together in a synergistic manner. All too often, parts of healthcare systems and practices operate as separate silos. Information stays locked within and people do not work collaboratively across organizational boundaries. For example, the contracting team that is negotiating a contract for a multispecialty practice to provide services to a large regional employer does not know that the orthopedic surgeons have just revised their critical care path for a hip replacement. The surgeons do not know that the contracting team is negotiating a contract that is very sensitive to cost issues, which their new care path affects directly.
- *Managing Change*: all organizations are confronted with the need to change. Changing medical procedures, information technology, competition, and legal issues, to name a few, all result in healthcare organizations having to change. Often, people resist change, because it threatens their own self-interest. Physician leaders must be able to recognize the need to change and be able to prevent or overcome resistance that may hinder them from putting needed changes into effect.
- *Negotiation*: physicians are constantly negotiating with patients, employees, partners, vendors, landlords, and colleagues.

- *Quality Improvement*: understanding that a primary component of the physician manager's job description is managing systems as well as people. These systems may include the employment system, collection system, management information system, clinical treatment systems, and others. Quality improvement is a management philosophy that emphasizes fixing processes and creating incentives for employees to point out problems and look for ways to improve processes. It uses statistical control and charting methods to document and plan for improvement.

## Marketing

Most physicians assume that marketing is simply a different word for advertising. This is not the case. Marketing begins with identifying customers' needs and then proceeds to identify internal and external factors when determining services offered, location, promotion, and pricing. Advertising, which is a form of promotion, is one small part of the marketing process.

The marketing concept is distinctly different from that of selling, which is the process of persuading patients, for example, that they need a particular service. Sellers ask, "Where and how can I find patients to buy the services that I currently offer?" In contrast, physicians and health providers that adopt a marketing approach begin with customers, determine what they need, can afford, where they would like to access the service, and then design, promote, price, and provide services so that customers will have a natural affinity for them.

A fundamental change that has occurred in health care is the nature of the customer. Healthcare providers have a very complex definition of a *customer* that generally includes, but is not limited to, the patient. Another customer is often the purchaser of health care, who may be employers, insurers, and governments. Often, the incentives of these different customers are not aligned. For example, patients may want unrestricted access to services, whereas an employer or payer may wish to restrict that access in order to obtain lower prices. This complicates the picture for the physician who accepts the marketing model, because he or she now must carefully determine how to balance these needs.

Some physicians question the ethics of including marketing considerations in medical decision making. The reality is that marketing considerations *are* very much involved in healthcare decision making these days.

## Financial Management

Financial management is the process of using accounting and financial information to make management decisions. Practices, hospitals, and all other organizations create a lot of financial information in the normal course of their daily operation. It is critical for the physician manager to *use* this information to make management decisions. Often, physicians use financial information in an autopsy mode. They consider financial outcomes two years after a decision was made, and use the financial data to describe the financial hemorrhage: "That sure was a costly decision we made two years ago!" A better approach is to use the financial information *proactively*, before making a decision. By doing this, the physician manager can reduce the chance of failure and identify critical success factors that can be actively managed, so one can redirect a project *before* it becomes a failure. Similarly, a physician manager can redirect a succeeding project to achieve even more success by refining it as new opportunities arise.

Financial management skills will help a physician leader answer the following kinds of questions:

- If I increase the size of my practice, what effect will this have on my profit?
- If I introduce a new program or procedure, how much volume must I have at a given fee before I break even or achieve a profit target?
- How do I evaluate a capital investment, such as building a new hospital wing, purchasing a second MRI, or acquiring two primary care practices?

### Business Law

Physician managers constantly interact with other entities, such as patients, insurance companies, landlords, suppliers, employees, and contractors. Many of these interactions have legal implications. Ideally, the time to address the legal implications of an arrangement is *before* the arrangement goes into effect. Agreements must anticipate anything that can go wrong, provide for what the physician manager would like to have occur if something does go wrong, and be legally binding. The physician leader certainly will want to consult an attorney during this process and have him or her draft all written agreements. There also will be situations that occur on a daily basis, when a physician manager makes decisions with legal implications. He or she will not want to or be able to contact an attorney for every negotiation with a vendor or for every employee hired. This book will acquaint you with basic business law concepts, so you will be able to appropriately respond to these daily business encounters, and know when and how to utilize your attorney.

### PROBLEMS FOR THE PHYSICIAN MANAGER

Those physician managers who also have some clinical responsibilities are probably thinking, "Easy for him to say! When am I supposed to do this? In the 60th through the 65th hour of each week?" This response does point out a challenge that physician managers have in attending to these management responsibilities. Many physician managers have a full-time job as a clinician and have to be a manager on top of that. To put this in perspective, however, this is the same challenge faced by all professions. Lawyers, accountants, and architects, for example, similarly must either reduce their professional hours or work additional hours to handle the management part of their business.

Another difficulty is that acquiring business skills requires learning a new language and developing new skills, which take time and effort. Physicians have several options for acquiring these skills. For those to whom a formal degree can add career value, an MBA from a business school can make sense. Some MBA programs offer the equivalent of a subspecialty in health care, and these programs are particularly appropriate for a physician.[3] If a formal degree is less significant, then certificate programs from organizations such as the American College of Physician Executives (ACPE) may provide a good balance between cost, time, and skills outcome. This book is a good supplemental source to physicians pursuing either of these alternatives, as well as a primary source of information to those who are trying to acquire some "just-in-time" knowledge on their own. It does not deliver the full content of an MBA program, but it does present some of the most powerful ideas that are contained in an MBA program, and certainly the ones that are most useful to physicians.

Another difficulty is that occasionally clinical and business issues come into conflict. For example, several years ago I had the opportunity to work with physicians in an oncology practice who understood that their costs were an important business consideration. One particular cost of about $3,500, which was never reimbursed, kept recurring. I asked one of the physicians about this, and he commented that this was for an antinausea medication that Blue Cross and many other insurers would not pay for. "Their attitude is that the patient will be sick as a dog for a few days, but 6 months from now they will not remember it," he commented. He then went on to say that he and his colleagues decided to supply the medication to their patients in order to provide the standard of care with which they were comfortable.

As a consultant who is not a physician, I could not advise these physicians one way or another on whether to provide the medication. By teaching them how to evaluate financial issues, however, the physicians *could* appropriately balance both the medical and business aspects of the decision. As business-skilled physicians, they were in the *best* position to decide whether to stop supplying the medication, selectively supply it, or provide it to all appropriate patients. In this case, the medical and financial considerations *did* come into conflict. I suggest, however, that the conflict was there all along. Acquiring financial *knowledge* simply brought it to the surface, and allowed the physicians to make a conscious, considered decision, as opposed to a decision without knowledge and by default.

Finally, it is important to recognize that providing medical services is not the same as producing computer software or selling soap. There *are* important qualitative considerations to health care that would be lost by simply transferring accepted business practices to the healthcare setting. This uniqueness is a result of several factors. The close, personal relationship that often exists between the patient and the physician removes many of the adversarial boundaries normally defining a customer's relationship to a business. If the nature of the physician-patient relationship is not properly addressed, a conflict can arise between the humanitarian and ethical aspects of health care, and the financial considerations that are necessary for organizational survival. Physician managers often make decisions that involve the quality and quantity of patient life, and these are interwoven with the cost of services, the history of accepted medical practice, and the welfare of their organization. Few managers in other industries face challenges with this magnitude of professional, ethical, legal, and organizational complexity.

## THE BUSINESS CONTEXT

What would Apple Inc.'s CEO and top managers do before making a decision about the "next generation" iPod, *if–*

- They thought that price competition would force down the price of "MP3" (iPod) players?
- Consumers continue to demand ever-higher quality and more capable products?
- Technology continues to evolve rapidly—hard drives keep getting smaller while capacity increases, flash memory costs continue to decrease, power consumption improves, and video technology evolves?

What questions would they ask and what data would they want to see before proceeding?

I have presented many groups of physicians with this situation and these two questions. Invariably, they come up with many excellent suggestions that include considering market factors, customer desires including their perception of quality; evaluating competitors' products; financial considerations such as component costs, return on investment, cost of new production equipment, production strengths, and so forth. It is obvious to them that in a situation such as this, some business analysis is *essential* before proceeding. Interestingly enough, these are the same three challenges—price pressure, customer demand for higher quality, and rapidly evolving technology—that confront health care at all levels today.

Logically, therefore, the same types of business analyses should be used by healthcare providers prior to acting, as would be used by Apple executives.

- If you are living in an unforgiving financial environment, then you need financial skills to anticipate the financial consequences of your decisions. You need marketing skills to be certain that new services address real customer wants and needs. Finally, you need effective leadership, because there will be lots of contention about how to use limited human and financial resources and you cannot afford to be indecisive or wasteful.
- If there is pressure to increase quality, then you need financial skills to *selectively* limit costs by eliminating fat and not muscle. One aspect of quality is what the customer defines it to be, so we need marketing skills to assess this. Finally, the most basic aspect of quality is the quality that your employees provide on the job. Managing by using performance appraisal and quality improvement methods is basic.
- If new technology is endemic to health care, then you need financial skills to evaluate the consequences of buying this piece or developing that service line. You need marketing skills to be certain that the new wiz-bang technology actually satisfies some real customer need, and you need management skills to overcome the inevitable resistance that goes along with change.

Stated another way, healthcare organizations and physicians routinely encounter *business* problems, and they are amenable to the same types of business analyses and solutions as any other business problem. The real problem is change, and the real question is, "How will *you* respond to the changing rules of this game?"

Physicians who acquire business skills can make unique contributions. They are the only constituency that can balance the medical perspective with the business perspective. Consider what it tells administrators when physician managers can sit at the table and converse using *their* language? At a minimum, it tells them that they can't fool you—but, more importantly it tells them that they can't discount your ideas simply because you are a physician, and "don't understand their world." More positively, it means that you can be a *participant* in all those decisions, which have both business implications and medical consequences. It means that you can be an effective representative of physicians' and patients' interests. It means that you can help others to make medically informed business decisions. It means that you can foster integration between the parts of the medical delivery system, break down barriers and adversarial boundaries, and thereby improve both business and clinical performance.

1. Smith, C., Cowan, C., Heffler, S., Catlin, A. "National Health Spending in 2004: Recent Slowdown Led By Prescription Drug Spending," *Health Affairs,* 2006, 25(1), 186–196.

2. An exception might be if the position is directly reporting to you, such as a surgical assistant in which case you probably would want some significant involvement.

3. Some MBA programs offer an executive MBA curriculum. Typically, these meet one day each week on Fridays or weekends for 12 to 18 months. They offer the practicing physician a more feasible schedule than the typical full-time MBA curriculum.

# CHAPTER 1

# Financial Management

### Chapter Objectives

The goal of this chapter is to help you become an informed *consumer* and *user* of financial and accounting information. When you have completed this chapter, you will be able to:

1. Use financial information, such as for practice expansion or new program development, to help you make decisions.
2. Assess the financial health of your practice or organization, and determine how well it is doing in comparison with past years.
3. Utilize cash and accrual accounting information to better understand the financial status of your practice or organization.
4. Evaluate the financial impact of capital decisions, such as purchasing additional clinical equipment.
5. Determine whether you should lease or purchase equipment.
6. Use a budget to help you plan, evaluate, and guide performance.

Physician leaders are in a unique position in the healthcare system. By virtue of their medical training, they are capable of understanding the medical implications of management decisions. Physician leaders who have acquired financial skills then can combine this medical perspective with their understanding of the financial implications of a decision. This ability to consider both the medical and financial components of a decision is unique to financially literate physician leaders, and provides them with the opportunity to make unique contributions to system decision making.

As noted, all too often physicians, practices, and healthcare systems use financial information as if it were an autopsy. Two years after the expansion was undertaken, or

after the new physician was hired, or after the outpatient surgery center was initiated, the financial reports are examined, and the conclusion is "Oops! This sure isn't working well, is it?" Financially literate physician leaders can use their financial skills *proactively*; that is, they can consider the financial implications and risks *before* proceeding with a project or decision. This not only reduces the chance that a poor decision will be made, but it also results in identifying what things must occur for both the financial and clinical outcomes to be achieved. Then, by tracking progress against those scheduled goals, changes can be made before financial disaster ensues.

To use financial data proactively, physician leaders need to know what financial information they need in order to make an informed decision. Consistent with the physician leader's appropriate role, assembling data, constructing spreadsheets, and undertaking other data collection and basic analysis tasks generally should be done by others. Physicians should not be replacing their accountants or chief financial officers. There is a direct analogy here to the physician's clinical role, which includes identifying tests to be performed but does not encompass personally conducting the laboratory analysis on a patient's blood. Similarly, the physician leader's critical financial role is to know what financial information to ask for, understand how to interpret the data, and make medically and financially informed recommendations and decisions.

The emphasis in this chapter is to describe financial tools and show how they apply to decision-making situations that physician leaders routinely encounter. The primary financial tools used by physician leaders include the following:

1. *Cost-Volume-Profit (CVP) Analysis*—this provides understanding of costs and how different types of costs along with volume affect profit. Understanding and managing CVP relationships is fundamental to the success of any medical organization.
2. *Capital Asset Planning*—evaluating the financial impact of major capital acquisitions, such as buildings, office equipment, and medical equipment, and using time value of money concepts, such as net present value (NPV) and internal rate of return (IRR) to evaluate capital projects.
3. *Statements, Reports, and Systems*—understanding the use and significance of standard financial statements, such as the income statement, balance sheet, and cash flow statement. Understanding the appro-

priate uses of cash and accrual accounting methods are fundamental to evaluating the strength of any health care organization.
4. *Control and Budgeting*—developing financial plans and using them to evaluate the performance of operations, using budgets to benchmark goals for financial performance. These help the physician leader to plan for the future, track progress, and made changes to avoid problems or take advantage of opportunities.
5. *Short-Term Financial and Cash Control*—accounting for cash, so that it is not diverted; converting receivables into cash; knowing what reports to examine so the organization meets its cash obligations. Having timely access to cash is necessary for all organizations. These reports and methods provide critical cash knowledge and deterrence.

Physician leaders in all settings should be proficient in the first four categories. The fifth category is covered in a separate chapter (Chapter 2), because it is most directly applicable to physician leaders who are working in a practice setting.

## CVP ANALYSIS

CVP analysis examines how different kinds of costs interact with the volume of business to affect profit. It can help you to answer such questions as the following:

- How many procedures will have to be conducted in order to break even or to hit a targeted profit level?
- How would combining several primary care practices into a group affect profitability?
- What would happen to profitability if a partner were to leave the practice?

- What would happen to an integrated healthcare system, if it sells its psychiatric hospital?
- If a group of orthopedic surgeons starts an outpatient surgery center and takes 20 percent of our inpatient volume, how might this affect hospital costs and profitability?
- If I make an investment in education and equipment to learn a new procedure, how many procedures will I need to conduct to break even or to reach a profitability target?

As you can see, the issues raised in these questions are critical to the financial viability of any healthcare organization. CVP analysis, therefore, is one of the most powerful financial analysis tools available, and it should be routinely performed whenever decisions will be made that may affect cost, volume, or profitability.

To perform a CVP analysis, you must understand the nature of costs. Costs are expenditures of cash, such as for supplies, personnel, interest, and rent. Costs, however, can behave in different ways. Fixed costs remain the same irrespective of the number of procedures conducted, patients treated, hospital beds filled, and so forth. In contrast, variable costs change with the amount of service provided. As more patients are treated or hospital beds are filled, these costs change. Mixed costs have features of both fixed and variable costs. Understanding these distinctions is important, because the nature of a cost has a profound effect on how you manage it, and on the profitability of any healthcare organization.

Fixed costs remain stable as services vary. Typical examples include rent, compensation for salaried personnel, interest on equipment (computers, laboratory equipment, etc.), and property taxes. This notion of a cost being truly fixed, however, is a convenient convention. In reality, no cost is truly fixed. Over a period of years, rent may increase, salaries may change as personnel come and go and job performance changes, loans may be paid off, and taxes may increase. In addition, if volume changes enough, fixed costs may change. For example, if a health system obtains a new contract with an employer to cover an additional 20,000 lives, new physicians, nurses, and nonmedical personnel may have to be hired. As volume increases beyond a certain level, a hospital may have to build an additional wing, which will generate many additional fixed costs. Similarly, if volume decreases substantially, a hospital may be able to close a wing, downsize its personnel, and thereby reduce its fixed costs. Fixed costs, however, remain stable within a broad band of business activity, which is called the *relevant range*.

Fixed costs represent the risk of doing business. Irrespective of whether the patients come, the fixed costs will be there. Practices, programs, hospitals, and healthcare systems that have high fixed costs, generally speaking, have high risk. When you are negotiating the terms of a contract, for example, one of the important issues to consider is who has the fixed cost. Often, a negotiating objective will be to try to get the other party to take the fixed cost and, with it, the risk.

There are two strategies for controlling fixed costs. The first is procurement. The maxim "Don't buy a Mercedes if a Honda Civic will do the job" is appropriate. This statement assumes that the job to be done is basic transportation; getting from point A to point B. If the job, however, was defined as "doing this in a safe manner in the event of an accident, providing superior comfort (because we have a lot of work to do and need to arrive rested), and conveying a certain image (because that communicates a message of success, and success begets success)," then a Honda Civic would be the wrong procurement decision. By effective procurement, I mean that we don't waste money on attributes that don't relate to our mission.

The second strategy for controlling fixed costs is *"Use it, use it, use it!"* Keep salaried personnel busy, keep treatment rooms full, expand office hours, and so on. All these tactics get more use out of costs that will be there anyway. This strategy is the economic driver behind the increased number of group practices that occurred in the 1980s and 1990s, the growth in the size of group practices, the amalgamation of individual hospitals into large healthcare systems, and the growth in the size of healthcare systems. One secretary, one nurse, one computer, and often one office suite can all service more than one physician. As the second physician is acquired, *the fixed costs remain the same,* but the second physician is generating additional revenue, so the *fixed cost as a percentage of*

*revenue generated* is obviously lower. In effect, the practice has become more efficient.

Graphically, fixed costs plot as a series of stair steps, such as in **Figure 1–1**. Here, salary costs for intake at an imaging center remains the same for the first 300 patients per week. Once this relevant range is exceeded, additional salary cost is incurred, and we go up to a new cost plateau. When you examine this fixed cost–volume relationship, it is clear that you always want to be at the far right side of any fixed cost plateau, because this will give you the most revenue generated for the given level of fixed cost. In fact, it should be apparent that your net income (net revenue minus expenses) probably will go *down* as a result of taking on the 301st patient and the associated additional fixed cost. Obviously, you would not want to take on the 301st patient and move to the higher cost plateau if you didn't have good reason to believe that you could push the volume up well beyond this level.

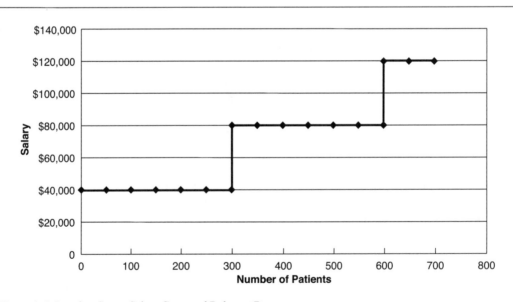

**Figure 1–1**  Imaging Center Salary Costs and Relevant Ranges.

This relationship between fixed cost and volume underlies the failure of many businesses and projects. Take, for example, the restaurant that given the opportunity to expand into adjacent space does so to address overbooked weekends during the summer. As a result, it greatly increases its fixed costs. These costs are present during weekdays and in slower seasons. The owner never comprehended that the expansion was perhaps tantamount to moving from the right end of a lower cost plateau to the left end of a higher cost plateau. Sometimes ill-informed decisions such as these translate into working harder just to stay in place. Sometimes they lead to lower profits and even failure. Uninformed decisions such as this may mean that you are betting the business on a large increase in volume.

Variable costs vary in total as activity varies. Typical examples include medical supplies, office supplies, postage, and the salaries of hourly personnel who can be called in or not called based on need. When more patients are treated, total variable costs increase; when fewer patients are treated, total variable costs decrease. Because total variable costs are obviously affected by volume, we need to think of them in terms of variable cost per unit, such as the variable cost per procedure, per patient, per DRG, or per minute of machine time. The unit of analysis (procedure, patient, DRG, etc.) is often called a *cost driver*, because this variable drives the total variable cost up or down. Another way to think of this is that the cost driver is an independent variable, with the variable cost being a dependent variable. Once I know the level of the independent variable, I can predict the level of the dependent variable. If my variable cost per patient is $30, then I know with some certainty that if I treat 100 patients my total variable cost will be $3,000.

As with fixed costs, there are two fundamental strategies to control variable costs. The first is procurement. The goal is to purchase at the lowest per unit cost. To do this, however, I must clearly specify the quality and characteristics that I need. Otherwise, suppliers will translate "lowest possible cost" into "cheap." A low variable cost that changes the nature of your product or service in ways that are unfavorable to the customer or the healthcare organization is a false economy. On the other hand, reducing variable costs that don't affect real or perceived quality is a legitimate cost control.

For example, Sutter Health in Sacramento, California, and Piedmont Hospital in Atlanta, Georgia, evaluated the cost of vegetables served to patients.[1] The cost of vegetables ranged from $2.22 per pound for asparagus to $0.69 per pound for baby carrots. Quality was controlled by specifying USDA Grade "A" frozen vegetables. An analysis of the costs showed that the annual expenditure for frozen vegetables was $45,468, of which $26,707 was for asparagus. By completely eliminating asparagus and consolidating all frozen vegetable purchases into a mix, they achieved a 54 percent savings while maintaining the prescribed quality standard. In addition, patients were not expecting a five-star meal anyway, and indicated equivalent levels of satisfaction on opinion surveys. In this case, the hospitals used three aspects of effective procurement to control variable costs. They specified a quality standard, they eliminated unneeded cost (asparagus), and they used their purchasing power to purchase a standard mix at the lowest possible cost per unit.

Another strategy for controlling variable costs is conservation. The goal is to eliminate waste and unnecessary usage. The cardiologist who without thinking asks to have an extra package of balloons opened "just in case we need them" is a case in point. For example, an analysis of sutures used for total abdominal hysterectomy at Memorial Hospital in Houston, Texas, indicated that 27 percent of the sutures pulled were not used.[2] The hospital developed an education and conservation plan, and reduced the rate of unutilized sutures to 8 percent, for an annual savings of $5,625 for this one procedure.

With both fixed and variable costs, physician leaders should be very concerned with purchasing wisely and clearly specifying the quality that is needed. However, the prescription for utilizing fixed and variable costs is diametrically opposite. When we incur fixed costs, the goal is "use it, use it, use it," whereas with variable costs the goal is to conserve, eliminate waste, and restrict usage to when it is really necessary.

We have discussed fixed and variable costs as though items were intrinsically in one category or the other. Often, this is not the case. Employees can be compensated on the basis of an annual salary (fixed), or on a commission (variable), or for call-in hours worked (variable). In fact, some employees receive both forms of compensation. Similarly, rent can be fixed for a time period or taken as a percentage of sales, or both. One of the goals of good financial management is to try to take costs in their most favorable form. For example, if you believe that you can get high volume, then it may be advantageous to take costs such as salary and rent as fixed. If, however, you are uncertain of your volume level, then you can pass the risk to others by negotiating salary and rent as a percentage of revenues collected. A reasonable strategy if you are seeing about 300 patients given the data in Figure 1–1 would be to hire part-time help until you move further to the right on that cost plateau. The part-time staffing is called in only when needed. Another example of gaining efficiency by choosing how you take your costs would be to routinely collect patient e-mail addresses at intake, obtain appropriate written releases, and replace some patient mail (variable cost) with e-mail (fixed cost).

Finally, some items have characteristics of both fixed and variable costs. These are called *mixed costs*. Some cell phone contracts, for example, have a fixed component for in-network calls and minutes per month, and a variable component for roaming or exceeding your monthly minutes budget. Employee compensation may be composed of a fixed salary plus a commission based on volume. Similarly, rent can be a fixed monthly base plus a percentage of sales. Mixed costs must be broken into their fixed and variable components to control them effectively and to perform the calculations described later.

*Contribution margin* is defined as the excess of net revenue per unit over variable costs per unit.[3]

$$\text{Contribution Margin} = \text{Net Revenue per Unit} - \text{Variable Cost per Unit} \quad (1\text{--}1)$$

For example, if a hospital collects average net revenue of $170 on a panel of outpatient diagnostic tests, and if its variable cost for consumable supplies (e.g., reagents, disposable syringes, report paper, etc.) is $20, then the contribution margin is $150. This contribution margin of $150 is not profit! Remember, we still haven't paid for the fixed costs (e.g., the building, salaries, etc.). The contribution margin can then be used to *contribute* to paying these fixed costs. Once the fixed costs are paid, then the contribution margin goes to the bottom line, meaning that it all becomes profit.

Different products and services have different contribution margins. For a gastroenterologist a flexible sigmoidoscopy generally has a higher contribution margin than an office visit, and a colonoscopy a higher contribution margin than a flexible sigmoidoscopy. Variability of margins occurs in all industries. In the fast food industry, the biggest margins are on soft drinks, and the margins on hamburgers are much smaller. When the order taker asks you whether you want fries and a deep-fried pie with your burger, that question is not necessarily directed at achieving a nutritionally balanced meal. The fries and the pie each add higher margin items to your order, with no increase in fixed costs.

The portfolio of services offered by a healthcare organization or a practicing physician has varying margins. A healthcare system's outpatient chemotherapy center may have higher margins than the emergency department or maternity center. As a physician or healthcare system leader, you need to offer those services that are medically necessary. As a business, however, you need to understand *where* the margins are, and be certain that the mix produces a financially acceptable outcome. For example, immunizations may have negative margins (variable cost is greater than net revenue), especially if they are administered by a physician. This is not to suggest that you should stop providing immunizations. This service, however, must be balanced somewhere else in your portfolio. Similarly, you might want to examine your portfolio of services and their margins to consider how the services that are being promoted relate to their margins. Do you really want to develop a high-profile promotion campaign around a low-margin service? Correspondingly, is there something that you could do to vari-able costs to change a low-margin service that must be provided into one with more favorable margins?

Once we understand which costs are fixed and variable, and what our contribution margin is for a service, we can make some calculations that will tell us the volume necessary to break even and the volume necessary to achieve a stated level of profitability. We will do this with two forms of CVP analysis called *Break-Even Analysis* and *Target Analysis:*

$$\text{Break Even (in Units)} = \text{(Total Fixed Costs)}$$
$$\div \text{(Contribution Margin per Unit)} \quad (1\text{--}2)$$

For example, if a dialysis center receives on average $150 for a dialysis, and variable costs average $40 per dialysis this would result in a contribution margin of $110 per dialysis ($150–$40). If monthly total dialysis center fixed costs are $40,000, then the break-even point would be 363.64 dialyses per month ($40,000 ÷ $110). If each patient on average received 13 dialyses a month, this would mean that the facility would break even with 28 full-time equivalent (FTE) patients per month (363.64 ÷ 13). Conducting a break-even analysis is appropriate when you can make the following assumptions: You can determine whether a given cost is fixed or variable, you can break mixed costs into their fixed and variable components, and there is a consistent linear relationship between costs and some measure of activity, such as the number of patients treated or the amount of revenue.

Generally, we are in business not just to break even, but also to achieve a certain profit level. Target Analysis allows you to state the volume level that must be achieved to achieve a net income target:

$$\text{Target Volume} = \text{(Fixed Costs + Net Income Target)}$$
$$\div \text{(Contribution Margin per Unit)} \quad (1\text{--}3)$$

In this dialysis center example, if the center wishes to make $10,000 of net income per month, then this would be achieved with 455 dialyses or 35 FTE patients if patients average 13 monthly dialyses:

$$\text{Target Volume} = (\$40,000 + \$10,000)$$
$$\div (\$110) = 455 \qquad (1\text{--}4)$$

### Case: General Hospital MRI System[4]

General Hospital is the flagship hospital in a system that includes four other hospitals. The staff of General Hospital was asked to evaluate a proposal to acquire a second MRI system. At the request of the hospital president, the following financial data were accumulated.

### Equipment Cost and Useful Life

The estimated total cost of the installed system is $2,800,000. The expected useful life is 5 years, and depreciation[5] is accounted for by recording one fifth of the system cost each year (the straight line method). Warranty coverage for equipment maintenance and repairs includes the first 2 years of operation. Repairs and maintenance costs for year 3 are projected at $248,000.

### Revenue Projections

The average gross revenue per MRI scan before subtracting bad debt and contractual adjustments is expected to be $625. Based on past experience, bad debt and contractual adjustments average 25 percent of gross revenue. Volume projections take into consideration that volume for the first year of operation will be unusually high because of an existing backlog. The estimate for the first year of operation is 2,260 MRI scans from new demand plus 940 scans from the existing backlog. After the first year, volume is projected to grow at the annual rate of approximately 15 percent. Thus,

Year 2 volume is projected to be 2,599 (115% × 2,260), Year 3 volume is projected to be 2,989, Year 4 volume is projected to be 3,437, and Year 5 volume is projected to be 3,953.

### Operating Costs

**Supplies and film.** These expenses are based on historical expense information and include film, developer, contrast media, chemicals, and other miscellaneous expenses. In Year 1 the cost is estimated at $30 per MRI scan.

**Salaries.** Salary expense for Year 1 is projected at $120,000 based on four technicians and one receptionist for 10 hours per day, 5 days per week. Additional staffing costs of $20,000 are required when the volume approaches 3,800 MRI scans. Employee benefits, including the employer's share of payroll taxes, health insurance, life insurance, and other benefits, are estimated at 25 percent of wages.

**Cryogens.** Cryogen expense is based on historical information. This cost is estimated at $40,000 for Year 1.

**Indirect expenses.** Indirect expenses are allocated to the MRI facility by General Hospital. Indirect expenses are charges to the MRI facility for costs that don't directly relate to treatment, such as hospital administration, parking lot, cafeteria, and the like. The allocated indirect expenses for Year 1 are $142,000.

### Inflation

Based on past experience, cash operating costs (with the exception of salaries) are expected to increase at the rate of 5 percent per year. Salary costs include a provision for inflation and merit raises that are expected to total 8 percent per year.

## Case Analysis: Building and Using a CVP Model

This case describes a typical situation in which physician leaders may be asked to participate with professional administrators to make a decision that has both financial and medical implications. Without a way to organize the information, you may find the task to be confusing, if not overwhelming. Without an idea of how to use the information, you may not answer, or even ask, the important questions. The CVP model provides a way of organizing the information and provides answers to some of the most critical financial questions. To construct the model, the following data are required:

- net revenue per MRI scan
- variable cost per MRI scan
- projected volume
- total fixed costs

**Exhibit 1–1** MRI Facility CVP Analysis

| | |
|---|---:|
| Gross Fee per MRI Scan | $625 |
| Less Adjustments (25%) | $156 |
| Net Fee per MRI Scan | $469 |
| Variable Costs per MRI Scan | $30 |
| Contribution Margin per MRI Scan | $439 |
| Fixed Costs | |
|   Salaries | $120,000 |
|   Benefits | $30,000 |
|   Cryogens | $40,000 |
|   Indirect Expenses | $142,000 |
|   Depreciation | $560,000 |
| Total Fixed Costs | $892,000 |
| Break-Even Calculation | |
|   Units at Break Even | 2033 |
|   Net Revenue | $952,991 |
|   Total Fixed Cost | $892,000 |
|   Total Variable Cost | $ 60,991 |
|   Total Cost | $952,991 |
|   Net Income | $0 |

*Source:* © William T. Geary, Ph.D., and Robert J. Solomon, Ph.D. 2007. All Rights Reserved.

The model that we will build will provide a description of the cost, volume, and profit relationships within the MRI project. We can use this model to compute the break-even point, determine a safety margin, perform target analysis, and gain a better understanding of the financial risks involved.

The cup model is in **Exhibit 1–1**. The gross fee per MRI scan is $625, which is reduced by contractual adjustments and bad debt to result in a net revenue per MRI scan of $469. Next, we identify our variable costs, which in this case are $30 per MRI scan. We then calculate the contribution margin by subtracting variable cost per scan from net revenue per scan, for a contribution margin of $439. This $439 now is available first to cover fixed costs and then, once they are paid, to contribute to net income. Total Fixed Costs are $892,000. We can now calculate the break-even point by

dividing the Total Fixed Costs by Contribution Margin per MRI Scan. If we have $439 left over after we pay the variable costs for each MRI scan, then we must conduct 2,033 scans to break even. Exhibit 1–1 also reports revenue and cost totals at breakeven.

**Exhibit 1–2** column A uses the CVP model that we developed to project the outcome for the first year when we anticipate a total of 3,200 MRI scans. The projected net income (profit) is $512,000, with a safety margin or cushion above breakeven of 1,167 MRI scans. **Exhibit 1–2** column B contains a projection for the second year. We can see that variable costs are projected to grow, and fixed costs have increased as a result of salaries, benefits, and cryogens, with a large increase due to maintenance. As a result, the break-even point has increased to 2,717 MRI scans, and the safety margin is down to 283 scans over the projected volume. At this level of operation, the projected net income will be down to $123,410.

Once this model has been built in a spreadsheet, it is then easy to run a "what-if" analysis, which is also called a *sensitivity analysis*. For example, what if increased competition and other market factors increase the average adjustment to gross fees from 25 percent to 35 percent in Year 3? The answer (**Exhibit 1–2** column C) is that projected net income would be a *negative* $64,090. In effect, we sensitize the spreadsheet to alternative scenarios and see what happens. Using our model, we can see how

susceptible this project is to changes in fees, fixed costs, variable costs, and volume.

If we decide that we don't want to purchase an additional MRI machine unless we can generate $500,000 of net income per year by the third year, then we can conduct a target analysis using Formula 1-3 (**Exhibit 1–2** column D) to determine that this would require conducting 3,592 MRI scans:

$$(\$1,183,615 + \$500,000) \div (\$625 - \$156)$$
$$= 3,592 \text{ scans}$$

CVP analysis and its variants break-even analysis, target analysis, and sensitivity

**Exhibit 1–2** MRI FacilityProjections

| | A | B | C | D |
|---|---|---|---|---|
| | | | 35% Adjustment | |
| | Year 1 | Year 2 | Year 3 | Target Analysis |
| Projected MRI Scans | 3,200 | 3,000 | 3,000 | |
| Fee per MRI Scan | $625 | $625 | $625 | $625 |
| Gross Fees | $2,000,000 | $1,875,000 | $1,875,000 | |
| Less Adjustments | $500,000 | $468,750 | $656,250 | $156 |
| Net Fees | $1,500,000 | $1,406,250 | $1,218,750 | |
| Variable Cost per MRI | $30 | $33 | $33 | |
| Total Variable Costs | $96,000 | $99,225 | $99,225 | |
| Contribution Margin | $1,404,000 | $1,307,025 | $1,119,525 | $469 |
| Fixed Costs | | | | |
| Salaries | $120,000 | $139,968 | $139,968 | |
| Benefits | $30,000 | $34,992 | $34,992 | |
| Cryogens | $40,000 | $44,100 | $44,100 | |
| Indirect Expenses | $142,000 | $156,555 | $156,555 | |
| Depreciation | $560,000 | $560,000 | $560,000 | |
| Maintenance | $— | $248,000 | $248,000 | |
| Total Fixed Costs | $892,000 | $1,183,615 | $1,183,615 | $1,183,615 |
| Projected Net Income | $512,000 | $123,410 | $(64,090) | $500,000 |
| Break-Even Point | 2,033 | 2,717 | 3,172 | |
| Safety Margin | 1,167 | 283 | (172) | |
| Target Volume | | | | 3,592 |

*Source:* © William T. Geary, Ph.D., and Robert J. Solomon, Ph.D. 2007. All Rights Reserved.

analysis is fundamental to understanding the finances of any healthcare organization irrespective of its size or mission. For example, suppose a physician in a solo practice was considering enlarging his or her facility, hiring an additional secretary, and bringing on an associate. By adding the projected additional fixed costs to current fixed costs and using current variable costs to estimate the variable costs associated with the new associate's production, the physician then could project how much revenue the new associate would have to produce for the practice to break even or to reach a profit goal.

As the product mix becomes more complex, the calculations may become longer, but they remain fundamentally the same. For example, if fixed costs are common to a range of services with different contribution margins, then a weighted average variable cost must be calculated. Suppose that fixed costs for three procedures are $100,000. The procedures are provided in the ratio of 5:3:1, and their contribution margins are respectively $100, $75, and $25. The weighted average contribution margin is [($100 $\times$ 5) + ($75 $\times$ 3) + ($25 $\times$ 1)] $\div$ 9 = $83.33. The break-even point would be calculated by dividing the total fixed cost of $100,000 by $83.33, or 1,200 procedures distributed in the projected 5:3:1 ratio. If you build a model such as this, then an important leadership role would be to review reports to see if productivity is occurring in the projected 5:3:1 ratio, and to adjust financial projections, if necessary, so there are no nasty surprises down the road.

As a physician leader, generally, you will not be assembling the spreadsheets and performing the calculations.[6] You should, however, cause them to be generated, examine the analyses, and ask "what-if" sensitivity analysis questions to better understand the financial impact of varying conditions. Your role is to *use* the financial data, along with your knowledge as a physician, to make decisions.

## CAPITAL ASSET PLANNING

*Capital purchasing* is the process of acquiring equipment, buildings, and other items with lives longer than 1 year. Examples include purchasing an electronic medical record system, laboratory and diagnostic equipment, a building to locate a practice, computer equipment, a new wing to a hospital, or a new hospital. Capital asset planning methods are used to evaluate the consequences of these purchase decisions. Consistent with the theme of this book, the physician leader's goal is to use financial data to anticipate these consequences before making the purchase decision.

Asset decisions are particularly important because, by definition, they involve major expenditures with long-term commitments. Resources that are unwisely invested in one area are unavailable for opportunities in another. Because most asset decisions in healthcare systems have both financial and medical consequences, asset planning is an area in which physician leaders can make major contributions. The ability of financially literate physicians to consider both the medical and financial consequences of capital asset decisions offers their organizations a uniquely insightful perspective. We will use three tools to evaluate the financial consequences of a capital asset decision: payback analysis, net present value (NPV), and internal rate of return (IRR).

### Payback Analysis

This method asks the very simple and direct question: "How long will it take to recover the original investment?" To calculate the payback period, you must first estimate the annual net revenue flow. This then is compared with the initial capital investment to determine the year and month in which it would be repaid. If the income stream is equal over the life of the project, the calculation is easy. For example, a surgery suite that costs $1,500,000 to construct and is estimated to generate $400,000 of net revenue per year has a payback period of 3 years and 9 months ($1,500,000 ÷ $400,000 = 3.75). If the revenue stream is projected to be uneven, then the calculation is somewhat more involved. For example, **Exhibit 1–3** contains a payback analysis of the General Hospital MRI facility. Payback will be reached at approximately 3 years and 4 months.[7]

Payback analysis is a very limited analytical tool because it does not take into account the *time value of money.* A dollar you receive a year from now is worth less to you than a dollar in hand today, because the latter can earn interest during the year. In addition, payback tells you nothing about profitability. Payback analysis is useful, however, to gain a sense of risk. If a piece of equipment has a useful life that is not much longer than it takes to pay it off, then this indicates a high level of risk. In the MRI machine example, there appears to be about a 2-year window of opportunity, given the 5 years to obsolescence stated in the case and the payback period of 3 years 4 months. Payback analysis can be useful, therefore, for a first, quick, but limited analysis of a project's financial implications.

### Net Present Value and Internal Rate of Return

Net Present Value (NPV) uses the time value of money concept to compare, or net, the projected financial benefits of a project against its projected financial costs. Internal Rate of Return (IRR) is the interest rate that

**Exhibit 1–3**  MRI Facility Payback Analysis

| Year | Projected Net Revenue | Cumulative Net Payback |
|------|------------------------|-------------------------|
| 1 | $1,072,000 | $1,072,000 |
| 2 | $783,313 | $1,855,313 |
| 3 | $678,552 | $2,533,865 |
| 4 | $831,764 | $3,365,628 |

Estimated Capital Cost: $2,800,000

Year 4: Average Monthly Revenue   $69,314
Year 4: Residual to Earn   $266,135
Year 4: Months to Break Even   3.84
Payback Period: 3 Years 4 Months (Approx.)

*Note:* See Exhibit 1–5 for projected net revenue source data.

a project returns when financial benefits are exactly balanced by the financial costs, and once again considers the time value of money. Because it is unlikely that two or more investment alternatives will have the same capital requirements, the IRR provides a way of directly comparing two otherwise disparate projects.

Both the NPV and the IRR concepts are based on the notion of present value (PV). PV is the value today of money received in the future. Money received in the future can't generate revenue for you between now and then, so the PV of the sum to be received in the future must be *discounted* to account for the lost opportunity. The present value of an amount received in the future is a function of the interest rate you could have earned if you could have invested the money, and the length of time between now and the receipt of the money.[8]

A hand-held calculator or computer spreadsheet program can be used to calculate the PV of an amount. Prior to the development of computers and calculators PVs were calculated by using a PV table, such as the one in **Table 1–1**. We are going to use the PV table, because it is helpful to actually see how the financial numbers are derived. The columns in Table 1–1 are for various interest rates, and the rows are for various time periods. The entries in the table tell you the present value of $1.00 given the time period and the interest rate. For example, you receive an offer today for a lot you own that would net you $48,000 after transaction costs. Your cousin Phil has told you that he will buy it from you in 1 year for $50,000, once again, net of all costs. The land market has been flat, so you have no reason to believe that your lot will increase in value during the next year. What should you do?

Family issues aside, first you need to determine an interest rate. You look at alternatives. A 1-year certificate of deposit from a bank will net you 5 percent. Your mutual fund has averaged 13 percent over the last 5 years. You feel confident that you could safely invest the money in a AAA corporate bond at 8 percent. You choose to use the 8 percent interest rate. You enter Table 1–1 in the 8 percent column and the 1-year row. The factor 0.9259 indicates that $1.00 that you have to wait a year to receive is worth 92.59 cents today. Stated another way, if you invest 92.59 cents at an 8 percent annual yield today, you will have $1.00 in a year. Therefore, your cousin's offer of $50,000 that you must wait a year to receive is equivalent to $46,295 today ($50,000 × 0.9259). The current offer of $48,000 is greater than $46,295, so if selling price is your only consideration, you should take the current offer.

The concept of an annuity also is useful for evaluating capital investments. An *annuity* is a series of equal payments that are received periodically. For example, how much would you be willing to pay right now for the right to receive $1,000 cash annually for 3 years? Let's assume that the prevailing interest rate is 10 percent. The value of this income stream would be equivalent to the PV of the stream of payments. **Table 1–2** is a PV annuity table. It is used in a similar manner to Table 1–1. The columns are for various interest rates, and the rows are for the number of payments. In the example just stated, each dollar invested has a PV of 2.4869, so the $1,000 revenue stream for 3 years has a present value of $2,486.90. Stated another way, $2,486.90 invested today at 10 percent is equivalent to three annual payments of $1,000. An annuity calculation is a shorthand way of doing a series of PV calculations. In fact, you

**Table 1–1** PV Figures

| Periods | 6% | 7% | 8% | 9% | 10% | 11% | 12% |
|---|---|---|---|---|---|---|---|
| 1 | 0.9434 | 0.9346 | 0.9259 | 0.9174 | 0.9091 | 0.9009 | 0.8929 |
| 2 | 0.8900 | 0.8734 | 0.8573 | 0.8417 | 0.8264 | 0.8116 | 0.7972 |
| 3 | 0.8638 | 0.8163 | 0.7938 | 0.7722 | 0.7513 | 0.7312 | 0.7118 |
| 4 | 0.7921 | 0.7629 | 0.7350 | 0.7084 | 0.6830 | 0.6587 | 0.6355 |
| 5 | 0.7473 | 0.7130 | 0.6806 | 0.6499 | 0.6209 | 0.5935 | 0.5674 |
| 6 | 0.7050 | 0.6663 | 0.6302 | 0.5963 | 0.5645 | 0.5346 | 0.5066 |
| 7 | 0.6651 | 0.6227 | 0.5835 | 0.5470 | 0.5132 | 0.4817 | 0.4523 |
| 8 | 0.6274 | 0.5820 | 0.5403 | 0.5019 | 0.4665 | 0.4339 | 0.4039 |
| 9 | 0.5919 | 0.5439 | 0.5002 | 0.4604 | 0.4241 | 0.3909 | 0.3606 |
| 10 | 0.5584 | 0.5083 | 0.4632 | 0.4224 | 0.3855 | 0.3522 | 0.3220 |

**Table 1–2** PV Annuities

| Periods | 6% | 7% | 8% | 9% | 10% | 11% | 12% |
|---|---|---|---|---|---|---|---|
| 1 | 0.9434 | 0.9346 | 0.9259 | 0.9170 | 0.9091 | 0.9009 | 0.8929 |
| 2 | 1.8334 | 1.8080 | 1.7833 | 1.7590 | 1.7355 | 1.7125 | 1.6901 |
| 3 | 2.6730 | 2.6243 | 2.5771 | 2.5310 | 2.4869 | 2.4437 | 2.4018 |
| 4 | 3.4651 | 3.3872 | 3.3121 | 3.2400 | 3.1699 | 3.1024 | 3.0373 |
| 5 | 4.2124 | 4.1002 | 3.9927 | 3.8900 | 3.7908 | 3.6959 | 3.6048 |
| 6 | 4.9173 | 4.7665 | 4.6229 | 4.4860 | 4.3553 | 4.2305 | 4.1114 |
| 7 | 5.5824 | 5.3893 | 5.2064 | 5.0330 | 4.8684 | 4.7122 | 4.5638 |
| 8 | 6.2098 | 5.9713 | 5.7466 | 5.5350 | 5.3349 | 5.1461 | 4.9676 |
| 9 | 6.8017 | 6.5152 | 6.2469 | 5.9950 | 5.7590 | 5.5370 | 5.3282 |

will notice that the entries for a single time period (the top row) are the same in both Tables 1–1 and 1–2. In effect, the PV of an amount is equivalent to a one-period annuity. In addition, the entry in Table 1–2 for any given interest rate and number of payments is equal to the sum of the entries for an equivalent number of time periods in Table 1–1. For example, the sum of the entries in Table 1–1 for three periods at 10 percent is 2.4869 (0.9091 + 0.8264 + 0.7513), which is the same as the entry for the three-period annuity at 10 percent as noted previously.

It is also possible to calculate the future value of a dollar received today. For example, suppose that you invested $10,000 today in a certificate of deposit that pays 10 percent annually for 3 years. A future value table provides a factor of 1.3310, so the future value of the $10,000 is equivalent to $13,310 in 3 years at 10 percent interest. Generally, future value calculations should *not* be used for making capital acquisition decisions, because psychologically we tend to have difficulty judging the effects of inflation. Stated another way, you have a better sense of what a dollar is worth today than tomorrow. Therefore, the methods that we will use to evaluate capital decisions will "bring back" future financial effects into today's dollars.

Let's now use these time value of money concepts to evaluate an investment in new equipment. This equipment will require an initial investment of $30,000. You estimate that its useful life to you is 5 years, and that you may then be able to resell it for $4,000. In addition, you must keep $5,000 worth of parts and supplies available to keep the machine in operation. These parts and supplies, however, can be easily resold, so when you sell the machine you can recover your parts and supplies inventory costs. Finally, you estimate that if you purchase the machine, you will be able to generate an additional $12,000 in net revenue each year as a result of providing additional services. Is this a desirable investment from a financial perspective?

A payback analysis indicates that payback will be achieved in 2.5 years ($30,000 ÷ $12,000). Another simple analysis that does not take into account the time value of money indicates that the equipment will generate $64,000 of revenue ($12,000 × 5 years + $4,000 for the resale of the equipment) and $35,000 of costs, for a net revenue of $29,000 and a total return of 183 percent ($64,000 ÷ $35,000). Given the 5-year useful life, the equipment is looking promising.

We will now use NPV and IRR, to gain a better understanding of the financial consequences of this decision. **Exhibit 1–4** lists the various elements of this problem as either a benefit or a cost. Some of the elements, such as the $12,000 of net revenue (gross revenue – expenses) that the machine will generate each year, are currently stated in future value terms and will have to be "brought back" to the present. Other elements, however, such as the initial capital investment of $30,000, are currently stated in PV terms.

To evaluate this investment, all the elements should first be converted into PV terms. This also has been done in Exhibit 1–4 in the "PV Equivalent" column. Let's examine the benefits first. We will assume that the going interest or discount rate is 10 percent. The $12,000 annual revenue for 5 years has been treated as an annuity at an interest rate of 10 percent. This is the equivalent of $45,490 in today's dollars (Table 1–2: $12,000 × 3.7908). The resale price of $4,000 will not be realized for 5 years, so this number currently is being expressed as a future value. It is necessary, therefore, to convert this into

today's dollars, which is accomplished by calculating the PV of $4,000. At 10 percent interest, each dollar in 5 years is worth 0.6209 of today's dollars (Table 1–1), which equates to $2,484. The PV of the total benefits is, therefore, $47,973.

Examining the costs, the capital investment of $30,000 is already expressed as a PV, because the equipment is being purchased today. The $5,000 for parts and supplies inventory is currently expressed as a PV, because these must be purchased when the machine is purchased. The resale of these parts and supplies in 5 years when the equipment is sold currently is expressed as a future value and must, therefore, be converted into PV terms. The PV of $5,000 in 5 years at a discount rate of 10 percent is $3,105 ($5,000 × .6209). Because we will be selling these parts, they are listed as a reduction in cost by $3,105. The PV, therefore, of the total costs is $31,896.

The *net* present value (NPV) of this investment, $16,078, is defined as the PV of the total benefits ($47,973) minus the PV of

**Exhibit 1–4** NPV and IRR Analyses of Equipment Acquisition

| | Amount | PV Equivalent |
|---|---|---|
| Benefits | | |
| Net Revenue ($12,000 per Yr. × 5 Years) | $60,000 | $45,490 |
| Resale of Equipment | $4,000 | $2,484 |
| Total Benefits | $64,000 | $47,973 |
| Costs | | |
| Capital Equipment | $30,000 | $30,000 |
| Parts and Supply Inventory | $5,000 | $5,000 |
| Inventory Recouped in 5 Years | | $(3,105) |
| Total Costs | $35,000 | $31,896 |
| Discount Rate | 10% | |
| PV of Total Benefits | $47,973 | |
| PV of Total Costs | $31,896 | |
| NPV | $16,078 | |
| IRR | 27.47% | |

the total costs ($31,896). Because the NPV is positive, this indicates that the investment will exceed the 10 percent hurdle rate or the return that we want from this investment in order to proceed. If the NPV had been negative, that would mean that the investment would not meet our 10 percent criterion.

The IRR is the discount rate at which the PV of the projected benefits is equal to the PV of the projected costs. It is calculated through trial and error by using different discount rates and observing the effect on NPV. When NPV is zero, the IRR has been found. Alternatively, computer spreadsheet programs[9] and hand-held calculators can determine IRR using this same trial-and-error approach. In this example, the IRR is 27.47 percent. The IRR is useful if you are comparing this project with other projects and trying to determine which one to finance. If, for example, you had an office expansion alternative with an IRR of 20 percent, this would tell you that it would be an inferior *financial* investment compared to the project generating a 27.47 percent IRR.

Given that you have no other projects with a more favorable IRR, and the NPV of this investment is a positive number at a hurdle rate that you find acceptable, purchasing the equipment is worthy of consideration. Remember, however, that as a physician leader the financial considerations are only *one* aspect of your total decision-making process. For example, you might decide to purchase the equipment for ethical, convenience, or quality of care considerations even if the financial return is projected to be lower than another alternative. This thinking strikes back to one of the advantages of having physician leaders involved in the decision-making process. Performing the financial analysis first will tell you what your ethics, quality, or convenience considerations would be costing you.

Next, we will apply these tools to a more complex problem by revisiting the General Hospital MRI facility case. **Exhibit 1–5** contains an evaluation of the MRI facility based on expected volumes. With a discount rate of 12 percent, the NPV is $352,091.32. This indicates that the project passes the selected hurdle rate of 12 percent, since the NPV is positive, and that the PV of the benefits exceeds the PV of the costs by $352,091.32. The IRR is 17.08 percent, so this number could be used to compare the MRI project with other hospital projects competing for the same investment funds. The data in Exhibit 1–5 are simply the financial information provided in the preceding MRI discussion, extrapolated forward through year 5. The NPV and IRR are calculated using the NPV and IRR functions in Microsoft Excel. These financial data are one set of information that the physician leader can qualitatively consider along with expected clinical impact when evaluating this project, as well as from other projects competing for the same funds.

Here is a more detailed look at the NPV and IRR analyses in Exhibit 1–5. Begin by looking at the column Year 1. This presents the financial facts of the case, such as the projected volume (3,200 cases), average charge ($625), and so forth. The projected net revenue is $1,500,000, contribution margin is $1,404,000 and total fixed costs before depreciation are $332,000, which results in cash generated by operations of $1,072,000. Year 2 is simply based on a projected volume of 115 percent (stated in the case) of the 2,260 Year 1 base cases (remember, there was a 940 case backlog projected for Year 1). Following the rows down under Year 2, this results in a projected cash generated by operations for Year 2 of $783,313. This is then repeated for each of the remaining years covered in the projection.

**Exhibit 1–5**  General Hospital MRI Proposal: NPV and IRR Analysis

| | Year 1 | Year 2 | Year 3 | Year 4 | Year 5 | Total |
|---|---|---|---|---|---|---|
| Volume | 3,200 | 2,599 | 2,989 | 3,437 | 3,953 | 16,178 |
| Average Charge | $625 | $625 | $625 | $625 | $625 | $625 |
| Gross Revenue | $2,000,000 | $1,624,375 | $1,868,031 | $2,148,236 | $2,470,471 | $10,111,114 |
| Less Bad Debt and Contractual Adj. (25%) | $500,000 | $406,094 | $467,008 | $537,059 | $617,618 | $2,527,778 |
| Net Revenue | $1,500,000 | $1,218,281 | $1,401,023 | $1,611,177 | $1,852,853 | $7,583,335 |
| Less Variable Expenses | | | | | | |
| Supplies and Film | $96,000 | $81,869 | $98,856 | $119,369 | $144,138 | $540,232 |
| Contribution Margin | $1,404,000 | $1,136,413 | $1,302,167 | $1,491,808 | $1,708,716 | $7,043,104 |
| Less Fixed Expenses | | | | | | |
| Salaries | $120,000 | $129,600 | $139,968 | $151,165 | $183,259 | $723,992 |
| Employee Benefits | $30,000 | $32,400 | $34,992 | $37,791 | $45,815 | $180,998 |
| Cryogens | $40,000 | $42,000 | $44,100 | $46,305 | $48,620 | $221,025 |
| Indirect Expenses | $142,000 | $149,100 | $156,555 | $164,383 | $172,602 | $784,640 |
| Maintenance | $— | $— | $248,000 | $260,400 | $273,420 | $781,820 |
| Total Fixed Costs Before Depreciation | $332,000 | $353,100 | $623,615 | $660,045 | $723,715 | $2,692,475 |
| Cash Generated by Operations | $1,072,000 | $783,313 | $678,552 | $831,764 | $985,000 | $4,350,629 |
| Less Depreciation | $560,000 | $560,000 | $560,000 | $560,000 | $560,000 | $2,800,000 |
| Net Income | $512,000 | $223,313 | $118,552 | $271,764 | $425,000 | $1,550,629 |

| | | Year 1 | Year 2 | Year 3 | Year 4 | Year 5 | Total |
|---|---|---|---|---|---|---|---|
| Discount Rate | 0.12 | | | | | | |
| Cash Flows | (2,800,000) | $1,072,000 | $783,313 | $678,552 | $831,764 | $985,000 | $4,350,629 |
| IRR | 17.08% | | | | | | |
| NPV | $352,091.32 | | | | | | |
| Break-Even Point | | 2,033 | 2,088 | 2,717 | 2,811 | 2,970 | |

The cash generated by operations row contains the values that will be used in the NPV and IRR calculations, and these are simply copied into the cash flows row so that all of the variables used for the NPV and IRR analyses are located in the same part of the spreadsheet for the sake of clarity. The case states a discount rate of 12 percent. The initial investment is stated as a negative cash flow of $2,800,000, so this appears as a negative number in the Cash Flows row.

The Microsoft Excel formula for calculating IRR is:

IRR (Value1, Value2, Value3, . . . ValueN)

or in this case,

IRR (−$2,800,000, $1,072,000, $783,313, $678,552, $831,764, $985,000)

which returns a value of 17.08%.

The Microsoft Excel formula for calculating NPV[10] in this instance is:

NPV (Rate, Value1, Value2, . . . ValueN) + Original Investment

The original investment in this case is occurring at the *start* of the first period and this is indicated to Microsoft Excel by adding it to the NPV results, or in this case,

NPV (.12, $1,072,000, $783,313, $678,552, $831,764, $985,000) + −2,800,000

which returns a value of $352,091.32.

You can obtain a feel for how these formulae work and develop a sense of how the variables interact by opening a Microsoft Excel spreadsheet, entering the cash flows and discount rate data into cells, and then calculating IRR and NPV. Change a few of the variables, such as the discount rate, ini-

tial investment, or a cash flow and see the effects on NPV and IRR. Then, imagine what would be necessary in order to achieve this change. This type of "what if" sensitivity analysis is illustrated in detail in Exhibits 1–6 and 1–7.

Once a model like this is created in a spreadsheet, it becomes easy to test the project's sensitivity to various assumptions. For example, an analysis at the 85th volume percentile (**Exhibit 1–6**) paints a very different picture. A drop of 15 percent in volume results in a decrease of more than 41 percent ($512,000 − $301,400 = $210,600) in year 1 net income. The reason that a 15 percent volume reduction can cause a 41 percent drop in net income is that this operation has a high proportion of fixed to variable costs. Each dollar in contribution margin is, therefore, very important. The NPV at the 85 percent volume level is −$384,324.77, which indicates that the costs exceed the benefits by this amount if we need to obtain a 12 percent return on our investment. In addition, the IRR is now 6.12 percent, which is the return that we will receive when benefits equal costs at the 85 percent volume level.

Finally, **Exhibit 1–7** shows the analysis at 115 percent of expected volume. NPV is $1,085,670.27, with an IRR of 26.98 percent. Once again, a modest change in volume has a large impact on net income, NPV, and IRR.

After an examination of these statistics, it becomes very clear that the financial success of this project is highly dependent on the volume level. A physician leader considering this project should question very closely how the volume projections were derived. In addition, he or she should look at the marketing plan to see whether there is a concrete strategy to obtain the needed volume. The model also could be sensitized to other critical assumptions, such as the average charge

**Exhibit 1–6** General Hospital MRI Proposal: NPV and IRR Analysis at 85th Percentile of Projected Volume

| | Year 1 | Year 2 | Year 3 | Year 4 | Year 5 | Total |
|---|---|---|---|---|---|---|
| Volume | 2,720 | 2,209 | 2,541 | 2,922 | 3,360 | 13,751 |
| Average Charge | $625 | $625 | $625 | $625 | $625 | $625 |
| Gross Revenue | $1,700,000 | $1,380,719 | $1,587,827 | $1,826,001 | $2,099,901 | $8,594,446 |
| Less Bad Debt and Contractual Adj. (25%) | $425,000 | $345,180 | $396,957 | $456,500 | $524,975 | $2,148,612 |
| Net Revenue | $1,275,000 | $1,035,539 | $1,190,870 | $1,369,500 | $1,574,925 | $6,445,835 |
| Less Variable Expenses | | | | | | |
| Supplies and Film | $81,600 | $69,588 | $84,028 | $101,464 | $122,517 | $459,197 |
| Contribution Margin | $1,193,400 | $965,951 | $1,106,842 | $1,268,037 | $1,452,408 | $5,986,638 |
| Less Fixed Expenses | | | | | | |
| Salaries | $120,000 | $129,600 | $139,968 | $151,165 | $163,259 | $703,992 |
| Employee Benefits | $30,000 | $32,400 | $34,992 | $37,791 | $40,815 | $175,998 |
| Cryogens | $40,000 | $42,000 | $44,100 | $46,305 | $48,620 | $221,025 |
| Indirect Expenses | $142,000 | $149,100 | $156,555 | $164,383 | $172,602 | $784,640 |
| Maintenance | $0 | $0 | $248,000 | $260,400 | $273,420 | $781,820 |
| Total Fixed Costs Before Depreciation | $332,000 | $353,100 | $623,615 | $660,045 | $698,715 | $2,667,475 |
| Cash Generated by Operations | $861,400 | $612,851 | $483,227 | $607,992 | $753,693 | $3,319,163 |
| Less Depreciation | $560,000 | $560,000 | $560,000 | $560,000 | $560,000 | $2,800,000 |
| Net Income | $301,400 | $52,851 | ($76,773) | $47,992 | $193,693 | $519,163 |

| Discount Rate | 0.12 |
|---|---|
| Cash Flows | (2,800,000) |
| IRR | 6.12% |
| NPV | ($384,324.77) |

| | Year 1 | Year 2 | Year 3 | Year 4 | Year 5 | Total |
|---|---|---|---|---|---|---|
| Cash Flows | $861,400 | $612,851 | $483,227 | $607,992 | $753,693 | $3,319,163 |
| Break-Even Point | 2,033 | 2,088 | 2,717 | 2,811 | 2,912 | |

**Exhibit 1–7** General Hospital MRI Proposal: NPV and IRR Analysis at 115% of Projected Volume

|  | Year 1 | Year 2 | Year 3 | Year 4 | Year 5 | Total |
|---|---|---|---|---|---|---|
| Volume | 3,680 | 2,989 | 3,437 | 3,953 | 4,546 | 18,604 |
| Average Charge | $625 | $625 | $625 | $625 | $625 | $625 |
| Gross Revenue | $2,300,000 | $1,868,031 | $2,148,236 | $2,470,471 | $2,841,042 | $11,627,781 |
| Less Bad Debt and Contractual Adj. (25%) | $575,000 | $467,008 | $537,059 | $617,618 | $710,261 | $2,906,945 |
| Net Revenue | $1,725,000 | $1,401,023 | $1,611,177 | $1,852,853 | $2,130,782 | $8,720,835 |
| Less Variable Expenses |  |  |  |  |  |  |
| Supplies and Film | $110,400 | $94,149 | $113,685 | $137,274 | $165,759 | $621,266 |
| Contribution Margin | $1,614,600 | $1,306,875 | $1,497,492 | $1,715,579 | $1,965,023 | $8,099,569 |
| Less Fixed Expenses |  |  |  |  |  |  |
| Salaries | $120,000 | $129,600 | $139,968 | $171,165 | $184,859 | $745,592 |
| Employee Benefits | $30,000 | $32,400 | $34,992 | $42,791 | $46,215 | $186,398 |
| Cryogens | $40,000 | $42,000 | $44,100 | $46,305 | $48,620 | $221,025 |
| Indirect Expenses | $142,000 | $149,100 | $156,555 | $164,383 | $172,602 | $784,640 |
| Maintenance | $0 | $0 | $248,000 | $260,400 | $273,420 | $781,820 |
| Total Fixed Costs Before Depreciation | $332,000 | $353,100 | $623,615 | $685,045 | $725,715 | $2,719,475 |
| Cash Generated by Operations | $1,282,600 | $953,775 | $873,877 | $1,030,535 | $1,239,307 | $5,380,094 |
| Less Depreciation: | $560,000 | $560,000 | $560,000 | $560,000 | $560,000 | $2,800,000 |
| Net Income | $722,600 | $393,775 | $313,877 | $470,535 | $679,307 | $2,580,094 |
| Discount Rate | 0.12 |  |  |  |  |  |
| Cash Flows | (2,800,000) | $1,282,600 | $953,775 | $873,877 | $1,030,535 | $1,239,307 | $5,380,094 |
| IRR | 26.98% |  |  |  |  |  |
| NPV | $1,085,670.27 |  |  |  |  |  |
| Break-Even Point | 2,033 | 2,088 | 2,717 | 2,869 | 2,974 |  |

and bad debt assumptions. We would expect that, given the sensitivity to changes in net revenue, controlling these other two variables also would be critical to the project's success. Once again, making certain that the business plan for this project makes reasonable volume, fee, and collection assumptions, and that there will be a plan to manage these variables after project implementation will be critical to the project's success. The physician leader who asks these questions, who ensures that reasonable assumptions are being made, and who ascertains that the business plan makes reasonable provision for achieving and monitoring critical success these factors is making a very positive contribution to his or her organization.

## LEASE VERSUS PURCHASE DECISIONS

Another capital asset decision that healthcare organizations often need to make is whether to purchase equipment outright or through a lease. Once again, the technique of pulling all financial considerations back to

the present through a PV analysis provides a time-consistent method of addressing this problem. For example, suppose that you either could buy an office networked computer system for $10,000 or lease it with the following terms: an initial payment of $1,000, three annual payments of $2,500 at the end of each year, and an option to buy the computer system at the end of the lease for $3,500. In addition, you feel that the value of the system in 3 years will be $4,000. Under both arrangements, you will have to maintain it. The prevailing interest rate is 10 percent.

The real cost of the lease can be determined through a PV analysis, as shown in **Exhibit 1–8**. The initial payment of $1,000 is stated as a PV. The PV of the three $2,500 payments is evaluated as an annuity at 10 percent, which has a PV of $6,217 (Table 1–2: $2,500 × 2.4869). Assuming that you want to keep the computer at the end of the lease, the PV of the $3,500 payment is $2,630 (Table 1–1: $3,500 × .7513). The total PV for the lease comes to $9,847 ($1,000 + $6,217 + $2,630). The purchase alternative costs $10,000, so that leasing the computer is $153 less expensive.

---

**Exhibit 1–8**  Analysis of a Lease versus Purchase Decision

| Item | Amount | Lease PV Equivalent | Purchase PV Equivalent | Difference |
|------|--------|--------------------|-----------------------|-----------|
| *Purchase After 3 Years* | | | | |
|   Initial Payment | $1,000 | $1,000 | $10,000 | |
|   3 Annual Payments @ $2,500 | $7,500 | $6,217 | $   — | |
|   Purchase at End of Lease | $3,500 | $2,630 | $   — | |
|   Total | | $9,847 | $10,000 | $(153) |
| | | | | |
| *Do Not Purchase After 3 Years* | | | | |
|   Initial Payment | $1,000 | $1,000 | $10,000 | |
|   3 Annual Payments @ $2,500 | $7,500 | $6,216 | $   — | |
|   Est. Selling Price | $4,000 | $   — | $(3,005) | |
|   Total | | $7,216 | $ 6,995 | $222 |
| Discount Rate: 10% | | | | |

If you do not buy the computer system at the end of the lease, the PV analysis in Exhibit 1–8 indicates that leasing will be $222 more expensive than purchasing. Note that the purchase choice includes selling the computer, so the outcome for both the lease and purchase is that you no longer own the computer system. Obviously, this analysis is very sensitive to the resale price of the computer in 3 years. It could be performed, however, for any level of equipment value, and the physician then could make a decision to lease or buy based on the subjective probability of various resale values. This analysis also excludes the cost and inconvenience of selling the computer.

## FINANCIAL STATEMENTS, REPORTS, AND ACCOUNTING SYSTEMS

Three financial statements form the basis for describing the financial status of any organization, whether it is a solo private practice or a large healthcare system. They are the balance sheet, income statement, and cash flow statement. They provide a standard, accepted way of presenting and summarizing important and fundamental financial information. They are informative in their own right, but they can also be used as the basis for additional analyses. The *balance sheet* is a listing of the organization's assets and claims against the assets at a point in time. The *income statement* compares the wealth generated by the organization against the expenses incurred as a result of generating that wealth during a time period. The *cash flow statement* describes cash receipts and cash disbursements that have occurred during a time period.

**Exhibit 1–9** contains a balance sheet for a private practice as of December 31, 20XX. A balance sheet shows the financial condition of an organization on a given day, and it is based on the following financial model:

$$\text{Assets} = \text{Liabilities} + \text{Owner's Equity}$$

The items in Exhibit 1–9 under the heading "Assets" delineate all the wealth owned by the practice. This can be cash, office equipment, medical equipment, receivables, and the like. Generally, they are listed in order of their liquidity, or the ability to turn the asset into cash. The liabilities are a listing of the claims against the assets. Examples include accounts payable (unpaid bills), salaries owed, taxes due, and loans payable. Owner's equity is that part of the assets that exceeds the liabilities. In effect, the owner(s) own whatever is left over after creditors have been assigned their claims against the assets.

Owner's equity can occur in various ways. Retained earnings represent the earnings over the life of the organization that have not been distributed to the owners. When the organization generates earnings but keeps them in the company, perhaps in anticipation of financing additional growth, this constitutes retained earnings. Contributed capital is wealth that the owner has put into the organization in the form of cash, equipment, or some other asset. In this case, most of the owner's equity has resulted from retained earnings ($184,412) due to operational activity, and only $20,000 is due to contributed capital. If the situation were reversed, it would provide a very different economic picture. In a private practice, retained earnings are usually distributed to the owner each year to avoid double taxation.[11]

*Balance sheets always must balance.* The sum of liabilities and owner's equity always must be equal to assets. Someone always has a claim against the assets, whether it is creditors or owners of the organization. If liabilities exceed assets, then there will be a negative

**Exhibit 1–9**  Balance Sheet: Arnold Bennett, MD, PC

| | | | |
|---|---|---|---|
| *December 31, 20XX* | | | |
| ASSETS | | | |
|   Current Assets | | | |
|     Cash | $40,589 | | |
|     Accounts Receivable | $145,664 | | |
|     Adj. Participating Contracts and Bad Debt | $(43,699) | | |
|     Marketable Securities | $3,572 | | |
|     Prepaid Expenses | $7,325 | | |
|     Inventory: Medical and Office Supplies | $3,589 | | |
|     Total | | $157,040 | |
|   Property and Equipment | | | |
|     Building | $109,237 | | |
|     Land | $40,896 | | |
|     Medical and Office Equipment, Furniture | $87,567 | | |
|     Less Accumulated Depreciation | $(23,879) | | |
|     Total | | $213,821 | |
|   Total Assets | | | $370,861 |
| LIABILITIES | | | |
|   Current Liabilities | | | |
|     Accounts Payable | $28,479 | | |
|     Refunds Due Patients | $879 | | |
|     Salaries Due | $29,875 | | |
|     Prepaid Patient Fees | $527 | | |
|     Payroll Taxes Due | $5,010 | | |
|     Salaries Due on Accounts Receivable | $61,179 | | |
|     Total | | $125,949 | |
|   Long-Term Debt | | | |
|     Bank Loan Capital Equipment | $40,500 | | |
|     Total | | $40,500 | |
|   Total Liabilities | | | $166,449 |
| OWNERS EQUITY | | | |
|   Contributed Capital at Start-Up | $20,000 | | |
|   Retained Earnings | $184,412 | | |
|   Total Owner's Equity | | | $204,412 |
| TOTAL LIABILITIES AND OWNER'S EQUITY | | | $370,861 |

owner's equity. A negative owner's equity indicates that the organization is insolvent.

At this point, it is appropriate to say a few words about depreciation. Depreciation is an adjustment for capital items, such as office equipment, surgical lasers, computers, buildings, and the like, which are consumed through their use. All capital except land wears out with use and over time. An estimate is made of an item's useful life, and its cost is depreciated on that basis. If a lithotripsy machine has an expected useful life of 6 years and costs $300,000, then we would take $50,000 ($300,000 ÷ 6) each year, if we are using straight-line depreciation.[12] Depreciation appears on the balance sheet as a negative value under assets. This indicates that the full value of the asset is being reduced by the amount of the depreciation.

If depreciation of capital equipment is not provided for, then it is possible that when the equipment does wear out, there will not be cash available to purchase a replacement. Imagine, for example, a self-employed trucker who does not set aside cash every year for the day that his rig wears out. If this trucker makes no provision for depreciation and treats all his net income as profit available for spending, he may well be living off his depreciation. When the inevitable happens and the rig does wear out, he may not have the cash available to purchase a replacement.

Cities, such as New York in the 1970s, and countries, such as Great Britain after World War II, found themselves in the predicament of not being able to tax their citizens at a sufficiently high rate to renew their capital infrastructure and pursue all the other initiatives that were politically desirable. As a result, both these entities did to some degree live off their depreciation, which ultimately resulted in near bankruptcy for New York, along with potholed roads and crumbling bridges.

The income statement compares the wealth generated by an organization with the expenses incurred as a result of generating the revenue for a particular time period, such as a month or year. The income statement is built on the following financial model:

$$Income = Revenues - Expenses$$

**Exhibit 1–10** contains an income statement for a private practice. Revenues reflect the acquisition of wealth. They can be generated by clinical services, laboratory fees, patient beds, the gift shop, consultations, or any other product or service that the organization provides. Expenses are all the costs incurred by the organization to generate those revenues. These could include clerical and professional salaries, rent, medical supplies, and so on. Net income is what is left over after expenses have been subtracted from revenues.

Both the balance sheet and the income statement are examples of *accrual basis accounting*. Accrual accounting records events when wealth is generated, as opposed to when cash is received. Similarly, it records expenses when the wealth that they are associated with is generated, as opposed to when a check is written to pay for the expense. By pairing the wealth generated with the expense of generating that wealth, it is possible to determine whether the practice, program, or hospital, is operating at a profit or loss.

This should be contrasted with *cash basis accounting* (also called *checkbook accounting*), in which revenues are recorded when they are received and expenses are recorded when they are paid. With cash basis accounting, there is no attempt to match revenues with the specific expenses that they generated to determine income. As a result, if cash disbursements lag or precede the collection of cash, you cannot determine your true profit or loss position.

The cash flow statement is a cash-based analysis of cash receipts and cash disbursements for a given time period. **Exhibit 1–11** shows a cash flow statement. It begins in the first column with the current cash balance. Cash receipts and cash disbursements for the period then are noted, and a net income for the period is calculated. This then is added to the entering cash balance to calculate an ending cash balance for the period. This ending cash balance then becomes the entering cash balance for the next time period. The cash flow statement tracks cash, which is very important, because creditors have to be paid in cash. An organization can have wealth, but if

**Exhibit 1–10**  Income Statement: Arnold Bennett, MD, PC

| | | | |
|---|---|---|---|
| *January 1, 20XX, to December 31, 20XX* | | | |
| REVENUE | | | |
| | Clinical Services | $1,056,825 | |
| | Bad Debt and Adjustments | $(264,206) | |
| | Consultation Fees | $12,587 | |
| | Speakers Fees | $8,655 | |
| | Total Revenue | | $813,861 |
| EXPENSES | | | |
| | Clerical Salaries | $103,667 | |
| | Professional Compensation | $296,438 | |
| | Payroll Taxes | $118,575 | |
| | Rent | $48,000 | |
| | Advertising | $8,995 | |
| | Office Supplies | $37,889 | |
| | Medical Supplies | $56,551 | |
| | Interest Expense | $1,229 | |
| | Local Taxes | $4,670 | |
| | Insurance | $67,889 | |
| | Education | $8,977 | |
| | Telephone—Land Line | $1,320 | |
| | Telephone—Cell | $1,200 | |
| | Depreciation | $14,278 | |
| | Total Expenses | | $769,678 |
| NET INCOME | | | $44,183 |

it is not present in the form of cash when the bills need to be paid, it will have a serious liquidity problem.

Organizations need both cash and accrual information. Each serves a different purpose. Cash accounting is necessary to pay the bills. It is the financial minimum that all organizations need. Cash management is important, because bills must be paid with cash, checking accounts need to be balanced, and cash should be managed so it is in the most favorable place to earn interest and be available to pay expenses. Accrual-based accounting information is used for making decisions. It provides a more complete picture of the financial situation by controlling for when bills *happen* to be presented, and when payments *happen* to be received. Both cash in-

formation and accrual information are necessary to effectively manage an organization's finances.

For example, suppose that you pay an annual liability insurance premium of $12,000 in April. You need to record the full amount in a cash disbursements journal in April, because it reflects the reality that your checking account has $12,000 less in it. If other total disbursements for April were $38,000 and total monthly receipts were $45,000, then on a cash basis you would be showing a $5,000 loss for the month ($45,000 − $12,000 − $38,000 = −$5,000). The full $12,000 will appear in the cash basis cash flow statement. This cash basis information, however, would provide a misleading picture of how well you did financially in April. The

**Exhibit 1–11**  Cash Flow Statement: Arnold Bennett, MD, PC

|  | January | February | March | Year to Date |
|---|---|---|---|---|
| ENTERING CASH BALANCE | $10,237.67 | $49,434.44 | $27,328.36 | $10,237.67 |
| **CASH RECEIPTS** | | | | |
| Fees Collected | $60,046.06 | $33,082.35 | $68,746.74 | $161,875.15 |
| Interest Income | $61.49 | $59.73 | $48.56 | $169.78 |
| TOTAL INCOME | $60,107.55 | $33,142.08 | $68,795.30 | $162,044.93 |
| **CASH DISBURSEMENTS** | | | | |
| Salaries—Management | $0.00 | $6,812.22 | $7,322.70 | $14,134.92 |
| Salaries—Administrative | $1,735.79 | $4,016.14 | $6,429.97 | $12,181.90 |
| Salaries—Physician | $7,536.15 | $30,723.40 | $22,976.23 | $61,235.78 |
| Temporary Help | $401.85 | $619.20 | $0.00 | $1,021.05 |
| Employee Benefits | $236.98 | $445.70 | $440.00 | $1,122.68 |
| Building Rent | $5,789.95 | $7,021.41 | $5,492.48 | $18,303.84 |
| Equipment Rental | $0.00 | $836.74 | $418.37 | $1,255.11 |
| Utilities | $447.95 | $381.69 | $626.91 | $1,456.55 |
| Maintenance and Repairs | $0.00 | $46.25 | $40.50 | $86.75 |
| Advertising | $0.00 | $570.25 | $407.34 | $977.59 |
| Office Overhead | $1,409.03 | $656.80 | $1,804.09 | $3,869.92 |
| Professional Services | $500.00 | $700.00 | $250.00 | $1,450.00 |
| Service | $0.00 | $0.00 | $321.00 | $321.00 |
| Insurance | $1,060.01 | $455.06 | $877.99 | $2,393.06 |
| Interest | $0.00 | $0.00 | $0.00 | $0.00 |
| Credit Card Discounts | $30.50 | $84.29 | $53.53 | $168.32 |
| Bank Service Charges | $25.68 | $25.68 | $25.68 | $77.04 |
| Dues and Subscriptions | $97.47 | $58.00 | $51.47 | $206.94 |
| Auto and Travel | $0.00 | $0.00 | $178.00 | $178.00 |
| Meals and Entertainment | $626.49 | $146.35 | $318.99 | $1,091.83 |
| Taxes and Licenses | $739.03 | $1,375.27 | $1,969.83 | $4,084.13 |
| Fines and Penalties | $0.00 | $0.00 | $10.00 | $10.00 |
| Depreciation | $294.00 | $294.00 | $294.00 | $882.00 |
| Amortization | $5.00 | $5.00 | $5.00 | $15.00 |
| TOTAL DISBURSEMENTS | $20,935.88 | $55,273.45 | $50,314.08 | $126,523.41 |
| NET INCOME | $39,171.67 | ($22,131.37) | $18,481.22 | $35,521.52 |
| ENDING CASH BALANCE | $49,409.34 | $27,303.07 | $45,809.58 | $45,759.19 |

insurance payment is an annual premium, and you are distorting the April results by dumping all the insurance expense into that month. To gain a better understanding of how the practice really performed in April, you should recognize that you really only used one twelfth of the premium ($1,000) during April. An accrual analysis, such as found in an income statement, would show net income for April of $6,000 ($45,000 − $1,000 − $38,000 = $6,000). Both perspectives are important. You need cash accounting to be certain that the cash is available to pay the insurance premium. You need accrual information to understand the financial position of the organization and for planning purposes.

Accrual-based accounting utilizes the following adjustments that otherwise would distort the financial picture:

- *Revenue collected in advance, but not yet earned (deferred revenue)*—Mr. Chandhari sees you on January 23 for a sinus infection. You treat him and tell him to return in 2 weeks. Mr. Chandhari's copayment is $25, but he makes a $50 payment to cover today's appointment and the future visit. In this case, the cash that was collected for the future visit preceded the recognition of revenue, because you have not yet provided the service. Mr. Chandhari's payment for the future appointment would appear as a balance sheet liability, because it is a debt or obligation that you owe to Mr. Chandhari. It might appear under a category such as "Prepaid Patient Fees." This second $25.00 payment would not affect the income statement because the activity that generates the recognition of wealth (the follow-up visit) has not yet occurred. Both $25.00 transactions would be logged as a cash receipt in the cash flow statement, because cash was received.

Prepayment of fees to cover a panel of patients for a future time period also falls into this category. Failure to treat the prepaid fees in this manner could lead to disbursements of cash to physicians because cash would be available. Unfortunately, the expenses (patients coming in for services) would then follow. In addition, the fixed expenses associated with these future time periods would also become payable. The result could be that cash might not be available to cover them.

- *Revenue earned, but not yet collected (accrued revenue)*—When you provide services today but patients or insurance carriers pay at a future time, the moneys are recorded *now* as revenue. Revenue is recorded when you provide the service irrespective of whether the service is paid for immediately in cash, whether you extend credit in the form of a promise to pay, or whether you bill an insurance company. Some revenue will translate into future cash, and some will not, such as bad debt or insurance company contractual adjustments. Revenue that will be paid at a future time can be listed as an asset in the form of an accounts receivable item, such as on the balance sheet in Exhibit 1–9. Notice also that this balance sheet makes a provision for bad debt and contractual write-offs. Wealth in this category will appear on the income statement under revenue (See Exhibit 1–10). Once again, it would be appropriate to make an adjustment for expected bad debt and contractual write-offs. Items in this category would not affect the cash flow statement because no cash has been received.

- *Expenses paid in advance, but not yet incurred (deferred expenses)*—Expenses that are paid in advance must be deferred to the future time periods to which they apply. These prepaid items appear as assets on the balance sheet. Prepaid expenses could include annual insurance premiums, computer service contracts, rent, and so on. Prepaid expenses appear on the balance sheet as an asset. They don't affect the income statement because the activity that generates the recognition of wealth has not occurred yet. They do appear on the cash flow statement, because cash has been expended. From a cash receipts and disbursements perspective, deferred expenses can create cash flow problems. Usually, you will have no choice regarding the prepayment of these items. The malpractice insurance company, for example, may want the whole annual premium now. Examining this situation from an accrual perspective will not make the insurance company's "bite" any less painful. It will put it into perspective, however, so that you can see the real relationship between your assets and your liabilities, and between your revenues and expenses. Obviously, from a time value of money perspective, this category of expense should be avoided.

Prepaid expenses do not affect the income statement. Once again, the activity that generates the wealth, and therefore its associated expenses, has not occurred yet. Prepaid expenses *do* appear on the cash flow statement. In this case the whole prepayment is entered, because that was the actual amount of cash that was disbursed.

- *Expenses incurred but not yet paid (accrued expenses)*—Expenses in this category must be recorded in the time period in which they were incurred irrespective of when you actually pay them. For example, suppose your local government assesses a 0.58 percent annual tax on gross receipts in arrears. Your cash flow statements and your checkbook will show no local tax payments for 12 months, and one large payment in the 13th month. Accrual-based accounting, however, would recognize 0.58 percent of gross receipts as they are earned. The balance sheet, therefore, will show a tax liability and the income statement will show an expense. The cash flow statement would not be affected because no cash has been disbursed. Once again, cash-based accounting would be deceptive of the true economic situation. If you are deceived and don't make a provision for the taxes you have incurred, a cash flow problem may appear when the tax is due.[13]
- *Allocation of the cost of long-term assets considered used up in the current period to help generate revenues*—An example is the requirement that a hospital record monthly depreciation charges (expenses) for a portion of the property, plant, and equipment that is considered to be consumed each month. The effect on the balance sheet is to reduce assets, such as capital equipment, along with retained earnings on the liability side. This item also affects the income statement, since the asset has been consumed or depreciated in value in the process of generating revenue. It does not affect the cash flow statement, because no disbursement of cash has taken place.

### Case Analysis: Angus McLeod, MD[14]

Angus McLeod, MD, was perplexed. "I can't figure it out," he said. "I've run my own practice for almost a year now, and I have more patients by far than I have ever had. Yet here I am, just before Christmas, and I don't have enough cash in the bank to pay for that new HDTV for my family. What has gone wrong?"

Dr. McLeod started his own practice on January 1, after leaving a seven-physician group psychiatric practice, where he had worked for 3 years. He left the group because he did not like the "politics." He took $80,000 from savings, rented office space, purchased the necessary furniture and supplies, and hired a secretary/business manager.

By midyear, his practice had grown substantially, and he hired a clinical psychologist to take his overflow. He also hired an insurance/collection clerk to deal with the volume, upgraded his computer system for billing and word processing, and signed a lease for adjacent office space for the new staff. "Other than this, I don't recall any other major changes," he added. It seemed to him, however, that the better his practice became, the less cash he had in the bank.

Dr. McLeod was confident that his December work would bring in enough cash to meet the December 31 payroll. Even so, he had far less cash in the bank at the end of the year than when he started his practice. This disturbed him because, as he put it:

> I have sunk a lot into this practice—given up the security of a large group practice, and have worked day and night to make a go of it. If this isn't going to pay off, I'd like to know it soon, so that I can make other plans. Recently, for example, a health system asked me if I would like to join them in a salaried position. I've made a lot of sacrifices in this past year, and I'd like to know whether it was all worthwhile.

A balance sheet for Dr. McLeod's practice dated October 1, 20XX, is shown in **Exhibit 1–12.** The top row of data in the spreadsheet in **Exhibit 1–13** is the same as the data in the balance sheet in Exhibit 1–12, but turned on its side so we can use them more easily to do calculations. We will use this spreadsheet to construct a new income statement, bal-

---

**Exhibit 1–12** Balance Sheet: Angus McLeod, MD

*Balance Sheet: October 1, 20XX*

ASSETS
| | | |
|---|---|---|
| Cash | $10 | |
| Accounts Receivable | $60,000 | |
| Prepaid Insurance | $1,000 | |
| Equipment | $24,000 | |
| Total | | $85,010 |

LIABILITIES
| | | |
|---|---|---|
| Accounts Payable | $2,000 | |
| Total | | $2,000 |

OWNER'S EQUITY
| | | |
|---|---|---|
| Capital Contributed | $80,000 | |
| Retained Earnings | $3,010 | |
| Total | | $83,010 |

| | |
|---|---|
| LIABILITIES AND OWNER'S EQUITY | $85,010 |

*Source:* © William T. Geary, Ph.D., and Robert J. Solomon, Ph.D. 2007. All Rights Reserved.

---

ance sheet, and cash flow statement based on the following events that occurred in October. The numbers of the following items pertain to the Items column in Exhibit 1–13:

1. The total revenue generated in October through therapy sessions, medication evaluations, hospital rounds, and his employed psychologist is $60,000. Of this amount, $10,000 is received in cash or check, and the remainder is billed. *Effect:* We add $10,000 to the cash account and $50,000 to the receivables account. Because balance sheets always must balance, we must add $60,000 to the retained earnings account. *Notice that all the wealth is recorded at the time it was generated,* not when it happens to be converted into cash collected.

2. $38,000 in cash is collected on old accounts. *Effect:* Add $38,000 to the cash account and subtract $38,000 from the receivables account. Notice that nothing needs to be done to the right side of the spreadsheet because the wealth was recorded at the time that it was generated. What has happened is that the form of the wealth has shifted from receivables to cash, which is of course a welcome shift.

3. Dr. McLeod pays an annual insurance premium, due November 15, of $6,000. *Effect:* We move $6,000 from cash into prepaid insurance. Once again, nothing needs to be done to the right side of the statement, because we are simply changing how we are holding wealth that has already been accounted for. Note also that none of the value of the insurance has been consumed yet.

4. $8,000 cash is paid for monthly operating expenses exclusive of salaries. *Effect:* Cash is disbursed, so the cash account is reduced by $8,000. The balance sheet must remain in balance, so retained earnings must also be reduced by $8,000. The

**Exhibit 1–13** Spreadsheet Analysis: Angus McLeod, MD

*Transactions for October 20XX*

| Item | ASSETS | | | | = | | LIABILITIES + OWNER'S EQUITY | | |
| | Cash | Accounts Receivable | Prepaid Insurance | Equipment | = | | Accounts Payable | Contributed Capital | Retained Earnings |
|---|---|---|---|---|---|---|---|---|---|
| | $10 | $60,000 | $1,000 | $24,000 | = | $85,010 | $2,000 | $80,000 | $3,010 | = | $85,010 |
| 1 | $10,000 | $50,000 | | | | | | | $60,000 |
| 2 | $38,000 | $(38,000) | | | | | | | |
| 3 | $(6,000) | | $6,000 | | | | | | |
| 4 | $(8,000) | | | | | | | | $(8,000) |
| 5 | $(22,000) | | | | | | | | $(22,000) |
| 6 | $(8,000) | | | $8,000 | | | | | |
| 7 | $(3,000) | | | | | | | | $(3,000) |
| 8 | | | $(800) | $(500) | | | | | $(1,300) |
| 9 | | $(15,000) | | | | | | | $(15,000) |
| | $1,010 | $57,000 | $6,200 | $31,500 | = | $95,710 | $2,000 | $80,000 | $13,710 | = | $95,710 |

*Note:* Item numbers refer to description in the text.

*Source:* © William T. Geary, Ph.D., and Robert J. Solomon, Ph.D. 2007. All Rights Reserved.

distinction between this disbursement and the preceding one is that this time the disbursement is for items that have been consumed in this month. Retained earnings represent the wealth retained in the organization. The $8,000 cash is gone, as is the value of what it purchased. Retained earnings, therefore, must be reduced by this amount.

5. Cash is paid to employees for salaries of $22,000. *Effect:* Once again, we have a disbursement for work that was fully utilized in this month, so both the cash account and the retained earnings account are reduced by $22,000.

6. $8,000 cash is paid for new computer equipment and upgrades in office furnishings. *Effect:* This transaction simply changes the form in which we are holding this wealth. As a result, we decrease the cash account by $8,000 and increase the equipment account by $8,000. Our balance sheet remains in balance.

7. Dr. McLeod pays himself $3,000 in salary for the month. *Effect:* We reduce the cash account by $3,000. Because this is a transfer of wealth outside the practice, we also must reduce the retained earnings account by $3,000, and our balance sheet remains in balance.

8. Monthly adjustments are made of $800 for expired insurance and $500 for depreciation. *Effect:* We reduce the prepaid insurance account by $800 and the equipment account by $500 because we have consumed a month's worth of insurance and equipment life. The retained earnings account must also be reduced by these amounts because this wealth has been consumed. The balance sheet remains in balance.

9. During this month, Dr. McLeod writes off $15,000 of his outstanding receivables as uncollectible. *Effect:* Both the accounts receivable and retained earnings accounts are reduced by $15,000. The balance sheet remains in balance.

If we now examine our final spreadsheet, the bottom row constitutes our new balance sheet. We can construct an income statement for October 20XX by looking at the new revenues and expenses that have been incurred during October 20XX. Finally, we can construct a cash flow statement from the cash account by noting the beginning balance, the cash transactions that occurred, and the ending balance.

A new set of financial statements appears in **Exhibit 1–14**. What conclusions can we draw about Dr. McLeod's practice? We can see from the cash flow statement that he is short on cash. Things are better, however, than they were at the beginning of the month. The income statement tells us that he had a very good month for generating wealth. Unfortunately, much of the wealth is not in cash but in receivables. The balance sheet tells us that his assets are largely in receivables and equipment. In addition, the retained earnings are largely due to his original investment, not economic growth. The last month, however, has seen his retained earnings due to economic growth increase by $10,700. This is hopeful.

In summary, Dr. McLeod has put the pieces in place to generate wealth. The question now is whether he can convert the wealth that exists in his receivables and equipment into cash and continue to do this in the future. The cash picture is not rosy. He must manage his cash very carefully, stop all spending on equipment unless it is absolutely essential—perhaps use leasing—and motivate his staff to effectively collect on the accounts receivable.

This case illustrates how financial information can help describe the financial status

**Exhibit 1–14**  October 20XX Financial Statements for Angus McLeod, MD

*Cash Flow Statement: October 1–30, 20XX*

| | | |
|---|---:|---:|
| Opening Balance | $10 | |
| Cash Received | $10,000 | |
| Cash Collected on Accounts | $38,000 | |
| Insurance Premium | $(6,000) | |
| Operating Expenses | $(8,000) | |
| Employee Salaries | $(22,000) | |
| Computer, Etc. | $(8,000) | |
| Angus' Salary | $(3,000) | |
| Closing Balance | | $1,010 |

*Income Statement: October 1–30, 20XX*

REVENUES

| | | |
|---|---:|---:|
| Cash | $10,000 | |
| Receivables | $50,000 | |
| Total | | $60,000 |

EXPENSES

| | | |
|---|---:|---:|
| Operating | $8,000 | |
| Salaries | $22,000 | |
| Angus' Salary | $3,000 | |
| Insurance | $800 | |
| Depreciation | $500 | |
| Bad Debts and Write-Offs | $15,000 | |
| Total | | $49,300 |

| | |
|---|---:|
| NET INCOME | $10,700 |

Balance Sheet: October 30, 20XX

ASSETS

| | | |
|---|---:|---:|
| Cash | $1,010 | |
| Accounts Receivable | $57,000 | |
| Prepaid Insurance | $6,200 | |
| Equipment | $31,500 | |
| Total | | $95,710 |

LIABILITIES

| | | |
|---|---:|---:|
| Accounts Payable | $2,000 | |
| Total | | $2,000 |

OWNER'S EQUITY

| | | |
|---|---:|---:|
| Capital Contributed | $80,000 | |
| Retained Earnings | $13,710 | |
| Total | | $93,710 |

| | |
|---|---:|
| LIABILITIES AND OWNER'S EQUITY | $95,710 |

*Source:* © William T. Geary, Ph.D., and Robert J. Solomon, Ph.D. 2007. All Rights Reserved.

of an organization. It also illustrates how financial information can be used to guide management decision making. The financial data from the balance sheet, income statement, and cash flow statement tell Dr. McLeod where he needs to focus his attention in his capacity as a physician leader. Finally, they also provide him with some insight into his decision about the health system job offer. This practice clearly needs management attention, specifically Dr. McLeod's attention. If he decides that the management part of being a physician leader is not for him, then he probably will be best off to accept the health system's offer. The use of financial information to aid in making management decisions is further illustrated by the case of Oregon Sports Medicine, which is discussed at the end of this chapter.

### Ratio Analysis

Data from the balance sheet and the income statement can be used to assess an organization's liquidity, solvency, and profitability by constructing ratios. Ratios also can be used to help examine an organization's financial performance over time and to observe developing financial trends.

*Liquidity* is the ability to use assets to meet currently maturing debts. Tests of liquidity evaluate the degree to which an organization's current liabilities can be met using its current assets. *Current liabilities* are defined as obligations or services that a practice owes or will have to fulfill within the next year. Examples include wages payable, income taxes payable, and credit card balances. *Current assets* are resources owned by the organization that are currently in cash form, or could be converted into cash within the next year. Examples include cash savings, shares in publicly traded common stock, and

a reasonable (defined as likely to be collected) proportion of accounts receivable. Dr. Arnold Bennett's balance sheet (Exhibit 1–9) and income statement (Exhibit 1–10) will be used to illustrate examples of ratio analysis.

### Liquidity Ratios

A commonly used test of liquidity is called the *current ratio*, which is defined as follows:

$$\text{Current Ratio} = \text{Current Assets} \div \text{Current Liabilities} \qquad (1\text{--}5)$$

Referring to the data in Exhibit 1–9, the current ratio for Dr. Bennett's practice is:

$$\text{Current Ratio} = \$157,040 \div \$125,949 = 1.25$$

This indicates that Dr. Bennett has $1.25 of current assets for each dollar of current liabilities. Stated another way, this indicates that Dr. Bennett has a 25 percent "cushion" to deal with his liabilities. This cushion is helpful given that cash may flow unevenly into his practice. If Dr. Bennett's current ratio was 2.00 at this time last year, then he should consider investigating the change.

A more demanding test of a practice's liquidity is called the *quick ratio* or the *acid test ratio*:

$$\text{Quick Ratio} = \text{Quick Assets} \div \text{Current Liabilities} \qquad (1\text{--}6)$$

Quick assets are cash or other current assets that can be easily converted into cash, such as stocks, bonds, certificates of deposit, and accounts receivable adjusted for bad debt and write-offs. Dr. Bennett's quick ratio is as follows:

$$\text{Quick Ratio} = \$146,126 \div \$125,949 = 1.16$$

All Dr. Bennett's current assets, except his inventory and prepaid expenses, are considered quick assets, because they could be readily converted into cash. Dr. Bennett's quick ratio indicates that his practice has $1.16 worth of readily available assets for each dollar of current debt.

An additional perspective on liquidity is gained by considering how quickly a practice's receivables are turned into cash. An index of this can be calculated by examining the average daily billings and the average collection period, which are defined as follows:

$$\text{Average Daily Billings} = \text{Net Billings} \div 365 \text{ Days} \quad (1\text{--}7)$$

$$\text{Average Collection Period} = \text{Accounts Receivable} \div \text{Average Daily Billings} \quad (1\text{--}8)$$

By using the data in Exhibits 1–9 and 1–10, we can calculate these ratios for Dr. Bennett's practice:

$$\text{Average Daily Billings} = \$792,619^{15} \div 365 = \$2,172$$

$$\text{Average Collection Period} = \$101,965^{16} \div \$2,171 = 47 \text{ Days}$$

This indicates that, on average, Dr. Bennett collects his receivables in 47 days. This figure can be used in two ways. First, it can help determine whether the collection performance is acceptable. What is required is a qualitative evaluation in which Dr. Bennett examines the 47-day average in the context of his revenue sources. If, for example, he does a large amount of insurance work, then an average collection period of 47 days might indicate acceptable effectiveness. On the other hand, if a large proportion of Dr. Bennett's patients are cash patients and are supposed to pay at the time of service or are prepaid, such as in a concierge practice, then 47 days might indicate a collection problem. Collection assessment and methods will be discussed in Chapter 2.

A second use of the average collection period ratio is as a gauge of liquidity over time. By tracking this ratio over the years, Dr. Bennett can assess how his practice's liquidity is changing and examine whether changes in his clientele, the services he provides, insurance company policies and procedures, and so on may be affecting its liquidity.

### Solvency Ratio

An organization's solvency is its ability to meet its debt obligations. A common statistic used to assess solvency is the debt-to-equity ratio (DER). The data used to compute the DER are contained in the balance sheet (Exhibit 1–9). The ratio is computed as follows:

$$\text{DER} = \text{Total Liabilities} \div \text{Owner's Equity} \quad (1\text{--}9)$$

Both current and long-term practice liabilities are included in this ratio. Dr. Bennett's DER is as follows:

$$\text{DER} = \$166,449 \div \$204,412 = 0.81$$

This means that, for every dollar of equity owned by Dr. Bennett, there are 81 cents worth of liabilities. The use of debt may involve risk, because interest will have to be paid on some of it, and eventually the principal must be repaid. Typically, young organizations have high DERs, because large capital expenditures are required for equipment, and revenue levels are relatively low at start-up.

### Profitability Ratios

Return on owner's investment (ROI) is a measure of an organization's profitability. It indicates how well the owner's equity is being used to generate income. Stated another way, the organization's equity could be "cashed in" and invested in other ways, such as in treasury bills or the stock market. Given that this money is invested in your organization (practice, hospital, etc.), what return are you receiving on this investment? In a sense, evaluating your profitability involves taking off your physician's hat and looking at your organization as a stockholder. Are your invested funds being well used? Return on owner's investment is calculated using the following formula:

$$\text{ROI} = (\text{Pretax Income} + \text{Interest Expense}) \div \text{Owner's Equity} \quad (1\text{--}10)$$

$$\text{ROI} = (\$44,183 + \$1,229) \div \$204,412 = 22\%$$

It is important to remember when examining Dr. Bennett's return on investment that his salary and his net income are inversely related. If Dr. Bennett increases his salary, then the net income of his practice will decline and vice versa. To evaluate the profitability of a practice as a *business,* a fair market rate must be paid to the physician/owner for professional and administrative services. Looking at it another way, Dr. Bennett wears two hats. Wearing one hat, he is an employee-physician-administrator; wearing the other, he is a stockholder-investor. To evaluate his success as a stockholder-investor, he must compensate himself fairly as an employee, just as he would fairly compensate any other employee who would perform the same administrative and medical duties with the same level of competence. Dr. Bennett's return on investment of 22 percent is meaningful only to the extent that his compensation as an employee-physician-administrator is equitable. A tax reality is that many physicians will pay their practice's profit to themselves before the end of a tax year to avoid double taxation. To the extent that this occurs, ROI can still be meaningful if the calculations are made taking this tax adjustment into consideration. Once again, to small closely held medical practices tracking this ratio over time may be a meaningful way to track changes and identify relevant financial questions.

Another way of assessing profitability is to examine the relationship between total assets and the income used to generate them. This ratio is called *return on total investment* (ROI-T) and is defined as follows:

$$\text{ROI-T} = (\text{Pretax Income} + \text{Interest Expense}) \div \text{Total Assets} \quad (1\text{--}11)$$

Dr. Bennett's return on total investment is:

$$\text{ROI-T} = (\$44,183 + \$1,229) \div \$370,861 = 12\%$$

Stated another way, Dr. Bennett's practice earned 12 percent on the total resources that it used during the year. Conceptualized in this manner, investment is defined as the total resources provided by both the owner(s) and the creditors.

Another gauge of profitability is the profit margin. The profit margin is defined as follows:

$$\text{Profit Margin} = \text{Net Income} \div \text{Total Net Revenue} \quad (1\text{--}12)$$

Dr. Bennett's profit margin is as follows:

$$\text{Profit Margin} = \$44,183 \div \$813,861 = 5.4\%$$

This says, in effect, that for each dollar of service provided by Dr. Bennett's practice, the practice makes an average of 5.4 cents profit. It is important to remember when evaluating the profit margin that this statistic does not take into account the amount of resources invested to generate this profit. Obviously, a practice that has a 5.4 percent profit margin but has required only a $20,000 investment is in one sense performing better than a practice that has the same profit margin but has required a $100,000 investment. Profit margin is a part of the profitability picture, but because it omits the very important investment component, it should be considered in conjunction with return on investment statistics.

## USES FOR RATIOS

After examining these ratios, you may well be wondering how to use them. Ratios are useful as screening devices to highlight possible problems and strengths. They are particularly useful for making internal comparisons over time. If you notice, for example, that your profit margin has declined from the previous year, this should stimulate you to investigate why this happened. Have expenses risen without an adjustment to fees? Are insurers' participation contracts forcing revenue down? Is your product mix changing so that you are conducting a greater proportion of lower-profit procedures?

If you find that your quick ratio is more favorable this year than it was last year, then you might give yourself a pat on the back. On the other hand, perhaps your quick ratio is too high! You might conclude that you could be investing your funds in other, more profitable ways, which might make the funds less liquid and could reduce your quick ratio. Ratios, therefore, are useful tools for stimulating thinking. They do not provide answers by themselves. Instead, they allow you to focus and direct your inquiries.

## CONTROL AND BUDGETING

*Control* is the process of measuring, evaluating, and correcting actual performance to ensure that goals and plans are accomplished. The control issues that will affect a physician leader will vary depending on the physician leader's job description. Physician leaders working in larger healthcare organizations will be working on control issues in response to plans and budgets. For example, the financial analysis of the MRI acquisition decision discussed above can be used as a basis to generate a budget and evaluate subsequent performance against that budget. Based on how results compare with projections, the MRI project could be modified to better achieve target net income, NPV, and IRR goals. Oversight can be an ongoing process so that adjustments can be made if the project is getting off track.

Physician leaders working in smaller organizations, such as solo and small group practices, similarly can use plans and budgets to implement controls. In addition, they should also be interested in cash control to deter theft, and to be certain that office operations are complying with practice policy and guidelines.

### Using a Postacquisition Analysis to Achieve Control

We will revisit the General Hospital MRI facility case to demonstrate how the financial projections already discussed can be used as the basis of a control process for the project. **Exhibit 1–15** contains a postacquisition analysis performed 1 year after the new MRI machine was put into operation. The data in Exhibit 1–15 indicate that net revenue is 5.07 percent above projections. Examination of the volume level, however, provides some disturbing information. Volume was 242 (7.56 percent) MRI scans *lower* than expected. Fortunately, the average gross charge had a favorable variance of $115, or 18.40 percent above expectations. The bad debts and adjustments rate was 28 percent

**Exhibit 1–15**  MRI Facility Postaquisition Analysis after Year 1

---

*Executive Summary*

A postacquisition analysis was performed for MRI system 2 for the year ended June 30, 1991, after the first year of service. Net income exceeded projections for year 1 by $29,513 and cash generated by operations exceeded plan by $47,513. Volume, however, was 242 MRI scans fewer than projected. Downward revisions for years 2 through 5 result in a corresponding downward revision of the internal rate of return to approximately 6 percent.

GENERAL HOSPITAL
MR Imaging System 2
POSTACQUISITION ANALYSIS for the Year Ended June 30, 1991

| | Year 1 Actual | Year 1 Projected | Variance Favorable (Unfavorable) | Change |
|---|---|---|---|---|
| Volume | 2,958 | 3,200 | −242 | −7.56% |
| Average Charge | $740 | $625 | $115 | 18.40% |
| Gross Revenue | $2,188,920 | $2,000,000 | $188,920 | 9.45% |
| Less Bad Debts and Contractual Adjustment (25%) | $612,898 | $500,000 | $(112,898) | −22.58% |
| Net Revenue | $1,576,022 | $1,500,000 | $76,022 | 5.07% |
| Less Variable Expenses | | | | |
| Supplies and Film | $121,870 | $96,000 | $(25,870) | −26.95% |
| Contribution Margin | $1,454,152 | $1,404,000 | $50,152 | 3.57% |
| Less Fixed Expenses | | | | |
| Salaries | $121,300 | $120,000 | $(1,300) | −1.08% |
| Employee Benefits | $33,964 | $30,000 | $(3,964) | −13.21% |
| Cryogens | $40,825 | $40,000 | $(825) | −2.06% |
| Indirect Expenses | $138,550 | $142,000 | $3,450 | 2.43% |
| Maintenance | $0 | $0 | $0 | |
| Fixed Expenses Before Depreciation | $334,639 | $332,000 | $(2,639) | −0.79% |
| Cash Generated by Operations | $1,119,513 | $1,072,000 | $47,513 | 4.43% |
| Less Depreciation | $578,000 | $560,000 | $(18,000) | −3.21% |
| Net Income | $541,513 | $512,000 | $29,513 | 5.76% |

Revised Projections

| | Year 1—Actual | Year 2—Proj. | Year 3—Proj. | Year 4—Proj. | Year 5—Proj |
|---|---|---|---|---|---|
| Volume | 2,958 | 2,200 | 2,420 | 2,662 | 2,928 |
| Average Charge | $740 | $740 | $650 | $625 | $625 |
| % Collectible | 72% | 75% | 75% | 75% | 75% |
| Average Variable Cost | $41.20 | $42 | $44 | $46 | $49 |
| Net Revenue | $1,576,022 | $1,221,000 | $1,179,750 | $1,247,813 | $1,372,594 |
| Variable Costs | $121,870 | $92,400 | $106,722 | $123,264 | $142,370 |

*continues*

**Exhibit 1–15** continued

| | | | | | |
|---|---|---|---|---|---|
| Fixed Costs Before Depreciation | $334,639 | $353,100 | $623,615 | $660,045 | $698,715 |
| Cash Generated by Operations | $1,119,513 | $775,500 | $449,413 | $464,504 | $531,509 |
| Discount Rate | 12.00% | | | | |
| Cash Flows | | | | | |
| | ($2,890,000) | $1,119,513 | $775,500 | $449,413 | $464,504 | $531,509 |
| IRR | 5.98% | | | | |
| NPV | ($355,534.50) | | | | |

*Notes*

1. The cost to acquire and install the equipment was $90,000 more than plan (total cost: $2,890,000). This results in an increase in the annual depreciation charge of $18,000.
2. The rate of growth in volume projections for years 3 through 5 has been revised downward from 15 percent to 10 percent.
3. Projected average charges reflect recent experiences and current expectations. For the year ended June 30, 1991, the bad debt and contractual adjustment were 28 percent of gross revenue.
4. Variable costs for supplies and film averaged $41.20 during the year ended June 30, 1991.

*Source:* © William T. Geary, Ph.D. 2007. All Rights Reserved. Used with permission.

($612,898 ÷ $2,188,920) versus a projected 25 percent. Variable costs were expected to average $30 per MRI scan, but actually were more than $41 ($121,870 ÷ 2,958 MRIs = $41.20) per scan. Fixed costs were about what was expected.

The fact that the volume estimates were below expectations is very disturbing, because our previous analyses have demonstrated the volume sensitivity of this project. In addition, the unfavorable variable cost variance compounds the problem for a volume-sensitive project. As a result of the first-year experience, the projections for years 2 through 5 were revised. The primary changes are a reduced volume level and an increased variable cost to $40 per MRI scan, plus inflation. The effects of these changes on NPV and IRR are disconcerting. NPV now is negative, which means that we will miss our 12 percent profit goal by $355,534.50. The IRR is now at 5.98 percent. At this point, management has the opportunity to change this unfavorable outcome. The postacquisition analysis

pointed out where the problem areas are, and indicates where management must make changes to turn this project around.

A second postacquisition analysis was conducted after the second year of operation. Unfortunately, it contained more bad news. Volume was 1,909 MRI scans, which was well below the original projection of 2,599 scans and also below the revised projection of 2,200 scans. Average variable costs rose to $43.10 and exceeded the revised projection of $42. Fixed costs were almost 30 percent above expectations, due largely to cryogens, which were 293 percent ($123,231) above expectations. The impact on NPV was dramatic. Given the desire for a 12 percent return, the projected NPV was a *negative* $737,294. The IRR was a dismal 0.83 percent—and to make matters worse these number were only achieved *by extending the project out to 7 years*! If they retained the original 5-year payback, the projected NPV would be under the target 12 percent return by $1,058,698.18, with a *negative* IRR of 10.07

percent. After the second post-acquisition analysis the MRI facility was projected to generate net cash of $2,293,306 versus the initial projection of $4,350,629 (Exhibit 1–5). Once again, we can see the volume sensitivity of this project.

At this point management has another opportunity to intervene. One major problem is volume. Devoting more marketing resources and restructuring management positions to emphasize critical parts of the marketing mix (Chapter 7) are options that could increase MRI volume. A second major problem is cost control. Fixed costs are 30 percent above expectations by year 2. Because volume is down, there should be excess capacity, and management needs to think creatively of ways to reduce fixed costs. One strategy would be to try to convert some to variable costs. Perhaps there are some positions that could be changed from full time to part time and ideally part time on-call. The major fixed cost variance has been cryogens. Greater efficiency in purchasing has to be examined. Perhaps General Hospital can form a purchasing alliance with other hospitals to gain purchasing power and a lower price.

The sudden rise in the cost of cryogens was largely due to federal regulation of ozone-depleting chemicals. One must question why this somewhat predictable event was not considered in the original financial analysis. It turns out that radiologists, who might well have been more aware of this issue, were *not* an integral part of the original financial analysis team. This illustrates the importance of having financially literate physicians fully involved in the decision-making process.

## Using Budgets for Financial Control

A *budget* is simply a formal statement of your financial plans for a specific time period. It is a statement about what should happen financially to your practice or healthcare organization. You then can compare actual events with the budget to see whether you are behind, matching, or exceeding your expectations. Often, budgets are viewed as constraints. Viewed more positively, however, they can be an important part of a control process to identify when the unexpected has occurred, and to create an opportunity to proactively deal with it. Budgets are not essential to the operation of a small medical practice. They are a step above the minimum financial cash accounting methods that often characterize small private practices. Budgets, however, can be important for even a small practice if it must demonstrate a degree of financial planning so that a lending institution will lend it money.

The sophistication that budgets can add to the process of identifying financial problems early enough to take effective action must be balanced against the time that they take to construct and utilize. Budgeting is very consistent, however, with the notion that as a physician leader you are a consumer of financial information and will use it to plan and make management decisions. Budgets are most useful when they stimulate you to think ahead, anticipate future conditions, prepare for them, and take action if things are not going according to plan.

Budgets can be established for virtually any quantifiable issue, including cash receipts and disbursements, procedures, DRGs, revenues, and expenses. Some organizations may find the budgeting process useful for tackling very specific financial problems. For example, if an evaluation of office supply expenses indicates substantial waste, then budgeting for office supplies and closely examining variances would be an effective cost-control procedure. Similarly, other expense or revenue items can be selectively targeted and brought into line through the budgeting process.

Let's examine how a budget could be used to help manage a group practice. Dr. Brandon Jones has two colleagues. He is undertaking the budgeting process because he expects that his practice will be growing. He wants to plan for this growth so it takes place in an orderly, efficient manner. As a result, he has decided to construct a budget for the next 3 months.

Because many costs vary with the activity level of a business, the budgeting process often begins with the development of an index of sales. Dr. Jones and his two colleagues each estimated their mix and number of procedures that they believed they would conduct over the next 3 months. They did this by obtaining reports containing historical data from the practice's medical office management system, which they adjusted where appropriate using their judgment. Associated revenues were projected using historical write off and adjustment data. They chose not to consider special consultation fees and speaking fees, because they were minor. The physicians' forecasts are shown in **Exhibit 1–16** in the column headed "Budget January–March."

Next, Dr. Jones projected the following expenses:

- Rent, interest, and insurance expenses were fixed, so he simply carried over the monthly amounts from the previous year.
- Clerical salaries would remain the same for the first 3 months, because all performance appraisals and probable pay raises should occur in the second half of the year.
- Professional compensation would remain proportionally the same, so Dr. Jones took the percentage of revenue paid to physicians in the previous year and multiplied the projected net revenue by this percentage.

- Payroll taxes would remain proportional to compensation.
- Dr. Jones reviewed the expenditures for office supplies for the previous year with the practice business manager. He concluded that supplies were not being wasted. He assumed that supplies would be used at the same rate as last year, so he budgeted for 25 percent (3 months) of the previous annual expenditure. If he thought that there had been waste, he could have used the budget to try to reduce the utilization of supplies by budgeting at a level below the previous year's expenditures.
- Education expenses were calculated by estimating the amount Dr. Jones and his colleagues were likely to spend at the conferences they were planning to attend during the 3-month period.
- Telephone expenses were fairly consistent across the previous year, and Dr. Jones saw no reason for there to be a change. In addition, he reviewed the cell phone "overage" charges and determined that they were reasonable. As a result, he budgeted 25 percent of last year's cell phone and land line bills for each month.
- Advertising consisted of two display ads each month in the "Science and Medicine" section of the daily newspaper plus Yellow Pages listings. Dr. Jones planned to continue this practice for the next 3 months.
- All other expenditure categories were entered into the budget at the rate of 25 percent of the previous year expenditure.

The "Actual" column in Exhibit 1–16 is a performance report comparing first quarter revenues and expenses with the budgeted amounts. The data indicate that the practice had lower net income than had been planned for the first quarter. Fortunately, total expenses were also lower than the budget. Advertising, insurance, and education had

**Exhibit 1–16**  Static Budget: Dr. Jones

| | Budget Jan.–Mar. | Actual | Variance | Direction |
|---|---|---|---|---|
| **REVENUES** | | | | |
| Dr. Jones | $100,000 | $95,468 | $(4,532) | U |
| Dr. Warren | $80,000 | $85,684 | $5,684 | F |
| Dr. Stewart | $90,000 | $75,698 | $(14,302) | U |
| Total | $270,000 | $256,850 | $(13,150) | U |
| **EXPENSES** | | | | |
| Clerical Salaries | $39,057 | $39,057 | $— | — |
| Professional Compensation | $118,800 | $113,674 | $(5,126) | F |
| Payroll Taxes | $14,207 | $13,746 | $(461) | F |
| Rent | $12,000 | $12,000 | $— | — |
| Advertising | $2,249 | $2,732 | $483 | U |
| Office Supplies | $10,500 | $9,375 | $(1,125) | F |
| Medical Supplies | $14,138 | $14,101 | $(37) | F |
| Interest Expense | $307 | $307 | $— | — |
| Local Taxes | $1,575 | $1,498 | $(77) | F |
| Insurance | $16,975 | $17,250 | $275 | U |
| Education | $2,249 | $2,800 | $551 | U |
| Telephone—Land Lines | $489 | $489 | $— | — |
| Telephone—Cellular | $981 | $929 | $(52) | F |
| Total | $233,527 | $227,958 | $(5,569) | F |
| **NET INCOME** | $36,473 | $28,892 | $(7,581) | U |

*Note:*
U = Unfavorable
F = Favorable

unfavorable variances. They were compensated for, however, by favorable variances in professional compensation (although Dr. Jones might not take pleasure in this "favorable" variance) and the related payroll taxes and local taxes, office supplies, medical supplies, and cell phone.

Dr. Jones now could use the performance report to examine the causes of this situation. After talking with Dr. Stewart, Dr. Jones determined that his variance was due to a combination of illness and an unexpected "product mix" in terms of Dr. Stewart's procedures for the quarter. Examination of the unfavorable variances in advertising and ed-

ucation both revealed explanations. The advertising variance resulted from an additional display ad in a local newspaper in a special local high blood pressure awareness week section. Dr. Jones felt, after a review, that advertising in this edition of the paper was well justified. The education variance was explained by Dr. Warren exceeding his budgeted education amount. Dr. Jones concluded that Dr. Warren's actual expenditures were questionable and planned to have a collegial discussion with Dr. Warren.

Dr. Jones may encounter some difficulties, however, in evaluating some of the other variances. For example, office supplies and medical supplies both show favorable variances. The practice's activity level, however, was below expectations, so it really isn't clear whether the lower utilization of office and medical supplies was due to treating fewer patients or to more efficient operations or for that matter whether they should have been even more favorable than they were! Unfortunately, such questions cannot be easily answered with the static budget used by Dr. Jones. They *can* be addressed, however, with a flexible budget.

A *flexible budget* utilizes a budget formula to express the relationship between variable costs and an index of activity level, such as revenue or number of procedures. Flexible budgets adjust to reflect the *actual* volume as opposed to the *projected* or budgeted volume. Based on the previous year's data, Dr. Jones expected that the following budget items would vary with physician revenues:

- professional compensation, because Dr. Jones and his colleagues pay themselves a percentage of the revenues
- payroll taxes, because these are a function of professional and clerical compensation
- office and medical supplies, because their consumption should vary with the practice's activity level
- local taxes, because these are a direct function of revenue level

Dr. Jones determined the flexible budget amounts by examining the relationship between these variables and clinical revenue for the previous year. Each dollar of clinical service revenue resulted in the generation of 44.0 cents of professional compensation expense, 9.0 cents of payroll tax expense, 3.8 cents of office supply expense, 5.2 cents of medical supply expense, and so forth. These relationships are indicated in the "Flexible Formula" column in **Exhibit 1–17**.

Differences between flexible budgets and static budgets that are due to variance in activity level are an index of *effectiveness*. Differences between flexible budgets and actual results are due to *efficiency*, meaning that the amount of inputs used for a given level of output is less (or more) than expected, and *price efficiency*, if the cost or price per unit of service differs from that expressed in the flexible budget formula.

The relationship between effectiveness and efficiency is important to understand. For example, you may have an objective of generating $30,000 in revenues in a month. You only generate $25,000, but you do this with the inputs specified in the flexible budget. Your production has been ineffective, but it has also been efficient. Alternatively, you could have a $30,000 revenue month but have unfavorable variances on several flexible budget items, in which case you have been effective, but inefficient.

Several conclusions can be reached after examining both Dr. Jones's flexible and static budgets:

- Revenues were $13,150 less than expected. Expenses, however, were $5,569 less than expected, for a net income of $7,581 below expectations. Net variance across both static and flexible budgets was a −$6,553, which was in the favorable direction. Most of this ($5,664) was due to lower professional compensation and associated taxes. However, the flexible budget indicated that an additional $660 was paid to a physician. Dr. Jones determined that he needed to find out how this error occurred.
- Office supplies were efficiently used, because actual consumption was less than that in the flexible budget (−$385).
- The cost of medical supplies was less than what had been statically budgeted, but not as low as would be expected in the flexible

**Exhibit 1–17** Flexible Budget: Dr. Jones

| | Budget Jan.–Mar. | Actual | Variance | Direction | Flexible Formula | Flexible Budget | Flexible Variance | Flexible Direction |
|---|---|---|---|---|---|---|---|---|
| **REVENUES** | | | | | | | | |
| Dr. Jones | $100,000 | $95,468 | $(4,532) | U | | | $(4,532) | |
| Dr. Warren | $80,000 | $85,684 | $5,684 | F | | | $5,684 | |
| Dr. Stewart | $90,000 | $75,698 | $(14,302) | U | | | $(14,302) | |
| Total | $270,000 | $256,850 | $(13,150) | — | | | $(13,150) | |
| **EXPENSES** | | | | | | | | |
| Clerical Salaries | $39,057 | $39,057 | $— | — | | | | |
| Professional Compensation | $118,800 | $113,674 | $(5,126) | F | 44% × Total Revenue | $113,014 | $660 | U |
| Payroll Taxes | $14,207 | $13,746 | $(461) | F | 9% × (Cler. Sal. + Prof. Comp.) | $13,746 | $0 | |
| Rent | $12,000 | $12,000 | $— | — | | | | |
| Advertising | $2,249 | $2,732 | $483 | U | | | | |
| Office Supplies | $10,500 | $9,375 | $(1,125) | F | 3.8% × Total Revenue | $9,760 | $(385) | F |
| Medical Supplies | $14,138 | $14,101 | $(37) | F | 5.2% × Total Revenue | $13,356 | $745 | U |
| Interest Expense | $307 | $307 | $— | — | | | | |
| Local Taxes | $1,575 | $1,498 | $(77) | F | .58% × Total Revenue | $1,490 | $8 | U |
| Insurance | $16,975 | $17,250 | $275 | U | | | | |
| Education | $2,249 | $2,800 | $551 | U | | | | |
| Telephone—Land Lines | $489 | $489 | $— | U | | | | |
| Telephone—Cellular | $981 | $929 | $(52) | F | | | | |
| Total | $233,527 | $227,958 | $(5,569) | F | | | | |
| NET INCOME | $36,473 | $28,892 | $(7,581) | F | | | $1,028 | U |
| NET VARIANCE | $(6,553) | F | | | $(5,664) | | | |

*Note:*
U = Unfavorable
F = Favorable

budget. This implies inefficient utilization ($14,101 − $13,356 = $745). This also, however, could have resulted from an unexpected change in procedure mix.

• Dr. Jones needs to reevaluate the issue of discipline. Advertising and education had unfavorable variances because someone *chose* to exceed the budget. These choices could have been good decisions or wasteful decisions. A budget should not be viewed as inviolate, because situations change and organizations must have enough flexibility to adapt. On the other hand, a lack of discipline will almost always be clad in the armor of necessity. The effective manager will be able to determine when a variance is truly in the organization's best interest, and when it is simply the result of extravagance.

The concept of flexible budgeting can be applied to the MRI facility year 1 postacquisition analysis (**Exhibit 1–18**). Volume and charge are drivers. One flexible formula evaluates actual average charge to expected average charge ($740 − $625), which indicates a $115 favorable efficiency variance. This results in a gross revenue favorable efficiency of $340,170, meaning that *for the volume achieved,* the facility efficiently generated revenue from the 2,958 MRI scans. Overall effectiveness, however, is unfavorable by $151,250, which is due to lower-than-expected volume. These two effects net to the static favorable gross revenue variance of $188,920.

Of the $112,898 unfavorable static collection variance, $65,668 was due to inefficient collection as a result of exceeding the 25 percent uncollectible target. The remaining $47,230 was due to the higher-than-expected gross revenues. This finding indicates that if management could improve the collection efficiency (i.e., get it back down to a projected

25 percent rate), then about 58 percent of the unfavorable collection variation could be eliminated. Finally, it can be seen that the unfavorable static supply variance (−$25,870) was actually worse than it first appears. There was an inefficiency of −$33,130 that was partially obscured by the positive effectiveness variance ($7,260) of conducting 242 fewer-than-projected MRI scans.

In summary, the budgeting process can be used to help evaluate whether an organization is proceeding according to plan. It comes, however, at a price in both effort and time. This issue is especially relevant for smaller practices. In a practice setting, someone such as Dr. Jones or his business manager or accountant must construct the budget and look for and investigate variances. Only Dr. Jones can determine whether this was or will be worthwhile in his particular situation. Some might believe that the variances that Dr. Jones discovered hardly justify the effort expended. Dr. Jones, however, may feel that the budgeting process was worthwhile, if it gives him some assurance that things are generally going according to plan, and that he has the capability of identifying specific variances as they grow, thereby providing the opportunity to control them before they reach critical levels.

In larger healthcare organizations, the use of budgets and projections as controls are essential. The numbers are simply too large and the consequences too great to "fly by the seat of your pants" in an unforgiving cost-conscious healthcare environment. We have seen how badly a project, such as the MRI facility, can go. To forego the opportunity to change the course of events in midstream would be foolish. Finally, the budgeting process conveys an image of financial competence, if not sophistication. Both large and small healthcare organizations that are seeking financing will have to demonstrate their financial competence to lending institutions.

Exhibit 1-18  MRI Facility Flexible Budget Analysis

| | Year 1 | | Static Variance | Change | Flexible Formula | Flexible Efficiency | Flexible Effectiveness |
|---|---|---|---|---|---|---|---|
| | Actual | Projected | | | | | |
| Volume | 2,958 | 3,200 | −242 | −7.56% | =740−625 | | |
| Average Charge | $740 | $625 | $115 | 18.40% | | $115 | |
| Gross Revenue | $2,188,920 | $2,000,000 | $188,920 | 9.45% | | $340,170 | $(151,250) |
| Less Bad Debts and Contractual Adjustment (25%) | $612,898 | $500,000 | $(112,898) | −22.58% | 25% × Gross Revenue | $(65,668) | $(47,230) |
| Net Revenue | $1,576,022 | $1,500,000 | $76,022 | 5.07% | | | |
| Less Variable Expenses Supplies and Film | $121,870 | $96,000 | $(25,870) | −26.95% | $30 × Volume | $(33,130) | |
| Contribution Margin | $1,454,152 | $1,404,000 | $50,152 | 3.57% | | | $7,260 |

Source: Copyright © William T. Geary, Ph.D. 2007. All Rights Reserved. Used with permission.

Almost without exception, this will imply presenting a budget and a management plan to effectively implement it.

## ACTIVITY-BASED COSTING

One of the major challenges currently facing healthcare organizations is determining what it costs them to provide a service. It is difficult to knowledgeably or confidently bid on a contract to provide services, for example, unless you know what it costs you to provide the service. Activity-based costing (ABC) is a method for attaching costs to activities, such as a procedure, DRG, diagnosis, or the like. Once you know what it costs to provide the procedure or DRG, then you can negotiate more effectively to provide medical care in a cost-conscious environment. If you know, for example, that it costs you, on average, $18,369 to provide a cardiac artery bypass graft (CABG), then you can add margin over this level to determine a price. Sometimes, the market price for a service may be above your own cost. You then may have to make a decision about whether to provide the service at a negative margin,[17] or to decline the opportunity. You will, however, be making this decision from a point of knowledge as opposed to ignorance.

An effective ABC system captures both direct financial information and behavioral information that has financial consequences. Often in health care, the value that is added is provided by the human, such as when a nurse, laboratory technician, or physician provides a service. It is essential, therefore, to attach a cost to this activity. The difficulty arises when we observe that much of the human behavior that occurs in healthcare systems is quite variable.

For example, think of the activities of a nurse working in an outpatient oncology practice. Much of the activity involves responding to the needs of patients receiving chemotherapy. Some of this activity is quite predictable and easily assessed, such as preparing and administering an infusion. If nurses are paid at $20 per hour, and one nurse prepares and monitors on average six patients over a 2-hour infusion, then the personnel cost per patient per infusion would be $6.67 ($20 × 2 Hours/6 Patients). Adding the cost of variable cost items (infusion drugs, syringes, tubing, etc.), and charges for use of the facility, capital equipment, and so forth for the time involved then provides a cost for the activity. Determining the cost of the activity becomes more problematic, if there is significant "off-the-record" activity. Ms. Smith calls the next day. She is running a fever, doesn't feel well, and wishes to talk to a nurse about her symptoms. Nurse Diaz responds to the call and talks with the patient for 9 minutes. Mr. Jackson calls later that afternoon. He received a similar infusion the previous day. Nurse Li takes the call and talks with him for 26 minutes. Two things of significance just occurred. First, an additional 35 minutes of nursing time needs to be allocated to the cost of the procedure. Second, there was significant variance in the time allocated across patients by nurses. Unless we know enough about the procedure to understand that there will be nursing time consumed in subsequent days as a result of the procedure, and unless we know how much this time can vary, we may fail to capture a significant amount of the procedure's cost.

The process for capturing behavioral cost information utilizes interviews, questionnaires, and sampling methods to determine what activities are performed by particular jobs and how much time it takes to perform the activities. Obviously, this can be an intrusive process. In this example, nurses would fill out activity questionnaires or enter their time directly into a computer over a period of days or weeks to get an assessment of their activities that would have some statistical stability. In addition, job analysts may observe nurses performing their tasks to be certain that the questionnaires were assessing the full range of activities. The validity of the data will be influenced by the organization's internal climate. If employees perceive that the data will be used to affect their pay, their discretion to act as they see fit, or their ability to provide the quality of care that they feel is appropriate, then the data may be biased. In more extreme cases, employees may resist the measurement process. Generally, this resistance will be covert as opposed to overt, such as when assessment questionnaires aren't completed for a myriad of reasons, all of which are *somewhat* legitimate.

It should be apparent that developing ABC systems can be very expensive and time consuming and may require skills not currently possessed by the healthcare organization. Given the current state of the art, these systems are probably most appropriately applied only to high value procedures and programs. A practice, therefore, might develop ABC models of its most important procedures. A hospital might develop ABC models for the most important parts of its most financially important programs, such as CABG, normal delivery, Caesarian delivery, hip replacement surgery, and so forth.

**Exhibit 1–19** shows a case example of an ABC model developed by a gastroenterology practice. This model focuses on the practice's outpatient services.[18] Practice leadership determined that the most appropriate way to organize the ABC analysis was around their most important procedures and procedure codes. These are the columns in Exhibit 1–19. The rows represent medical and business costs. The medical and business cost totals were obtained from the practice's prior year

income statement. The ABC task, therefore, was to fully allocate these income statement costs across the procedures. The cost data then can be used by the practice to evaluate insurer proposals, prepare for negotiations, and determine where to provide services.

For example, an insurer provides a physician fee of $300 for a colonoscopy (45378). Alternatively, if the endoscopy is conducted in the hospital, they will pay the physician $200. The ABC data in Exhibit 1–19 indicates that conducting the endoscopy in this office will cost the physician $206.98, so the physician's net income for the office based procedure would be $93.02 (**Exhibit 1–20**). The physician now knows that she has to negotiate a facility fee[19] of at least $106.98 to break even with doing the work in the hospital setting.[20] When preparing to negotiate with the insurer, the physician learned that the insurer pays the hospital "about $700" for a facility fee, so the physician estimates that the insurer's practice delivered costs are $300 and hospital delivered costs are $900 (Exhibit 1–20). The negotiation zone, therefore, is for the insurer to pay the physician a facilities fee somewhere between $106.98 and $600.00.[21] Any negotiated solution within this range mutually benefits both the physician and the insurer (See Chapter 8 on integrative negotiating).

**Effectively Using Financial Advisors**

The relationship that a physician leader has with financial professionals should be analogous to that between an architect and an informed client who has opinions regarding the qualities and characteristics of his or her home. By having a very clear understanding of your specific financial needs, you will be able to work most effectively with financial advisors. In practices and smaller healthcare organizations, the financial advisor may be

**Exhibit 1–19** Gastroenterology Practice: Outpatient ABC Analysis of Procedures

| | New Patient Consultation | Follow-Up Office Visit | 43235 EGD | 43239 EGD Biop. | 45330 Flex. Sig. | 45331 Flex Sig. Biop. | 45333 Flex. Sig. Polyp Rem. | 45378 Colon. | 45380 Colon. Biopsy | 45384 Colon. Polyp Rem. |
|---|---|---|---|---|---|---|---|---|---|---|
| Number of services rendered in 19XX | 967 | 1,287 | 9 | 32 | 169 | 66 | 4 | 23 | 17 | 15 |
| Total time for procedure in minutes | 20 | 10 | 95 | 110 | 35 | 50 | 50 | 65 | 80 | 80 |
| Physician time spent with patients in min. (see Table 1) | 20 | 10 | 10 | 12 | 5 | 10 | 15 | 25 | 35 | 35 |
| Nursing time spent with patient in min. (see Table 1) | | 8 | 90 | 105 | 30 | 45 | 45 | 60 | 75 | 75 |
| MEDICAL EXPENSES | | | | | | | | | | |
| Physician cost per procedure-min./cost per min. (see Table 2) | $30.86 | $15.43 | $15.43 | $18.52 | $7.72 | $15.43 | $23.15 | $38.58 | $54.01 | $54.01 |
| Nursing cost per procedure-min./cost per min. (see Table 2) | $7.47 | $2.99 | $33.62 | $39.22 | $11.21 | $16.81 | $16.81 | $22.41 | $28.02 | $28.02 |
| Medical supplies | $4.32 | $3.75 | $37.79 | $41.47 | $21.78 | $25.46 | $25.46 | $35.99 | $39.67 | $39.67 |
| Equip maint. and rep. - cost per procedure (see Table 7) | | | $8.06 | $8.06 | $8.06 | $8.06 | $8.06 | $8.06 | $8.06 | $8.06 |
| Endo suite space rent-total time rent per proc. min. (see Table 6) | | | $46.69 | $54.06 | $17.20 | $24.57 | $24.57 | $31.94 | $39.31 | $39.31 |
| Exam room rent cost per use (see Table 4) | $2.96 | $2.96 | | | | | | | | |
| Equipment cost (see Table 7) | | | $21.95 | $21.95 | $0.98 | $0.98 | $0.98 | $18.18 | $18.18 | $18.18 |
| TOTAL | $45.62 | $25.13 | $163.54 | $183.28 | $66.94 | $91.31 | $99.03 | $155.17 | $187.26 | $187.26 |
| BUSINESS EXPENSES | | | | | | | | | | |
| Administration and Advertising | | | | | | | | | | |
| Administration-annual salaries (see Table 9)/total number of services rendered | $13.53 | $13.53 | $13.53 | $13.53 | $13.53 | $13.53 | $13.53 | $13.53 | $13.53 | $13.53 |
| Telephone/advertising cost per procedure-cost per year (see Table 8) / total number of services | $5.61 | $5.61 | $5.61 | $5.61 | $5.61 | $5.61 | $5.61 | $5.61 | $5.61 | $5.61 |
| Equipment rental cost per procedure-cost per year (see Table 8) / total number of services | $1.50 | $1.50 | $1.50 | $1.50 | $1.50 | $1.50 | $1.50 | $1.50 | $1.50 | $1.50 |
| Office space rent (see Table 5) | $10.16 | $10.16 | $10.16 | $10.16 | $10.16 | $10.16 | $10.16 | $10.16 | $10.16 | $10.16 |
| Billing and Collection | | | | | | | | | | |
| Office supplies-annual cost (see Table 8)/total number of services | $1.64 | $1.64 | $1.64 | $1.64 | $1.64 | $1.64 | $1.64 | $1.64 | $1.64 | $1.64 |
| Postage-annual cost (see Table 8) / total number of services | $1.85 | $1.85 | $1.85 | $1.85 | $1.85 | $1.85 | $1.85 | $1.85 | $1.85 | $1.85 |
| Salary and benefit cost per procedure-cost per procedure (see Table 9) | $5.80 | $5.80 | $5.80 | $5.80 | $5.80 | $5.80 | $5.80 | $5.80 | $5.80 | $5.80 |

| Reception. Scheduling, Med. Records and Transcription | | | | | | | | | | |
|---|---|---|---|---|---|---|---|---|---|---|
| Minutes per procedure | 63 | 15 | 37 | 37 | 37 | 37 | 37 | 37 | 37 | 37 |
| Receptionists' cost per procedure-Reception wage per minute (see Table 8)/minutes per procedure | $9.06 | $2.16 | $5.32 | $5.32 | $5.32 | $5.32 | $5.32 | $5.32 | $5.32 | $5.32 |
| Office supplies-annual cost (see Table 8)/total number of services | $3.28 | $3.28 | $3.28 | $3.28 | $3.28 | $3.28 | $3.28 | $3.28 | $3.28 | $3.28 |
| Postage-annual cost (see Table 8)/total number of services | $0.87 | $0.87 | $0.87 | $0.87 | $0.87 | $0.87 | $0.87 | $0.87 | $0.87 | $0.87 |
| Transcriptionist-annual cost (see Table 8)/total number of services | $2.25 | $2.25 | $2.25 | $2.25 | $2.25 | $2.25 | $2.25 | $2.25 | $2.25 | $2.25 |
| TOTAL | $55.55 | $48.65 | $51.81 | $51.81 | $51.81 | $51.81 | $51.81 | $51.81 | $51.81 | $51.81 |
| Cost per Procedure Rendered | $101.17 | $73.79 | $215.35 | $235.09 | $118.75 | $143.12 | $150.84 | $206.98 | $239.07 | $239.07 |

*Note:* Supporting tables are not provided.

*Note:* The figures contained in this exhibit are specific to one practice at one point in time. They should not be generalized to another practice.

*Source:* © Sentara Health System, William T. Geary, Ph.D., and Robert J. Solomon, Ph.D. 2007. All rights reserved. Used with permission.

**Exhibit 1–20** Negotiation Analysis Using ABC Data

|  | Location | | |
|  | Office | Hospital | Differential |
| --- | --- | --- | --- |
| Physician's Analysis | | | |
| Physician Revenue | $300.00 | $200.00 | |
| Physician's Cost | $206.98 | $— | |
| Net Revenue | $93.02 | $200.00 | $(106.98) |
| Insurer's Analysis | | | |
| Physician Fee | $300.00 | $200.00 | |
| Hospital Facility Fee | | $700.00 | |
| Total Costs | $300.00 | $900.00 | $(600.00) |

a consulting accountant or perhaps an employed business manager with an MBA. In larger healthcare organizations financial information and support may come from a finance department headed by a chief financial officer.

Accounting data are to your healthcare organization what current and historical medical test data are to a clinician treating a patient. They indicate the current and past states of the organization and allow you to make rational management decisions about future courses of action. The goal of using financial information is to manage your organization proactively and to make appropriate changes that take into account both financial and medical considerations. A knowledgeable financial professional can further this goal by providing you with the appropriate information that you need to be part of the decision process.

Generally, it will be a misuse of your time and your staff's time to perform specialized financial tasks in which accountants and financial professionals develop efficiency and proficiency over a period of years. For example, use an accountant for tasks that require skilled or timely financial or accounting knowledge, such as the preparation of tax returns or the development of a pension

or profit-sharing plan. Use financial professionals to build financial models in spreadsheets and to perform the initial financial analyses for developing a new service line, practice expansion, significant equipment purchase, practice acquisition, and the like. Use financial professionals to get an expert's perspective. Similarly, you will want to use a financial professional to create your financial procedures and set up your cash and accrual accounts, so you produce accounting data in a form that is most useful for tax, reporting, and planning purposes.

### Case Analysis: Oregon Sports Medicine

The use of financial information to aid in making management decisions is illustrated by the case of Oregon Sports Medicine. Performance appraisal and compensation issues are central to the concept of control, and these issues are at the heart of the challenge facing the physicians at Oregon Sports Medicine. The data that they will use to help them make the critical decision that they face come from their income statement. The analytical method they will use employs the CVP model. Finally, the projections that they make can be used to develop static and flexible budgets to monitor progress toward financial goals and to modify management actions to achieve these goals.

Oregon Sports Medicine is composed of three physicians, Drs. Able, Baker, and Cane, along with several nurses, secretaries, and assistants. Drs. Able and Baker are partners; Dr. Cane is an employed associate. **Exhibit 1–21** contains an income statement at the top. Below the income statement is an analysis of each physician's net revenue. Dr. Able has generated 30.58 percent percent of the net revenue, Dr. Baker has generated 41 percent of the net revenue, and Dr. Cane has generated 28.42 percent of the net revenue. Next, they assign 40 percent ($250,822.33) of the total practice expenses ($627,055.22) equally to each physician ($83,607.44). Then, they take the remaining 60 percent of the expenses and divide them based on each physician's percentage of net revenue. Baker, the high producer, therefore takes $154,267.64 of additional expenses based on her volume, Able takes $115,053.26, and Cane, the low producer, takes an additional $106,912.60 of expenses. Each physician's annual salary is the sum of his or her net revenue minus his or her assigned expenses.

This case is not presented as an endorsement of how to structure compensation and incentive arrangements. Rather, it is presented as a case study of how one practice wrestled with the issues of how to tie work to rewards, control expenses, create equity so that those who incurred expenses would pay for them, and create incentives so that physicians would want to work harder and smarter.

As we examine this plan, it does have some logic to it. The sharing of a proportion of the expenses equally recognizes that some expenses are present irrespective of utilization. They are opportunity costs that occur as soon as the door is opened, and they will be there largely irrespective of the number of patients who walk in the door. In effect,

these are fixed expenses given the practice's current size (relevant range). Recognition that some expenses are tied to activity level, and that those who use more should pay more, and those who use less should pay less, is also encompassed in their compensation formula. This notion of variable cost is operationalized by the 60 percent of expenses assigned based on physician net revenue. Net revenue in this instance is being used as a surrogate for activity, probably because it is easily measurable. It is a cost driver. Intuitively, the physicians seemed to have had an appreciation of the concepts of fixed and variable expenses. Finally, this system creates an incentive for all to try to reduce both fixed and variable expenses, because each physician will receive some portion of the cost savings back through a higher salary.

Where did the 40 percent and 60 percent numbers in the expense allocation formula come from? Who knows? However, we are not in a position to be critical. If the physicians are happy with this division and if it creates equity in their minds, then that is good enough. An alternative, however, would be to go down the list of expenses and classify each one as fixed or variable (mixed expenses would have to be broken into their fixed and variable components). The difficulty with changing an existing compensation formula such as this is that someone will be a winner and someone will be a loser. For example, if an analysis of the costs indicates that more than 40 percent is fixed, then Dr. Baker, the high producer, would gain at the expense of both Drs. Able and Cane.

Dr. Baker is a partner in the practice. She is young, raising a family, and still paying off education loans, and she has a significant mortgage. Dr. Able is the other partner. He is in his early 60s and he has been reducing his involvement with the practice. Because he would like to retire in 3 to 5 years, Dr. Able

**Exhibit 1–21**  Oregon Sports Medicine: Income Statement, Revenue Analysis, and Salary Calculation

| INCOME STATEMENT JANUARY–DECEMBER 20XX | | |
|---|---|---|
| NET REVENUE | | % |
| Dr. Able | $390,109.27 | 30.58 |
| Dr. Baker | $523,072.85 | 41.00 |
| Dr. Cane | $362,506.86 | 28.42 |
| Total | $1,275,688.98 | 100.00 |
| | | |
| EXPENSES | | |
| Nonphysician Gross Payroll | $151,943.11 | 11.91 |
| FICA (Includes Physicians) | $26,699.61 | 2.09 |
| Advertising | $26,601.83 | 2.09 |
| Maintenance | $6,619.63 | 0.52 |
| Telephone | $8,415.60 | 0.66 |
| Radiology | $12,106.81 | 0.95 |
| Postage | $6,942.50 | 0.54 |
| Licenses | $175.00 | 0.01 |
| Janitorial | $3,400.00 | 0.27 |
| Contributions/Gifts | $16,800.05 | 1.32 |
| Petty Cash | $3,132.76 | 0.25 |
| Accounting/Legal | $10,847.10 | 0.85 |
| Taxes—Corporate | $— | 0.00 |
| Personal Property | $2,920.07 | 0.23 |
| State Unemployment | $76.02 | 0.01 |
| Fed. Unemployment | $2,288.80 | 0.18 |
| Gross Receipts | $6,872.54 | 0.54 |
| Office Supplies | $25,103.24 | 1.97 |
| Medical Supplies | $35,498.29 | 2.78 |
| Dues | $10,540.50 | 0.83 |
| Books | $8,775.59 | 0.69 |
| Meetings | $18,239.11 | 1.43 |
| Insurance | $68,138.58 | 5.34 |
| Rent | $65,832.00 | 5.16 |
| Christmas Parties | $1,039.01 | 0.08 |
| Equipment Lease | $50,429.97 | 3.95 |
| Interest Bank Note | $7,488.87 | 0.59 |
| Interest to Owners | $10,265.79 | 0.80 |
| Electricity | $7,150.98 | 0.56 |
| Depreciation | $25,113.00 | 1.97 |
| Miscellanous | $954.46 | 0.07 |
| Transcription Service | $6,645.00 | 0.52 |
| Total Expenses | $627,055.82 | 49.15 |
| | | |
| Net Income Before Physician Salaries | $648,633.16 | 50.85 |
| | | |
| PHYSICIAN NET REVENUE ANALYSIS | | |
| Dr. Able—Net Revenue | $390,109.27 | 30.58 |
| Dr. Baker—Net Revenue | $523,072.85 | 41.00 |
| Dr. Cane—Net Revenue | $362,506.86 | 28.42 |
| Total | $1,275,688.98 | |

*continues*

**Exhibit 1–21** continued

| DISTRIBUTION OF EXPENSES | | |
|---|---|---|
| 40% Equally | $250,822.33 | |
| 60% Based On Net Revenue | $376,233.49 | |
| Total | $627,055.82 | |

| | Equally | By Revenue |
|---|---|---|
| Dr. Able | $83,607.44 | $115,053.26 |
| Dr. Baker | $83,607.44 | $154,267.64 |
| Dr. Cane | $83,607.44 | $106,912.60 |
| | $250,822.32 | $376,233.50 |

| PHYSICIANS' INCOMES | | % of Net Revenue |
|---|---|---|
| Dr. Able | $191,448.57 | 15.01 |
| Dr. Baker | $285,197.77 | 22.36 |
| Dr. Cane | $171,986.82 | 13.48 |
| Total | $648,633.16 | 50.85 |

*Source:* © William T. Geary, Ph.D., and Robert J. Solomon, Ph.D. 2007. All Rights Reserved.

is concerned about the value of the practice and who will purchase his interest. Dr. Cane has started the fourth year of a 4-year contract. A partnership decision must be made in the next 2 months. Dr. Cane has made it clear that if he is not admitted to partnership, he will leave at the end of his contract. Unfortunately, all is not going well at Oregon Sports Medicine. Drs. Baker and Cane do not get along. Although Baker has expressed concerns about some of Cane's treatment decisions, she is quick to admit that the fundamental problem is a personality conflict. As she put it, "The thought of working together and managing a practice together for the next 20 years with him is truly depressing. He is not collegial. It will be constant conflict. We just look at the world differently." Dr. Able is less critical of Dr. Cane. He describes the situation differently:

He can be tough to get along with on some days, but his manner doesn't really bother me that much. His technique is good. He has good clinical skills, and he is a competent diagnos-

tician—not a superstar, but well within the bounds of accepted practice. The patients like him. He will do well. I certainly can live with him for a few more years.

Dr. Able commented on the difficulty of replacing Dr. Cane:

If we decide not to offer partnership, we will have a major problem replacing him in the short run. We are out of synch with the recruitment cycle. It will probably take us at least 18 months to get a replacement in here. In addition, we may have to provide some significant financial incentives and subsidies.

Given the information in Exhibit 1–21 we can see that it would not be too difficult to develop a model to see what would happen if Dr. Cane were to leave. This model is presented in **Exhibit 1–22** and a supporting spreadsheet in **Exhibit 1–23**. The model construction began with the current income statement in Exhibit 1–21. It was assumed that all Dr. Cane's revenues would be lost, because Dr. Baker's schedule already was

**Exhibit 1–22** Oregon Sports Medicine: What if Dr. Cane Leaves?

| | With Cane | Without Cane | Variance |
|---|---|---|---|
| **NET REVENUE** | | | |
| Dr. Able | $390,109.27 | $390,109.27 | |
| Dr. Baker | $523,072.85 | $523,072.85 | |
| Dr. Cane | $362,506.86 | $— | |
| Total | $1,275,688.98 | $913,182.12 | $362,506.86 |
| **EXPENSES** | | | |
| Nonphysician Gross Payroll | $151,943.11 | $136,914.32 | $15,028.79 |
| FICA (Includes Physicians) | $26,699.61 | $21,090.67 | $5,608.94 |
| Advertising | $26,601.83 | $26,601.83 | $— |
| Maintenance | $6,619.63 | $6,619.63 | $— |
| Telephone | $8,415.60 | $8,415.60 | $— |
| Radiology | $12,106.81 | $8,666.47 | $3,440.34 |
| Postage | $6,942.50 | $4,969.68 | $1,972.82 |
| Licenses | $175.00 | $155.00 | $20.00 |
| Janitorial | $3,400.00 | $3,400.00 | $— |
| Contributions/Gifts | $16,800.05 | $10,000.00 | $6,800.05 |
| Petty Cash | $3,132.76 | $3,132.76 | $— |
| Accounting/Legal | $10,847.10 | $10,847.10 | $— |
| Taxes—Corporate | $— | $— | $— |
| Personal Property | $2,920.07 | $2,920.07 | $— |
| State Unemployment | $76.02 | $68.50 | $7.52 |
| Fed. Unemployment | $2,288.80 | $2,062.41 | $226.39 |
| Gross Receipts | $6,872.54 | $5,296.46 | $1,576.08 |
| Office Supplies | $25,103.24 | $17,969.76 | $7,133.48 |
| Medical Supplies | $35,498.29 | $25,410.90 | $10,087.39 |
| Dues | $10,540.50 | $8,250.50 | $2,290.00 |
| Books | $8,775.59 | $8,775.59 | $— |
| Meetings | $18,239.11 | $16,955.40 | $1,283.71 |
| Insurance | $68,138.58 | $50,179.44 | $17,959.14 |
| Rent | $65,832.00 | $65,832.00 | $— |
| Christmas Parties | $1,039.01 | $1,039.01 | $— |
| Equipment Lease | $50,429.97 | $50,429.97 | $— |
| Interest Bank Note | $7,488.87 | $7,488.87 | $— |
| Interest to Owners | $10,265.79 | $10,265.79 | $— |
| Electricity | $7,150.98 | $7,150.98 | $— |
| Depreciation | $25,113.00 | $25,113.00 | $— |
| Miscellanous | $954.46 | $954.46 | $— |
| Transcription Service | $6,645.00 | $4,756.72 | $1,888.28 |
| Total Expenses | $627,055.82 | $551,732.90 | $75,322.92 |
| Net Income Before Physician Salaries | $648,633.16 | $361,449.23 | $287,183.94 |
| **PHYSICIAN NET REVENUE ANALYSIS** | | | |
| Dr. Able—Net Revenue | $390,109.27 | $390,109.27 | |
| Dr. Baker—Net Revenue | $523,072.85 | $523,072.85 | |
| Dr. Cane—Net Revenue | $362,506.86 | $— | |
| Total | $1,275,688.98 | $913,182.12 | |

*continues*

**Exhibit 1–22** continued

**DISTRIBUTION OF EXPENSES**

| | | |
|---|---|---|
| 40% Equally | $220,693.16 | |
| 60% Based On Net Revenue | $331,039.74 | |
| Total Expenses | $551,732.90 | |

| | Equally | By Revenue |
|---|---|---|
| Dr. Able | $110,346.58 | $141,419.40 |
| Dr. Baker | $110,346.58 | $189,620.33 |
| Dr. Cane | $— | $— |
| | $220,693.16 | $331,039.74 |

**PHYSICIANS' INCOMES**

| | | % of Net Revenue |
|---|---|---|
| Dr. Able | $138,343.29 | 15.15% |
| Dr. Baker | $223,105.94 | 24.43% |
| Dr. Cane | $— | 0.00% |
| Total | $361,449.23 | 39.58% |

| | Before | After | Variance |
|---|---|---|---|
| Dr. Able | $191,448.57 | $138,343.29 | $(53,105.28) |
| Dr. Baker | $285,197.77 | $223,105.94 | $(62,091.83) |
| Dr. Cane | $171,986.82 | $— | $(171,986.82) |
| Total | $648,633.16 | $361,449.23 | $(287,183.93) |

*Source:* © William T. Geary, Ph.D., and Robert J. Solomon, Ph.D. 2007. All Rights Reserved.

full and Dr. Able was winding down and not interested in increasing his workload. Variable expenses were adjusted by using a flexible budget formula using total revenue as a cost driver. These adjustments were made on the supporting spreadsheet (Exhibit 1–23). For example, current radiology expense was divided by total net revenue, so that radiology expense could be expressed as a percentage of net revenue; in this case, 0.95 percent. This factor then could be used to project the future radiology expense after Cane's revenues have been removed. Fixed expenses were adjusted by asking: Do we still need it? Could it be eliminated or at least cut back? For example, Irene's position (Exhibit 1–23) was eliminated.

After these adjustments were completed, a projected income statement was produced, which is the "without Cane" column of Exhibit 1–22. The results are sobering. They indicate that Dr. Baker's salary is likely to drop by about $62,000 and Dr. Able is projected to make about $53,000 less. Examination of the projected income statement reveals why the salary decreases are so large. If Cane goes, he will take with him his variable expenses, but he will leave his share of the fixed expenses. Unfortunately, this practice is largely a fixed expense operation. Once a model such as this is produced, it can easily be sensitized to other scenarios. If Drs. Able and Baker don't like the outcome or the assumptions,[22] then they can try other "what-ifs." Perhaps one of the other radiology technician positions could be converted to part time. Perhaps other fixed expenses could be reduced or eliminated. Perhaps they should recruit two new associates instead of one. Perhaps Dr. Baker may conclude that Dr. Cane is not so bad after all! Modeling such as this does not solve the problem. It simply attaches a financial cost to the modeled outcome. It provides an opportunity to explore

**Exhibit 1–23**  Oregon Sports Medicine: Projection Calculation Worksheet

| ADJUSTMENTS | | WITH CANE | WITHOUT CANE |
|---|---|---|---|
| Personnel Salaries | | | |
| Office Manager | Ann | $23,410.66 | $23,410.66 |
| Computer Input | Bryan | $20,207.85 | $20,207.85 |
| Receptionist | Charlotte | $18,100.39 | $18,100.39 |
| Insurance/Collections | Dean | $17,898.07 | $17,898.07 |
| Medical Secretary | Elvira | $14,600.00 | $14,600.00 |
| Radiology Technician (Dr. Able) | Georgina | $20,984.24 | $20,984.24 |
| Radiology Technician (Dr. Baker) | Harry | $21,713.11 | $21,713.11 |
| Radiology Technician (Eliminated) | Irene | $15,028.79 | $— |
| | | $151,943.11 | $136,914.32 |
| X-RAYS (Percentage of projected net revenue) | | 0.95% | $8,666.47 |
| POSTAGE (Percentage of projected net revenue) | | 0.54% | $4,969.68 |
| BUSINESS LICENSES | | | |
| Dr. Able | | $60.00 | $60.00 |
| Dr. Baker | | $20.00 | $20.00 |
| Dr. Cane | | $20.00 | $— |
| Oregon Sports Medicine | | $75.00 | $75.00 |
| Total | | $175.00 | $155.00 |
| GROSS RECEIPTS TAX | | $7,399.00 | $5,296.46 |
| CONTRIBUTIONS/GIFTS (Estimated) | | $16,800.05 | $10,000.00 |
| OFFICE SUPPLIES (Percentage of projected net revenue) | | 1.97% | $17,969.76 |
| MEDICAL SUPPLIES (Percentage of projected net revenue) | | 2.78% | $25,410.90 |
| DUES | | | |
| Dr. Able | | $4,173.50 | $4,173.50 |
| Dr. Baker | | $4,077.00 | $4,077.00 |
| Dr. Cane | | $2,290.00 | $— |
| Total | | $10,540.50 | $8,250.50 |
| MEETINGS | | | |
| Dr. Able | | $6,221.58 | $6,221.58 |
| Dr. Baker | | $9,836.78 | $9,836.78 |
| Dr. Cane | | $1,283.71 | $— |
| Staff | | $897.04 | $897.04 |
| Total | | $18,239.11 | $16,955.40 |
| INSURANCE | | | |
| Dr. Able—Dis, OH, Life, HIV | | $2,475.34 | $2,475.34 |
| Dr. Baker—Dis, OH, Life, HIV | | $2,807.50 | $2,807.50 |
| Dr. Cane—Dis, OH, Life, HIV | | $4,844.14 | $— |
| Business Ins. | | $4,657.00 | $4,657.00 |

*continues*

**Exhibit 1–23** continued

| | | |
|---|---|---|
| Dr. Able -Malpractice | $15,642.00 | $15,642.00 |
| Dr. Baker—Malpractice | $15,642.00 | $15,642.00 |
| Dr. Cane—Malpractice | $13,115.00 | $— |
| Corporate | $8,955.60 | $8,955.60 |
| Total | $68,138.58 | $50,179.44 |
| TRANSCRIPTION (Percentage of projected net revenue) | 0.52% | $4,756.72 |

*Source:* © William T. Geary, Ph.D., and Robert J. Solomon, Ph.D. 2007. All Rights Reserved.

the financial consequences of alternative outcomes, and attaches a cost to behavioral choices.

If Dr. Cane does depart, there will be little room for financial errors until he can be replaced. The projected income statement can form the basis for static and flexible budgets, so that Drs. Able and Baker can track how they are proceeding against expectations. This may allow them to detect unfavorable trends before they become crises, and manage the practice through a time when there will probably be little margin for error.

Cases such as Oregon Sports Medicine reinforce the importance of a number of other issues discussed in this book. The goal of management should be to prevent a situation such as this from occurring by carefully selecting partners and then guiding their development through a performance appraisal and goal-setting process, so that antagonisms such as have occurred at OSM are managed, if not prevented.

## CONCLUSION

The strength of the material discussed in this chapter is that it really does work. The problem, however, is that it can work too well. When leaders who are motivated primarily by financial considerations make critical decisions in an organization with a healthcare mission, it can result in the medical mission being subordinated to the financial mission. The underlying message in this chapter is that financial considerations in healthcare organizations are too important to be left entirely to financial leaders. Physician leaders must intercede and contribute a medically based perspective to decision making. To do this, they must understand the financial mind set, as well as how to use financial data as an aid to decision making.

The current healthcare environment places a premium on creating and operating financially sound healthcare organizations, hospitals, and practices. The financial orientation to managing healthcare organizations is analogous to the camel whose nose was under the tent and who now has every intention of moving in and taking over. Pretending that this is not happening by ignoring it will not work. Simply leaving decisions totally to financial professionals ignores the problem. If a healthcare organization's medical mission is to be well served, financially literate physicians must participate in the decision-making process.

## NOTES

1. *Utilization: A guide to reducing variations to improve outcomes.* Irving TX: VHA Inc., (1994) 9–10.
2. Ibid, 13–16.
3. *Net revenue* is being defined as the fee as stated in a fee schedule less contractual write-offs, adjustments, and an average provision for account delinquency. For example, the fee for a panel of laboratory tests might be $200, but the insurance company contract may specify a contractual write-off of 15 percent ($30). If the insurance company and/or the patient paid the $170, it would be called net revenue.
4. This case was written by William T. Geary, Ph.D., Mason School of Business, College of William & Mary, Williamsburg Virginia. Used with permission.
5. *Depreciation* is the accounting term that is used to recognize that assets have a limited useful life. Sometimes, this is due to literally using them until they no longer work, but depreciation can also be used to recognize technological obsolescence.
6. Some physicians really enjoy working with spreadsheets, doing the sensitivity analyses, and modifying the assumptions contained in the spreadsheet formulas. If this is true for you, I am not suggesting that you forgo this activity, only that you consider what is the best use of your time.
7. Note that the Projected Net Revenue in Exhibit 1–3 and Projected Net Income in Exhibit 1–2 are different. Payback analysis is examining actual cash in versus cash out so Net Revenue does not reflect an adjustment for depreciation, which is a noncash expense. If you add the Depreciation and the Projected Net Income in Exhibit 1–2, it will equal the Projected Net Revenue in Exhibit 1–3.
8. The interest rate reflects three components: risk, the rate of inflation, and real profit that is needed to bring money into investment markets. For example, if a company offers a bond at 10 percent, inflation is 3 percent, and U.S. government securities, which are generally considered risk free, are selling for 5 percent, then the cost of capital is 2 percent.
9. Use the IRR function in Microsoft Excel.
10. If you are following this example by building a spreadsheet and using the spreadsheet formula note the following. In Excel, the NPV formula is NPV = (Rate, Value1, Value2, . . . ) . Because the capital investment of $2,800,000 occurs at the beginning of the first period, it is *not* included as a value, but is instead added to NPV, so the appropriate formula is NPV = (Rate, Value1, Value2, . . .) + Capital Investment.
11. Often, this is done as salary at the end of the tax year. One must be careful to justify this distribution based on job content, such as management responsibilities, or to show that the total salary is in line with the amount of clinical work. Otherwise, the Internal Revenue Service (IRS) might consider the distribution a dividend, in which case both the corporation and the recipient would be taxed on the distribution.
12. There are many ways to calculate depreciation. The IRS prescribes some given particular factual circumstances. Often, what is advantageous for tax reasons may not be the most descriptive of economic reality. You might, therefore, want to consider examining different balance sheets for different purposes, such as one required by IRS for tax purposes and another for financial planning purposes.
13. It is likely that you intuitively understand the concept of accrual-based accounting. For example, if during the course of the year you say to yourself "I've got a big malpractice insurance bill due at the end of the year, and I should reserve some cash each month so that I will be able to pay it," then you are making a provision for an expense incurred but not yet paid.
14. This case was prepared in collaboration with William T. Geary, Ph.D., Mason School of Business, College of William & Mary, Williamsburg, Virginia.
15. Exhibit 1–10: Clinical Services—Bad Debt and Adjustments.
16. Exhibit 1–9: Accounts Receivable adjusted for write-offs and bad debt.
17. Justifications for offering a service with a negative margin include ethics, such as perhaps immunizations, free clinic, and "cross fertilization," such as when a negative margin service such as obstetrics in some hospitals creates an affiliation between the hospital and the community, thereby supporting other positive margin procedures in other areas such as cardiology.
18. Additional procedures were performed at hospital's endoscopy facilities.
19. Sometimes this is called a *tray fee*. It is designed to cover facility costs and variable costs.

20. This analysis leaves aside issues of travel time, schedule control, and work satisfaction issues. It also does not address the likelihood of the patient having a lower copayment for the office-based procedure.
21. For a more detailed analysis of a similar case, see Pike, I. (2002). Outpatient endoscopy possibilities for the office. *Gastrointestinal Endoscopy Clinics of North America*. 12: 245–258.
22. Perhaps, for example, given the outcome in Exhibit 1–22 Drs. Able and Baker decide that they each will take on more patients after all. The model then can be sensitized to the new volume levels.

## CHAPTER 2

# Cash Management and Collection in Private Practices

## Chapter Objectives

The items covered in this chapter pertain most directly to physician leaders working in private practices. This chapter will address two broad cash management issues. The first is to identify management reports that a physician leader should routinely examine in order to ensure the validity of a practice's financial data and to deter and identify theft. The second category is to lead and manage the collection process. Leading the collection process involves developing an effective collection process including collection reports and a collection database. Managing the collection process involves supervising the practice's collection manager and regularly reviewing reports that assess collection performance.

Successful cash control involves generating financial and production reports that tell the physician leader how well the organization is functioning. These reports are easily generated by computer directly from the practice's medical office management software (MOMS), so it is feasible to examine them on a routine basis. Many of these reports will be used on a daily basis by the business staff. Nevertheless, the physician leader must be familiar with their significance and use for two reasons. First, to ensure that subordinates are fully utilizing the information they contain, and second so medical leadership can use this information to make management decisions. The names that are used for the following reports are somewhat arbitrary and may differ from those in your specific office software. The important consideration is the information they provide.

*Collection* is the process of converting the potential wealth that is generated through practicing medicine into cash. This issue is too important to exclude physician leadership in the design and management of this process. Specifically, we will examine:

1. The physician leader's appropriate role in the collection process
2. What employees can do to increase collection effectiveness
3. Methods for increasing patient payments, including education and collection methods
4. Methods to manage insurance collection
5. Selecting and using a collection agent
6. What to do if your collection process is in disarray

## CASH MANAGEMENT

Reports that form the basis of an effective cash management process are described here.

### Daily Receipts/Adjustments

This report (**Exhibit 2–1**) provides the information necessary to determine whether the posting of payments to patient accounts is accurate. It should be run either at the very end of each day, or at the beginning of each day on the transactions for the previous day. It provides the information necessary to audit, or verify, the accuracy of the following critical pieces of information:

- the amount of each payment to an account
- the account it is posted to
- the type of each payment (e.g., insurance payment, check, cash, credit card)
- the totals for each type of payment

The contents of this report should be checked against the actual cash receipts for that day. Receipts in hand (cash, checks, credit card slips) must *exactly* match the totals reported in the daily receipts/adjustments report. If there is a discrepancy, it must be resolved immediately.

This report is important for several reasons. First, if the accuracy of accounts is secured on a daily basis, problems are more easily resolvable, because the problem must have occurred on one date. If the report is run less frequently, such as every week, the auditing and correction tasks become much more complex. Second, using this report on a daily basis acts as a deterrent to some types of theft. If cash, primarily currency and checks, is being diverted, then this will be detected when the cash and checks posted to accounts does not balance against the cash and checks on hand. For this control to be effective, both the posting of cash and the verification of the posting

must be separated from the task of receiving cash. This involves dividing these responsibilities across different front office positions. Running this report each day ensures that any employee whose theft could be detected by this report will only have access to cash from one day before it would be detected. This report should be run daily. The users will generally be front office personnel.

### Daily Activity by Provider

This report (**Exhibit 2–2**) provides a summary of clinical work performed each day. If your practice has more than one provider, this report also will ensure that the correct physicians have been credited for their work. This report should be run either at the end of each day or at the beginning of each day for the previous day. This report should indicate the name of the patient, the procedure that was performed, the provider who performed the procedure, and the fee that was charged. The contents of this report should be validated against an independent record, such as a day sheet or encounter form, to ensure that all services have been properly entered.

This report also can be used to deter theft. An employee might try to hide the diversion of cash by simply not entering the cash and the associated procedures that generated them into the MOMS. Comparison of this report with an independent record of procedures, such as encounter forms, could defeat this strategy. For this control to be effective, the person reviewing the report should be someone other than the person who collects cash. Once again, carefully dividing duties across front office positions can increase the difficulty of theft. Users will generally be front office personnel, although ideally physicians should receive their own reports for deterrence and quality control purposes.

**Exhibit 2–1** Daily Receipts and Adjustments for January 23, 20XX

| Number | Name | Transaction | Amount |
|--------|------|-------------|--------|
| 21–G | Mills Joe | ››Check Payment | $500.00 |
| 21–G | Mills Joe | ››Cash Payment | $310.00 |
| 21–2 | Mills Candace | Full-thick. skin graft to lip/mouth | |
| 21–G | Mills Joe | ››Card Payment | $600.00 |
| 21–3 | Mills Jeff | Closure of nasal sinus fistula | |
| 23–G | Hernandes Tim | ››Positive Adjustment | $150.00 |
| 23–G | Hernandes Tim | ››Positive Adjustment | |
| 23–G | Hernandes Tim | ››Uncollectible Write-Off | $191.80 |
| 23–2 | Hernandes Christine | Corneal transplant—not other. spec. | |
| 23–2 | Hernandes Christine | Tattooing of cornea | |
| 10–G | Snyder David | ››Card Payment | $85.00 |
| 10–G | Snyder David | Cisternal Puncture | |
| 10–G | Snyder David | [DELTA] Aetna Life & Casualty | $210.00 |
| 10–G | Snyder David | Other diagnostic procedures on skull | |
| 10–G | Snyder David | ››Money Express | $45.00 |
| 10–G | Snyder Shari | Other cranial puncture | |
| 10–G | Snyder David | ››Cash Payment | $35.00 |
| 10–G | Snyder David | ››Welfare Check | $50.00 |
| 20–G | James Jim | ››Check Payment | $90.00 |
| 20–1 | James Jim | Suture of corneal laceration | |
| 20–G | James Jim | ››Negative Adjustment | $96.80 |
| 20–G | James Jim | ››Welfare Check | $126.55 |
| 20–1 | James Jim | Thermokeratoplasty | |
| .... | .......... | .......... | $... |
| .... | .......... | .......... | $... |
| .... | .......... | .......... | $... |
| .... | .......... | .......... | $... |
| 2–G | Prokesh David | ››Cash Payment | $55.00 |
| 2–G | Prokesh David Jr. | Myringotomy w/insert of tube | |
| 2–G | Prokesh David | ››Welfare Check | $150.50 |
| 2–G | Prokesh David | ››Negative Adjustment | $90.00 |

| | |
|--|--|
| Total Checks | $1,367.76 |
| Total Cash | $347.50 |
| Total Credit Cards | $885.75 |
| Total Insurance | $4,332.98 |
| Total Uncollectible Write-Offs | $987.76 |
| Total Adjustments (+) | $558.94 |
| Total Adjustments (−) | $186.80 |
| Total Deposit | $6,933.99 |

## Gross Receipts Report

This report (**Exhibit 2–3**) provides a summary of receipts for any given time period. The gross receipts report is primarily useful as another deterrent to theft. The practice gross receipts for a month should balance exactly against bank deposits over the same time period. If the gross receipts report does

**Exhibit 2–2** Daily Activity by Provider: April 12, 20XX

| Number | Patient Name | Chart # | Diagnosis | Procedure | Producer | Fee | Balance |
|---|---|---|---|---|---|---|---|
| 21–4 | Mills Heather | 21–4 | 995.5 | 21.22 | D6A6 | $250.60 | $250.60 |
| 21–4 | Mills Heather | 21–4 | 682.2a | 21.71 | D4A4 | $382.98 | $633.58 |
| 21–3 | Mills Jeff | 21–3 | | 22.71 | D1A1 | $600.00 | $600.00 |
| 21–3 | Mills Jeff | 21–3 | | 22.11 | D1A1 | $274.60 | $874.60 |
| 21–2 | Mills Candace | 21–2 | 781.2 | 27.55 | D3A3 | $306.32 | $306.32 |
| 23–2 | Hernandes Christine | 23–2 | 303.93 | 11.6 | D2A2 | $91.80 | $91.80 |
| 23–2 | Hernandes Christine | 23–2 | | 11.91 | D2A2 | $100.00 | $191.80 |
| 10–1 | Snyder David | 10–1 | 793.2 | 1.01 | D3A3 | $83.75 | $83.75 |
| 10–1 | Snyder David | 10–1 | | 1.19 | D3A3 | $210.00 | $293.75 |
| 10–1 | Snyder David | 10–1 | | 1.24 | D3A3 | $150.00 | $443.75 |
| 10–2 | Snyder Shari | 10–2 | 781.2 | 1.12 | D2A2 | $284.75 | $284.75 |
| 10–2 | Snyder Shari | 10–2 | | 1.09 | D2A2 | $45.00 | $329.75 |
| 20–1 | James Jim | 20–1 | 303.9 | 11.51 | D5A5 | $89.25 | $89.25 |
| 20–1 | James Jim | 20–1 | | 11.74 | D5A5 | $126.55 | $215.80 |
| 20–2 | James Bonnie | 20–2 | 704 | 2.02 | D5A5 | $471.00 | $471.00 |
| 2–3 | Prokesh David Jr. | 2–3 | 272.2 | 20.01 | D2A2 | $205.50 | $205.50 |
| 2–3 | Prokesh David Jr. | 2–3 | | 20.22 | D2A2 | $390.00 | $595.50 |

Total for Producer(s)  $7,468.33
D1A1 Joe Carter  $1,537.96
D2A2 Carl Yates  $2,379.34
D3A3 Stephen Webb  $750.07
D4A4 Keith Jergens  $864.90
D5A5 Joseph Harris  $1,685.46
D6A6 Bob Lovette  $250.60

*Source:* Courtesy of Health Care Communications, Inc., Lincoln, Nebraska.

**Exhibit 2–3** Gross Receipts Report

| Posted Date: 06/01/20XX–06/30/20XX | |
| --- | --- |
| Description | Amount Received |
| Check | $8,188.26 |
| Cash | $898.00 |
| Credit Card | $305.00 |
| Insurance | $11,054.03 |
| User 1 Payment >>Joseph Jones, JD | $– |
| User 2 Payment >>Smith and Wesson, JD | $456.07 |
| Total Receipts | $20,901.36 |
| | |
| Uncollectible Write-Offs | $2,483.80 |
| Self-Pay Write-Offs | |
| Workers Compensation Write-Offs | |
| Medicare Write-Offs | |
| Medicaid Write-Offs | |
| Other Federal Program Write-Offs | $546.89 |
| Commercial Insurance Write-Offs | 2,308.87 |
| Blue Cross/Blue Shield Write-Offs | $2,398.70 |
| Other Write-Offs | $543.98 |
| Positive Adjustments | $227.97 |
| Negative Adjustments | $45.98 |

not reconcile against the deposits to the bank account as indicated on your monthly bank statement, then it is possible that the person responsible for managing your checking account or making deposits is diverting funds.

To make this reconciliation easier, the posting of payments to patient accounts should be coordinated with deposits into the bank account, so that all payments posted into the MOMS for a calendar month or the time period to be reconciled are deposited in a timely manner and will appear on the bank statement for the same month. If this goal is not achieved, the balance can be reconciled by adjusting the gross receipts or the bank balance for cash posted to MOMS but not

yet deposited to checking. This report should be run at the end of each month, but could be run more frequently and reconciled with an online checking account register and balance. Users of this report will generally be front office personnel and the practice's physician manager. The physician manager should receive a copy of the checking account statement, the report as it is produced by the computer, and any reconciliation calculations.

## REVENUE AND PROCEDURE DATABASE

Revenue generated is an indicator of the financial status of the practice, especially if you do a lot of work that is billed to insurance. These revenue figures tell you what you are putting into the "pipeline." Unless you put revenues into the pipeline, you cannot get cash out. This truism is important because it will allow you to spot changes in practice patterns well before their cash impact. For example, if you are tracking revenues and notice that they suddenly decline, then you can be certain that cash will decline several weeks later. This lag can be predicted with some accuracy by knowing the normal delay in payment by your insurance companies. If you know that revenues are down now, then you can plan for the decline in cash by curtailing and delaying spending, arranging for credit, and so on.

A significant revenue decline can be due to many causes, and it should always generate an investigation. For example, revenues will decline if there has been a shift from higher-paying to lower-paying procedures. Examining MOMS reports that provide distribution of procedures over time would be a place to look. Similarly, a decline in the absolute level of work also will generate reduced revenues. One practice identified a billing software problem by noting a decline in revenues. The billing program was not recognizing some procedures as billable, and as a result it did not post insurance transactions and send bills (insurance forms) that also would have increased revenue.

Lower revenues also can be a symptom of theft. If someone is diverting cash, they may try to hide the theft either by not entering procedures or by entering lower paying procedures in the medical management software, and then billing the procedures manually or with a personal copy of the software. The result may appear as a decline in revenue. If you have split the fee collection and posting duties, then a diversion scheme such as this may indicate collusion between two or more employees.

Revenue data can be assembled into a separate database to more easily detect changes in revenue. An example of a report produced from such a database is found in **Exhibit 2–4**. It can be seen that this practice is undergoing very rapid growth in terms of both revenues and procedures. The 90801 procedure is an initial evaluation. Because this code is only used for the patient's first visit, it is a precursor of growth in other procedures. In this case, the practice's revenue growth is driven by an increase in demand for the 90806 procedure. The revenue growth could be predicted, however, by the 90801 growth. Similarly, revenue growth is a precursor to cash growth and a decline in revenue for a period will be a precursor to declining cash several weeks hence. A revenues database should be revised and examined each month. The users will generally be top-level front office personnel and the physician leader. The focus will be on detecting revenue trends, anticipating cash trends and needs, and longer term planning and adjustment to change.

## CASH RECEIPTS AND DISBURSEMENTS

Cash receipts and disbursements journals are records of original entries into your accounting software. The receipts and disbursements can be tabulated into a number of separate accounts. **Exhibit 2–5** contains a chart of accounts for a private practice. Typical disbursement accounts for a medical practice include office expenses (rent, electricity, water, etc.), advertising, office supplies, medical supplies, interest payments, laboratory fees, legal and accounting fees, payroll, payroll taxes, corporate taxes, and so on. Receipt accounts might include receipts for medical services, hospital services, and laboratory tests. Work with your ac-

**Exhibit 2–4** Revenue and Procedure Database Report

| Month | Revenue | Procedure Codes | | | |
| | | 90801 | 90806 | 90853 | 90862 |
| --- | --- | --- | --- | --- | --- |
| January | $75,940 | 78 | 608 | 47 | 102 |
| February | $81,705 | 84 | 652 | 49 | 115 |
| March | $88,165 | 93 | 705 | 65 | 103 |
| April | $94,495 | 101 | 751 | 59 | 127 |
| May | $100,880 | 125 | 792 | 45 | 133 |
| June | $106,540 | 137 | 823 | 57 | 142 |

**Exhibit 2–5**  Chart of Accounts

<u>**Assets**</u>
1010 Cash—Checking Accouint
1020 Cash—Savings Account
1100 Accounts Receivable
1200 Prepaid Expenses
1600 Furniture
1700 Medical Equipment
1800 Accumulated Depreciation

<u>**Liabilities**</u>
2100 FICA Tax Payable—Employer
2210 FICA Tax Payable—Employee
2220 Federal Withholding Tax Payable
2230 State Withholding Tax Payable
2240 Federal Unemployment Tax Payable
2250 State Unemployment Tax Payable
2300 Employee Deductions
2400 Stockholder Loans Payable

<u>**Owner's Equity**</u>
3000 Common Stock
3100 Retained Earnings

<u>**Income**</u>
4000 Hospital Income
4100 Practice Income
4200 Capitated Income
4300 Interest Income
4400 Office Rental Income
4500 Other Income

<u>**Operating Expenses**</u>
6100 Advertising—Marketing
6150 Advertising—Personnel
6180 Advertising—Yellow Pages
6200 Credit Card Discounts
6250 Bank Service Charges
6275 Interest Expense
6280 Tax Penalties
6300 Conference Expenses/Education
6350 Travel—Business Related
6360 Travel—Not Business Related
6370 Professional Dues
6380 Licenses—Professional
6390 Licenses—Business
6395 Other Taxes and Licenses

<u>**Operating Expenses**</u> (cont.)
6500 Business Meals
6550 Food—Entertainment
6600 Legal Expenses
6625 Legal Expenses—Collections
6650 Accounting Expenses
6670 Other Professional Expenses
6700 Rent—Office Space
6750 Rent—Equipment
6800 Office Supplies
6801 Medical Supplies
6802 Laboratory Fees
6803 Pharmaceuticals
6804 Transcription Services
6810 Gifts
6820 General Overhead
6830 Computer Repair/Maintenance
6835 General Repair and Maintenance
6850 Payroll Taxes—Employer Total
6860 Electricity
6870 Cleaning
6900 Postage
7100 Health Insurance
7150 Professional Liability Insurance
7175 Insurance—Other
7200 Repairs
7300 Salaries—Professional Staff
7400 Salaries—Front Office Staff
7600 Payroll—Front Office Staff
7700 Telephone—Verizon
7750 Telephone—AT&T Wireless
7760 Telephone—Answering Service
7800 Depreciation
7900 Donations
8000 Retirement Plan—Dr. Able
8100 Retirement Plan—Dr. Baker
8200 Retirement Plan—Dr. Cane
8300 Retirement Plan—Staff

countant to develop a system of accounts that will provide you with the most useful reports. In addition, the Medical Group Management Association has developed a chart of accounts for medical practices, and most accounting software will come with a suggested chart of accounts.

**Exhibit 2–6** contains an example of a practice's cash receipts journal. The document column is used to record the deposit slip number. The accounts column lists the accounts that have been debited and credited in the transaction. All transactions always affect two sides of the accounting system,

**Exhibit 2–6** Cash Receipts Journal

| 8/1/20XX to 8/31/20XX | | | | |
|---|---|---|---|---|
| Document | Date | Acct | Debits | Credits |
| 126 | 8/1 | 1010 | $1,102.00 | |
| | | 4000 | | $547.87 |
| | | 4100 | | $554.13 |
| 130 | 8/7 | 1010 | $2,368.00 | |
| | | 4100 | | $2,368.00 |
| 131 | 8/7 | 1010 | $52.95 | |
| | | 4400 | | $52.95 |
| 132 | 8/12 | 1010 | $459.35 | |
| | | 4100 | | $459.35 |
| 133 | 8/12 | 1010 | $1,818.21 | |
| | | 4100 | | $1,818.21 |
| 134 | 8/12 | 1010 | $1,682.03 | |
| | | 4100 | | $1,682.03 |
| 135 | 8/15 | 1010 | $1,616.22 | |
| | | 4100 | | $1,616.22 |
| 136 | 8/15 | 1010 | $1,209.45 | |
| | | 4100 | | $1,209.45 |
| 137 | 8/15 | 1010 | $738.24 | |
| | | 4100 | | $738.24 |
| 138 | 8/15 | 1010 | $2,219.25 | |
| | | 4100 | | $2,219.25 |
| 139 | 8/15 | 1010 | $3,229.38 | |
| | | 4100 | | $3,229.38 |
| 140 | 8/20 | 1010 | $831.80 | |
| | | 4100 | | $831.80 |
| 141 | 8/21 | 1010 | $3,187.50 | |
| | | 4000 | | $2,137.50 |
| | | 4100 | | $1,050.00 |
| 1010 Cash–Checking Account | | | $20,514.38 | |
| 4000 Hospital Income | | | | $2,685.37 |
| 4100 Practice Income | | | | $17,776.06 |
| 4400 Office Rental Income | | | | $52.95 |
| | | | $20,514.38 | $20,514.38 |

which always must be in balance. The left side is referred to as the debit side, and the right side is the credit side. Assets are increased by a debit and decreased by a credit; liability accounts are increased by a credit and decreased by a debit. Therefore, when you add funds to checking (an asset account), these funds are listed as debits, and they show as a credit in the liability account to which they are also posted. For example, for deposit 126, the checking account (1010 Cash in Checking) has been debited $1,102.00 because this amount was added to it, and the income accounts (4100 Practice

Income and 4000 Hospital Income from Exhibit 2–5) have been credited a total of $1,102.00, because they are the source of the cash.

**Exhibit 2–7** contains a practice's cash disbursements journal (abridged). The documents column contains the check number, or electronic funds transfer number, and the account column indicates the accounts that were credited and debited as a result of each transaction. For example, check 6043 was written on (or credited to) account 1010 (Cash-Checking Account) and used to pay (or debit) account 6800 (Office Supplies). Check

**Exhibit 2–7** Cash Disbursements Journal (Abridged)

| 9/1/20XX to 9/30/20XX | | | | | |
|---|---|---|---|---|---|
| Document | Date | Acct | Item Description | Debits | Credits |
| 6043 | Sep-9 | 1010 | Polar Water Company | | $32.85 |
| | | 6800 | Polar Water Company | $32.85 | |
| 6051 | Sep-10 | 1020 | Bank of Portsmouth | | $5,502.94 |
| | | 2100 | Bank of Portsmouth | $1,048.07 | |
| | | 2210 | Bank of Portsmouth | $1,048.08 | |
| | | 2220 | Bank of Portsmouth | $3,406.79 | |
| 6052 | Sep-11 | 1010 | Our Own Community Press | | $162.00 |
| | | 6100 | Our Own Community Press | $162.00 | |
| 6055 | Sep-11 | 1010 | Postmaster | | $75.50 |
| | | 6900 | Postmaster | $75.50 | |
| 6054 | Sep-12 | 1010 | Fidelity Magellan | | $370.81 |
| | | 8100 | Fidelity Magellan | $370.81 | |
| EFT-23 | Sep-14 | 1010 | United Family Practices | | $800.00 |
| | | 1020 | United Family Practices | $800.00 | |
| 1010 Cash–Checking Account | | | | | $1,441.16 |
| 1020 Cash–Savings Account | | | | $800.00 | $5,502.94 |
| 2100 FICA Tax Payable–Employer | | | | $1,048.07 | |
| 2210 FICA Tax Payable–Employee | | | | $1,048.08 | |
| 2220 Federal W/H Taxes Payable | | | | $3,406.79 | |
| 6100 Advertising–Marketing | | | | | $162.00 |
| 6800 Office Supplies | | | | | $32.85 |
| 6900 Postage | | | | | $75.50 |
| 8100 Retirement Plan— Dr. Baker | | | | $370.81 | |
| TOTAL | | | | $6,944.10 | 6,944.10 |

6051 was credited against cash and used to debit, or pay for several tax liability accounts (2100, 2210, and 2220). By classifying transactions in this manner, it is possible to track where your receipts and disbursements come from and go to. The accounts that you choose to use are entirely up to you. In the extreme you only need two accounts: receipts and disbursements. The goal, however, is to create a more precise set of receipt and disbursement classifications for greater understanding and control of your practice's finances.

Examining monthly cash receipts and disbursements can help you control the flow of cash through your practice by allowing you to see in detail the sources of your receipts and disbursements. A cash receipts and disbursements report, such as the cash flow statement in Exhibit 1–11 combines the cash receipts data and the cash disbursements data into one report. This report can be used to assess receipt and disbursement trends over time and to evaluate the cash position of the practice. A cash receipts and disbursements report tells you how well you are meeting your cash needs.

Many excellent personal computer-based cash accounting software packages are available that will allow your business manager to track and manage your cash receipts and disbursements. As was previously discussed in Chapter 1, accrual-level accounting can provide additional information that is beyond the scope of cash-level accounting. When you are using accrual-level software, cash-based reports are virtually a no-cost byproduct of paying bills and collecting receipts. If the person using the software is capable of making accrual decisions, or if the software is sophisticated enough to be programmed for accrual decisions, then useful accrual-based reports can be produced within a practice as part of the cash accounting process at virtually any time.

## APPLIED CASH MANAGEMENT PROCEDURES

To some degree, the size of your front office staff and your own possible unwillingness to involve yourself in some of the cash management responsibilities may require that you compromise on some of the cash management guidelines that are proposed here. These guidelines are offered, therefore, as objectives, and the impracticality of implementing some of them in your practice should not preclude you from implementing as many others as is feasible. At a minimum, however, you will understand where your cash control procedures are weak, and, hopefully you will be especially vigilant in those areas.

The basic principle in controlling cash is to separate various functions and responsibilities, so they are performed by different persons. In this way, you prevent theft by employees by reducing their ability to hide their actions. Procedures that facilitate the internal control of cash include the following.

1. **Keep the Physical Handling of Cash Separate from All Phases of the Accounting and Record-Keeping Function.** The reason for this is obvious. If a person handling the cash also controls the function that can disclose a diversion, then hiding a theft becomes easy. This means, for example, that if your receptionist is collecting cash at the window, then he or she should not be involved in posting to MOMS or balancing the cash against MOMS cash receipts. If your business manager manages your checking account and also posts insurance payments, then the posting should be done from the insurance company remits, and the manager should not have access to unendorsed checks or cash. Similarly, the person post-

ing payments to accounts should not open the incoming mail (thereby having easy access to unendorsed checks) to avoid the possibility of this person taking the check and simply writing off that amount on the appropriate patient account.

The practical reality in a small medical practice is that some cash handling and accounting functions may overlap as a result of the small staff size. In this case, you might want to institute procedures that create additional "audit trails." For example, you might inform patients and post a sign to the effect that anyone who pays in currency *must* receive a written receipt from a receipt book that leaves a copy. Require that all checks that come into the office be immediately stamped "For Deposit Only to Account Number . . ."

2. **Separate the Posting of Procedures and Payments to Patient Accounts from Management of the Checkbook.** Because checkbook receipts and the receipts as recorded in your patient accounts must balance, these functions must be separate if each is to serve as a control for the other.

3. **Make Deposits to Your Checking Account on a Daily Basis.** If cash is not physically present, then it cannot be stolen.

4. **Make All Cash Disbursements for Practice Expenses with Prenumbered Checks.** If all disbursements are made by check, then your checking account contains a complete record, and there is no opportunity for funds to be "lost" in petty cash. If you pay for some bills with a credit card, then the credit card statement should be posted to the checkbook software by debiting and crediting the appropriate accounts. You may choose to have more than one cash account. For example, you may have a savings account to store operating cash at a more favorable

interest rate while retaining liquidity. Cash can be moved easily from one account to another by check or by on-line transfer if you are using electronic banking.

5. **Establish a Petty Cash Account.** Petty cash is the cash that you need to provide change for patient transactions. Keep this petty cash fund as small as possible, locate it in a lockable cash box, use it only for providing patient change, and always fund the petty cash box by cashing a company check. Do not use the petty cash fund for small expenses, such as stamps or a business lunch. Once the notion of making unrecorded withdrawals from petty cash as a convenience has been established, it will be impossible to reconcile this account. An irreconcilable account is an invitation to exploitation. In addition, include the petty cash account in your cash receipts and disbursements journals.

6. **Keep Check Signing Authority in the Hands of a Practice Owner.** Never give employees signature power on your checking account. Trustworthiness and loyalty are difficult to assess and apt to change. If an employee forges your signature, then you potentially have recourse with the bank, because the bank is responsible for recognizing authorized signatures. In addition, forgery is a crime, which can be used as leverage to recover stolen funds. If the employee has check signing authority, then the question of whether an employee issued a check for an appropriate reason can be problematic (e.g., "I bought copier paper last February as a convenience to you, and you never did pay me back."). In any event, the bank is off the hook, and all your recovery options probably will be lengthy or complicated. Larger practices may find this suggestion to be cumbersome, and they may have to resort to giving an employee

check signing authority. If this is the case, then have the employee bonded, and limit the balance in this "operational" checking account.

7. **All Employees Must Take Vacations.** Often, cash diversion schemes rely on someone being present at the right time to cover the previous diversion of funds.

## CASE ILLUSTRATIONS

The following cases illustrate the ease with which an employee can divert funds and cover it up if the proper controls are not in place:

- *Case A:* The business manager of a small practice posts all payments to patient accounts, manages the checkbook, and opens the mail. A cash payment is received for $100 on the Jones account. The business manager pockets the cash and writes off or adjusts $100 on the Jones account.
- *Case B:* The business manager has check signing authority as well as the responsibility for paying all the practice's bills. She issues a check to a fictitious creditor, such as an office supply store, and then cashes the check herself.
- *Case* C: A secretary posts all procedures to patient accounts and verifies his own work the next day by comparing postings to the appointment book. No one else validates his work. He fails to post some procedures and keeps the payments.
- *Case D:* A business manager posts all procedures and opens the mail. She posts a procedure, bills the insurance company, corrects the ledger to show a posting error, and then intercepts the insurance check when it arrives in the mail.
- *Case E:* The business manager collects patient payments and posts all payments to patient accounts. Accounts are loosely

managed, and the physician manager normally doesn't get concerned about an account until it is 150 days old. Patient Smith pays off a $200 balance on her account, which is 30 days old. Patient Jones pays off a $100 balance on his account, which is 120 days old. The business manager posts $100 from Smith's payment to the Jones account and pockets the remaining $100. He then continues to post money across accounts, always covering older diversions with newly received payments. Employees who use this strategy to divert funds don't take many vacations, and when they do they don't return!

All the safeguards to theft that have been discussed can be overcome if employees act in collusion. The probability of collusion, however, is obviously less than the probability of having one employee who is willing to steal if the opportunity presents itself.

## THE SMALL PRACTICE PHYSICIAN MANAGER'S ROLE IN CASH CONTROL

The physician manager's role in the accounting and financial affairs of a practice is crucial. This role will vary somewhat with the size of the practice. In smaller practices, the physician manager is regularly involved in cash control procedures. The physician manager, for example, should be the only one with the authority to sign checks, although an employee should prepare the checks for signature. The solo practice physician manager also should be ultimately responsible for managing the checkbook and reconciling it with the bank statement. Because balancing a checking account is almost certainly not a good use of a physician manager's time, this task should probably be contracted out to a bookkeeper or an accountant. Even if the task is contracted out, the physician manager retains the ultimate responsibility and should routinely review the consultant's work.

Physician managers in all practices, irrespective of their size, should use financial, accounting, and production data extensively in their role as practice manager. Physician managers are ultimately responsible for the financial health of the practice and have a duty both to themselves and to their employees to use these data to ensure that the practice will survive and prosper. The following are some suggestions regarding the physician manager's role:

- The physician manager should determine which financial tasks will be performed by the various front office personnel. The business manager should be consulted about appropriate roles, but the ultimate decision must reside with the physician manager. This is essential to ensure financial control and reduce the possibilities of embezzlement or collusion.
- The daily receipts and adjustments and daily activity reports should be forwarded to the physician manager each day after they have been reconciled. The degree to which the physician manager should examine these reports on a daily basis can vary. The most important thing, as far as cash control is concerned, is that the physician manager *has* the report and that employees *know* it. Spot checks by the physician manager on a random basis can be used to detect sloppy, misleading, or deceitful posting practices.
- Cash receipt and disbursement reports and various other reports, including gross receipt, write-off, and aging reports and aging history reports (see the following section in this chapter) should be examined by the physician manager. These reports also should be examined by the

business manager, but this is never a substitute for close review by the physician manager. The business manager should be using these reports to direct day-to-day activities. Part of the physician manager's job, however, is to ensure that the business manager is performing adequately, which requires that the physician manager be personally familiar with the data in these reports. In addition, the physician manager should be using these data to provide guidance regarding practice growth and direction. Personal familiarity with practice finances is essential for the physician manager to make intelligent, rational choices. In this regard, it is always important to remember that the physician manager is the best guardian of his or her own welfare.

- The physician manager and the practice's accountant should review the financial status of the practice annually. A logical time for this review is after the accountant has prepared the annual tax return.
- The physician manager should determine which of the various accounting and financial reports will be useful for management purposes. The physician manager should direct employees to gather the appropriate information so that it will be available when it is needed.

Unfortunately, the task of managing a practice's finances takes time, which will be obtained by working more total hours or by sacrificing clinical hours. Administrative responsibilities such as these are simply part of the baggage that goes along with any business organization, whether it's medicine, law, architecture, or whatever. Furthermore, your work as an administrator will have an impact on your patients. It will assure them that you and your practice will be available when they need your services. Practices do fail as a result of mismanagement, fraud, and poor planning.

Bankruptcy can occur even if you have first-rate clinical skills. Your role as a vigilant, involved administrator is essential if these problems are not to befall your practice.

Physician managers in private practice should remember that this is *their* practice and that they are the only ones who will consistently look out for their own welfare. Relying on another party to examine financial data might be more efficient, but it might also be ineffective or even disastrous if the other party is incompetent or has a self-interest inconsistent with your own. For example, a business manager with an incentive compensation contract might benefit if you bring in additional colleagues and hence might interpret the financial data in a biased manner. Similarly, a business manager who is on a flat salary might have an interest in keeping the practice small to minimize work. Your bookkeeper might be diverting funds and would be only too pleased to tell you that the accounting reports indicate that all is well. A consulting accountant may simply be uninterested in why expenditures for supplies have been steadily growing over the last 2 years. He or she might assume that it is a result of practice growth, whereas you would be more likely to wonder whether your staff has been wasteful.

## COLLECTION MANAGEMENT

*Collection* is the process of converting receivables owed to the practice by insurers and patients into cash. It may seem like a mundane topic, when most of the financial discussions in health care these days are focusing on national debates of providing universal coverage, insurance premium costs, controlling provider costs, and the impact of high technology. Nevertheless, most incarnations of the current payment process still require filing claims with insurers and collecting co-

payments from patients. In addition, some specialties, such as cosmetic plastic surgery, ophthalmology, and dermatology can have a significant number of self-pay patients.

The foundation for effective collection is having an effective collection plan. A collection plan describes in detail how accounts will be handled, what actions will be taken, when these actions will occur, and the reports and databases that will be used to manage the collection process. Once you have a formal written plan, failures to collect can be used to modify the plan, so the plan over time continues to improve and adapt to new delinquency tactics on the part of patients and insurers, and to changes in collection law. Effective collection, then, is the result of consistently applying a well-conceived collection process, learning from collection failures, and using these experiences to improve the collection process.

## COLLECTION ROLES
## AND RESPONSIBILITIES

A cornerstone of effective collection is having the right personnel undertaking the right collection activities. Effective collection occurs when the physician leader, collection administrator, and front office staff work together as an effective team. **Exhibit 2–8** describes how the responsibilities of the physician, collection administrator, and front office staff interact with the collection process plan, collecting from patients, and collecting from insurers. The ideas presented in Exhibit 2–8 are a starting point that you should consider modifying based on your own experience and practice circumstances. At various points in the following discussion, I will use the term "you." Generally, the context will clearly indicate whether the "you" refers to the physician leader or the collection administrator. That said, effective collection is

**Exhibit 2–8** Collection Roles and Problem Areas

| Role | Collection Process Plan | Problem Areas | |
|---|---|---|---|
| | | Patient | Insurance Company |
| Physician | Design/Modify Collection Process<br>Design controls<br>Supervise and motivate<br>Receive and give process feedback | No direct negotiation<br>Determine billing strategy<br>Design patient education<br>Monitor controls<br>Supervise | Monitor controls<br>Supervise |
| Collection Administrator | Design/Modify Collection Process<br>Design controls<br>Supervise<br>Receive and give process feedback | Use collection plan<br>Provide patient education information<br>Provide patient education information<br>Use controls<br>Supervise<br>Receive and give feedback | Use collection plan<br>Use controls<br>Supervise<br>Receive and give feedback |
| Front Office Staff | Use collection plan<br>Provide process feedback | Use collection plan<br>Provide patient education information<br>Use controls<br>Give feedback<br>Provide patient education information | Use collection plan<br>Use controls<br>Give feedback |

the outcome of a true team effort and this is most likely to occur when each team member is aware of all other members' duties and responsibilities.

Let's begin with the physician's role. There are three themes to the physician leader's collection role. The first theme is to ensure that the practice has the appropriate collection procedures in place. The process by which revenue is collected is far too important to delegate to others without physician input. The second theme is control. This means that the physician leader is instrumental in ensuring through oversight that collection activity is achieving desired results. This is achieved primarily by physician review of critical reports and supervising the collection administrator. (The term *collection administrator* is used to refer to the front office position primarily responsible for revenue collection. This position may in fact be titled *office manager, accounts receivable manager,* or have some other job title.). The third theme of the physician leader's role is motivating employees to collect fees. Many employees think that they and the physician will be unaffected by a few dollars that are not collected here and there. It is important for employees to understand that this is not the case, and that inattention to collection could jeopardize everyone's job. Many employees never seem to make the connection between their paychecks, their job security, and their role in collecting fees and turning revenue into cash. Physician leaders reinforce this link through face-to-face meetings and practice documents, such as in the employee handbook. Physician managers also can affect employee motivation by making collection effectiveness an important factor in employees' performance evaluations. Revenue collection should be an evaluation factor for any position with a role in the collection process. This includes the secretary who takes pay-

ments at the front desk, as well as the collection administrator. An employee's evaluation on this factor should be tied to subsequent pay raises, rewards, discipline, or promotions in the same manner as any other important evaluation issue. This statement does *not* imply that you should implement a merit system in which pay is directly driven by the performance evaluation. It simply suggests that collection effectiveness should be considered in the same manner as any other important job performance issue. This issue of performance appraisal is discussed in detail in Chapter 3.

Physicians should have no involvement in day-to-day collection activities. Generally, physicians also should stay out of direct financial negotiations with patients. Physicians should not discuss payments with patients because:

- they usually aren't aware of all the financial considerations regarding a given case.
- they may allow their feelings for a patient to interfere with what is essentially a business matter.
- their involvement is likely to be perceived as interference that may frustrate the collection administrator, who as a result may hesitate to act for fear of being overruled.

This does not mean that physicians can't be involved in particular cases, but it does mean that this involvement should occur behind the scenes and *through* the collection administrator.

The physician should be very involved in designing patient education information. A major reason for patient delinquency is ignorance of financial responsibility, insurance benefits, and the like. Development of these materials is too important to delegate entirely to the collection administrator. The physician manager should review patient pamphlets, intake forms, and other materials relevant to patient financial responsibilities for completeness and clarity.

Controls are reports and measures that provide information about whether a process, such as collection, is working according to plan. The physician leader needs to routinely review control reports that describe the state of patient collection. The aging analysis is the most critical control report. An example of an aging analysis is found in **Exhibit 2–9**. Each day uncollected revenue becomes a day older. The aging analysis ages receivables so the physician manager can get a picture of the state of accounts. Because a practice will probably have several hundred patient accounts in the aging process most of which are not problem accounts, it is critical that your MOMS be capable of selecting and sorting accounts so that the worst ones stand out. The data in Exhibit 2–9 was exported from the MOMS into an Excel spreadsheet. This practice considered money that got into 90 days[1] as "out of tolerance." As a result, a new column defined as 90+ days was created in Excel, which was the sum of the 90, 120, and 150 days columns. The cases then were sorted in descending order on the 90+ days column, thereby highlighting those accounts that need immediate attention.

An important point to consider is what constitutes an unacceptable aging. One way to address this consideration is to refer to external data sources. For example, you can compare your practice's data with national or regional data by specialty, such as can be obtained from the Medical Group Management Association and other medical professional associations. Use this approach with care. First, some published databases have small sample sizes. Second, the data are generally national or regional, so their relevance to your local situation is problematic at best. Third, unless stated otherwise, participants self-select into the database and this may af-

fect the quality of information. Finally, and arguably most importantly, why limit yourself to what your colleagues are doing?

A better strategy is to utilize Total Quality Management (TQM) thinking (see Chapter 11) and methods. Consider collection to be a process that is amenable to statistical analysis and continuous quality improvement. Start from where you are now, and manage against this performance level. Analyze cases (accounts) to look for process failures. Use this information to correct the defects in the collection process. Set specific improvement goals in target categories, such as 150+ days and 90+ days. When those are reached, look at the failed cases, and see where you can improve the process again. If 150+ gets down to 1 percent of receivables, what changes can be implemented to bring it down to 0.5 percent? Managing your collection process with the goal of continuous improvement from where you are now is a far superior solution than relying on external and perhaps questionable databases.

The sorted aging report will be used by both the collection administrator and the physician leader, but for different purposes. The collection administrator will use the report to identify those accounts to work first. The physician leader will use the report to supervise the collection administrator, and also to lead the change process by working with the collection administrator to improve the collection process. The physician leader should meet on a regular basis with the collection administrator to discuss the collection process. During these meetings, the physician should ask for a synopsis of some of the worst aging cases. If it is obvious that the collection administrator is knowledgeable about these cases and is effectively applying practice collection standards, then this is an indication that the collection process is being effectively managed. If, on the other

**Exhibit 2–9**  Sorted Aging Analysis: April 30, 20XX (Abridged)

| Acct. | Guarantor | Current | 30 Days | 60 Days | 90 Days | 120 Days | 150+ Days | Total | 90+ Days |
|---|---|---|---|---|---|---|---|---|---|
| 2203–G | XXXXXXXXX | $0.00 | $90.00 | $0.00 | $270.00 | $90.00 | $450.00 | $900.00 | $810.00 |
| 2189–G | XXXXXXXXX | $37.85 | $165.00 | $90.00 | $360.00 | $90.00 | $320.00 | $1,062.85 | $770.00 |
| 2182–G | XXXXXXXXX | $25.00 | $90.00 | $153.74 | $90.00 | $127.48 | $467.16 | $953.38 | $684.64 |
| 2163–G | XXXXXXXXX | $4,536.00 | $90.00 | $180.00 | $532.30 | $0.00 | $0.00 | $5,338.30 | $532.30 |
| 1855–G | XXXXXXXXX | $235.68 | $159.30 | $0.00 | $0.00 | $0.00 | $315.10 | $710.08 | $315.10 |
| 2208–G | XXXXXXXXX | $0.00 | $111.00 | $21.00 | $201.00 | $55.50 | $0.00 | $388.50 | $256.50 |
| 2214–G | XXXXXXXXX | $0.00 | $0.00 | $22.50 | $45.00 | $165.00 | $37.50 | $270.00 | $247.50 |
| 2262–G | XXXXXXXXX | $56.98 | $0.00 | $0.00 | $180.00 | $0.00 | $0.00 | $236.98 | $180.00 |
| 2001–G | XXXXXXXXX | $0.00 | $90.00 | $90.00 | $90.00 | $90.00 | $0.00 | $360.00 | $180.00 |
| 2134–G | XXXXXXXXX | $0.00 | $0.00 | $0.00 | $0.00 | $0.00 | $180.00 | $180.00 | $180.00 |
| 945–G | XXXXXXXXX | $0.00 | $0.00 | $150.00 | $175.00 | $0.00 | $0.00 | $325.00 | $175.00 |
| 1996–G | XXXXXXXXX | $366.57 | $0.00 | $0.00 | $0.00 | $0.00 | $170.00 | $536.57 | $170.00 |
| 1979–G | XXXXXXXXX | $0.00 | $0.00 | $0.00 | $0.00 | $0.00 | $168.00 | $168.00 | $168.00 |
| 2178–G | XXXXXXXXX | $0.00 | $75.00 | $150.00 | $88.00 | $75.00 | $0.00 | $388.00 | $163.00 |
| 2157–G | XXXXXXXXX | $5,225.30 | $0.00 | $105.00 | $130.00 | $10.00 | $0.00 | $5,470.30 | $140.00 |
| 2244–G | XXXXXXXXX | $10.00 | $0.00 | $0.00 | $45.00 | $90.00 | $0.00 | $145.00 | $135.00 |
| 1858–G | XXXXXXXXX | $25.36 | $0.00 | $45.00 | $0.00 | $0.00 | $126.00 | $196.36 | $126.00 |
| 2213–G | XXXXXXXXX | $687.36 | $118.00 | $0.00 | $97.00 | $0.00 | $0.00 | $902.36 | $97.00 |
| 743–G | XXXXXXXXX | $0.00 | $270.00 | $41.40 | $0.00 | $90.00 | $0.00 | $401.40 | $90.00 |
| 2266–G | XXXXXXXXX | $0.00 | $45.00 | $0.00 | $90.00 | $0.00 | $0.00 | $135.00 | $90.00 |
| 2173–G | XXXXXXXXX | $0.00 | $0.00 | $0.00 | $0.00 | $0.00 | $89.27 | $89.27 | $89.27 |
| 1268–G | XXXXXXXXX | $56.35 | $243.60 | $162.40 | $86.20 | $0.00 | $0.00 | $548.55 | $86.20 |
| 2253–G | XXXXXXXXX | $56.36 | $0.00 | $0.00 | $0.00 | $80.00 | $0.00 | $136.36 | $80.00 |
| 2097–G | XXXXXXXXX | $123.65 | $247.20 | $235.80 | $74.80 | $0.00 | $0.00 | $681.45 | $74.80 |
| 2147–G | XXXXXXXXX | $274.35 | $90.00 | $27.60 | $53.88 | $13.80 | $0.00 | $459.63 | $67.68 |
| 1862–G | XXXXXXXXX | $15.00 | $65.00 | $270.00 | $65.00 | $0.00 | $0.00 | $415.00 | $65.00 |

| | | | | | | | | | |
|---|---|---|---|---|---|---|---|---|---|
| 2222–G | xxxxxxxx | $3,623.36 | $0.00 | $67.50 | $0.00 | $45.00 | $17.50 | $3,753.36 | $62.50 |
| 2227–G | xxxxxxxx | $56.98 | $0.00 | $0.00 | $0.00 | $0.00 | $62.50 | $119.48 | $62.50 |
| 1997–G | xxxxxxxx | $98.67 | $79.65 | $0.00 | $0.00 | $6.59 | $48.65 | $233.56 | $55.24 |
| 2180–G | xxxxxxxx | $552.37 | $270.00 | $41.40 | $53.80 | $0.00 | $0.00 | $917.57 | $53.80 |
| 2028–G | xxxxxxxx | $65.98 | $124.00 | $152.00 | $51.25 | $0.00 | $0.00 | $393.23 | $51.25 |
| 1170–G | xxxxxxxx | $10.00 | $0.00 | $0.00 | $0.00 | $9.17 | $40.95 | $60.12 | $50.12 |
| 1478–G | xxxxxxxx | $0.00 | $0.00 | $0.00 | $0.00 | $8.87 | $39.31 | $48.18 | $48.18 |

| | | |
|---|---|---|
| Net Current | $16,139.17 | 59.94% |
| Net 30 Days | $2,422.75 | 9.00% |
| Net 60 Days | $2,005.34 | 7.45% |
| Net 90 Days | $2,778.23 | 10.32% |
| Net 120 Days | $1,046.41 | 3.89% |
| Net 150+ Days | $2,531.94 | 9.40% |
| Total | $26,923.84 | |
| | | |
| Net 90+ Days | $6,356.58 | 23.61% |

hand, the collection administrator's response is frequently "I'll have to get back to you on that one," or if it appears that practice collection standards are not being *consistently* applied, then there is a job performance problem, which the physician leader must address (See Chapter 3 on performance appraisal). In addition, both the collection administrator and the physician leader should be looking for "themes" in the bad collection cases. These themes can be used to revise collection procedures, so the process continually improves. The physician leader has a crucial role in facilitating this TQM approach to the collection process.

Each monthly aging analysis should be recorded as a row in an aging history database. The aging history database is used to track collection performance over time. **Exhibit 2–10** contains an aging history database that was assembled retrospectively for a practice that lost control of its collection process. The increase in the current column indicates that the practice grew in size, however, the out-of-tolerance column of 120 to 180+ days grew far more rapidly. In a situation such as this, it is possible for the practice's growth to mask the collection problem because cash receipts may remain stable or even grow (see Cash Versus Accrual Accounting in Chapter 1). If the practice had been keeping an aging history database, it would have seen that something was going wrong in September, if not before.

The aging history database is useful for seeing trends over time and judging whether the collection process is responding to changes in procedures and personnel. It and the aging analysis are the two most fundamental control reports that the physician leader has for managing the collection process. Generally, MOMS do not have aging history databases. They are easy to construct, however, using spreadsheet programs

such as Excel. The physician leader should review the aging history database at least once each month and review trends and causes with the collection administrator. It is also appropriate to ask the collection administrator to make brief verbal reports on selected significant collection accounts; reason for delinquency, last action taken, next action, process implications, and so forth. This can be made analogous to a grand rounds, in which the emphasis of the case discussion is understanding, collegial discussion, and process revision.

All too often, the physician manager will avoid the responsibility of looking at aging analyses, using the rationalization that it is really the collection administrator's job to identify and resolve receivable problems. The physician's objective, however, is different from that of the collection administrator. The collection administrator reviews aging analyses to determine which accounts need immediate action. The physician manager reviews aging analyses to determine whether the collection administrator is doing his or her job and to evaluate overall collection process success. This is a critical physician manager responsibility. Failure to perform this control function exposes the practice to collection failure and eventual cash problems that otherwise could have been detected and corrected.

On occasion, a collection administrator may not want physician leadership to regularly review aging analyses, the aging history database, and other management reports. The collection administrator may pander to the physician's ego, and imply that this task is beneath the physician. Physician review of these reports is critical, however, to the physician's ultimate responsibility, which is to ensure the financial soundness of the practice. A good collection administrator will be proud of his or her achievements, and

**Exhibit 2-10** Aging History Database

| Date | Current | 90 Days | 120 Days | 150 Days | 180+ Days | 120 –180+ Days |
|---|---|---|---|---|---|---|
| 8/19/20XX | $50,337.71 | $10,848.94 | $7,808.98 | $7,367.05 | $13,133.66 | $28,309.69 |
| 9/1/20XX | $50,662.18 | $12,553.90 | $9,316.42 | $5,821.28 | $16,796.44 | $27,691.60 |
| 9/8/20XX | $45,168.16 | $11,917.86 | $10,072.02 | $6,188.59 | $17,316.72 | $33,577.33 |
| 9/16/20XX | $44,391.19 | $11,100.43 | $10,558.39 | $6,448.95 | $17,404.32 | $34,411.66 |
| 9/23/20XX | $46,590.00 | $11,261.68 | $11,392.22 | $7,220.92 | $17,900.17 | $36,513.31 |
| 10/1/20XX | $44,213.02 | $12,888.17 | $10,106.40 | $8,144.31 | $17,650.38 | $35,901.09 |
| 10/8/20XX | $50,995.77 | $13,960.67 | $10,278.99 | $8,887.63 | $16,988.79 | $36,155.41 |
| 10/20/20XX | $52,224.71 | $15,564.54 | $8,929.06 | $8,673.35 | $17,979.17 | $35,581.58 |
| 10/31/20XX | $52,893.07 | $13,872.83 | $10,933.86 | $7,764.96 | $18,678.98 | $37,377.80 |
| 11/11/20XX | $51,042.84 | $11,861.86 | $12,372.18 | $8,545.72 | $19,477.86 | $40,395.76 |
| 11/16/20XX | $56,353.12 | $11,233.73 | $13,329.26 | $7,880.51 | $18,820.92 | $40,030.69 |
| 11/23/20XX | $56,918.49 | $10,269.26 | $12,861.16 | $5,818.36 | $19,801.99 | $38,481.51 |
| 11/30/20XX | $54,111.96 | $10,368.25 | $11,315.71 | $7,339.91 | $20,091.09 | $38,746.71 |
| 12/7/20XX | $56,878.04 | $9,530.61 | $12,226.70 | $7,419.02 | $21,086.99 | $40,732.71 |
| 12/21/20XX | $58,209.00 | $9,699.90 | $9,558.29 | $9,991.87 | $19,730.74 | $39,280.90 |
| 12/28/20XX | $56,851.92 | $10,561.54 | $9,861.57 | $9,251.78 | $23,662.41 | $42,775.76 |
| 1/11/20XY | $44,365.88 | $15,368.72 | $8,017.26 | $8,312.27 | $24,480.69 | $40,810.22 |
| 1/25/20XY | $51,291.50 | $17,920.38 | $9,215.53 | $7,672.12 | $25,599.25 | $42,486.90 |
| 2/2/20XY | $52,428.12 | $19,180.18 | $10,213.47 | $7,690.16 | $27,296.92 | $45,200.55 |
| 2/22/20XY | $56,697.74 | $15,610.55 | $15,598.89 | $7,075.35 | $25,485.00 | $48,159.24 |
| 3/8/20XY | $53,696.79 | $16,538.98 | $16,055.50 | $9,189.50 | $27,179.17 | $52,424.17 |
| 5/11/20XY | $57,707.94 | $11,786.93 | $8,260.40 | $10,561.27 | $34,407.16 | $53,228.83 |
| 5/24/20XY | $52,550.12 | $12,584.63 | $8,089.75 | $9,761.48 | $36,362.00 | $54,213.23 |
| 6/20/20XY | $62,099.38 | $13,994.78 | $9,657.96 | $6,154.00 | $40,096.60 | $55,908.56 |
| 7/6/20XY | $63,470.52 | $14,751.89 | $9,494.78 | $7,456.28 | $41,387.89 | $58,338.95 |
| 7/10/20XY | $60,828.01 | $16,570.60 | $9,129.24 | $8,190.20 | $42,778.60 | $60,098.04 |
| 7/19/20XY | $58,256.31 | $14,958.84 | $10,003.03 | $7,688.08 | $42,295.48 | $59,986.59 |
| 8/11/20XY | $48,444.09 | $11,753.63 | $10,831.80 | $5,795.95 | $34,785.62 | $51,413.37 |
| 8/19/20XY | $62,533.46 | $14,226.72 | $9,193.01 | $6,449.50 | $34,508.65 | $50,151.16 |

these achievements ultimately appear in the collection and financial reports. Whenever a collection administrator in any way suggests that the physician should not routinely review collection and financial reports, the physician should become concerned.

The physician manager's responsibility regarding the collection process is to work with the collection administrator on its design. This is an area that is too critical to delegate to the collection administrator. A reasonable division of effort might be for the collection administrator to create initial drafts of policies, procedures, and timetables and for the physician leader to respond to and modify the proposals. Similarly, the physician should be involved in the identification of controls that will be used to monitor collection process success.

The collection administrator's responsibilities involve working with the physician manager to design the collection plan, patient education information, and control systems. In addition, this position is primarily responsible for using these systems on a daily basis. The collection administrator is also the primary conduit for information from front line personnel, such as secretaries and insurance clerks.

Finally, it is the responsibility of front office staff to put the collection policies and procedures into operation. Because two of the keys to effective collection are consistency and timeliness, we don't want a whole lot of unguided creativity going on in the front line. We do want, however, front-line personnel's ideas to be evaluated and acted on where appropriate. It is important, therefore, to encourage front-line employees to think creatively about collection problems, and to communicate their ideas to the collection administrator. From the collection administrator's perspective, an important goal is to encourage communication, provide

feedback, and put reasonable suggestions offered by front-line personnel into operation.

All employees with some collection responsibility must be held accountable for successfully completing their tasks. Accountability is achieved by ensuring that there are undesirable consequences for failing to collect fees, as well as desirable ones when it is done effectively. Whenever there is a collection problem that can be traced back to a particular employee or job, it is important to analyze the reward contingencies. Does the employee benefit by a failure to collect? What happens when the collection does not take place? The following case illustrates the application of these ideas.

## CASE ANALYSIS: REWARDS AND BEHAVIORS

Nan was a receptionist for a group family practice that was having difficulty collecting copayments and deductibles. She reported to the collection administrator. Nan's collection responsibilities consisted of collecting payments, copayments, and deductibles at the time of service. She had a copayment database for commercial insurance, HMO, and preferred provider organization (PPO) plans for patients who were returning for treatment.

On occasion, Nan simply did not collect the fees. Her excuses included "I didn't see the patient leave," and "The patient told me he forgot his checkbook." The collection administrator routinely responded to these collection lapses by sending a bill to the patient or calling the patient and asking for payment by mail. The net effect, however, was that the collection administrator was devoting time to collection tasks that properly belonged to Nan. When the collection administrator was asked why Nan's behavior was tolerated, she stated, "Generally, Nan does a very good job.

Revenue collection is an exception. Besides, once the patient leaves without paying, I can follow through faster than she can."

Nan suffered no bad consequences when a patient avoided payment. On the contrary, if Nan didn't do her job, the collection administrator would do it for her. In effect, the collection administrator was rewarding Nan for not doing her job.

Once the collection administrator understood that she was rewarding undesirable behavior, she changed Nan's responsibilities. She told her that she was responsible for one *effective* collection attempt for each visit. If a patient managed to leave unnoticed, or Nan dealt ineffectively with a patient's unacceptable excuse, she would be responsible for contacting the patient by telephone that day and asking the patient to put a check in the mail. Nan quickly learned that it was easier to collect from patients before they left the practice. This had two effects. First, Nan greatly improved her collection rate. Second, the collection administrator now had more time available to pursue other tasks.

## COLLECTING FROM PATIENTS

One way to conceptualize collection from patients is as follows: There is a line of creditors at the patient's front door. Unfortunately, the patient does not have enough money to pay everyone in the line, and the line is growing longer day-by-day, week-by-week. Your practice must be assertive enough to jump to the front of the line, so that it will be one of the few creditors that will be paid.

Sometimes it is helpful to understand the reasons for delinquency when you are formulating a strategy to collect on accounts. Patients don't pay bills for an almost infinite number of specific reasons. Almost all, however, are variations on three themes:

1. Economic hardships or misfortune
2. Perceptions of inequity
3. Irresponsibility

Unexpected economic hardship can befall anyone. Unfortunately, you are probably not the patient's only creditor. Moving to the front of the line is particularly important when you are dealing with this class of delinquency. You can do this in a number of ways:

- *Be assertive.* The squeaky wheel does tend to get greased first. If your practice is visible through letters, telephone calls, collection procedures, and so on, you will be paid before the creditor who blends into the background.
- *Give the patient a solution.* Remind the patient that he or she can use a credit card. Suggest that the patient get a part-time job or obtain a loan from a bank, sibling, or parent. Have the patient complete a new financial information form. This may reveal some previously undisclosed assets as well as help your staff to develop a payment plan. Propose a plan that will pay off the debt over a short period of time. If the amount is small, try to get the patient to make a payment *now* and close the account with a second payment. The patient may not follow through with the plan, but you may collect some of the debt. Your suggestions may not be in the patient's best financial interests. This is, however, an adversarial situation, and solutions here are intended to maximize your revenue collection. This said, you should assess these solutions in light of your views regarding what is ethical or socially responsible.
- *Consider giving the patient a deal.* For example, if Sarah has a $500 balance, tell her that it will be turned over for collection on Friday, at which time legal fees of $250

will be added to the balance. If, however, she pays $400 by Thursday, the account will be closed, thereby saving her $350. Once Friday arrives, the matter will be out of your hands.

- *Don't be intimidated by threats of bankruptcy.* If a patient truly is insolvent, then bankruptcy protects the creditor as well as the debtor. In addition, it is unlikely that aggressively acting on the patient's debt will be the final act that pushes the patient into bankruptcy.
- *Accept known financial hardship cases with open eyes.* Intake procedures should be designed to identify potential financial hardship cases. For example, patients without insurance or without a job are likely to be hardship cases. You then can decide whether to take potential hardship cases that are likely to require ongoing treatment. If you do, be certain that the payment terms are agreed to in writing. If you feel that you have an obligation to take hardship cases or treat some patients at reduced fees, be certain that you closely monitor the proportion of these patients in your practice. You also have an obligation to your employees, your other patients, and your family to stay in business.

Some patients don't pay because they feel that a fee is unreasonable given the quality or quantity of service. Equity problems can be reduced, although not eliminated, by providing sufficient information to patients. Be certain that patients understand that fees are for services rendered and *are not contingent upon the success of treatment.* Educating patients concerning fees, their insurance coverage, probable clinical outcomes, and so on will allow them to make informed decisions regarding whether to seek services. Generally, a patient is less likely to feel that a fee is unfairly high when all the facts are known

and the patient seeks treatment fully appraised of the probable clinical outcomes and financial implications.

Finally, irresponsibility is another delinquency theme. Some people are ineffective at managing their lives and their responsibilities. Generally, these peoples' lives are characterized by unorganized and inappropriately directed activity. Obligations are not acted upon using objective, rational considerations. A major debt, such as a $300 gynecology fee, has no greater importance than a minor luxury, such as going out to dinner. Irresponsible patients fail to pay for a number of reasons, including the following:

- *Paying is inconvenient.* The inconvenience, however, may be perceived as trivial by most people. Watching a basketball game on television, for example, may be more important than using this time to pay 2 months of back bills.
- *Irresponsible patients are often disorganized.* Bills are lost, misplaced, or never opened. Payments may sit on a desk for weeks, because there are no stamps or envelopes in the house.
- *They often don't plan ahead.* The end of the month may well reveal debts in excess of available cash. In addition, these patients are usually responsible for a disproportionate number of appointment cancellations.
- *They impulse buy.* A patient with a $300 balance buys a "cute, irresistible" puppy for $500, even though your bill remains unpaid.
- *They devise reasons why they can't pay now.* Rationalizations such as "Physicians are rich anyway," "I'll pay after my next paycheck," and "It's inconvenient to draw money out of savings" are sufficient justification for delinquency in the mind of the irresponsible patient.
- *They tend to deny the significance of their debts.* Irresponsible patients often feel that

their obligations will disappear if they can postpone them long enough. Unfortunately, this belief is grounded in reality. Some creditors do in fact go away, either out of exhaustion or as a result of disorganized or inefficient collection methods.

The irresponsible patient often responds to personal impulse and to the most immediate or salient force in the environment. Therefore, the primary objective when dealing with an irresponsible patient is to provide structure and consistency. When the irresponsible patient addresses financial commitments, you want to be the first creditor to come to mind. Providing constant reminders is an effective strategy. Collection letters and telephone calls with very direct messages will give you a salient presence. It also is essential to provide structure by enforcing cancellation fees, late payment charges, and, ultimately, termination of treatment for failure to meet financial obligations. Obviously, this last alternative needs to be done in a medically appropriate manner to avoid an abandonment tort.

Patients with personality disorders may at first appear to be simply irresponsible. The distinction is one of degree, with the depth, persistence, and creativeness of the irresponsible behavior being markers. Unfortunately, there are no clear indicators that will differentiate irresponsible patients who have personality disorders from those who do not. There are several types of personality disorders, but all of them are characterized by a high degree of self-centeredness and limitless ability to deny personal obligations. Patients with personality disorders have either no conscience or only a minimally developed conscience. Some are incapable of feeling guilt, obligation, or remorse and tend to view the world as existing solely to meet their needs. If lying or deception is necessary to

satisfy a personal need, then that is what will be done. Another characteristic of people with personality disorders is that they have an uncanny ability to involve others in their disputes. They are adept at "triangling," or passing on their responsibility to another party. For example, the patient who manages to get your collection administrator to agree to charge her estranged husband for your services has adeptly removed herself from the collection process. The husband may or may not be estranged, and he may or may not have any legal obligations in the matter.

## Case Example 1

Mrs. Phlegmatic brought her youngest child to Dr. Phillips for treatment of allergies. She was poor, but she had insurance, and she told Dr. Phillips' collection administrator that social services had agreed to cover the copayment and deductible. After several visits and no sign of payment from social services, the collection administrator contacted the agency and was informed that Mrs. Phlegmatic already had exhausted her benefits.

At her next visit, Mrs. Phlegmatic was told that she would have to make payments on the account. She made payments for 2 weeks, at which time they stopped, and the collection administrator received a call from Reverend Mooney. He told the collection administrator that Dr. Phillips was inhumane, uncaring, and trying to take advantage of this poor woman. Reverend Mooney then stated that he would try to obtain the money for Mrs. Phlegmatic. Several weeks passed, and the collection administrator had several additional discussions with Reverend Mooney regarding the account. During this time, Mrs. Phlegmatic's child continued treatment, and the personal balance approached $1,000. The contacts between the practice and Reverend Mooney became increasingly strained and adversarial. On several occasions, the collection administrator delayed calling Reverend Mooney, because the conversations had become so unpleasant. Finally, Reverend Mooney informed the collection administrator that he would not be able to obtain the funds. The practice then looked to Mrs. Phlegmatic for payment, who responded, "I've paid enough, and I'm not going to pay anymore. I'm leaving, and I'm not coming back!"

Mrs. Phlegmatic was very successful at triangling the collection administrator. She also was no fool. She chose well when she selected Reverend Mooney to champion her cause. She deflected her responsibility to Reverend Mooney, who was more than happy to adopt her cause and confound it with his own agenda—trying to get physicians to behave in more socially responsible ways. Unfortunately, the collection administrator took the bait and focused his attention on Reverend Mooney instead of Mrs. Phlegmatic. The net result was that Dr. Phillips was not paid, Reverend Mooney had more fuel for his indignation, and Mrs. Phlegmatic had taught her child another valuable lesson regarding how easy it is to manipulate others and evade personal responsibility.

Logic, rationality, equity, and guilt are useless when you are trying to collect from a patient with a personality disorder. Success will depend on power. Sanctions, legal procedures, and collection attorneys are the only alternatives when such a patient does not want to pay.

Often, the personality disorder patient will threaten to file a malpractice suit if the physician attempts to collect on the account. If this happens, the physician must balance the outstanding fee, the real probability of litigation, and the principle of resisting what amounts to extortion against the time and effort that could be expended in a legal defense.

**Case Example 2**

Rose was a medical secretary for Dr. Jonathan, a general surgeon. When she needed surgery, Dr. Jonathan recommended her to Dr. Apple, who performed a rhinoplasty and billed Rose's commercial insurance carrier for $1,800. The carrier directly reimbursed Rose $1,000, but Rose never forwarded the payment to Dr. Apple. After several months, Dr. Apple sent her a collection letter. At that point, Rose forwarded Dr. Apple two bad checks for the insurance amount of $1,000. Finally, after a call from Dr. Apple's collection administrator, Rose forwarded a good check. Dr. Apple's office then attempted to collect the personal balance. After several fruitless phone calls and collection letters, the office obtained a warrant in debt on Rose, and she was served with papers by a uniformed sheriff at work. Rose immediately responded by calling Dr. Apple's office. She stated that Dr. Apple had not taken good care of her, that she had a poor clinical outcome, and that she was thinking about filing a malpractice suit. In addition, she conveyed this information using abusive and defamatory language. Dr. Apple decided to write off the account. Rose was obviously a "loose cannon," and her threat to file a malpractice suit was sufficient to intimidate him.

## THE PATIENT INTAKE PROCESS

Successful collection begins with the patient intake process. The intake process will provide you with the legal authority to render treatment as well as the information and the legal standing necessary to pursue collection. Insurance information may be taken over the telephone when the patient schedules the initial office visit. This task can be performed by a clerical employee after brief training by the collection administrator. Practices with high "no-show" rates may find it a waste of time to verify coverage before the initial appointment. These practices should conduct the verification at the time of service. Upon arrival, the new patient should complete an intake form that solicits biographical information that could be useful for collection purposes and for initially evaluating the patient's credit worthiness. This form should also contain wording approved by your attorney that commits the patient to:

- seek treatment voluntarily
- be responsible for the fee, including any co-payments, deductibles, or insurance denials
- cooperate in the filing of insurance claims by providing any necessary information
- be responsible for any collection fees, court costs, legal fees, or finance charges if the account becomes delinquent

In many states, finance charges are not worth the bother to collect. They do have a deterrent value, however, and once again they represent a way to convey the message that the practice is serious about collecting its fees. Note that state laws vary regarding provisions of this nature, so it is advisable to consult your attorney to obtain appropriate language for the assignment of collection fees, court costs, and finance charges.

If the patient is going to receive some form of extensive or ongoing care, such as repeated psychiatric visits or cancer treatments, it also is desirable to have the patient sign a method of payment form. Patients undergoing recurrent treatment have more potential to incur large balances, so the additional educational value of a method of payment form makes it worthwhile. This form contains detailed information about specific payment arrangements, what the practice expects of the patient, and other patient responsibilities. It also contains any specific payment plans,

including payment schedules and copayments (if known and applicable). A sample method of payment form is found in **Exhibit 2–11**. Any time a special payment arrangement is negotiated with a patient, it should be put in writing on a method of payment form. Placing provisions for legal fees, court costs, collection fees, and finance charges in the method of payment form achieves three objectives:

1. It puts the patient on notice that you have procedures for dealing with delinquent accounts.
2. It informs the patient that he or she will bear any costs of delinquency by creating a legal agreement that will allow you to pass delinquency costs on to the patient (the language required will vary with state law; consult your attorney for the most favorable language).
3. It communicates this information in a tactful and socially appropriate manner. Most of your patients will not become collection problems, and they will view this wording as a necessary condition of doing business in our times, not as specifically directed at them.

## PATIENT EDUCATION

Educating patients regarding their financial obligations lets them make informed choices and avoid misconceptions and reinforces your legal standing if you eventually must resort to collection proceedings. Patient education, at a minimum, should include information about the patient's insurance coverage and probable fees and terms of payment. The practice also should indicate its expectations regarding payment and emphasize that the ultimate responsibility for settlement of the account lies with the patient.

**Exhibit 2–11** Sample Method of Payment Form

Medical Associates, P.C.
123 Main St., Suite 123
Virginia Beach, VA 23456

STATEMENT OF FEE AND METHOD OF PAYMENT

This form is utilized to establish a clear understanding regarding the details of your financial account with this practice. Please read it, and do not hesitate to ask any questions. Your signature is an acknowledgment of your understanding and agreement with the provisions of this agreement.

Name of Patient: _____   Date:_____

Name of Responsible Party: _____   SSN:_____

Relationship to Patient:

I, _____, agree to be responsible for payment in full of the charges for professional services which have been rendered to the above mentioned patient by Medical Associates, P.C. I also understand and agree to the following provisions regarding the fee and method of payment:

1. Medical Associates, P.C., will file primary insurance claims on behalf of the patient for rendered services. Insurance payment shall be made directly to the practice. Should any payment be made to the Responsible Party or any other individual, the Responsible Party agrees to promptly forward payment to the Practice.
2. The patient or Responsible Party will supply to the Practice any forms or documents that may be necessary to expedite the insurance filing process.
3. The Responsible Party shall pay the coinsurance payment (copayment) at the time of each service. The copayment is that part of the fee which is not covered by insurance after the deductible has been paid, or it is the amount that your insurer (HMO, PPO, etc.) specifies as your personal payment for each appointment.
4. Based on the information provided by your insurance company, we estimate your copayment for each visit to be $_____. Please call your insurance company to verify your copayment.
5. The deductible is the amount that you must personally pay each year for covered services, before your insurance begins to provide coverage. Your insurance company has told us that your annual deductible is _____ and that your current unpaid deductible is $_____. Please call your insurance company to verify these numbers.
6. The Responsible Party shall pay any outstanding balance, which is not covered by insurance. The Responsible Party shall also pay claims or any part thereof which are denied or unpaid by an insurance company for any reason, such as for deductibles, copayments, unfiled claims, preexisting conditions, etc., irrespective of who is responsible for the denied claim or the uncovered service. The patient or Responsible Party may receive a statement whenever there is an outstanding balance. The Responsible Party, not the insurance company, is ultimately responsible for payment for the rendered services.
7. It is understood that the usual and customary collection procedures may be initiated should the account become delinquent. It is also understood that any collection fees, including any reasonable court costs, and an attorney's fee of thirty-three and one-third percent (33⅓ percent) will be payable by the Responsible Party.
8. If for any reason the account becomes 90 days past due, the Responsible Party or the patient may be billed and expected to bring the account current. Please remember that we file insurance as a courtesy to our patients, and that your insurance contract is between you and your insurance company. We consider payment, therefore, to be the responsibility of the patient if a delay occurs from the insurance com-

*continues*

**Exhibit 2–11** continued

pany. You will be expected to pay *any balance not paid by your insurance company, or which your insurance company delays beyond 90 days after the date of service.*

9. A fee of $15.00 will be charged for any returned checks. An interest charge of 18% per annum may be added to any balance which is not paid within 30 days of the date that it is billed to you.
10. Only the business manager is authorized to modify this agreement, or to make any financial arrangements between the practice and the patient. Physicians are specifically excluded from making any financial arrangements with patients.
11. I hereby authorize Medical Associates, P.C., to provide my insurance company with any clinical or financial information that they may require.
12. Additional details or considerations regarding the method of payment may be outlined below:

_____        _____
Signature of Responsible Party                                Date

_____        _____
Signature of Business Manager                                 Date

Patient education can proceed somewhat differently for patients who will be receiving long-term or repeated treatment as opposed to walk-ins or patients who will receive infrequent treatment. Both infrequent and recurrent treatment patients should receive written patient educational material. Patients who are identified as infrequent should receive a standard patient education pamphlet. This pamphlet should describe billing methods, emphasize the patient's responsibility for the account, outline expectations (e.g., the practice's appointment cancellation policy), indicate where to call during an emergency, and so on. Infrequent treatment patients also should meet with the collection administrator if either party has any questions regarding insurance coverage or payment arrangements.

Recurrent treatment patients should meet with the collection administrator, who should review the topics covered in the patient education pamphlet; answer any questions regarding insurance coverage; discuss payment and copayment arrangements, deductibles, and so on; and review all appropriate practice policies. The collection administrator should also negotiate a payment schedule, if necessary and appropriate. All these arrangements then should be written into the method of payment form, which the patient should sign. The method of payment form then becomes a contract between the practice and the patient. It also gives the patient a written document to refer to regarding expectations and financial commitments.

Large fees should always be discussed with patients before treatment is provided. The physician may want to discuss a large fee directly with the patient. If this turns into a negotiation, however, the physician should turn it over to the collection administrator and orchestrate it from behind the scenes. If the physician feels uncomfortable discussing the fee, he or she should discuss the clinical aspects of the treatment and then direct the patient to the collection administrator, who will discuss the financial arrangements. If the procedure involves a standard fee, the collection administrator will be able to handle this as a routine matter. If the fee is not standard, the physician can explain the contingency issues to the collection administrator, who will then make payment arrangements with the patient. This approach has the added advantage that the collection administrator, who is knowledgeable about insurance matters and the patient's coverage, will handle all the financial arrangements.

## BILLING STRATEGIES

A *billing strategy* is a plan for how and when to collect fees. In fee-for-service situations, there are two widely used strategies and several less-frequently used strategies.

### Insurance Pay-Patient Statement Strategy

This strategy is characterized by the following sequence of events:

1. The patient receives services.
2. The physician bills the insurance company.
3. When the physician receives an insurance company payment or denial, the patient is mailed a statement indicating their personal balance.

This is one of the most commonly used billing strategies. The advantage of this strategy is that it results in uncomplicated patient billing. Because the patient is not billed until the insurance company's obligation is resolved, the balance owed by the patient is clarified before the patient receives a statement. The patient receives statements on a regular basis, such as each month or each time that an insurance claim reaches resolution. This system is particularly effective when the physician's services are largely covered by insurance or when patients receive infrequent treatment.

This strategy becomes more expensive and cumbersome when patients receive frequent treatment. When a physician supplies patients with weekly services or with several services per week over a period of time, the physician can be carrying large receivables on many patient accounts. This strategy also requires the mailing of a large number of statements. Because each mailing incurs postage, supply, and labor costs, this strategy becomes less efficient as the number of patients treated increases and as insurance coverage for typical services decreases. It also becomes complicated and time consuming when patients are covered by more than one insurer, because the practice then must coordinate the payment of benefits among the carriers before issuing a statement to the patient.

### Patient Payment-File Insurance Strategy

When this strategy is used, the patient pays for the estimated share of the fee plus any copayment and deductible at the time of service, and the insurance company is simultaneously billed. This strategy is particularly appropriate when patients will receive continuing, frequent treatment. This approach is advantageous because the practice collects the estimated personal balance at the time of service, thereby taking advantage of the time value of money. In addition, this strategy reduces the expenses associated with mailing statements, because statements are only mailed when the insurance benefit for a procedure has been overestimated or underestimated, when a patient misses a payment, or upon termination of treatment if the account closes with either a positive or negative balance.

**Modified Strategies**

With both of these strategies, the practice assumes the risk that insurance companies will be slow to pay. In some cases, insurance companies will classify a claim as pending for several months. As a result, a medical practice's business office must constantly monitor the status of claims, refile lost or improperly denied claims, and call or send interrogatories regarding claims. Available cash is reduced because revenue is tied up in receivables. In addition, the eventual day of reckoning with the patient is delayed. Patients who do not receive a final statement for several months are less likely to pay, and tend to consume more collection effort on the part of the practice.

Both of the first two strategies can become particularly burdensome to a practice when patients have more than one insurance carrier. When this occurs, all claims must be filed with the primary carrier, and copies of the explanation of benefits for each payment or denial from the primary carrier must accompany claims sent to the secondary carrier. Needless to say, this has the potential to become a protracted process. Unless the claims are large, practices whenever possible should not accept the responsibility of filing secondary insurance. Whether you can do this depends on whether you have signed a participating agreement contract with the secondary provider. Whenever possible, shift this burden to the patient. If you do this, then when the primary carrier pays or denies a claim, the patient becomes responsible for payment and the patient can file the secondary claim.

Some practices have adopted a strategy in which they will try to collect from an insurance carrier for a stated period of time, such as 90 days. Delayed or denied claims are then billed to the patient irrespective of whether the practice could continue to pursue the claim with the insurance carrier. Patients are instructed to contact the insurance carrier if they have any questions. If the insurance company subsequently pays the claim to the practice, the practice then sends a refund to the patient. When practices use this approach, they should inform the patient before the "90-day clock" expires on a claim. Often, including the patient in the process will get quicker action from the insurer. Once again, contracting with the insurer may preclude this option.

**Full-Payment Strategy**

With this strategy, the patient is expected to pay the full fee at the time of service. Insurance may be filed as a courtesy to the patient, with the payment going directly to the patient. The practice, of course, can choose not to file insurance. Filing the claim, however, is a reasonable act of goodwill toward the patient. This strategy has the advantage of increasing the practice's immediate cash flow, and places the burden of insurance company collection on the patient. It is consistent with the idea that insurance coverage is based on a contractual agreement between a patient and an insurance carrier. It is also obviously the most advantageous strategy for the practice and the least favorable one for the patient.

The full-payment strategy may be appropriate if there is more demand for services than a physician can supply. Even if this strategy is not feasible for most patients and practices, it may be feasible for certain niches. Examples might include cosmetic plastic surgery, psychoanalysis, and foreign nationals who are willing to pay cash for high-quality immediate services in the United States.

A variation on this strategy is to use it for procedures below a certain amount, such as

$300 for indemnity insurance patients. Fees above this amount are billed using the patient payment-file insurance strategy.

### Patient Prepayment Strategy

In this strategy, the patient prepays for services. The prepayment can take a number of forms. For physicians in very high demand, the prepayment can be for reserving an initial appointment. Patients who have ongoing but standard treatment plans can prepay according to a regular payment schedule. For example, a patient who receives a routine course of allergy desensitization injections can be billed before treatment on a quarterly basis, with insurance being filed as a courtesy to the patient at the time of treatment.

A recent trend is the growth in "concierge" practices. In the typical concierge arrangement, the patient pays an annual fee, which may be payable in monthly or quarterly installments. Typically, the physician provides same-day or next-day access, with the emphasis being on providing quick, intensive, and personalized service. The practice does not accept insurance, and does not charge a copayment at the time of service. The concierge approach allows the practice to eliminate fixed and variable costs associated with billing insurance companies and patient collection. When properly managed, it has the potential to provide a predictable cash flow, and the opportunity to deliver more individualized patient-focused medical care.

### Preventing Patient Payment Problems

One tactic that is essential for successful revenue collection is collecting personal fees at the time of service. Front office staff must be trained to respond appropriately to the typical payment problems presented by patients. The collection administrator should provide this training. Appropriate responses include suggesting credit cards when checkbooks and cash are forgotten and giving the patient an addressed envelope with instructions to mail the payment today. In addition, the receptionist should approach the patient with the *expectation* of payment, not offer the patient excuses for failure to pay, and direct any patient who will be missing a second consecutive payment to the collection administrator. As we have seen, examination of the reward contingencies for employees with cash collection responsibilities is also important.

Patients who repeatedly fail to make payments should meet with the collection administrator. Some patients test how far they can go before there will be consequences. Other patients may truly not have the funds. In either case, the collection administrator needs to ascertain the *reason* for the delinquency and reiterate and enforce the agreement as stated in the method of payment form or patient pamphlet, negotiate new terms (taking into account any change in the patient's financial circumstances), or recommend suspension of the patient's treatment to the physician.

### COLLECTING OVERDUE PATIENT BALANCES

Success in collecting overdue patient balances depends on consistency and timeliness. Consistency means that there is a plan and that it is followed in an automatic, relentless manner. The collection process should progress step by predetermined step with clockwork regularity. There should be *no* exceptions. Timeliness is important, because as accounts age they become less collectible. This is true for a number of reasons, including:

- *Patients move and thereby become difficult to locate.* If a patient moves to another jurisdiction or state, the collection mechanics become more difficult and expensive.

- *As a debt becomes older, you will move farther toward the back of the line in the mind of the patient.* The longer you wait, the more time the patient will have to go even further into debt. In addition, other creditors will have time to collect, thereby depleting the patient's assets and decreasing your chances of collecting.
- *Patients are more likely to consider older debts "ancient history."* The anxiety, fear, or pain you alleviated will become less salient with time, and thus any feelings of guilt and the associated motivation to pay the debt will be reduced.

Perhaps the simplest initial step, and the most appropriate one when failure to pay is truly an oversight, is to send a bill in a timely manner. Next, consider a collection letter. Some physicians attach a special mystique to collection letters. They assume that, if they could only assemble the right combination of words, they would be able to convince even the most irresponsible patients to settle their account. Remember, however, that the irresponsible patient is probably well aware of the debt and has *chosen* not to pay, so the ability of collection letters to produce positive results is limited. Collection letters, however, will be more effective if they follow these guidelines:

- A collection letter should be short. This will focus the patient's attention on the overdue balance.
- Don't dissipate your strength by giving the patient excuses or alternatives to payment ("I know that times are hard . . . ," etc.).
- The *initial* contact should assume that the patient is not malevolent. The overdue balance could be due to lost mail or to an oversight. Don't give excuses to the pa-

tient, but don't preclude them either. If the patient wants to save face and at the same time pay the bill, that shouldn't make any difference to you.
- Command the patient to action. Clearly state that the patient *must do something,* either pay the bill or contact the office, and do it *by a stated date.*
- Always enclose a statement of the account with any collection letter.

**Exhibits 2–12** and **2–13** contain sample first and second collection letters. The first letter should contain an action date, which is the date by which you tell the patient you should receive the payment; 10 days from the date of your letter. If the first letter is unsuccessful, then send the second and final letter on the day after the action date. The second letter should state that if the bill is not paid within 10 days, legal action will result. The content of the second collection letter in (Exhibit 2–13) is based on a research study, which compared it with other letters containing less-direct content. This letter produced statistically superior results when compared to two other content strategies.[2] Both letters should command the patient to action by stating what to do and by when, as well as provide a reason why the patient should act. Two letters are sufficient. Adding additional letters is a waste of time, because the patient has already made a clear choice not to pay. If a patient does not respond to the second letter by the action date +2, then either write off the balance or give the account to a collection attorney. With either choice, your staff can move on to cases with higher chances of success.

There are other techniques that should be used in addition to collection letters. The first and most obvious is to suspend services. This tactic is most effective when the patient is receiving continuing treatment, because it creates immediate consequences for the patient.

**Exhibit 2–12** Sample First Collection Letter

---

(Date)

(Guarantor Name)
(Billing Address)          Acct. # (Account Number)
(Billing Address)          (Patient Name)

Dear (Guarantor):

Recently, we sent you a bill for your outstanding personal balance of $(Balance). We asked for payment by (Enter Date), and we have not yet received it. I ask that you pay this balance, so that it is received no later than (Enter Date).

We have provided services in good faith, and we rely on the good faith of our patients to promptly pay their bills. If you have any questions regarding your account, please contact me at (Phone Number). Thank you for your attention to this matter.

Sincerely,

(Name of Business Manager)
Business Manager

Enclosure: Account Statement

(*Note:* This letter is provided as an example. State laws vary regarding the methods that you can use in pursuing a delinquent account. Consult your attorney regarding specific content in your state.)

---

Naturally, termination must be done in a medically and legally appropriate manner to avoid a malpractice charge of abandonment (see Chapter 10). Physicians with high proportions of continuing patients, such as psychiatrists, gynecologists, family physicians, and allergists, should systematically apply this tactic using established rules. These rules should be communicated to patients through patient pamphlets or method of payment forms. For example, failure to make two payments or failure to pay two consecutive mailed statements will automatically result in the suspension of treatment. At a minimum, suspending services will put a cap on the outstanding balance. Once again, appropriately terminating treatment is absolutely critical to avoid a charge of abandonment.

The telephone can be a very effective collection tool, because it is both intrusive and selective. The telephone places your collec-tion administrator in the patient's office, living room, bedroom, or kitchen (consult your attorney regarding state laws governing collection methods; some states have laws precluding collection calls outside certain hours and to certain locations). Practices often delay using the telephone, either out of fear of a direct confrontation with the patient, or because of a feeling that it is inappropriate to make such a personal intrusion except as a last resort. Instead, the telephone should be used *early* in the collection process, because it lets the collection administrator evaluate why the patient is delinquent. If the patient has a grievance, this can be determined, and the collection administrator can begin resolving the problem. If there is an economic hardship, then it becomes possible to arrange a payment schedule. If the patient is irresponsible, then some structure can be applied to direct and motivate payment. If the pa-

**Exhibit 2–13** Sample Second Collection Letter

---

(Date)

(Guarantor Name)   Acct. #: (Account Number)
(Billing Address)    (Patient Name)
(Billing Address)

Dear (Guarantor):

This is your final notification that you have an outstanding personal balance of $(Balance). As you will recall, you signed an agreement with this practice to pay for our services. We have provided services in good faith. We assumed good faith on your part, and that you would live up to your responsibility to pay for these services.

If complete payment is not received by (Enter Date), your account will be turned over to our attorney for legal action, which can include a hearing in general district court, garnishment of wages, and attachment of bank funds. This will result in additional costs to you, because collection fees, attorney's fees, court costs, and finance charges will be added to your balance.

Once an account is turned over to our attorney for collection, we cannot call it back, and you will be assessed these additional charges.

Sincerely,

(Name of Business Manager) Business Manager

(*Note:* This letter is provided as an example. State laws vary regarding the methods that you can use in pursuing a delinquent account. Consult your attorney regarding specific content in your state.)

---

tient's behavior suggests a personality disorder or simple intransigence, then aggressive collection strategies can be implemented more quickly than normally would be the case.

Here is a sequence of steps for the collection administrator to follow when using the telephone:

1. *First, identify the answering party, and only talk to the patient (or whoever is responsible for the debt).* If Mr. Smith is the guarantor of the account, then you are wasting your time discussing the matter with Mrs. Smith. In addition, talking to the wrong person may breach confidentiality.
2. *Try to determine the patient's state of mind regarding the debt.* The collection administrator needs to determine whether he or she is confronting someone who accepts this as a legitimate debt, someone who will be aggressive, or someone who will seek sympathy. One tactic for determining this is to identify yourself, state the nature of the debt, and then listen. Listen for both *what* the patient says and the *way* in which it is said.
3. *Control the conversation by offering the patient alternatives that meet your objectives.* Phrases such as "How large a payment can you make?", "When will you make your next payment?", or "What would be a good time for you to come to the office to discuss this?" convey weakness. Determine what *you* need. Make a proposal, and let the patient accept it or make a counterproposal. You then can accept or reject the counterproposal. These

questions could be replaced with "I need a payment of $200" (determine a level that will be satisfactory and propose it), "I expect to receive your final payment by Friday, February 18" (let the patient tell you if that is not possible), and "Let's meet this Friday at 10:00 A.M." (you can always state an alternative if the patient objects).

4. *Get to the point.* Brief conversations allow your collection administrator more time to contact more patients. Brief, no-nonsense contacts also communicate the serious nature of the discussion to the patient.

5. *Obtain specific commitments from the patient.* Do this by getting specific agreements regarding amounts and time: "I'll send you a substantial payment in a few days" is worthless. In addition, the collection administrator always should restate the agreement to the patient and tell him or her that a note will be entered in the financial record (e.g., "You agree, then, that you will mail a check for $200 so that I will receive it by Monday, March 23, and I am noting this in your financial record."). Whenever a payment arrangement is negotiated over the phone, it also should be mailed to the patient.

6. *Be persistent, and follow through with your promises.* If a patient does not meet a commitment, immediately contact the patient. This tells the patient that you will not go away, and it also provides validity to future promises. For example, consider the following statement: "Mr. Johnson, I did not receive your payment for $200. If I don't receive it by Wednesday, I will turn your case over to our lawyer for collection on Thursday." Is Mr. Johnson more likely to respond to this message if it is communicated on the day that the $200 had been due or if it is communicated 3 weeks later? The telephone offers you the

ability to provide immediate follow-through on broken promises.

## PLACING AN ACCOUNT IN COLLECTION

Some patients will not respond to statements, collection letters, or telephone calls. When this happens, you will need to implement collection proceedings. The first step is to write off any account that will cost more to collect than it will generate in cash. The automatic write-off criterion for your practice should be determined by looking at the time, effort, and cost that are likely to be expended by your staff. Next, you must decide whether the practice will institute the legal process or whether you want to turn the account over to a collection agent.

If you are not faced with large numbers of accounts that must be placed in collection, you may want to consider undertaking collection in small claims court. The advantages of pursuing this course are that you will retain control over your cases, and you will keep all the money that you collect. Generally, patients who are employed and for whom you have good addresses are good bets. In about 75 percent of these cases, obtaining a warrant in debt will result in a quick settling of the account.

The small claims process varies from state to state, but generally it proceeds in the following manner. The practice obtains a warrant in debt against the patient. Some jurisdictions will let a practice obtain a warrant by mail, whereas others require that this be done in person at the courthouse. The warrant specifies the delinquent amount and sets a court date. The cost is usually nominal (typically, $15 to $35), and it generally can be added to the patient's account. The patient then is served with a copy of the warrant by the sheriff and/or through the mail. At this point, many patients contact the office and arrange to make payment. It is amazing how a legal notice delivered by a uniformed sheriff will get a patient's attention! When the patient contacts the office, negotiate payment arrangements that will close the account *before* the court date. This will leave you with the option to pursue legal action if the patient breaks the agreement. If the patient does not arrange to make payment, the collection administrator will have to appear in court and present evidence that the services were provided and that the patient's account is still unpaid. The court will grant a judgment against the patient. If the patient still refuses to pay, you will then be faced with the challenge of collecting on the judgment. Once again, your options will be determined by state law, but the normal choices involve garnishing wages and attaching assets such as bank accounts, cars, and so on. Generally, these actions will require additional legal action.

Medical practices should not routinely use small claims court. You "win" in those cases that pay off the account as a result of the warrant in debt, because you will obtain payment with relatively little expenditure of time, effort, or money. The other cases, however, will require considerable collection effort. Some patients will contest the case in court. Many patients, however, will simply fail to appear, and in essence they will challenge you to collect on the judgment. Most of these cases will be hard-core collection veterans. It will be difficult to locate their bank accounts and employers, and they may well have falsified some of the information on the intake form with the objective of misleading you. These people can be abusive and vindictive. Your personnel are not trained to collect from these types of people, nor do they have the time or the resources available to track them down and force them to pay. As a result, the small claims procedure should only be con-

sidered for those cases in which there is a very high probability that the patient will pay as a result of receiving the warrant in debt. The collection administrator will have to make an educated guess based on the type of patient (hardship, equity, irresponsible, or personality disorder) and the patient's response to the initial collection attempts.

The alternative to small claims court is to utilize a collection agent, which can be a collection agency or an attorney who specializes in this type of work. In either case, you should select a collection agent based on cost, recovery rate, and methods employed. Cost and recovery rate are interrelated. An agent with a recovery rate of 70 percent and a fee of 50 percent returns 35 percent of the revenue to the practice. An agent with a recovery rate of 50 percent and a fee of 40 percent only returns 20 percent of the revenue to the practice. Obviously, you must simultaneously consider both the fee and the recovery rate when selecting a collection agent.

Collection methods used by an attorney or agent are a legitimate concern. Generally, attorneys are less tempted to use abusive tactics, because they have direct access to the court system and are more likely to pursue that route than an agent who is not an attorney. An attorney or agent will be representing your practice to the community. Illegal or particularly inappropriate, inhumane, or disproportionate collection methods can damage your reputation. It is important, therefore, to contact several professional references when you are evaluating attorneys and agents. Question the references about customer or patient complaints, the actual level of recovered revenue, and the time that it takes to collect on accounts. Also, inquire about how cooperative and responsive the agent's staff has been in responding to clients' questions.

Generally, a collection attorney offers the best possibility of successful collection. Most patients who have refused to pay after receiving a bill, telephone call, and two collection letters are *choosing* not to pay. When an account reaches this point, the only thing that will get a patient to pay is force. An attorney has the ultimate weapon: access to the legal system and the ability to obtain a legal judgment. Even if a judgment cannot be collected on immediately, it will sit out there for years like a mine floating in the ocean. It is not unusual for one to "go off" several years later. The routine credit checks associated with legal transactions, such as mortgages, car loans, and the like, will reveal the judgment, and suddenly the patient will be quite interested in settling the account.

Once you have retained a collection attorney, it is important to monitor results. Does the attorney successfully collect on your accounts, or have the accounts simply been moved into another black hole? If patients complain about collection methods, it is important to discuss this with the attorney. Probably, these patients are objecting to legitimate, appropriate, and successful tactics. It is important, however, for you to protect your reputation and to feel comfortable with the methods used by your attorney.

Another element of successfully using an attorney is to forward your delinquent accounts in a timely manner. If your final collection letter says that the account will be placed in collection if the balance isn't paid by a specific date, then be certain to turn the account over to the attorney on the day after the due date. Some attorneys will give you better terms for younger accounts, and there are good reasons for this. As we have seen, old accounts are more difficult to collect.

Once an account has been placed with a collection attorney, never take the account back from the attorney because a patient says that he or she will pay. Also, never accept a payment from a patient whose account is

with an attorney. Some patients will contact the practice in an attempt to avoid collection fees or attorney's fees after the attorney has applied pressure. If you take a patient's payment, you may be responsible for paying these fees. In addition, the patient will invariably renege on promises made to you. Don't get caught in a triangle. If a patient sends you the check, forward it to the collection attorney.

## COLLECTING FROM INSURANCE COMPANIES

Insurance collection is the single largest revenue source for most practices. Exhibit 2–8 summarizes the insurance collection roles of the physician, collection administrator, and front office staff. Ensuring the validity and consistency of the insurance collection process is essential, therefore, to financial survival. Each claim that you file is a test of the validity of all aspects of your filing process. The delay between when you file a claim and receive a reply makes it possible for a significant problem to arise before it is perceived by the practice. For example, a change in insurance printing requirements or a bug in your software that goes unnoticed can result in the practice generating hundreds of claims that will be denied.[3] Using efficient insurance billing procedures, monitoring insurance billing results, and identifying and correcting problems as early as possible are essential to protect the practice's revenue stream and its financial viability. Using electronic claims submission is one way to reduce this exposure.

Effective insurance collection begins with effective insurance billing procedures. The objective should be to bill as often as possible, with daily insurance claim filing being the ultimate goal. Filing insurance daily or as frequently as feasible is analogous to dividing a ship into a honeycomb of compartments. A catastrophe in any one compartment can be localized and will not threaten the survival of the ship. Individual events, such as the post office losing a bundle of mail, e-claims software developing a bug, the power going off during an insurance billing run, an insurance check or electronic funds transfer being lost, a hardware failure, or incompetence on the part of a particular claims agent, will then only affect a small and limited part of your revenue. If you file insurance claims on a weekly or monthly basis, then the same events might affect a week or month of revenues.

Electronic claim submission has a number of advantages, including faster payment, quicker error detection, reduced practice postage and mailing costs, and reduced clerical labor. Some electronic claims systems immediately indicate whether the claim will be paid or denied, which provides greater integrity to the billing process. Often, electronic claims must be filed through clearinghouses, which charge a fee. You should evaluate the total cost of electronic submission, including the cost of additional equipment and access fees. Some physicians, however, have concluded that immediate problem detection and reduced paperwork in the front office are worth any extra cost.

The next important consideration is to file your claims correctly and comply with any authorization procedures. Normally, there will be a provider support office to help practices deal with denied claims and comply with claim-filing procedures. Some insurers are willing to send a training representative to your office to train your staff in correct filing procedures. This training can be particularly helpful if your office has had turnover in critical billing positions, and you don't have written procedure manuals.

Insurance companies are very large bureaucracies. One characteristic of a bureaucracy is that it solves problems by applying standards and rules. If you (collection administrator) find that you are not getting your problems resolved, you have to get the ear of a person who is high enough in the bureaucracy to make exceptions to the standards and rules. The way to do this is to speak with a supervisor. If you don't get resolution to your problem, ask "If you agreed with my position, would you be able to . . . ?" If the answer is no, then you need to ask for *that* person's supervisor. If the answer is yes, then you must determine whether continuing up the corporate ladder is worth the time and effort. Generally, ascending two levels of supervision above the normal claims representative will place you in middle management.

Some insurers are very unresponsive to claim inquiries or take an unreasonably long time to process a claim or forward a payment. If an insurer is particularly unresponsive, you may want to consider filing a complaint with your state's insurance commission. Each state has an insurance commission or an agency that regulates insurance company operations. The power of the commission or agency, and the degree to which insurers will be responsive to complaints filed with it, varies from state to state. If you feel that a claim has been unreasonably denied or has not been responded to in a reasonable amount of time, and you have exhausted all internal remedies, you have little to lose by writing a letter to your state's insurance commission.

Generally, the most effective tactic for dealing with an unresponsive insurer is to involve the patient. This is particularly effective if your practice's education procedures have instilled in the patient the idea that unpaid claims will be the patient's responsibility. Contact the patient and let him or her know that the claim has been unreasonably denied or delayed. Tell the patient that he or she will be billed if the claim is not paid in 30 days as well as whom to call and what to do to get involved.

Dealing with a rejected claim is arguably the collection administrator's *highest* priority. A rejected claim means that the wealth represented by the denied claim will *never* be paid unless action is taken, and it is therefore a higher priority than current claims, which may be paid. Second, the denial may be symptomatic of a larger billing problem. This may mean that many other claims for this patient and for other patients may be destined for denial. This circumstance can, if left unattended, threaten the financial soundness of the practice.

All rejected or denied claims must be examined to determine their causes. The collection administrator must always be thinking of the implications of denied claims for other outstanding claims. If there are implications for other claims, the collection administrator must immediately address them. Often, the first indication of a software or a filing procedure problem will be a denied claim. If the symptom is not immediately detected, many additional claims will be denied. This not only delays the receipt of cash, but also requires refiling for the denied claims and those in process, which can add up to a substantial amount of additional work.

## Using Collection Report Data: Case Example

Field Psychiatric Associates was a group psychiatric practice. In addition to providing psychiatric services, it employed several psychologists and clinical social workers who were paid on the basis of monthly collections. Monthly collection figures were obtained from earned receipts reports for each producer. Dr. James was the practice's man-

aging physician and took the physician lead on all business-related issues.

The February earned receipts by producer report indicated a large drop in collections, and as a result the subsequent payroll, which would be payable on March 10, would be roughly 60 percent of normal levels. The drop was uniform across all producers, with the exception of Dr. James, whose receipts were at normal levels. She did not participate with any insurance companies, and all her patients paid full fee at the time of treatment.

Dr. James was very concerned because her monthly fixed expenses would exceed the monthly gross receipts. She was also very concerned about the financial well-being of her employees. Dr. James's first reaction was panic. Where should she look for the cause of the problem? What information was available that could give her a clue regarding what had happened?

First, she focused her thoughts on the fact that this problem was not caused by magic or demons. It was solvable and the answer, or at least some indication of the problem's source, would be found in the practice's financial data. Dr. James began the investigative process to determine the cause of the cash problem. She identified six hypotheses:

1. Cash receipts had been lost or stolen.
2. Insurance claims had not been mailed on a regular basis.
3. There had been a precipitous decline in procedures due to vacations during the holiday season, resulting in reduced receipts several weeks later.
4. Insurance claims had been improperly completed as a result of software or personnel problems.
5. Insurance receipts had been lost or stolen.
6. One or more insurance companies were having a problem processing claims or were purposefully delaying payments.

Dr. James first determined that the shortage was approximately $15,000 by comparing a report of the practice's gross receipts for the month with the gross receipts for the previous 3 months. She then noted that the cash collections for February totaled $17,793, whereas the collections for the previous 3 months averaged $18,396. Because cash collections were stable, this largely eliminated hypothesis 1. It also suggested that the problem had to be associated in some manner with insurance collections.

Next, she examined hypothesis 2 by looking at a sample of accounts in the computer. Insurance claims were uniformly sent on either the day of treatment or the following day. In addition, all information relating to the patient computer accounts appeared to be correct. Finally, November through February monthly reports of revenues generated by insurance company did not indicate any substantial or unexpected monthly variability. These data in combination largely eliminated hypothesis 2. Wealth was being put into the pipeline, and the question was where and when it would come out.

Revenue reports and reports on the number of procedures for December revealed less than a 10 percent decline. This eliminated hypothesis 3.

Hypothesis 4 could be time consuming to fully investigate. The collection administrator stated that she had not received an unusual number of returned claims. Her word was accepted at face value, although it was recognized that in theory she could be covering up a problem. Examination of a sample of accounts in the computer and test runs of the computer's claims filing program across major insurers indicated that the practice was generating payable claims.

Hypothesis 5 would take time to investigate, although the strategy to do so would be easy to implement. Two insurers paid a large proportion of the practice's insurance claims. If insurance funds amounting to $15,000 were lost or diverted, at least some of the money would have to come from one or both of these carriers. These companies could be questioned by telephone about claims that should have been paid by now. If there were funds that had been diverted or lost, then one or both insurance companies would indicate that they had paid on claims that the practice's computer indicated were still unpaid or had been covered with an adjustment or write-off. Once again, this would be a personnel-intensive process that could be addressed by sampling cases. Dr. James postponed further investigation of this hypothesis until other more easily researchable alternatives had been eliminated.

Two sources of data would be used to examine hypothesis 6. An examination of an aging analysis by insurance company revealed that Insurer X's receivables in 30 days past current were much higher than normal. Reducing the revenue in this category by the approximate write-off and then estimating the proportion in the category that would be old enough to be payable resulted in an estimate that could account for $15,000. An examination of insurance receipts by insurance company revealed that Insurer X's February receipts were $6,399, whereas they had averaged $22,118 for the previous 3 months. These data directly pointed to a problem with Insurer X's claims.

Dr. James now knew that the source of the problem was probably associated with Insurer X, although she still did not know with certainty whether the fault lay in the claims that her practice was sending, whether Insurer X's funds had been lost or diverted, or whether the problem was with Insurer X's claims processing. She decided that she would first test the hypothesis that would create the least difficulty for her. She called an administrator at Insurer X and stated that her 30 days past current claims were very high and that her cash receipts were down. She asked him whether there had been a problem in processing her practice's claims. The administrator stated that someone would look at the practice's accounts. Later that day, a subordinate called back and told Dr. James that the processing department had gotten behind, that temporary and overtime help was being enlisted, and that the fault lay with the insurance company. The data that Dr. James had used to confront the insurance company were incontrovertible. Insurer X knew that if it denied that the problem existed, Dr. James would begin inquiring about specific accounts. To its credit, Insurer X quickly admitted the problem.

Dr. James then asked for a supervisor and stated that she and her employees should not have to suffer as a result of the insurer's problem, and she asked for a $15,000 advance against the outstanding claims. Insurer X's administrator countered with an offer to pull all Dr. James's claims and "put them on the top of the stack." Dr. James agreed, and 3 days later she began to receive payments.

## PROBLEM ACCOUNT DETECTION AND TIMING

It is critical to have time standards and a sequence for collection activities. This ensures that the process moves along as rapidly as possible and that the most effective procedures are used in the most effective order. The most basic timing consideration is posed by the question: When is an account overdue? For a missed copayment or deductible, the answer is easy. It is overdue when the service is provided. The first collection action should take place within 1 day. A more difficult circumstance is defining when a billed transaction is overdue. For ex-

ample, when should action be taken on an unpaid insurance claim?

These less clearly defined billing questions can often be answered with enough precision from past data to set performance standards. For example, if 90 percent of Blue Cross of XX payments are received within 50 days of submission, then a reasonable standard that won't generate too many false positives (taking action when none is required, i.e., the check truly *is* in the mail!) might be to audit Blue Cross accounts that have moved into 60 days on an aging analysis. If another carrier has a turnaround that averages 21 days, then its accounts that have gotten into the 30-day category would be appropriate to audit.

Actions also need to be paired with consistent time standards. For example, the sequence on a patient collection might have four actions: statement, first collection letter, second collection letter with two telephone attempts, refer to attorney. The timing for this whole sequence should be standard for the practice and consistently applied to all cases. An example of an aggressive but reasonable patient collection process is found in **Exhibit 2–14**. This illustrates that it is possible to complete the collection sequence from initial delinquency to final action in 53 days. Although this process may seem fast, consider for a moment that the

---

**Exhibit 2–14** Aggressive Patient Collection Sequence and Timing

| Action | Act Day | Close Day |
|---|---|---|
| Patient delinquency | 0 | 0 |
| Send statement | 1 | 30 |
| First collection letter | 31 | 41 |
| Second collection letter | 42 | 52 |
| Telephone call* | 42 | 52 |
| Account to attorney | 53 | |

*Business manager tries twice.

patient has received at least four communications (statement, two collection letters, and one and perhaps two phone contacts or voicemail messages) and has failed to respond. This is a clear indication that the patient has made a conscious *choice* not to respond. At this point, it is futile to make further requests. The account should be forwarded to the attorney for collection on the 53rd day.

I cannot emphasize strongly enough the importance of actually following time standards. If a first collection letter is to be sent on the 31st day, then this must occur on that day. It should not wait until the 32nd day. This consistency has two critical effects. First, it wrings slack out of your office operations. If it becomes accepted that time standards are just rough guides, then some accounts will get the second letter on the 31st day, and others may stretch out to the 51st day. You will have lost control *over the process*, and having an effective *process* is the key to successful collection. Second, many patients and some insurance carriers test systems. They look for slack and take advantage of it. If you promise that you will follow through on the 10th day and you do, then your adversary will take you more seriously than the practice across town that is inconsistent. In effect, you just moved closer to the front of the line.

## COLLECTION DATABASE

To operate a collection process using the rapid time frames just illustrated, effectively using collection reports and databases is critical. For example, if your collection administrator has 600 accounts to manage and 57 are in some stage of delinquency, how does he or she know that Fred Kringle should have responded to his second collection letter by today or that Anne Blert promised to get her payment in by yesterday?

The simplest solution to this problem is to use a daily computer-based calendar. Whenever an action is taken, a note is made at that time of what should happen by the deadline date in the calendar. If Fred Kringle is given until November 14 to respond to a second collection letter, an entry to that effect is made for November 14. On November 14, the collection administrator will check the status of the account, and if Fred has not responded adequately, the collection administrator will *immediately* initiate the next collection step.

The same objective can be achieved, but with greater efficiency, by creating a collection database. This approach has the added advantage of allowing the collection administrator to quickly determine the status of any account in the database, and easily track each account's history. An example of a screen from a collections database is shown in **Exhibit 2–15**. Cases can be selected and

---

**Exhibit 2–15** Collection Database Screen

| | |
|---:|---|
| Last: | Riverside |
| First: | Philip |
| Account Number: | 78339 |
| Physician: | Dr. Smith |
| Case Manaager: | Sonja |
| Bill Sent Date: | Feb-1 |
| First Letter Date: | Mar-1 |
| Second Letter Date: | |
| Last Action Date: | Mar-1 |
| Next Action Date: | Mar-10 |
| Next Action: | Send Second Letter |
| BALANCE: | $360.67 |

*Notes*
Patient owes $350.67 deductible. Claims he has already paid this amount at other practices.

Ins. co. has no record of this. Told him this was between him and ins. co.

Missed copay $10.00 on 1/16/20XX. Said he would mail it in. Never did. This was noted in First Collection Letter.

sorted by *any* variable or combination of variables, so it is easy, for example, to call up all accounts requiring:

1. Action on or before March 15th
2. Which are being evaluated by Sonja, and then
3. Sorting the cases by type (second collection letter, referral to collection attorney, etc.)

The key to effectively using a collection database is that when you take an action, such as sending a second collection letter, the *next action* and the *next action date are immediately entered into the database.* When the next action date occurs, the account manager then can take quick action if the balance has not been paid.

The collection database can be part of the MOMS. Most MOMS, however, don't possess an easy capability to segregate those accounts that are in collection or allow you to define customizable actions that characterize your practice's collection process. Generally, it is easier and more effective to create a separate collection database by using a database program, such as Filemaker. In this way, you can develop a screen that exactly parallels your collection sequence.

## THE COLLECTION PLAN

The collection plan integrates all the parts of the collection process. Having a plan will help ensure that problem accounts are quickly identified and that revenue collection is pursued with consistency. An example of a collection plan is given in Appendix 2A. The plan should provide an outline of the various parts of the collection process. At a minimum, the plan should cover the following eight areas:

1. Patient Intake Process
2. Patient Education Process
3. Payment Arrangement Process
4. Verification and Preauthorization
5. Copay and Deductible Collection Procedures
6. Insurance Billing Procedures
7. Problem Account Detection
8. Collection Steps and Sequencing

As indicated in Exhibit 2–8, it is important for the physician leader and the collection administrator to jointly develop a collection plan that is reasonable to operate, but fulfills physicians' needs. If the practice is large and collection is one of several front office functions that are assigned to different positions, then it may be necessary to have other functional leaders involved in developing the collection plan.

## WHAT TO DO IF YOUR ACCOUNTS ARE OUT OF CONTROL

"I don't know where to begin. The accounts are a mess. Some patients come and go and don't pay. I'm not even sure what some patients owe. It takes forever to collect from insurance companies. It seems like everything is out of control! What do I do?" At this point, some physicians throw their hands up in frustration, others fire the business manager, and still others hire a consultant[4] or subcontract the whole receivable function, and some quit private practice and work in another context.

Let's evaluate each of these alternatives. Ignoring the problem is a prescription for bankruptcy. Firing the business manager may be appropriate if he or she is the source of the problem. *Assuming* that this is the case may make you feel better, but if this is not the case, then you have neither solved the problem nor delayed the ultimate consequences. Although a knowledgeable consultant can be helpful, simply handing the problem to a consultant and saying "fix it" is not a permanent solution. Someday the consultant will leave, and if your practice has not acquired the skill to adjust its collection processes to changes in the collection environment, then collection problems will inevitably recur. Subcontracting can be effective if the subcontractor is effective. Many, unfortunately, are not. At a minimum, you still must closely monitor *their* performance. Giving up private practice? If you aren't willing to manage the collection process, then this may be a rational choice.

What do you do? Begin by accepting your own personal responsibility for these circumstances. Whenever events get out of control, the ultimate source of the problem is top management, and that is *you,* the physician leader. It may be true that you hired others to run the front office and if they had performed better or more conscientiously, your collection problem would not have occurred. It is also true, however, that you are responsible for the actions of your subordinates. You may delegate *authority* to bill and collect in your name, but you can never delegate ultimate *responsibility* for their actions. The first step to turning around your practice's collection process is to accept that you are partly responsible for the situation. Your management job as a physician leader is to know enough about all business aspects of your practice, so you will know when things are going well, and when they are drifting toward disorder.

All that is history, however. What should you do *now?* Here are some ideas:

- *Audit all overdue accounts.* Reassign secretaries, use overtime, or hire collection contractors to gain sufficient staffing to audit back accounts fast. Smart managers can use almost any employee to do some of the simpler tasks, such as calling insurance companies, searching remits for denials, pulling financial records, and the like. Find out the real size of your receivables.

- *Work smart.* Direct your personnel to "triage" the accounts. First, work those accounts with the greatest potential return. Write off truly uncollectable accounts and those not worth pursuing. If an account with a $180 balance would take 4 hours of a contractor's time at $20 per hour to audit and rebill, work it after resolving higher-value accounts.

- *Determine why your accounts have reached this state.* The reasons will become evident as the accounts are audited. Your collection personnel may have a self-interest in hiding the truth from you. If you suspect this to be the case, hire consultants, and have them report directly to you. The bottom line, however, is that if accounts are in disarray you will have to become personally involved for a period of time to understand the sources of the problem and be certain that it has been corrected. Possible sources include sloppy follow-up on denied or rejected claims, poor coding, inconsistent collection of copays and deductibles, and the like. Whatever the cause or causes, you must get to the bottom of it if you are to fix the underlying problem.

- *Contain the problem now.* Once the sources of the problem are identified, your *highest* priority is to implement immediate corrections to the faulty process. It does you little good to resolve old accounts if you are creating additional new problems each day. Implement necessary policies and procedures. Discipline, terminate, or train ineffective staff. Do whatever is necessary *now.* This point is particularly important for building staff morale. There are few things more demoralizing than working hard to solve old cases, only to see another tidal wave approaching.

- *Set standards, and enforce them.* Most practices' receivables should not move into 90 days past current. If money does get into 90 days, someone should explain why to *you*. Ordinarily, you should receive account aging reports at least monthly, and in a crisis it should be weekly. Use the reports to set goals for and evaluate the performance of collection personnel. Construct an aging history database (see Exhibit 2–10). This will allow you to track collection trends.

As a physician leader, you should be actively involved in the management of your practice. This doesn't mean that you should be performing your subordinates' work for them. It does mean, however, that you cannot ignore your critical management role. Routinely reviewing aging reports and trends, looking for indications of potential problems, and determining and reviewing collection policies and standards are all appropriate activities for a physician leader. Your collection personnel should know that you are highly informed and very interested in the state of your practice's finances.

## CONCLUSION

Cash management is not a headline-catching issue. Nevertheless, it is one of those essential processes that all businesses must do well. Physicians generate wealth by practicing medicine, not by developing cash management procedures or reviewing aging history databases. Nevertheless, if physicians don't get involved in cash control and collection oversight, then they may be leaving a lot of the wealth they generated on the table.

---

**NOTES**

1. This practice's MOMS defined Current as between 1 and 30 days old, so money that shows in 90 days is at least 120 days old.
2. Solomon, R., K. Locke. (1990). Improving collection performance: Structuring the collection letter. *Journal of Medical Practice Management.* 9(4);157–160.
3. A recent example, an insurer began requiring the use of four digits (1963) in the date of birth field on some of its contracts while still accepting two digits (63) on other contracts.
4. A version of this section appeared in Solomon, R. (1992). Getting a grip on collections that have gone out of control. *American Medical News*, 17:34.

# Sample Collection Plan (Partial)

Note: Specific content should vary by medical specialty, patient characteristics, and personal, ethical, and legal considerations.

## PATIENT INTAKE PROCESS

1. Patients will complete an intake form, which will provide sufficient biographical information to pursue collection should an account become delinquent.
2. The collection administrator (CA) will scan each intake form for obvious signs of financial hardship. If a patient is likely to be a hardship case, the CA will advise the physician of this possibility, so that the physician can inform the CA if long-term treatment is necessary.
3. The intake form will provide for authorization to bill the patient's insurance company.
4. The intake form will unequivocally state that the patient is ultimately responsible for settlement of the account.
5. New referrals that have been scheduled more than 1 day in advance will be reconfirmed 2 days before the scheduled appointment.

## PATIENT EDUCATION PROCESS

1. A sign will be posted at the receptionist's window stating that payment is expected at the time of service.
2. When new referrals are taken over the telephone, the receptionist will inform the patient that payment or copayment is expected at the time of service. If the referral has any questions, the call will be immediately forwarded to the CA.
3. Each new patient will be provided with a copy of the new patient pamphlet.
4. Patients who will be undergoing continuing treatment will be scheduled for a brief meeting with the CA. During this meeting, the CA will review the patient's insurance coverage and copayment arrangements, and answer any financial questions.

## VERIFICATIONS AND PREAUTHORIZATIONS

1. Insurance information will be obtained from referrals at the time they schedule the initial office visit. All patients with plans requiring preauthorization will be informed of their preauthorization responsibilities at this time.
2. All patients with a preauthorization responsibility will be flagged in the appointment book by the receptionist taking the referral.
3. Upon flagged patients' arrival for the initial office visit, the receptionist will verify that they have in fact received preauthorization.
4. If a patient has not been preauthorized, the receptionist will immediately inform the CA, who will determine the best way to handle the situation.

## COPAYMENT COLLECTION PROCEDURES

1. The receptionist is responsible for all initial payment, copayment, and deductible collections.
2. The receptionist is responsible for maintaining a current and accurate listing of any patients with copayments.
3. The receptionist is responsible for one collection attempt at the time of service. If the attempt is not made, the receptionist is responsible for contacting the patient that day and requesting payment by mail.
4. The CA is responsible for ensuring that the receptionist is effectively performing these collection activities. This responsibility includes developing collection methods for when patients cannot or will not pay, employee collection training, and guidelines for when to refer the patient to the CA.

## INSURANCE BILLING PROCEDURES

1. The CA is responsible for the accurate collection and transmission of all information necessary to receive insurance payment.
2. All procedures will be entered into the computer each day, and insurance claims will be generated and mailed at least three times each week. The objective, however, is daily insurance billing.
3. The CA will maintain a file of all changes in billing procedures or notices received from insurance companies.

## PROBLEM ACCOUNT DETECTION

1. Any denied insurance claim will be of the highest priority. The CA will immediately investigate the denial, resolve the situation, do any rebilling necessary, and correct any problems with practice procedures, software, and the like.
2. The CA will immediately inform the managing physician whenever there are any insurance billing problems that are related to computer software or have larger insurance billing implications.
3. The CA will generate both aging and write-off reports each week. These will be forwarded to the managing physician.
4. The CA is responsible for maintaining aging balances at acceptable levels as determined by the managing physician.
5. All accounts that have money in 90 days past current will be reviewed at least monthly by the CA. The patient will be billed for personal fees. Insurance fees will be pursued either with a tracer or by resubmission of a claim.

## COLLECTION STEPS AND SEQUENCING

1. Patients will be informed within 1 day that a missed copayment must be paid by the time of the next visit or within 7 days. They will also be reminded that copayments must be paid at the time of service.
2. If a patient misses two consecutive copayments, the CA will inform the physician, and, with the concurrence of the physician, appointments will be suspended until the fees have been paid. The collection sequence will begin.
3. Any fees that move into 90 days past current will enter the collection sequence.
4. The collection sequence is as follows: A detailed bill is sent with notice to pay in 21 days. On day 22, a first collection letter is sent with notice to pay in 14 days. On day 15, a second collection letter is sent with notice to pay in 10 days. Simultaneously, the CA will make two attempts to contact the patient by telephone. On day 11, the account is sent to the collection attorney.

# CHAPTER 3

# Evaluating Performance

## Chapter Objectives

In this chapter, you will learn how to evaluate the job performance of your employees and colleagues, including physicians, so you can improve their effectiveness and, as a result, improve organizational effectiveness. One goal will be for you to develop personal performance evaluation skills so that the direct management of your employees improves. In addition, you will learn how to develop performance appraisal systems that ensure the effectiveness of the performance appraisal skills of other physicians and managers. These performance appraisal systems provide internal control, so management can assess and improve overall organizational productivity.

Effective performance-appraisal methods focus on the eventual outcome: improving employee performance. All too often, organizations focus on performance-appraisal *methods* and become overly concerned with form over substance. As a result, they create rigid, time-consuming evaluation methods that both managers and subordinates dread. This chapter emphasizes the evaluation of employee *behavior* and *behaviorally* what you need to do to achieve this end. I will not offer, therefore, a set of forms for you to use, because they almost certainly would be inappropriate for your specific circumstance. What I will provide, instead, is a philosophy of performance appraisal and a strategy for you to develop methods that will work best in your practice hospital, or healthcare system.

## PERFORMANCE APPRAISAL: CONTEXT

The process of determining how well an employee, peer, or partner is performing their job is called *performance appraisal*. The performance appraisal process includes:

- identifying the appropriate issues on which to evaluate performance
- evaluating the quality and quantity of work performed
- constructing a performance appraisal document to record the conclusions reached as a result of the performance evaluation

- informing the employee of your observations
- using this information to improve job performance by setting goals and providing appropriate training, coaching, additional equipment, and so on

Not all employees will do what you want them to do. Reasons for this include:

- limitations in ability or technical skills that prevent an employee from properly performing the job
- personality characteristics that limit an employee's willingness to follow directions

- the widespread view that institutions and organizations, such as medical practices, hospitals, and healthcare systems, exist to serve the needs of the employee as opposed to the employer

There are several reasons for developing a performance appraisal system and then using it to evaluate job performance. First, the performance appraisal process is important, because it is the organization's formal way of changing and improving job performance. Inadequate employee job performance has the potential to lower the quality of health care provided, to reduce profits, and ultimately to jeopardize an organization's existence. It is essential, therefore, that physician leaders routinely and effectively evaluate job performance, change employee performance when it is inadequate, reassign employees when necessary and possible, and terminate employees who will not or cannot improve their performance. Performance appraisals also provide employees with direct guidance regarding how you wish them to perform their jobs in the future. If, for example, a business manager is devoting too much time to producing unused financial reports and not enough time to working old accounts, then comment on it *now*. In the absence of your comments, the business manager will assume that you approve of the current job performance. By documenting your dissatisfaction, stating new goals, and then evaluating and rewarding the business manager's future performance, you will tie behavior to rewards, thereby motivating the employee to perform in the interest of the organization.

Performance appraisals can also tell you what additional training, supervision, and task changes might be needed by your employees. For example, if you find that your accounting data are not being kept in a timely enough manner, this may indicate that the employee who is responsible needs more direction regarding when you expect the data to be available. It also may indicate that the employee needs some additional training in the use of your accounting software, or that the employee's workload is too heavy and some tasks should be transferred to another employee or to your accountant.

Second, in a positive sense, performance appraisal is a strong motivational tool. Just as most physicians take real satisfaction when they are complimented on a job well done, most other employees will be energized and motivated to perform well when their efforts are recognized. Similarly, absence of recognition when performance meets or exceeds expectations can be demoralizing. Many employees adopt the attitude "Why should I care if management doesn't care enough to notice." Self-actualized, internally motivated employees can be particularly demoralized when they see lower performers receiving the same compliments, pay raises, and promotions that they receive.

Finally, performance appraisal should be the basis for personnel actions. By basing pay raises, promotions, training, discipline, and termination decisions on performance appraisal, you create equity, so that employees perceive that the organization is treating them fairly. Also, you create a legal defense against any allegations of wrongful discharge and infractions of equal employment opportunity laws.

There are, however, costs to performance appraisal. As you will see, one critical physician leader role is to ensure that effective performance-appraisal systems are in place. It takes time and effort to develop these systems. It also takes time and effort to use the performance-appraisal system to evaluate job performance, whether we are talking about evaluating front office clericals, laboratory directors, or physicians. Finally, it can be personally difficult to discuss substandard performance. It can be an intimidating and distasteful process to sit across a table from someone and say, "George, there are some real problems with part of your work, and we need to talk about it."

All supervisors, physician leaders, and even many physicians without formal management responsibilities should be proficient in using performance appraisal methods. Outside of your practice, physicians may be involved in the evaluation of hospital nursing and support personnel with whom they work, but over whom they have no direct line authority. For example, a physician may provide a hospital's nursing supervisor with observations regarding a nurse's job performance, which the supervisor then will take into consideration when writing the nurse's performance evaluation using the hospital's appraisal system. Within your practice, physicians should have input to the evaluations of technical, clerical, and medical personnel, including other physicians.

## PERFORMANCE APPRAISAL: THE SHORT COURSE

The performance appraisal process that evolves in many organizations can be a bureaucratic, form-laden affair. It doesn't need to be that way. The following seven guidelines form the foundation for conducting effective performance appraisals. This is the place to begin in terms of both personally conducting appraisals and designing a performance-appraisal system for your practice or healthcare organization. Subsequent parts of this chapter will elaborate with additional details and refinements, but if you can really instill these 7 concepts into your own and your organization's evaluations, you will get the first 85 percent of the value to be gained from performance appraisal. Politically, you may find it advantageous to add these elements to your current appraisal system and adjusting it where needed instead of tearing apart the old system. These seven guidelines can take you a long way toward personally conducting effective performance appraisals, and they should form the foundation for your practice's performance appraisal methods.

### 1. Always Start with an Accurate Job Description

To effectively evaluate an employee's job performance, you must first understand the content of their job in detail. If you don't know what skills and abilities are needed to perform the job, then you can't determine how well the employee has performed or how to provide appropriate improvement plans and goals. Performance appraisal, therefore, always starts with collecting information about the job. The process of collecting this information is called job analysis, and the resulting document describing the job is called a *job description*. **Exhibit 3–1** contains a sample job description for a practice business manager position.

Job analysis can be performed in a number of different ways. If you are a physician leader in a large organization, such as a hospital or large group practice, then job descriptions may already exist. Similarly, your practice may already have job descriptions. If this is the case, these job descriptions are a good place to start. Never assume, however, that an existing job description, especially if it is several years old, is still valid. Job content can rapidly change, especially in a high-technology, rapidly changing environment such as healthcare. If the job description is wrong or incomplete, you might not assess the right job performance issues. Existing job descriptions can be validated by talking to current incumbents or their supervisors. If you have any doubt about the accuracy of the job description, reanalyze the job.

The "you" referred to in the following discussion of writing job descriptions is generally

**Exhibit 3–1**  Practice Business Manager Job Description

1. *Collection.* Supervise the collection of all revenue. This includes using current office procedures and developing new ones to insure the collection of all copayments and insurance. This will involve working with the other front office staff to develop these procedures, and to make them work. Responsible for making certain that all accounts are paid within a reasonable time, which is normally not to exceed 90 days past current.
2. *Insurance Billing Supervision.* Supervise the billing process to insure that insurance bills are accurate and mailed on a regular basis.
3. *Payroll.* Maintain and generate accurate payroll records including collection for each physician; determine physicians' monthly income based upon collection; calculate and assemble the physician payroll and front office payroll; calculate and pay retirement benefits to appropriate retirement plans.
4. *Taxes.* Calculate all federal (941, 940, etc.) and state taxes; insure proper withholding for each payroll; make tax deposits in a timely manner; file all tax reports such as 941 quarterly, VEC quarterly, and state monthly in a timely manner.
5. *Accounts Payable.* Pay all practice bills. Manage the practice bank accounts, including keeping an accurate running balance and monthly reconciliation. Forward all appropriate financial information to the practice accountant when necessary.
6. *Posting and Accounting for Payments.* Supervise posting all payments received into the medical office management system. Responsible for reconciling all payments made the previous day with cash, checks, insurance remits, credit card receipts, etc. to provide accuracy and accountability.
7. *Fee Negotiation.* Negotiate patient fees in a manner that achieves practice financial objectives and protects practice financial integrity, but makes provision for patients with real financial hardships.
8. *Management Reports and Database Management.* Generate or cause to be generated management reports that are necessary for conducting the daily operation of the practice and provide accountability and problem identification. Examples include, but are not limited to, aging analyses, earned receipts by producer, daily receipts, aging history, and database reports, etc. Insure the integrity of these databases including accuracy and backups.
9. *Problem Identification and Resolution.* Identify problems in any area of the practice, immediately bring them to the attention of the managing physician, and propose and implement solutions.
10. *Supervision.* Supervise and evaluate the job performance of all front office employees.
11. *Scheduling.* Ensure the validity of the patient scheduling system. Troubleshoot any problems and redesigning the system as necessary.
12. *Additional.* Additional duties and responsibilities and issues as they are determined to be appropriate by the managing physician.

the position's supervisor. For example, the business manager might be responsible for all front office positions, the nursing supervisor for all nursing positions, and so forth. As a physician, you may become involved in writing descriptions for those who report directly to you, such as for the practice business manager position. Given your time commitments, however, you may want to enlist others to do the initial information collection and writing, so you allocate your time to reviewing and revising the initial work. For example, if you are a practice-based physician with a nurse who works directly for you, you could ask the business manager and the job incumbent to write the initial job description, which you would then revise or perhaps send back to them for additional work before it is finalized.

If you are in a practice that doesn't have job descriptions, or if the ones that you have are obsolete, then there are several ways to conduct a job analysis. If there is an employee currently performing the job, that employee can be interviewed. You need to know exactly what the employee does and how often he or she does it. You might ask the employee to verbally walk you through a typical day. Also, have the employee describe any tasks that are performed only weekly or monthly. Talk to the employee's supervisor. He or she may have a somewhat different perspective on the position's content.

Another good way to obtain job analysis information is to observe the employee performing the job. Keep in mind that, because of your presence, the employee may change the job content, or speed up or slow down the performance of tasks. Although employees may tend to exaggerate the importance or frequency of some tasks, it is rare that they will fabricate or totally eliminate tasks. This is especially true in smaller organizations such as a medical practice, where the employee might reasonably expect that whomever is conducting the job analysis knows the general content of the job.

Finally, sometimes you can obtain important information about a job by briefly performing it yourself. This technique familiarizes you with the small points that might easily be missed in an interview. For example, when analyzing a secretarial position, I sat in for the secretary for a few hours. I discovered that it was not unusual for a patient to be at the window making a copayment, while another was waiting to schedule an appointment, the telephone was ringing, and someone else was asking for the computer keyboard to schedule an appointment. Performing the work conveyed an intensity that was not readily apparent from interviewing or observing the incumbent.

Once you have a good sense of what the job entails, write a job description. Job descriptions should be written in concise, clear language. There is no point to using excessive, flowery, or imprecise language. The goal is to identify the major job performance issues. It is not necessary for the job description to describe the position down to the last de-

tail. For example, you don't need to know how many times a day the business manager uses a computer, but it is important not to miss any major job performance issues, such as that computer use is important and the critical computer content areas (medical records, databases, etc.) and programs (Excel, MOMs, Word, etc.). Generally, you will find that the duties and responsibilities cluster into several larger categories or factors, so this can be an effective way to structure the job description. In Exhibit 3–1 these job performance factors are Collection, Insurance Billing, Supervision, Payroll, and so forth.

The whole job analysis and description process should not take much time. The job analyst should be able to interview a typical clerical incumbent in about 30 to 45 minutes. Perhaps observation of any critical or confusing parts of the job will take another 30 minutes. Writing the job description should take about an hour. Once the job description has been assembled, give it to the incumbent for his or her comments, and then revise it based on these comments.

Job descriptions should be written before you need them. As you will see in Chapter 4, these same job descriptions will be essential to develop effective employment procedures. When employees give notice or are fired, you must move as quickly as possible. In addition, terminated employees and employees who resign because they are unhappy tend not to be cooperative. It is best, therefore, to write the descriptions in advance, so they will be available in an emergency. You also will use job descriptions to develop a fair and equitable compensation system (Chapter 5), so having job descriptions on hand is a generally desirable goal. The cost associated with developing accurate job descriptions is minimal when you consider the value they add by improving employee performance through the performance appraisal, employment, and compensation processes. The job description only needs to be changed if the job changes. A good maintenance procedure is to have employees review their job descriptions annually just prior to their performance review.

Another alternative for developing job descriptions is to hire a consultant who can conduct job analysis studies. Often, consultants will utilize questionnaires to conduct job analyses. In addition to providing narrative job descriptions, such as in Exhibit 3–1, this approach can also provide a quantitative analysis of job content on commonly observed knowledge, skills, and abilities (KSAs). This may prove useful for identifying employment selection factors. Another advantage of outsourcing this process is that it moves the burden off of your staff. That said, it would be useful for the consultant to train your staff to maintain the job descriptions, so they are routinely and inexpensively kept up to date.

**Figure 3–1** summarizes the personnel management process. This chapter covers the

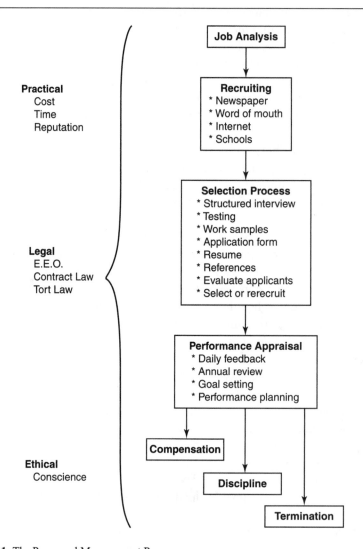

**Figure 3–1** The Personnel Management Process.

performance-appraisal process. Chapter 4 will discuss employee selection. Chapter 5 will cover compensation issues, and Chapter 10 (business law) will cover discipline and termination issues. Job analysis and the resulting job descriptions are the foundation necessary to conduct all of these processes in any organization including medical practices.

## 2. Immediate Feedback Is the Most Effective Form of Performance Appraisal

The single most effective performance appraisal procedure is to observe and comment on employee performance as it occurs. Immediate feedback has a number of benefits. If job performance is good, your comments will provide motivation and encouragement. If job performance needs improvement, you will immediately begin to change the substandard behavior. If an employee's performance is inadequate and you don't comment on it, you have implicitly told the employee that the performance is acceptable. For example, if a deadline for getting a radiology report out is missed by a day and you don't remark on this, then you have indicated that deadlines are not really that important. Delaying your comments until a periodic annual or semiannual performance review will probably result in many missed deadlines. In addition, if you don't comment on inadequate performance as it occurs, some employees may conclude that you are afraid of a confrontation. Employees who perceive that their supervisor is afraid of distasteful or confrontational situations may use this knowledge to achieve their own objectives at your expense or your practice's expense.

Some employees will be honestly confused by failure to immediately comment. For example, you review a report that indicates that there are a number of patients who are not making their copayments at the time

of service. You don't inquire or comment on this to the business manager, who is ultimately responsible for all financial matters in your practice. The business manager knows the practice's policy is that copayments must be made at the time of service, but assumes that because you have seen the report and haven't commented, you are satisfied with the current level of policy enforcement. In effect, not commenting has resulted in the business manager assuming that you concur with his or her actions, and that the policy has been changed.

Many physician leaders have difficulty providing immediate feedback, particularly when it is critical. It is much easier to be critical of an employee to your spouse or to your golfing partner, because he or she is likely to nod in agreement. All this does, however, is provide a safe outlet and temporarily relieve your frustration. It does not achieve the most important objective: changing the employee's behavior. On the other hand, some physician leaders are only too happy to be critical of an employee, but are slow to provide deserved compliments. This is a quick way to generate employee dissatisfaction and turnover. Effectively using immediate feedback is a difficult skill to master. It takes both experience and good judgment to distinguish between the occasional inconsequential error or achievement, and a failure or triumph of real significance. In effect it takes judgment, which for most of us is a learned skill. If you don't start making these judgments, however, you will never become proficient at it.

The meaning of the word *immediate* also should be understood. This does not mean providing comments in front of other employees, physicians, or peers. This, however, doesn't mean commenting 2 weeks from now. It probably *does* mean getting the employee aside, perhaps in the ensuing hours or in the next day or so, to provide the needed comments. It may mean providing your observations to the employee's direct supervisor, such as the nurse supervisor or business manager, so they provide the feedback because they are the employee's direct supervisor. Remember, the goal is to change behavior, not to embarrass or degrade an employee.

### 3. Review Your Direct Subordinates at Least Annually, and Have Your Managers Who Are Subordinate to You Review All Their Employees Annually

Periodic performance appraisals should be conducted regularly. Typically, these are done annually, although new employees should receive a review after 2 or 3 months on the job. By telling new employees at the time of employment that they will be formally evaluated in 2 or 3 months, you achieve two objectives. First, you give the new employee an extra incentive to learn the new job and to excel. Second, you emphasize that you are very concerned about job performance and will recognize when the employee's performance is inadequate, outstanding, or acceptable. In effect, this initial periodic review provides an opportunity to shape the new employee's development and set performance expectations.

Going forward, periodic reviews provide an opportunity to establish a coherent plan for improvement. Without periodic reviews, the feedback provided by daily supervision can simply amount to a series of unconnected comments. The review helps place these comments into a larger perspective and allow plans for improvement to be based on the employee's current strengths, weaknesses, and personal and practice goals.

An important tool to use in conjunction with a periodic review is a critical incident file (**Exhibit 3–2**). A critical incident file contains brief supervisor comments regard-

**Exhibit 3–2**  Critical Incident File Excerpts

| | |
|---|---|
| 2/11/07 | VISA bill not paid on time. $36.62 finance charge. |
| 4/29/07 | 941 tax form not prepared until the last day. Preparation done only after I happened to inquire. |
| 7/17/07 | Ran long computer reports during day instead of overnight, tying up billing computer during day. When asked, she had no reason for doing this. Poor time management. |
| 11/3/07 | Went out of her way to make Dr. Johnson feel welcome during his first week by taking him to lunch. |
| 12/9/07 | Got us a $6,000 advance from XXXXXX against insurance claims that insurance company is slow paying on. |

ing noteworthy events in the working life of an employee. Generally, if an event is significant enough for you to comment on it directly to the employee, then it is appropriate to put a note in the employee's critical incident file. The word *critical* in this instance means "out of the ordinary *and* important," not necessarily "bad." A critical incident file should include comments about praiseworthy as well as blameworthy incidents. The comments should be very brief. If they are not, then the time involved in documenting incidents will become burdensome, and the file will not be maintained.

Each employee should be able to review the contents of his or her own critical incident file. Remember, the goal is to improve job performance. You can't do that by keeping your comments, either positive or negative, secret. Correspondingly, any incident worthy of entering in a critical incident file is important enough to be discussed with the employee near the time of the occurrence. By commenting on performance as it occurs, and then documenting important deviations from the norm in a critical incident file, you make the assessment of performance an integral part of your management technique, and you construct a database for the annual review. It provides the supervisor with behavioral examples from the entire year, thus allowing a more balanced and accurate evaluation. Without a critical incident file, your memory may become selective. You may tend to remember only more recent events or may disproportionately recall positive (or negative) incidents. Critical incident files are maintained by the employee's direct supervisor, so you personally should maintain critical incident files only on those subordinates who report directly to you.

Next, be certain that those below you in the management hierarchy also similarly evaluate their employees on both immediate and periodic bases and keep critical incident files. Finally, be certain that all managers are evaluated on their ability to conduct performance appraisals. In this way, accountability cascades down the organization.

How do you know if a subordinate manager is doing a good job of performance appraisal? Obviously, you can't sit in on all of his or her evaluation interviews with subordinates, nor can you constantly observe the performance of the subordinates and compare this to his or her evaluations of their job performance! What you can do, however, is look at the documented evidence. If the business manager, for example, evaluates all his or her subordinates as "outstanding" but a sampling of critical incident files doesn't support this, then you have reason to believe that the manager isn't being totally accurate. Similarly, use a "reality check." If the business manager's subordinate evaluations seem inconsistent with the front office's perfor-

mance or with your personal observations of an employee, then you may also want to question the accuracy of the evaluation. Ultimately, of course, you can't judge your subordinates' ability to conduct performance appraisals with a micrometer. It's a judgment call. If there are inconsistencies, the goal is to improve the subordinate manager's observation and reporting skills. Additional training and, ultimately, tying raises and promotion opportunities to this factor, just like any other important area of job performance, should result in improved appraisals.

## 4. Set Goals for Those Who Report to You, and Have Them Set Goals for Those Who Report to Them

Goal setting is one of the most powerful tools available to managers. The simple act of telling an employee "This is what I want" or "This is where we are headed and how your performance can best help us get there" is a powerful way of directing and improving both employee and practice performance. When employees have specific goals, it gives them something concrete against which to match their daily actions. It also gives them predictability. There is nothing more frustrating to a subordinate than having to guess what a manager wants, especially if a wrong guess can result in criticism. Finally, setting difficult but realistically attainable goals stretches employees beyond where many would normally perform if they had no goals or a generalized goal such as "do the best you can."[1]

Setting goals for your subordinate managers and having them set goals for *their* subordinates result in coordinated goal setting cascading down through the organization. Those at the top, who are setting policy, will identify goals for their direct subordinates that are consistent with their view of where the organization is heading. These subordinate managers, in turn, will set even more specific goals for their subordinates that are consistent with the goals that they received from the highest levels. As this goal-setting process cascades down through the organization, it creates coordinated, directed behavior that coincides with top management's objectives. This top-down approach has the advantage that everyone is on the "same page" working in a coordinated integrated manner toward organizationally defined goals. The *potential* disadvantage is that policy and direction are being set by those who are furthest from the customer (patient, patient's family, referring physician, etc.). In order for this top-down coordination to work best, therefore, there needs to be significant *upward* communication between front-line personnel (physicians, nurses, clericals, etc.) to the top, so that top management is making *informed* market-based strategic decisions.

**Table 3–1** summarizes how a goal cascade might play out in a hospital. It begins with the chief executive officer (CEO) identifying cost reduction as one critical goal. The implications for each level below the CEO become more specific and operational as we

descend the organization's hierarchy, but each ties in with the policy goal set at the top.

Here's a goal-setting discussion between a physician leader and a practice business manager.

**Physician:** "We both agree that the money in the 61–90 day aging category is too high. I asked you to analyze the cases in those categories to see if there are any common themes that account for why we haven't collected on these accounts."

**Business Manager:** "I've found that 42 percent of the cases in this category are due to insurance companies simply not responding to our first billing. They are not denials; they simply aren't responding. Our current process just doesn't identify these cases soon enough. This goes down to 9 percent in the 91–120 day category, because we're catching these cases during the 61–90 day period. Nineteen percent of the cases are due to co-pays that we didn't collect at the time of service. It's a large volume of small amounts so we tend not to work them hard."

**Physician:** "Then we need to change our procedure. I want you to change our account

**Table 3–1**  Cascading Goals

| Position | Goal |
|---|---|
| Chief Executive Office | Reduce operating costs |
| V.P. Cardiac Services | Train staff physicians on cost issues<br>Develop activity-based costing of selected procedures |
| Director, Cardiac Surgical Care | Develop standard treatment protocols<br>Develop methods to assess clinical outcomes<br>Develop methods to "clean up" coding<br>Develop outcomes database |
| Director, Cardiac Care Case Managers | Develop/select case management software<br>Develop case management procedures<br>Identify sources of invalid coding<br>Specify outcomes database variables |

analysis and collection procedures so we'll catch the insurance no reply cases in the 31–60 day category so they never make it into 61 days. I would like to see you reduce them to less than 10 percent of the correct dollar amount in the 61–90 day category in 3 months and get copay defaults to less than 5 percent. If we do better at the time of service, then we won't have to deal with them later. In order to do this most effectively, develop guidelines and personal goals for those below you like Maria [billing supervisor] and Janet [front desk supervisor] that will help you to achieve these goals. Ask them to develop procedures that tie in their personnel into these objectives. As you are doing this, also be certain that our process includes getting everyone's ideas about how to change our procedures. This means right down to Bill sitting at the front desk."

## 5. You Will Get the Job Performance that You Are Willing to Accept. Don't Be a "Moab Manager"!

A few summers ago I was vacationing in the Moab, Utah, area visiting Canyonlands and Arches National Parks. One afternoon around 3:00 PM my wife and I returned to Moab after a hard day of hiking. My wife had burned up her breakfast with 4 hours to go to our dinner reservation. Solution: Get a quick burger at a brand-new outlet of a national hamburger chain.

We park in the lot. My wife waits in the car, and I go inside. There are two lines being worked by two servers. I get into a line with one couple in front of me. The server takes the couple's order: two burgers, two fries, two sodas. The server disappears.

Several additional people enter the restaurant. Some get in the line behind me, and some go to the other line. Eventually those behind me move into the other line. That line is moving; mine is not. I'm feeling relaxed—

after all, I'm on vacation and have just had a great day in a beautiful national park. After about 5 minutes, I realize that nothing is happening. People behind me in my line move to the other line. The other line is moving to some degree and is apparently being served by the store manager, who is running around frantically and obviously doing several jobs. I ask her "Is anyone serving this line?" She responds "Yes," drops her head, and continues working on the order in front of her.

Several more minutes go by. Nothing happens. At about this time I notice that to the manager's right there is another worker, who is drying a stack of trays with a towel—very, very slowly. A customer whom this worker knows enters the restaurant and begins to talk to her. She puts the trays and towel down and talks casually with her friend. The shop manager is working 5 feet to her left, yet neither seems concerned!

Then the drive-in clerk shouts back to the cook as he picks up a burger: "Last Double Belchfire Burger!" I'm distracted by the towel clerk again. She has picked up a tray now and continues to talk to her friend. Is she a mime doing slowness? Now the cook responds, about 2 minutes after the drive-in clerk's admonition. He mumbles in response to the drive-in clerk's comment "What did ya say?"

Ten minutes now in line. I'm beginning to feel trapped! I comment to the manager working the other line "Is anyone working this line?" She responds, with exasperation, "Yes, sir." A few moments go by, and she calls out "Where is Sherry?" The slow towel dryer mumbles (very, very slowly) "Dunnnnoohh." The manager calls out "Sherry, where are you?" Sherry now calls out from the back of the restaurant "I'm makin' fries!" Sherry is not making fries. The fry maker is in the front of the restaurant, and she is somewhere in the back. The manager goes scurrying off to finish some undone task, then rushes back to grab a handful of burgers and keep some movement in her line.

Finally, Sherry shuffles back to her line and completes the order for the couple. She then takes my order—very, very slowly. When I leave to take the food to my wife in the car, total elapsed time is *20* minutes. No exaggeration. *Twenty* minutes!

Incredible! I can't take it! My code of ethics as a management professor and consultant requires me to help! Besides, I'm madder than hell! I go back into the restaurant, walk to the front of the line, and state to the manager, in the calmest, quietest, most controlled voice that I can muster, "This is the *slowest* fast food restaurant that I've ever been in!" She immediately responds "We're short of help." I stare at her.

"That's not the problem!" I say. "The problem is that everyone, with the exception of you, is moving *SLOWLY*!" We both stare at each other. I turn and leave. I had not completed the consultation. Perhaps the pay was a little too low, and after all, I was on vacation. To complete the consultation, I should have added, ". . . and in addition to moving slowly, they are doing it in front of you, and your response is to do nothing other than compensate by working harder and faster yourself! You're the manager here but the only job that you are *not* doing is managing!"

This case is a good example of a basic management principle: You get what you are willing to accept. There are many employees who will give you the lowest level of performance that you will tolerate. This manager's employees worked slowly—*very, very slowly*—and did it right in front of her. Yet she didn't demand anything more of them, so naturally they didn't give more. The message that she gave her subordinates was, "That's OK." The message that she should have given is "If we're understaffed, we work that much harder and faster, and then some!" Instead, this "man-

ager" stopped managing, and tried to compensate personally for underperforming employees. Moab managing is often rationalized with the comment, "I can get it done better and faster if I do it myself." Unfortunately this may be true, *today*, but it is a slippery slope.

Be on the lookout for "Moab Management," both when you are personally supervising subordinates and in your subordinate managers. If you find yourself or your subordinate managers compensating for subordinates who don't meet standards, but you don't directly demand improvement, then you are a "Moab manager." The inevitable consequence is patient/customer dissatisfaction.

What should the manager have done? I would suggest closing the shop doors for 5 minutes and providing a clear explanation of performance expectations, assurance of training to those who haven't mastered skills yet, and an offer of resignation for those who can't or won't excel. What should you do if you find yourself Moab managing? The same thing. Let subordinates know what you need, train them if they are not adequately trained, and give them their notice if they choose not to perform.

## 6. People Do What They Want to Do: Hold Your Employees Responsible for Their Behavior

This is a corollary to Moab management, but nevertheless very important. As a manager, you do not have the luxury of excusing employee behavior as accidental or unintentional. Why did the tray dryer in Moab put the trays and towels down to talk with a friend? Because she *wanted* to! Her need to chat exceeded her work standards or her fear of retribution from her manager, who was working 5 feet to her left. Similarly, Sherry was slogging through the day in a fog because she (pick one):

- was hung over from the previous evening and didn't care enough about her work performance to drink in moderation the evening before
- was an underemployed college graduate and was thoroughly bored with her work
- was lazy and didn't want to give any more effort than was demanded
- had never been asked to perform any better

The reason that she was choosing to give substandard performance is *irrelevant*. The point is that she was doing it; customers didn't care why, and the supervisor was responsible for fixing this problem. Similarly, your patients don't care why the service is inadequate or slow, so as a manager that can't be your first concern either. You don't have the luxury to play psychiatrist. Stick to managing behavior, not intentions, explanations, or unconscious motivations. If you do otherwise, you will find yourself in a swamp of justifications and attempts to pass off responsibility to you and to others.

### 7. Have Realistic Expectations of Others. Is Getting that Last 5 Percent Really Worthwhile?

This is a *question*! If it is worthwhile, then go for it—if it's *not*, back off! There are two stereotypes of physicians. The first is the absentee physician leader. The absentee physician leader's attitude is often, "I'm paying for all of these professional managers around here. Managing is their job, mine is practicing medicine." The second is the martinet who overmanages and is always demanding more than what most would perceive as reasonable. This guideline applies to the latter stereotype. In a sense, it contradicts some of the earlier appraisal guidelines. The theme underlying the previous guidelines is "Hold employees strictly accountable, set high stan-

dards, and push, push, push!" There is a time, however, to back off.

Effective physician leaders set high standards but only ask for 110 percent when this is absolutely essential. Ineffective physician leaders continually ask for 110 percent, and generally they never get it. One aspect of the art of management is knowing what is reasonable. Become familiar with your subordinates' job descriptions—not only what's on paper but what they actually do on a day-to-day basis. Avoiding inequity requires judgement and becoming familiar with and considering as realistically as possible the level of demands that you place on your employees.

## CONDUCTING THE ANNUAL APPRAISAL

The goal of the annual appraisal is to evaluate incumbent performance in each major area of job performance. Without a good job description, there is a chance that you will miss some important aspect of performance. As the time for an employee's annual appraisal approaches, it is a good idea to give the incumbent a copy of his or her job description and ask whether anything of consequence has changed. If the job has changed, revise the description.

The first step is to schedule a date for the review. Provide enough notice so that you and the employee will have time to prepare. Next, ask the employee to write a *self-evaluation*. Have the employee organize his or her remarks around the major job performance issues noted in the job description. An example of a narrative self-evaluation by a practice business manager is found in **Exhibit 3–3**. Notice how this appraisal tracks the factors in the job description (Exhibit 3–1). This particular evaluation was written by a new business manager who was being evaluated after 90 days on the job. Generally, it is a good

**Exhibit 3–3** Self-Evaluation, December 3, 20XX

1. *Collection.* This is probably the area of most improvement from when I took over the job. Collection has gone extremely well. I have begun to tell patients more and more to call their insurance company themselves if there is a problem and then let me know if there is anything that I can do. I have felt overwhelmed by all the accounts that have needed my attention since I took over the position, but things are under better control now.

2. *Insurance Billing.* I am very confident in this area. I have developed procedures for Margie that have achieved consistency. Claims are sent out biweekly on Wednesdays and Fridays.

3. *Payroll.* Payroll has been a challenge because there is always something different to do, such as different deductions, phone charges, refunds, etc. I feel, overall, that I am mastering the process.

4. *Taxes.* The 941 taxes have gone smoothly. I have needed help coming up with the figures for state taxes. I have made a note on how to calculate state taxes, so this month it should not be a problem. Two concerns: Are the 940 taxes and the VEC taxes in my job description? Should I do these also, or are they the accountant's responsibility?

5. *Accounts Payable.* There have been no problems in this area that I am aware of. I have used George's system for keeping track of bill due dates and it is working well.

6. *Posting and Accounting.* I have not had any difficulty with posting payments and making deposits save the MEDWORK EAP checks. I have been clear about making EAP checks a separate deposit, but it seems to be confusing in the accounting system. We like to keep the check for office space rental on a separate deposit from patient payments, but at times MEDWORK puts both kinds of payments in the same check.

7. *Fee Negotiations.* I have negotiated fees for several patients. I feel comfortable with this area.

8. *Management Reports and Database Management.* I have had some difficulty with the aging analysis reports. Specifically, I am having trouble using the Excel spreadsheet to sort each physician's aging in the manner that you want. For the most part, I have mastered the reports that I need for my daily work, such as daily receipts and adjustments, insurance aging, production reports, adjustment reports, etc. I need some clarification on how to use the categories in the referrals database. Specifically, when do I use the "newspaper ad" and "generated by practice" categories. I get confused between these two.

9. *Problem Identification and Resolution.* I am skilled in the area of problem identification. We have constructed several office forms and eliminated others to make the office run more efficiently. "No pay" and "no show" bills are now sent out the next day. I have fixed the problem for getting timely releases signed by the physicians.

10. *Scheduling.* There have been a few errors with scheduling by Amanda for whatever reason. Overall this seems to be going well. Problems have been avoided by confirming patient visits. We have this up to almost 100 percent attempts within 2 days of scheduled appointments.

idea to formally evaluate all new employees after 60 to 90 days using your standard annual review process. Doing this with new employees helps to clarify responsibilities and identify where additional training is needed. This also tells the new employee that job performance is important. Instruct the employee to give you the written remarks several days prior to when you plan to write your performance evaluation.

The process of writing a self-evaluation causes the employee to think about his or her job performance, to examine it as a supervisor might, and to begin thinking about what needs to be done in the future. The self-evaluation also tells you how the employee has interpreted your feedback, and it gives you an indication of what to expect in the appraisal interview. Schedule the periodic review at a time during normal work hours, and explain to the employee that the purpose of the meeting is to review past performance and to begin planning for the next year.

The appraisal information that you will be discussing in the meeting and will be in your written appraisal should contain no surprises. If you are doing an adequate job of keeping the employee apprised of his or her performance on a daily basis, then the periodic review will simply be a reiteration of what has been said over the year.

Next, gather all relevant information. Review the employee's critical incident file. Classify incidents according to the factors noted on the job description. If some incidents need clarification, talk directly to the employee or others who were involved.

Many organizations use a 360-degree performance-appraisal process in which input on an employee's performance is obtained from peers at the same level, subordinates below the employee, and those above the employee. For example, when evaluating the business manager, you could obtain comments on performance factors from secretaries, the billing supervisor, nurse supervisor, and physicians. Obtaining information from various perspectives can provide a richer and more balanced perspective on performance. It's important to be clear that a 360-degree appraisal process should never be implemented just prior to an employee's appraisal. This makes both evaluators and the person being evaluated uneasy because the rules are being changed in the middle of the game. If you think that 360-degree information could be valuable, then this is a process change that should be implemented at the start of employees' appraisal year, and ideally should be implemented practice-wide including for physicians.

You are now ready to write the employee's performance evaluation report. Your evaluation should always be put in writing. A written report provides documentation that will be useful for tracking an employee's progress over the years. Written documentation also can be useful in defending against legal challenges to personnel decisions (see Chapter 10). **Exhibit 3–4** contains excerpts from a business manager's annual evaluation. This evaluation is based on the job description found in Exhibit 3–2, but it is for a different business manager than the one whose comments are found in Exhibit 3–3.

It is important to evaluate the employee separately on each job description factor. Be as specific as possible. Notice that the performance appraisal in Exhibit 3–4 directly parallels the job description factor by factor. Notice also that it focuses on job-relevant behaviors, not on personality characteristics or sweeping generalities. Finally, notice that it makes distinctions across factors. Performance on some factors is very good, while other areas need substantial improvement.

When writing an evaluation, it is important to use clear, concise language. This will save you time and will provide the subordinate with an unambiguous statement regarding strengths and weaknesses. Initially, you may find it difficult to be direct, especially if there are performance problems. It is important to remember, however, that careers can be ruined by supervisors who are kind and softhearted. *Avoiding the difficult issues until performance is so inadequate that you must discipline or fire the employee is not doing anyone a favor.* It is important that your comments remain related to job performance and are not condescending or personally derogatory. In summary, stick to the facts and work with the employee to develop reasonable solutions.

Next, meet with the employee to discuss your evaluation. Begin the performance-appraisal interview by giving the employee a copy of your written analysis. Then review

**Exhibit 3–4** Performance Evaluation (Excerpts) July 15, 20XX

1. *Collection.* The overall level of collection in the 120–180 day category is back into the acceptable range. This winter, however, collection totals exceeded $16,000 in this category, which was not acceptable. In addition, I had to supervise you closely to get the receivables back down. This should be a self-managing function. This pattern, however, of losing control and then having to be closely worked with to regain control has occurred consistently over the years. The fact that you can get the receivables back under control shows that you can do it. We want you to take more responsibility for dealing with this yourself, however, before it becomes a problem, and before it has to be addressed by me.

   You continue not to enforce the 90-day patient personal payment policy. Patients should be called when their balance reaches the 60-day category, encouraged to contact their insurance company on insurance balances, and told that they will have to pay personal balances immediately.

   In addition, each day you should review the next day's appointments, so that patients can be called before an appointment and reminded to bring in past due balances.

2. *Insurance Billing.* Insurance bills get out in a very timely manner. You have provided structure and procedure for Margie and this has really turned the posting and billing operations into a consistent and efficient process. This is a real strength. Generally, we generate insurance bills within 1 day of the patient encounter. In addition, all of the physicians report that the level of communication on coding questions has improved and is now fully acceptable. This occurred because you created a process to improve physician–front office communication.

3. *Payroll.* The basic payroll processing operates well in that we always pay the payroll on time. There have been some minor problems revolving around infrequent events. For example, you did not account accurately for physicians' Yellow Pages display ads. This was fixed only after I noted the error, because it affected me. It appears that personal long distance telephone charges have been dropped again. This was a problem that was noted last year. It got better for a while, but it is a problem again.

4. *Taxes.* There was one instance when a 941 payment was underpaid, but that was caught before the end of a quarter. With that exception, you did a lot better this past year.

5. *Accounts Payable.* This area has developed into a strength. You have consistently paid the bills on time without reminder. We incurred no interest expenses on our bills last year.

6. *Posting and Accounting for Payments.* This occurs in a timely and consistent manner. There have been no instances reported of incorrectly posted payments. In addition, you routinely handle the adjustments to payroll; bounced checks, insurance retractions, transfers, etc., correctly without the need for supervision. The documentation of adjustments is understandable to the physicians.

7. *Fee Negotiation.* The fee agreements that you negotiate with patients show good discretion in getting the best fee from patients who need a fee agreement. Your payment plans are highly structured and convey the message that we expect patients to meet their financial obligations. You have used good judgment in making decisions that protect the practice's revenue, yet are responsive to patients with real hardships. The McKlintock case in particular showed good judgment in setting a reasonable payment plan that respected the family's financial situation, yet still provides fairness for Dr. Johnson.

8. *Management Reports and Database Management.* I am routinely getting aging analyses now. This is an improvement from last year. Your consistency with write-off and adjustment reports and the aging database report could be improved. These should always be part of the package of reports that you give to me each month.

**Exhibit 3–4** continued

Patient records were put into storage and there was no update to the archived patient files database. In addition, some charts were in the wrong boxes. This caused several problems and delays during the Medicaid audit.

The referral database contains many omissions and errors. It is not a reliable source of information about referrals. Specifically, the categorizations of referrals has no consistency. In addition, data fields are often incomplete. We have talked about this several times over the last year. This is one of our most important databases. This is a major problem.

9. *Problem Identification and Resolution.* Thinking about the future consequences of events is still an area that needs attention. Generally, you react to problems once they occur and have been brought to your attention, but an important part of your job is to be looking for ways to improve things and prevent problems before they occur. For example, the growth in Insurance Company X's AR was rapid. You knew that we were considering not renewing our participation contract with them, yet you did not bring this to my attention until I requested a specific report. This situation should have been on your radar screen in March, and I should have been informed at that time.

Most of the physicians feel that we rarely get request sheets back in a timely manner. The request sheet process was developed by you to help you remember requests and to provide a process to return information to the physicians. If you feel that this system is too cumbersome or time consuming, then develop a better one. Responding to physicians' needs in a timely manner (typically on the same day) is important, and providing feedback is critical if we are to operate in a coordinated, integrated manner. If you can't get to something on the same day, then tell the physician, and estimate when you will be able to get to it.

10. *Supervision.* Your day-to-day supervision of the front office employees on routine activities is adequate. The duties and responsibility are logically assigned and the quality of your written appraisals of subordinates is behavioral and specific. Morale appears to be high.

It took longer than usual to get Janet fully trained. It appeared that the training program that you designed to train her in our medical office management software was not as complete as it could have been.

11. *Scheduling.* Scheduling has been a problem in the past. The new scheduling system software seems to have fixed most the overbookings and open slots issues. You did an excellent job of working with the staff after they were trained and ensuring that the transition to the new system worked smoothly.

12. *Additional.* None

## Areas of Improvement Since July 12, 20XX Evaluation

1. You consistently now use the financial warnings in the medical office management software and are compiling day sheets on this basis. This was a major goal and you succeeded in doing this.

2. You are doing a better job of utilizing our standard procedures including consistently verifying insurance and having all patients sign MOP forms.

### Summary

Overall, your job performance is good. You have some real strengths where your performance is excellent. Also, there are some areas that are important and need attention. Overall, the front office operates well. We get the patients through, we get the bills out; we get the money in, and the office operates in a generally effective manner.

My biggest concern is your ability to adapt to the changes that occur in the job and to identify and fix problems before they become serious. As cost issues and the need to work effectively as a team become increasingly important, anticipating problems and proposing solutions become more critical parts of your job.

the sources of data that you used to develop your evaluation, including critical incidents, observations of others, and objective measures (e.g., aging analyses). This tells the employee that your evaluation is based on fact, not conjecture, and that the appraisal is important enough for you to have taken time to assemble a written document based on data. Use the interview time to elaborate on your written appraisal and to begin planning for the future. Solicit employee comments, and explore any areas in which the employee has suggestions for how job performance might be improved. Although weaknesses and areas needing improvement should certainly be discussed, don't dwell on them. Most employees have strengths, and it is important to discuss these and build upon them.

At this point, you have reached a fork in the road. Quoting Yogi Berra, "Take it!" Less-effective organizations essentially tell the employee at this point "Go out there and continue what you are doing" or "Go out there and fix it!" More effective organizations do what is called *goal setting*. Goal setting is characterized by the following:

- Goals should be behavioral. This means that the goals should be observable job behavior as opposed to mentalistic impressions of improvement, such as "improve your leadership". Instead, say, "Improve your leadership. What I mean by this is that, based on the appraisal and our discussion of the events of the past year, you could solicit more input from your colleagues and subordinates. Publish agendas before meetings, so that everyone has time to prepare. Make conscious decisions about how you will involve others in decisions, such as the impending study that we will be conducting to determine whether to open a satellite clinic. Some of the work on this project might be best performed

through delegation, while in other parts consultation or joint consensus may work best. You should think about these leadership choices ahead of time, not as they are occurring in a meeting."

- You, perhaps with the employee's help, should identify a path for the employee to follow to achieve the goal. Don't leave this up to the employee. Many employees can't figure out how to get from here to there. Help them work through the details of that process. Similarly, there may be occasions where you don't know enough to identify the details of the path, but you can help the employee to find it. For example, suppose that you conclude that a business manager's collection problems are due to insufficient knowledge of how to use your medical office management software. You can't instruct the manager yourself, because you don't know the software in detail, but you can say "I want you to come back to me in a week with a plan for how you will acquire this knowledge. Be certain to include in this plan contacting the software provider to see what training is available. Also I would like you to schedule 1½ hours a week to go into a back room with the manual and work undisturbed to improve your skills. Finally, call Dr. Nakajima's office manager. We consulted her before we selected this software, and she appeared very knowledgeable. Perhaps, we could hire her after hours as a training consultant."

- There should be a time frame for completion. Always state deadlines for specific objectives. If you don't, then many employees will always find other things to do rather than deal with difficult objectives. Also, this gives you an "action date," so that you know that you can take another action as of a specific date.

• Periodically check to monitor the employee's progress. Don't assume that, just because performance has improved, it will remain that way. This, of course, ties in with the admonition to continuously observe and comment on job performance as it happens.

**Exhibit 3–5** contains goals set by the manager to follow up on the performance appraisal in Exhibit 3–4. Notice that the discussion is factual and that specific behavioral targets as well as time deadlines are identified.

## Start Evaluation Errors

There are a number of errors that physician leaders can make when evaluating job performance. Leniency errors occur when supervisors consistently rate employees either too high or too low. Some supervisors tend to evaluate subordinates consistently too favorably (positive leniency bias) because they think that a more accurate evaluation would have an adverse impact on morale. Some give high evaluations because they have not been paying close enough attention to subordinate performance, and no one ever

**Exhibit 3–5** Personal Goals Based on the Performance-Appraisal Interview

These are areas to work on. We will meet in late September to see how you are progressing in these areas.
1.  Respond to all physician request sheets on the day that you receive them. Begin doing this immediately.

2.  Call or have Margie call all patients with nonparticipatory insurance, when they have personal money in 60 days, and inform them that in 3–4 weeks they will have to pay unless their insurance company responds. The patient will not be surprised if you thoroughly review the method of payment with them at the time of the initial office visit. It is not sufficient simply to accept the patient's statement that he or she cannot pay. Failure to do this has delayed collecting funds that the office needs. Begin putting this policy into effect immediately.

    This was your number one goal last year. It really is important for you to make this a top priority.

3.  The referral database problem needs to be fixed. The target is zero errors. I want you to determine why referrals and fields are occasionally omitted and develop a solution to this problem. Also, it appears to me that we need to clarify the referral categorization guidelines. I want you to develop new written guidelines and forward them to me for my review. Please let me know your findings by August 15. In the interim, please carefully review all new referrals to be certain that they are entered into the database correctly. Once we agree on the new guidelines, design a training program for the front desk people.

4.  Work more closely with Margie to help her identify high-priority accounts. If necessary, work accounts aggressively on your own initiative to keep collection statistics at their current favorable levels. Review AR reports daily if possible, but certainly weekly. Begin doing this immediately.

5.  The nature of your job is changing. It is requiring you to look more inquisitively at the front office operation, identify problems and come up with solutions before they become serious problems. It is important for you to be continuously examining processes to see how they can be improved and to take a more proactive approach to your job. This should be a daily, ongoing part of your job. I want you to develop a list of practice management areas where our current methods could be improved. We will then discuss this list together, refine it, and develop improvement projects if appropriate. I want to see this list by September 15.

objected to a high evaluation! Other supervisors feel that a less-than-outstanding evaluation reflects poorly on their own leadership ability. Finally, some supervisors lack assertiveness, and they become overly dependent on acceptance and approval from their subordinates. Giving an accurate appraisal may threaten this approval.

Similarly, there are a number of reasons why some supervisors consistently downgrade subordinate performance. Some supervisors project their own failings onto their subordinates. If it is always a subordinate's fault, then the supervisor does not have to accept personal responsibility. Other supervisors have unreasonably high standards. It is important to remember that a medical practice owner or a physician in an executive management position will generally have a far greater degree of commitment to the organization than many other employees. It is important to be realistic about the degree of commitment and performance that can be expected from employees. Consistently giving low evaluations and demanding performance that employees perceive as unreasonable will only result in employee dissatisfaction and turnover.

Another common evaluation mistake is called a *halo error*. A halo error occurs when a supervisor allows an employee's performance on one job factor to influence the evaluation on another factor. For example, if Dr. Smith is outstanding at diagnosis, you should not allow this to influence your evaluation of her performance on communications with patients and "bedside manner." Similarly, if Vice President Andersen has developed an outstanding cost accounting system for oncology services, this should not raise his evaluation on supervisory skills if they in fact need improvement. These are separate, distinct issues and should be treated as such in the performance-appraisal process. A particularly insidious type of halo error occurs when the supervisor allows a factor that is not job relevant, such as physical attractiveness, to influence some or all of the evaluations of job-relevant factors. Sometimes this halo process can be very subtle, and it may occur at an unconscious or semiconscious level. Systematically conducting evaluations factor by factor based on job descriptions helps eliminate leniency and halo errors.

## PERFORMANCE EVALUATION DATA

The data that you will use to evaluate an employee can be classified as either quantitative or qualitative. Quantitative data are produced in the normal course of work activities. Examples include "reinfection rate," "percentage of insurance dollars collected within 90 days," "number of patients treated per week," "number of referrals generated per month," "average length of stay," and so on. Be very careful when using quantitative data. Unless you fully understand the numbers, they can be misleading. For example, suppose that you are evaluating a physician based on the number of referrals that he or she has generated over the past year. Can you separate referrals generated by the organization, such as those caused by a Yellow Pages ad that mentions your colleague's name, from referrals generated directly by the physician?

Similarly, mortality rates and other measures of physician performance can be very misleading, unless they take into account extenuating circumstances, such as comorbid conditions, sometimes referred to as illness burden or case-mix adjustment. Also, an increase in accounts receivable may be indicative of either a performance problem or organization growth. If the organization is growing, you may have to adjust the accounts receivable numbers to obtain a valid picture of a business manager's performance. You could, for example, take the accounts receivable money that is 90 days old as a percentage of the current accounts receivable. Quantitative data can be very useful for evaluating an employee's performance, *if the data truly reflect the performance.*

Another problem with using quantitative measures is that they can be "gamed." For example, a business manager who is evaluated on accounts receivable over 120 days could write off these balances. Unless you are observant and note or anticipate this behavior by being certain to review write-off reports (as you should!), the manager will look good on the performance evaluation *while at the same time producing a counterproductive outcome.* Similarly, a physician who is evaluated on the basis of clinical outcomes that are not properly adjusted for the illness burden of his or her patients may overrefer sicker patients. Once again, the performance-appraisal process will have generated counterproductive behavior.

Qualitative data include your personal interpretation of events, such as your judgment of an employee's ability to work with patients, diagnostic skills, supervisory skills, knowledge of software, and the like. Qualitative data are generally susceptible to the rating errors just mentioned. Most of the data available for evaluating healthcare employees are qualitative. Even those practices and hospitals that maintain databases on productivity and financial outcomes find that, in the final analysis, performance appraisals are largely qualitative, because the quantitative data are usually only relevant to part of each job.

As a physician leader, your challenge is to develop a set of evaluation criteria that draw on quantitative and qualitative data, and that in total will present a fair, complete picture of the employee's performance. When jobs contain evaluation issues that are both quantita-

tive and qualitative in nature, be especially vigilant for halo errors. It is very easy to let qualitative data bask in the halo of quantitative data. For example, you have good, hard evidence that Dr. Hoskins is an excellent surgeon. His reinfection and rework rates are low compared with those of his peers and national statistics. You may, unconsciously or semiconsciously, tend to allow these facts to bias your evaluations of other, less-measurable issues, such as his bedside manner, charting timeliness and quality, and treatment of staff. Similarly, Mr. Carney does a great job of collecting revenue, but he tends to look the other way when physicians provide incomplete documentation and notes. Once again, you may be inclined to overrate his ability to obtain physician compliance out of gratitude for his success in keeping the money flowing. It is important for supervisors to evaluate factors separately, because these independent evaluations are the basis for providing employees with the opportunity to improve in those areas that need development.

## PERFORMANCE STANDARDS

*Performance standards* (**Exhibit 3–6**) are statements that appear on rating forms that describe what any employee on a particular job must do to achieve that level of performance. Performance standards relate to the *job.* Irrespective of who occupies the position, the incumbent will be expected to meet the performance standards for that job. Performance standards should not be confused with employee goals. An employee's goal is a personal objective that may equal or exceed a particular performance standard. For example, a performance standard for the position of business manager may be to keep accounts receivable in 180+ days below 5 percent of total accounts receivable. By definition, any business manager who does this

**Exhibit 3–6** Typical Performance Standards

*Checkbook*
- Checkbook is reconciled with the bank statement no later than 5 days after the statement is received.
- Monthly income should always balance against the monthly collection for physicians plus other income.

*Accounts Receivable*
- Total accounts receivable should never exceed two times current accounts receivable.
- Accounts receivable report should be run each week.
- Cash box should be balanced against receipts printout each day.

- *Word Processing*
- Documents should contain no typing, spelling, or grammatical errors.
- Documents should be completed no later than 3 days after they are submitted for typing.

*Database Maintenance*
- Referral database should be revised at least weekly.
- All transactions should be entered into McNeal Office Management software daily.
- All other databases should be revised at least weekly.
- All databases should be backed up daily.

*Referrals*
- Twenty-five percent of a physician's referrals should be self-generated.
- Two public information seminars should be presented each year.
- Two network primary care physician training programs on new GI pharmaceuticals should be conducted each year.

is doing at least an adequate job on this factor. A specific goal for Mr. Carney, however, may be to reduce accounts receivable from its current 4.3 percent level to an average of 3.3 percent across the last 6 months of the year.

Many large organizations like to have written performance standards for virtually all factors on most jobs. This is a waste of time. It is difficult to write meaningful performance standards for some factors, and others are so obvious that it makes no sense to ponder the issue. For example, the following might be a performance standard for patient relations: "Employee is always courteous and attentive to patient needs." This statement is so bland that it is virtually meaningless. It states the obvious and provides no guidance to the employee. Don't waste your time or your employees' time writing or trying to apply meaningless performance standards.

On the other hand, if you have a clear standard of acceptable behavior and the job per-

formance issue is important, then it will be helpful to your employees if you share those standards with them. Performance standards should always be discussed with employees at the time of employment. They should also be communicated to employees in written form, either as part of the job description or the evaluation form for the job.

## RATING FORMS

Many supervisors consider completing a rating form (**Exhibit 3–7**) equivalent to doing a performance appraisal. As we have seen, performance appraisal is a much more broadly encompassing process than simply completing a form. Completing a rating form should instead be viewed as just a way to record the evaluation information and conclusions.

Evaluation forms such as in Exhibit 3–7 have their own special problems. Standardized rating forms take a lot of time and effort

**Exhibit 3–7** Typical Performance Appraisal Rating Scales

| | | | | | | |
|---|---|---|---|---|---|---|
| 1. When unsure about a problem, discusses it with supervisor. | | | | | | |
| Almost Always | 1 | 2 | 3 | 4 | 5 | Almost Never |
| 2. Has mastered the information provided in technical manuals for the office equipment and software used on the job. | | | | | | |
| Almost Always | I | 2 | 3 | 4 | 5 | Almost Never |
| 3. Has a sense of humor even with difficult patients. | | | | | | |
| Almost Always | 1 | 2 | 3 | 4 | 5 | Almost Never |
| 4. Accepts and adapts to change. | | | | | | |
| Almost Always | 1 | 2 | 3 | 4 | 5 | Almost Never |
| 5. Adequately delegates work. | | | | | | |
| Almost Always | 1 | 2 | 3 | 4 | 5 | Almost Never |
| 6. Gets written reports completed on time. | | | | | | |
| Almost Always | 1 | 2 | 3 | 4 | 5 | Almost Never |
| 7. Gets all appropriate paperwork signed by patients. | | | | | | |
| Almost Always | 1 | 2 | 3 | 4 | 5 | Almost Never |
| 8. Communicates appropriately with patients. | | | | | | |
| Almost Always | 1 | 2 | 3 | 4 | 5 | Almost Never |

to construct. As a result, some organizations use "one size fits all" appraisal factors across many, if not all, jobs. This approach is worthless. As we have seen, it is essential to identify specific aspects of performance *for each individual job*. Generic factors, such as quality, quantity, and willingness to follow directions, are not going to be appropriate or specific enough for many jobs. In addition, using standard forms allows managers to be lazy. If the factors to be evaluated are not job specific, the manager can complete the form without having to provide a lot of detail about the employee's performance.

Standardized rating forms can be useful, however, in larger organizations. Sometimes it is necessary to make comparisons across many employees, such as when a clerical supervisor position is being filled internally. It would be time consuming to try to equate the narrative performance appraisal reports across the several dozen applicants to determine who is most worthy of the promotion. Many large organizations, recognizing the critical importance of the performance appraisal process, have invested the time and money to develop performance appraisal forms for groups of jobs, although not necessarily for every single job in the organization. For example, all clerk/typist type positions have a custom-developed performance evaluation form, as do licensed practical nurses, registered nurses, pharmacists, nursing supervisors, and so forth. To do this effectively, supervisors of these positions—and ideally job incumbents—must be involved in the development of these evaluation forms. In addition, supervisors have as part of their job the responsibility to suggest changes to the standard evaluation form as the duties of the position change.

Because medical practices rarely need to make comparisons among large numbers of employees, rating forms such as the one in

Exhibit 3–7 generally are not necessary. Usually, performance appraisals in medical practices are aimed at assessing a few employees in great depth. The goal is to compare the employee against the demands of the job instead of with other employees. A narrative evaluation constructed around the job description factors for the position is the most appropriate type of evaluation to achieve this end. In effect, a blank piece of paper and an accurate job description are the key to conducting a superior performance evaluation, irrespective of the job.

## IMPROVING PERFORMANCE

Job performance can be improved by selectively using four techniques: training, incentives, discipline, and job restructuring. The choice of which method or methods to use depends on the employee's current circumstances. The performance-appraisal process will help you determine the best strategy. Training is appropriate for increasing an employee's skills if the low performance is due to limited ability *and if you believe that he or she has both the capacity and motivation to improve*. It is also beneficial in the case of an outstanding employee who still has some room to grow.

Incentives will be discussed more fully in Chapter 5. At this point, it is sufficient to say that providing an incentive, such as a pay raise or a bonus based on production, will only change behavior when the employee sees the incentive as valuable, and related to job performance, and if he or she has the ability to improve. If the employee lacks any of these elements, then incentives are not an appropriate behavioral change strategy. The same holds true for discipline. Threats and the removal of rewards only change performance when the threats are perceived as credible, the rewards are desired, each is per-

ceived as tied to achievement, and the employee has the skill to improve. If the employee really doesn't want the job or the rewards, or is unable to improve, then discipline will have no effect.

Job restructuring involves changing a job to compensate for an employee's strengths and weaknesses. For example, suppose an otherwise valuable secretary has difficulty collecting fees from patients at the time of service. Your business manager tries to improve performance by giving the secretary guidelines and having him work closely with another employee who is good at this task; the secretary reads articles on self-esteem, practices collection methods by role-playing with other employees, and so on. Performance, however, does not significantly improve. At this point, you may choose to rethink the tasks performed on this job and the other front office jobs.

If it is possible to restructure some of the jobs so this employee will spend little if any time collecting fees, then you will have solved the performance problem. Obviously, you must use this method carefully. If other employees perceive that they must bear an extra burden because of a coworker's incompetence or reluctance, you will simply be trading one kind of problem for another. Used skillfully, however, this can be an effective way to improve organizational performance while salvaging otherwise valuable employees.

## EVALUATING PHYSICIAN PERFORMANCE

As more physicians work in group practices, healthcare organizations, and salaried positions, the need to evaluate physician performance increases. Physicians are arguably in the best position to directly influence the quality and cost of the care delivered, which is central to the success of any practice or healthcare system.

Historically, physician evaluation has been handled through a peer-review process. For peer review to be effective, there must be a collegial atmosphere that supports an honest and thorough evaluation. All too often, peer review has meant "If you don't give me a hard time, I won't give you one when the roles are reversed." The current healthcare environment, however, is not supportive of this type of evaluation process. External forces, such as Medicare, insurers, employers, and increasingly patients and their families, are more broadly defining and examining physician performance. Physicians are being held accountable for such performance factors as quality defined in a multitude of ways, cost, rule compliance, clinical outcomes, effective communication, and the like, so internal practice and healthcare system evaluation systems must reflect this complexity. In a very real sense, a practice's or healthcare system's internal evaluation process prepares the physician, and through aggregation the organization, to deal effectively with the performance demands of external market forces.

Evaluation of physicians follows the same model as for any other type of job. Begin with the job description, and build the evaluation process around its content. What makes this a more challenging process for the physician leader is that many physicians have never been in positions where they were the subject of regular and thorough evaluations. As a result, personal sensitivities and the skill with which the process is managed become particularly important.

One very powerful way to address this problem is to involve the physicians affected by the evaluation system in the development of the appraisal system. This achieves two positive results. First, physicians who will be evaluated are in the best position to ensure that the appraisal plan actually captures all the complexity and nuances of their work. Their involvement can ensure that the evaluation plan is complete and realistic. Second, a general principle of management is that ownership increases acceptance. In this case, physicians who are instrumental in designing a plan are more likely to use it willingly, and to accept evaluations under it.

Some may counter that involving physicians in the evaluation plan's design gives them the power to produce an ineffectual plan. In a climate of distrust and adversarial scheming this certainly could be the case. If that is the nature of your internal practice climate, then there are more fundamental issues that must be resolved with physicians before the development of a performance-appraisal plan. In a somewhat healthier environment, the inclusion of line physicians in the design of the evaluation plan can help ensure teamwork and acceptance.

**Table 3–2** contains some generic physician evaluation factors to consider. **Exhibit 3–8** contains a 360-degree performance-appraisal form that a practice has developed to solicit information from a wide range of observers on relevant physician performance issues. As with any job, however, it is important to develop evaluation factors around your physicians' actual job description, and with a focus on what the practice is trying to achieve. Remember, identifying appropriate factor content and assessment methods will determine the ultimate success of the plan. Use of objective clinical outcome measures, surveys to assess professional (referring physician, ICU consultant, etc.) and patient satisfaction, and developing cost measures and management reports to quantify physician performance all are feasible. Does this level of monitoring cost something in terms of administrative overhead and physician leader time? Certainly. But what are the costs

**Table 3–2** Generic Physician Evaluation Factors

| *Factor* | *Description* |
|---|---|
| Productivity | Volume (patients, selected procedures), gross revenue, adjusted net revenue |
| Charting | Compliance with time standards, EMR utilization |
| Quality | Preventive care, protocol utilization, rework rate, mortality rate |
| Dependability | Patient continuity, colleague support, on-call compliance |
| Cost Control | Compliance with utilization standards |
| Patient Relations | Perception of treatment quality, patient relations, patient retention, waiting time |
| Teamwork | Flexibility and responsiveness to working with others including physicians, nurses, staff |
| Leadership | Training and motivating others to work toward practice goals |

*Source:* Adapted from Kongstvedt, P. R. (1993). *Formal Physician Performance Evaluations, the Managed Health Care Handbook*, 2nd Ed., pp. 189–197, © Aspen Publishers, Inc.

to a practice or health system when those who are instrumental in providing care and managing cost considerations do not have to live with the consequences of their actions? Also, what is the effect when the practice or health system across town *is* assessing these issues?

Introducing a physician appraisal process into a practice that has never had one can be difficult. Anticipate that there will be resistance. See Chapter 6 regarding the subject of change management and overcoming resistance to change. If this is your challenge, then I suggest that you approach this as a progressive task composed of three broad objectives:

- *Level I Goal—Develop a climate where it's OK to talk about performance.* This should be based on the use of collegiality where through protracted discussions all of the physicians in a practice agree to examine *themselves* on an agreed-upon set of clinical, governance, and management factors. In many small to moderate-sized practices, this may result in significant improvement. In essence, all physicians in the privacy of their own offices look at themselves on

those factors that all have agreed are important to practice success. Most physicians want to do the right thing and feel some level of obligation to their colleagues, so they will in fact follow through. Having this discussion of what each physician should be observing about themselves may take a long time—maybe 6 months or longer in a practice that is not used to doing these sorts of things. It is, however, a major breakthrough so don't rush it.

- *Level II Goal—Write narrative self-evaluations on each factor and develop a performance plan.* At this stage, each physician agrees to commit his or her observations to writing, and to develop improvement plans. There is no requirement, however, to share this with colleagues. The act of committing thoughts to paper will result in a much more thorough analysis of past behavior and needed future actions.
- *Level III Goal—Share observations with colleagues.* Once a degree of comfort has been achieved with Level II, then it's a relatively small step, which may naturally occur, to share your self-evaluation and

**Exhibit 3–8** 360-Degree Physician Performance Evaluation Form

PHYSICIAN PEER-REVIEW FORM

Please provide some observations of the physician under review. Specific comments will REMAIN CONFIDENTIAL, and will only be used as part of the overall evaluation process.

Physician Reviewed:                Evaluator:                Review Time Period:

1 = Not Acceptable 2 = Less than Satisfactory 3 = Satisfactory 4 = More than Satisfactory 5 = Outstanding. If you did not have the opportunity to observe a factor, enter ?.

Please comment on any scores of 5, 2, or 1.

Availability to Patients _____
Comments:

Appointment Timeliness_____
Comments:

Quality of Clinical Notes _____
Comments:

Medical Records Timeliness _____
Comments:

Medical Decision Making _____
Comments:

Technical Medical Skills _____
Comments:

Patient Communications _____
Comments:

Staff Interaction _____
Comments:

Overall Evaluation _____
Comments:

General comments:

_____
Signature

performance plan with those who may help you to achieve your stated goals. Alternatively, the practice physicians as a group may conclude after some time that everyone feels comfortable doing this, and so as a team everyone agrees to do this. For example, I note that I really could improve on some patient satisfaction issues. I've noted over the years that George just naturally seems to have "a way with patients"; it's common knowledge around the practice. I share my goal with George and ask him, in effect "how he does it." Once again the basis for this discussion is collegiality, but it's now a focused problem-oriented discussion.

## PERFORMANCE-APPRAISAL SUMMARY

Assessing job performance should be a continuous process. Formal appraisals provide an opportunity for you to review progress, solicit personal goals, and plan for the future. Performance appraisals help you motivate your employees, peers, and partners, and provide you with critical information for making management decisions, including training, job restructuring, compensation, and termination decisions.

You should personally conduct all performance appraisals of your direct subordinates. It is also desirable for you to occasionally observe the appraisal interviews conducted by subordinate managers of their subordinates. At a minimum, you should read their evaluations and review them with your subordinate managers. Reading evaluations will provide you with an efficient way of learning more about your employees and their strengths and weaknesses. Reading these evaluations is also critical to insuring the quality of these evaluations. If, for example, you are seeing lots of glowing reviews, but few critical incidents that support them, then question whether the evaluator is really doing a good job of appraisal. Similarly, if organizational performance is clearly lacking in an area, but individual appraisals are very positive in this area, then also begin to ask some questions. Finally, the key to an effective performance appraisal system is cascading this process down through all management levels. Familiarizing subordinate managers with the concepts in this chapter, and making their personal rewards dependent upon them doing a competent job of performance appraisal is essential to achieving effective clinical and business performance.

---

## NOTES

1.  Tubbs, M.E. (1986). Goal-setting: A meta-analysis examination of the empirical evidence. *Journal of Applied Psychology* 91:474–483.

## CHAPTER 4

# Employment Methods

---

### Chapter Objectives

This chapter will tell you how to hire front office and professional employees, including physicians, using empirical selection methods. By using these methods, you will reduce personnel costs due to turnover, absenteeism, and poor job performance, as well as legal costs associated with infractions of the equal employment opportunity laws. More importantly, you will have more capable employees who perform better, and are more likely to have positive work attitudes, work together more effectively, and relate better to your patients. You will learn how to:

1. use interviews, tests, references, résumés, and work samples to obtain the best available personnel
2. organize the employment process, so it is as inexpensive and time efficient as possible
3. define your appropriate role in the employment process, as well as the roles of others (managers, subordinates, and consultants)
4. recruit effectively, so you can apply the selection methods to a well-qualified pool of applicants

---

## INTRODUCTION

Whenever you hire someone, you are placing a bet. You are betting that the new employee *can* perform the job adequately, will *want* to perform the job adequately, and will *remain* with you for a reasonable amount of time. This chapter is about changing the odds on the employment bet so they become more favorable to you. No employment method works perfectly, but by using better ones you change the odds so they are significantly more in your favor.

As a physician leader, generally you will not be personally conducting interviews, ad-

ministering tests, and scanning résumés, with the possible exception of those times when you are hiring someone who will be working directly with you, such as a physician or nurse assistant. Instead, your business manager or human resources director will perform these tasks. Ultimately, however, you as a physician leader are responsible for the adequacy of the employment *process,* and you certainly will have to live with its consequences, so your involvement as a leader in its design and implementation is critical. Your appropriate role as a physician leader, therefore, is to ensure that those who will be doing the hiring know what to do. In order to do

137

this, you need a vision of what an effective employment process looks like.

In order to effectively use any of the employment methods that will be discussed, you first must determine which tasks are actually performed on the job. If you don't really understand what an employee does, then you won't know what selection hurdles to utilize in order to assess applicants' abilities. This process of discovering what employees really do is called *job analysis*, and it results in a document called a *job description*. As discussed in Chapter 3, accurate job descriptions are the raw data for developing effective performance appraisal, employee selection, and compensation plans.

Once you know the content of the job, you can choose appropriate tools for making the hiring decision. These tools include work samples, interviews, tests, references, and *résumés,* to name a few. Because each tool has distinct strengths and weaknesses, you will have to learn when to use each one. Many employers limit their choice of employment methods to interviews or, perhaps, to a particular test routinely used for all jobs. This strategy will result in less-than-ideal employment decisions. It is analogous to having only two tools in your garage, and using them for all jobs performed around the house. Try digging a ditch with a rake or cutting the lawn with a hedge trimmer. It *can* be done, but the costs are high in terms of time, effort, and the quality of the final product.

It also is important to generate a large pool of applicants. Even if you develop a very effective employment process, it will not help you much if competent applicants don't apply for your jobs. If, in the extreme, you only get one job applicant following a long diligent search, and you have to fill the job to keep your practice running, then there is no point interviewing or testing the applicant; you *must* hire that person! The process of

generating an applicant pool is called *recruiting*. It is important to know how to recruit a good applicant pool, as well as how to effectively select from it.

Finally, you will need a selection strategy for sifting through the applicant pool. The selection procedures that you will be using will generate data, so you must be able to quickly and accurately interpret the data to identify the best applicant. If you don't have a workable selection strategy, you will get bogged down in a swamp of applicants and information, and waste valuable time evaluating candidates who should have been eliminated at the beginning of the process.

In summary, instituting a selection process for a job proceeds in the following manner:

1. First, determine the tasks that are performed on the job.
2. Second, identify appropriate selection tools, and develop a strategy for how to efficiently and effectively sift through the applicants.
3. Third, develop a recruiting strategy so there will be many qualified applicants.
4. Fourth, recruit applicants.
5. Evaluate applicants.

Initially, I will cover these topics by focusing on hiring clerical, administrative, and supervisory personnel, such as secretaries, office managers, and computer operators. A significant proportion of medical practice and hospital employment is concerned with these types of positions. The strategy for hiring physicians and other professionals, such as nurses and technicians, is the same, although the details of the specific methods (interviews, work samples, etc.) will be different, because the nature of their work is different. The selection of physicians and other professionals is discussed in a separate section of this chapter.

One final note; I will be using the word "you" quite a bit in this chapter. Who the "you" is, however, will vary based on the context. Sometimes, "you" will mean literally *you,* the physician leader, such as when I'm discussing hiring someone who reports directly to *you*, or perhaps hiring a colleague physician. Sometimes, "you" will mean the person in charge of the hiring process, who often will not be you personally (physician leader), such as when a practice business manager is responsible for hiring a clerical or collection administrator. As the physician leader, you (personally) probably won't be directly involved in this latter situation, but you (the physician leader) will be indirectly involved, because you (the physician leader) will have previously ensured that the business manager has been appropriately trained to use the methods described in this chapter.

## USING THE JOB DESCRIPTION: IDENTIFYING SELECTION FACTORS

If you don't know what skills and abilities are needed to perform a job, then you can't determine whether an applicant has them. Employee selection, therefore, always starts with collecting information about the job. Once you have constructed a job description for a position or validated that the current one is accurate, distill it down to the major employment issues, which are called selection factors. Using the job description in Exhibit 3–2, the typical selection factors for this practice business manager might reduce down to supervision, collection, taxes, problem identification, and teamwork. Applicants, primarily, would be evaluated only on these factors. There are two reasons for this reduction process:

1. It would take too much time to evaluate applicants on their ability to perform *all*

tasks that make up a job, especially if the job is complex. Concentrate, therefore, on the most important job performance issues.

2. Many tasks cluster together, because they require the same underlying knowledge, skills, and abilities (KSAs). For example, it is not necessary to assess whether an applicant can word process letters as opposed to memos or address labels. There is an underlying factor here: the word-processing ability. Similarly, supervising the billing operation and supervising the front office crew is not a meaningful distinction from a selection perspective. If the applicant possesses supervisory skills, then it is reasonable to assume that this skill will generalize to a number of circumstances that only superficially differ.

**Exhibit 4–1** contains a job description for a computer operator/secretary position, and **Table 4–1** shows how this description can be reduced to a set of selection factors. Generally, you can adequately describe a job using between four and seven selection factors. If you draft more than eight selection factors, look at them carefully to see whether some factors can be combined. If you can't, then you should consider whether the job is too broad for any one person to perform adequately. It may be that a broad job can be performed if the workload is relatively light. As your organization grows and the workload increases, however, the employee may become overburdened.

The most appropriate person to perform the job-analysis task is the supervisor of the position to be filled. As a physician leader, you should only consider becoming personally involved in the job-analysis process for positions that report directly to you. If, for example, the position is your personal surgical assistant, then your business manager would probably conduct the job analysis and

**Exhibit 4–1** Job Description for Position of Computer Operator/Secretary

---

### Primary Duties

The Computer Operator/Secretary is the primary practice expert in the operation of the computer system. Duties include the operation of all computer hardware and software, troubleshooting problems with hardware and software, learning how to use new hardware and software, training new employees in the operation of hardware and software, making recommendations for the acquisition of new hardware and software, and developing procedures for and taking the responsibility for being certain that all databases are backed up on a regular basis.

In addition, it is the responsibility of the Computer Operator/Secretary to identify methods and procedures for the operation of the office in the event that the computer system becomes temporarily inoperative and to train appropriate personnel regarding these procedures.

The Computer Operator/Secretary must be proficient in the operation of *MediMac,* Microsoft *Office,* database (*Filemaker*), spreadsheet programs, e-mail, Web browsers, and any other applications necessary for the operation of the practice.

Secretarial duties include patient interaction, answering telephones, scheduling appointments, collecting fees, word processing, and other duties and responsibilities as assigned by the supervisor.

### Major Job Performance Factors

- Operate and troubleshoot computer hardware and software.
- Proficiency in various computer applications, including *MedMac,* Microsoft *Office (Word, Excel, Outlook) Filemaker,* scheduling software.
- Patient interaction: personal and telephone. Office activities: word processing, filing, scheduling appointments, etc.
- Collecting fees at time of service from patients.

### Supervision

Reports to the business manager.

---

draft the job description, but with substantial input from you and, ideally, from the current job incumbent. If you are a physician leader in a hospital or large healthcare organization, it is likely that the human resources department will conduct the job analysis. If this is the case, be certain that you are in the review process if the position reports to you, so you can add, delete, or modify content. Similarly, the business manager of a practice should conduct the job analysis and write the job description for secretarial, collection, and billing positions; the nurse supervisor should write the ones for nursing positions; and so

---

**Table 4–1** Selection Factors: Computer Operator/Secretary

| Factor | Description |
| --- | --- |
| Word Processing/Software | Ability to use Microsoft Office (Word, Excel, Outlook) and learn how to use proprietary medical office management and database programs |
| Typing Skills | Accuracy and speed |
| Interpersonal Skills | Ability to communication in socially appropriate ways with others |
| Anticipatory Skills | Ability to anticipate effects of actions on patients and peers |
| Language Skills | Appropriate use of grammar and syntax |

on. If you are a practice physician leader, and assuming that in most instances you will be delegating these tasks to someone else, you should occasionally interject yourself by examining the final list of selection factors and comparing them with the job description. You should be able to discern a logical relationship between the two documents. Occasionally, performing this personal check will serve as a control, providing some assurance that the job-analysis process is being properly performed.

In a private practice or smaller healthcare organization, all this work could easily be contracted out to a consultant. If you choose to use a consultant, it is a good idea to have the consultant simultaneously train one of your employees in job-analysis methods, because these skills are easily learned. A good private-practice candidate for learning these skills is the business manager. By doing this, you will reduce future consulting fees, create a self-maintaining job-analysis/job-description revision process, and probably get better job descriptions, because your staff will be very familiar with real job content.

## RECRUITING

*Recruiting* is the process of getting applicants to apply for a job. The objective is to attract those applicants who are likely to have the required skills, will find the job attractive, and will want to work for you.

The most commonly used recruiting tools are word of mouth and published advertisements, such as in general distribution newspapers, professional newspapers and journals, and on the Internet. Word-of-mouth recruiting has the advantage of quickly conveying information to people who have indicated to you or your employees that they are in the job market or enticing them into the job market. If your current employees are high performers, word-of-mouth recruiting may help

screen out unsuitable applicants. Usually, competent employees will not recruit those who they know are incompetent, because they will not want to work with them. Word-of-mouth recruiting also can result in your employees' persuading friends or associates to enter the job market and become applicants. Many people are not dissatisfied enough with their current job to take the risk or expend the effort to search for a new job. If opportunity knocks, however, they may respond. The danger of word-of-mouth recruiting is that the applicant who learns of a position from a friend may feel an allegiance to this friend that competes with the allegiance to the employer. Always be suspect of word-of-mouth referrals from low performing employees.

Perhaps the ultimate form of word-of-mouth recruiting is nepotism. I can sum up a lot of experiences that I've seen over the years with three words: *Never Do It!* The fundamental problem is one of boundaries. You won't be able to say the things that need to be said or take decisive actions in a timely manner, if you simultaneously have to balance family relationships and all of the other myriad complications that ensue when relatives become employees. If your brother-in-law really wants to be a practice business manager and has the skills to do this, then help him find a job with the practice across town.

Classified newspaper advertising is another way of generating an applicant pool for office and technical positions. The advertisement should clearly state the major duties of the job, the compensation level, and the work hours, so that applicants can self-select based on these considerations. Newspaper ads generate a low proportion of useful résumés. Expect between 50 and 75 percent of these applicants to be eliminated in the résumé-screening process. Historically, newspaper ads have compensated for this by generating large numbers of applicants.

Newspaper readership, however, especially among those under 40 is plummeting, whereas the "online lifestyle" is commonplace to this age demographic. Consider, therefore, online recruiting discussed below as your first line approach, which is selectively supplemented by other methods including newspaper.

Generally, employment agencies are not a desirable recruiting source for nonprofessional and nonmanagerial employees. If you hire one of their applicants, you will usually have to pay some form of fee. In addition, their screening methods often are ineffective, and you should *never* delegate a major part of the selection process to the employment agency. Employment agencies can be useful for supplying temporary replacements, thus allowing you enough time to find well-qualified applicants.

Employment agencies may be more helpful for executive and professional positions and positions with salaries exceeding $50,000. *Executive recruiters*, as they are called, may have access to successful managers who are not currently in the job market. Generally, these recruiters are more sophisticated in their screening methods than employment agencies that concentrate on lower-level positions. Here are some guidelines to consider if you plan to use an executive recruiter.[1]

1. Be certain that the agency you are choosing can conduct a thorough search. Does it have the resources and contacts in the healthcare industry to be successful?
2. Ask to meet the individual who will be handling your assignment. Would you be impressed with this person if he or she were trying to recruit you?
3. Clarify the search firm's fees, and get a signed contract. Be certain that contract-termination clauses and payment schedules are clearly stated. Generally, fees range from 25 percent to 35 percent of the salary of the position to be filled, plus expenses.
4. Choose a recruiter whom you can trust. This person will become aware of your practice's strengths and weaknesses, so you need to be able to trust this person with privileged information. If, during your conversations, the recruiter is revealing inappropriate information about other clients to you, he or she probably will not respect your confidentiality either.
5. Talk to some of the recruiter's clients. Ask these clients whether the consultant's appraisal of applicants was accurate.

A hybrid variation on the traditional employment agency and newspaper ad is to use an online recruiting firm, such as Monster. com. or Careerbuilder.com. These companies offer a number of advantages. You can post your ad faster, because you aren't limited by publication deadlines and schedules. You can instantaneously post your ad or search their applicant database. Generally, you will be able to provide a more complete description of the job than you could in a newspaper classified ad, and online sites also provide screening tools, so you can quickly identify more interesting candidates. You can utilize the online service two ways. One way is to post a job listing, so you will obtain applicants who find your listing and contact you. The second way is for you to search the résumés posted by applicants. Each approach has a separate cost associated with it. Using either approach, the cost is substantially lower than traditional employment agencies, because it is limited to an advertising fee for your listing or the search fee, with no residual payment based on salary. The downside of this approach is coverage. A national database for front office jobs is largely irrelevant to a medical practice.[2] The question, therefore, is whether you will receive sufficient exposure in *your* geographic region. If you practice in New York City, the answer to this question may be very different than if it's in Taos, New Mexico.

Other potential recruiting sources include local colleges and technical schools. In general, these sources are best used for jobs that require little or no previous experience. Schools have several distinct advantages:

- A school placement office can send you a large number of applicants with little effort on your part.
- Applicants with little or no experience will generally work for lower wages than experienced applicants. If the job doesn't require experience, why pay for it?
- A school may do some preliminary screening, so you only get the better applicants. One way to increase the chance of this happening is to tell the placement office that you will evaluate a few of their applicants, and will discontinue recruiting if applicant quality is low.

Finally, internal job posting is a useful method of recruiting in larger healthcare organizations. With this method, open positions are posted on a specific bulletin board, Web site, or distributed to all by e-mail. Initially, positions are only open to current employees. Job posting is good for employee morale, because it tells employees that the organization encourages career growth and that it is committed to working with current employees before searching elsewhere. This, in turn, generates employee commitment.

## DEVELOPING SELECTION PROCEDURES: THE BIG PICTURE

The quality of employees that you bring to your practice or healthcare system affects everything that subsequently occurs. Selection, or the process of hiring personnel for your practice, is the most complex human resource function and arguably the most important. That said, because there is extensive science-based empirical literature and applied technology in this area, it is possible to reduce this complexity down to some rather straightforward guidelines and procedures. The objective of this chapter, therefore, is to do exactly that; to provide you with clear ways to hire clerical, managerial, and professional employees. In order to provide you with an understanding of why the methods that I will discuss will work for you, I will begin by providing a general understanding of how to think about the employment process, and then discuss how to identify selection procedures for the specific jobs in your practice. This discussion will not be linear. I will need to introduce topics, then revisit some in greater detail or from a different perspective, but always the objective will be to develop additional practical understanding of a complex process, which when performed successfully can noticeably improve the clinical and business performance of your practice.

### Basic Principles

There are some selection concepts that you are probably intuitively aware of, but a more explicit understanding will help you to develop better ways to hire employees in your practice. One is that having more applicants for a position is better than having fewer applications. A statistic that quantifies this is the *selection ratio* (SR), which is the number of job openings divided by the number of applicants. Having 10 applicants for one opening (SR = 0.10), therefore, is more favorable than having only five applicants (SR = 0.20). *Validity* is the ability of any selection method (interview, test, reference, etc.) to predict job success. Validity is often measured by looking at the correlation between performance on tests, interviews, and the like and eventual job performance, such as supervisors' or patient satisfaction ratings. This is expressed as a number between 0.00 (no correlation) and 1.00 (perfect predictability).[3] If there is no correlation, then the selection method is worthless. It's equivalent to tossing a coin to determine whom to hire. Practically speaking, it is uncommon to find validities much above .60. Nevertheless, as you will see shortly, it's quite possible to use validities that are far less than perfect to dramatically improve your chances of finding good employees. What follows is an explanation of the reasons why these two intuitive observations of having favorable selection ratios and high validities are so important, and as an illustration, why you need to develop focused methods in your practice or healthcare system to effectively address both of these issues.

### An Example

Assume that the mean annual RN salary in your practice is $50,000. Two nurses performing the same job, however, may contribute different values of performance back to the practice. Stated another way, some nurses do a better job than others, and this variance can be expressed in terms of dollars. This issue of job-performance variability has been widely studied, and on average the standard deviation[4] of the value of performance for managerial and professional jobs expressed in dollars is 48 percent of the average salary. In this example, therefore, the standard deviation of performance is $24,000 ($50,000 × 48%). Another way of saying this is that a nurse who is performing one SD above the mean (84th percentile) is delivering $74,000 of value, while one performing one SD below the mean (16th percentile) is delivering $26,000 of value. For the purpose of this example, assume that the validity of

current selection methods is 0.25 (perhaps typical of a "somewhat structured" interview process), and you replace it with a new method with validity = 0.50, both of which are reasonable but conservative numbers. Assume also that the number of applicants versus openings (selection ratio) allows you to select at the 84th percentile of skills in the general population. A utility formula combines all of these statistics:

$$\Delta\$ \text{ value increase} = \Delta/\text{hire/year}$$
$$= \Delta r_{xy} \times SD_y \times Z_x$$

- where $\Delta r_{xy}$ is the difference between the validity coefficient of the new selection method and the old one
- $SD_y$ is the standard deviation of performance expressed in dollars
- $Z_x$ is the average score on the employment procedure expressed in terms of standard deviations above the selection procedure mean

This tells us that the average increase in $ value of improvement will be $6,000 per employee selected per year. Stated another way, the new employment method will result in an average 12 percent productivity improvement per year, per RN selected ($6,000 / $50,000) expressed in dollars. If 10 nurses are hired per year, than the $ value improvement is $60,000 per year. In 5 years, these 10 nurses will deliver approximately $300,000 of additional value. These numbers double if your current employment method has a validity near 0.00, which might characterize some unstructured interviewing processes. Similarly, moving to a more favorable SR also increases $ value improvement. For example, if SR only allows you to hire at the 50th percentile of skill, then these employees will deliver on average $6,000 less per employee per year than employees selected at the 84th percentile. If you combine these two effects and have recruiting methods that allow you to hire at the 84th percentile and improve the validity from 0.25 to 0.50, then each employee will deliver on average $12,000 more per year of value.

Let me illustrate these effects in a more graphic way using the concepts of false positives (saying applicants will be successful when in fact they fail) and false negatives (saying applicants will fail, when in fact they would succeed). **Figure 4-1** illustrates this relationship. The horizontal axis represents applicant performance on the employment method. This could be an interview, test, or work sample or a composite evaluation based on several employment procedures. The vertical axis represents employees' job performance.[5] Each dot in the scatter plot indicates how a particular applicant scored on both the employment method and job performance.[6] The oval encircling the scatter plot provides a visual summary of the employment method–job performance relationship. Notice that as employment method performance increases, job performance generally increases, although this does not happen in every instance, *because the validity of the employment method is not perfect*

*(1.00)*. Nevertheless, an applicant who performs higher on the employment method is *more likely* to perform better on the job than an applicant who performs lower on the employment method.

The vertical axis on Figure 4–1 is bisected to distinguish acceptable and unacceptable job performance. The effect of hiring at any given level of employment method performance can be observed by drawing a vertical line through the scatter plot. The scatter plot is now divided into four areas: the false-positive area, the false-negative area, the true-positive area, and the true-negative area.

True negatives occur when the employment method predicts that the applicant will fail, and the applicant does in fact fail. True positives occur when the employment method predicts that the applicant will succeed and the applicant does in fact succeed. False positives occur when the employment method predicts success, but the applicant fails. False negatives occur when the employment method predicts failure, but the applicant succeeds. Notice the size of the true-positive area relative to the size of the false-positive area in Figure 4–1. The ratio of these two areas is an index of the employment method's effectiveness, because all

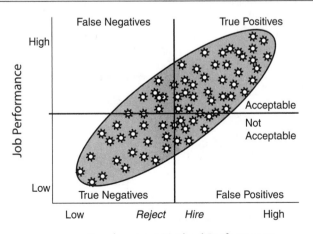

**Figure 4–1** False and True Positives and Negatives.

of these applicants would in fact be hired, since they are to the right of the reject-hire line.

Now, examine **Figure 4–2**. The only difference between Figure 4–1 and Figure 4–2 is that the reject-hire line is moved to the right. This means that the employer is demanding higher performance on the employment method, such as a higher test score or more favorable structured interview evaluation. Something has happened that has resulted in the practice's SR becoming more favorable, so the practice can require a higher test or interview performance, such as for example *improved recruiting effectiveness, which generates more applicants.*[7] Notice the effect that this has on the employment method's effectiveness. The ratio of the true-positive area to the false-positive area has decreased. Notice also that the ratio of the true-positive area to the false-negative area has increased. *Demanding higher applicant scores increases the probability that those hired will succeed, but at the cost of rejecting more applicants who would have been successful.*

From your perspective as an employer, a false-positive error is far more expensive and dangerous than a false-negative error. It is better not to hire someone who would succeed, and perhaps continue the selection process, than to hire someone who fails. Therefore, you want to bias your decision making so that you minimize the probability of making false-positive errors, even though that may increase the chance of making several false-negative errors. Obviously, applicants look at this situation very differently, but your duty is to yourself, your practice, and your current employees.

In addition, false negatives and false positives can be decreased and true negatives and true positives increased for any level of selection ratio by increasing validity—using a better selection method. This would be represented in Figures 4–1 and Figure 4–2 by making the oval containing the data points narrower, so there is less variance in the data. Imagine "squishing" the data points closer to a line running NE to SW through the data oval. You will see that many of the data points move from false positive to true negative and from false negative to true positive areas. If the validity is perfect (1.00), then the oval would collapse to a straight line running NE

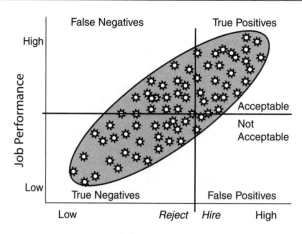

**Figure 4–2** Effect of Improving the Selection Ratio.

to SW with all of the data points falling exactly on this regression line, and there would be no predictability error.

It should be apparent that, theoretically, an employer could demand a selection procedure performance score so high that the probability of applicant success would be 100 percent. The limiting factor, however, is that the employer has to fill the position, and it may take a very long time to find an applicant who scores high enough for that degree of certainty. Stated another way, you have to have a favorable SR in order to push the accept/reject line further to the right and thereby increase the odds of picking a winner. This illustration also demonstrates that you should not jump at the first applicant whose selection-procedure performance scores are *acceptable*. Be patient enough to bring in sufficient applicants to give yourself a good chance of finding high-scoring applicants. This will increase the probability of success.

The implications of this illustration are as follows:

- Employment methods that are far less than perfect can nevertheless be very effective, *if you can require high enough applicant scores*.
- High applicant scores are more likely to occur if you recruit effectively. Your advertising, working conditions, compensation, and so on must help attract many qualified applicants.
- The value of finding high-scoring applicants must be balanced against the cost and time involved in evaluating larger numbers of applicants.

## SELECTION PROCEDURES

Employers use a wide range of selection procedures. Examples include interviews, tests, application forms, résumés, references, and the like. Unfortunately, some work much more effectively than others do, so choosing the *right* selection methods is critical. Industrial psychologists have been examining the validity of selection methods since the early 20th century and have reached some conclusions based on an extensive body of research. In a landmark paper published in 1998 Frank Schmidt and John Hunter[8] reviewed 85 years of selection research and offered a practical and rational approach to selection based on these research findings. They noted that the research literature has consistently identified general mental ability (GMA), also called IQ or intelligence, as the single best predictor of job success, irrespective of job content or context. also called IQ or intelligence. In addition, GMA was also the best predictor of performance in job-training programs. GMA is consistently the most valid predictor of job performance, because more intelligent people acquire more job-relevant skills in previous situations and in training programs, and acquire them more rapidly. They also have more ability to apply past knowledge to new circumstances, so they can take a principle, such as patient confidentiality, and appropriately apply it to a new unique situation better than someone with lower GMA. As a result of these widespread and consistent findings, Schmidt and Hunter conclude that GMA should be the *primary selection method for virtually all jobs*. So, how do you measure GMA? Fortunately, it's quite easy to do using short, inexpensive, easy-to-use published tests. I will describe how to do this in a later section after presenting the full picture of selection methods.

Schmidt and Hunter then raised the question of whether additional selection methods can add *incremental validity*, or validity over and above the predictability provided by GMA. They concluded that four other measures, when incrementally added to GMA, can appreciably increase the accuracy of hiring decisions. These methods and the percentage of increased validity that they provide, when each individually is incrementally added to GMA are:

1. integrity tests (27% increase)
2. work samples (24% increase)
3. structured interviews (24% increase)
4. personality factor of conscientiousness (18% increase)

Notably absent from this list are unstructured interviews and references, both of which are widely used by medical practices and healthcare systems.

Schmidt and Hunter limited their examination of selection methods to two-predictor pairs (GMA + Integrity tests; GMA + Structured Interview, etc.). Cortina, et al.,[9] however, looked at outcomes associated with the three predictor combination of GMA + Conscientiousness + Structured Interview. They confirmed the importance of the GMA + Conscientiousness combination, and also concluded that structured interviews do add incremental validity to the GMA + Conscientiousness combination, *to the extent that interviews are well structured*. Adding information from *highly* structured interviews contributed *substantially* to hiring better employees, while information from less-structured interviews helped less so. Unstructured interviews added no significant predictability to the GMA + Conscientiousness combination.

**What Does This Mean For You?**

The significance of these findings is that you can develop an effective employment process using empirically based selection methods for front office and administrative jobs in your practice that rely on assessing GMA, conscientiousness, and structured interview questions. The implications for filling very high-level professional positions, such as physicians, are somewhat different, but we will discuss physician selection in a separate part of this chapter. For now, let's focus on the majority of jobs in your practice, such as clerical (receptionist, word processor, scheduling), technical (lab technician), professional (nurse), and administrative (business manager) positions. The first element in your selection process should be GMA. There are many good GMA tests. The one I will use to illustrate this class of tests is called the Wonderlic Personnel Test, which is described in **Exhibit 4–2**. **Exhibit 4–3** contains the test's cover page, which provides an idea of the type of questions it contains. It is an inexpensive, fast, easily scored objective test of GMA that your office manager or a clerical can administer and score. Here's a personal example of the relevance of this type of testing. An applicant for a front office position, who was well dressed, and had good conversational English skills scored at the 12th percentile (88% of the general population would score higher than her) on the Wonderlic. As an example, she could not answer questions that were similar to the following:

An auto dealer bought some cars for $100,000. He sold them for $200,000, making $5,000 on each car. How many cars were involved?

Evaluation of her verbal skills and her motivation to get the job, as one would do in an interview, would never lead you to believe that she could not deal with simple reasoning problems, such as the one just given. In addition, if you asked her to divide 100,000 by

**Exhibit 4–2**  Wonderlic Personnel Test Description

---

**Purpose:** Measures level of mental ability that is relevant to business situations, such as jobs in a practice's front office as well as office management jobs such as practice business manager. The test will identify applicants who can generalize from principles, who can learn quickly, and who can adapt more quickly to unique situations. Similarly, it identifies applicants who will work more effectively at simpler more routine jobs.

**Description:** 50-item paper-pencil test measuring general learning ability in verbal, spatial, and numerical reasoning. Test items include simple arithmetic problems, rearrangement of words to form sentences, analogies, assembling geometric figures, logic problems, and following directions.

**Administration and Scoring:** 12 minutes. It can be easily scored with a scoring template placed next to the applicant's answers.

**Publisher:** E.F. Wonderlic Personnel Test, Inc.

*Source:* Adapted from Maddox, T. (Ed.). (1997). *Tests—A Comprehensive Reference for Assessments in Psychology, Education, and Business,* (4th ed.) Austin, TX: Pro-Ed.

---

5,000, she could give you the correct answer. What she was incapable of doing, however, was knowing *how* to analyze problems such as this and *when* to use certain arithmetical skills. This inability would show up on a frequent basis in any medical practice. If you think back to the discussion of false positives and false negatives, then it's obvious not to place a bet on this applicant.

The next element in your selection process will be to measure some relevant personality issues. Modern personality theory and research has concluded that there are five major personality factors, which are referred to as the Big 5. These are described in **Exhibit 4–4**. Integrity tests, which Schmidt and Hunter determined were highest in validity after GMA, are highly correlated with conscientiousness, and to some degree with agreeableness and emotional stability. Integrity tests, per se, are designed to identify those who are likely to steal or otherwise be "organizationally delinquent." I will discuss integrity tests in greater detail in a separate section, because there may be circumstances that would make you want to use them irre-

spective of other elements in your selection plan. Because integrity tests are strongly correlated with personality factors, the next element in your selection process should be a personality test. As one example, the Hogan Personality Inventory (HPI) is supported by numerous validity studies and is one company's own development of assessing a combination of Big 5 personality factors that they have found to predict job success.[10] The test is easily and quickly administered, can be scored online, and provides clear evaluations of applicants. An example of a partial Hogan Personality Inventory report is found in **Exhibit 4–5**. This graph indicates that the applicant has adequate adjustment, prudence, and inquisitiveness for the job. Ambition and interpersonal sensitivity are low, and the other scales are not relevant to success on this job.

If the job that you are filling requires some interpersonal or verbal communication skills, then the final element in your selection process should be, as Cortina et al. suggest, a structured interview. The interview is the most commonly used selection tool in the

**Exhibit 4–3**  Wonderlic Personnel Test Form

---

*WONDERLIC*

# PERSONNEL TEST

FORM V

NAME ................................................................................ Date ...............................

(Please Print)

Social Security Number    ⬜⬜⬜⬛⬜⬜⬛⬜⬜⬜

READ THIS PAGE CAREFULLY. DO EXACTLY AS YOU ARE TOLD.
DO NOT TURN OVER THIS PAGE UNTIL YOU ARE
INSTRUCTED TO DO SO.

PROBLEMS MUST BE WORKED WITHOUT THE AID OF A CALCULATOR
OR OTHER PROBLEM-SOLVING DEVICE.

This is a test of problem solving ability.  It contains various types of questions.  Below is a sample question correctly filled in:

PLACE ANSWERS HERE

REAP is the opposite of
   1 obtain,    2 cheer,    3 continue,    4 exist,    5 <u>sow</u> ................................................. [ 5 ]

The correct answer is "sow".  (It is helpful to underline the correct word.)  The correct word is numbered 5.  Then write the figure 5 in the brackets <u>at the end of the line.</u>

Answer the next sample question yourself.

Paper sells for 23 cents per pad.  What will 4 pads cost?.......................................................... [    ]

The correct answer is 92¢.  There is nothing to underline so just place "92¢" in the brackets.

Here is another example:

MINER    MINOR — Do these words
   1 have similar meanings,    2 have contradictory meanings,    3 mean neither the same nor opposite? [    ]

The correct answer is "mean neither same nor opposite" which is number 3 so all you have to do is place a figure "3" in the brackets <u>at the end of the line.</u>

When the answer to a question is a letter or a number, put the letter or number in the brackets.
All letters should be printed.

This test contains 50 questions.  It is unlikely that you will finish all of them, but do your best.  After the examiner tells you to begin, you will be given exactly 12 minutes to work as many as you can.  Do not go so fast that you make mistakes since you must try to get as many right as possible.  The questions become increasingly difficult, so do not skip about.  Do not spend too much time on any one problem.  The examiner will not answer any questions after the test begins.

Now, lay down your pencil and wait for the examiner to tell you to begin!

*Do not turn the page until you are told to do so.*      925714870

**Exhibit 4–4** Big 5 Personality Factors

Extroversion—relates to the quality and intensity of social interaction. Those high on this factor are sociable, assertive, and outward oriented. Those low on this factor are observed to be inward oriented, quiet, and reserved.

Openness To Experience—the degree to which the person is open to new experiences, intellectually curious, and broad-minded. Those high on this factor seek new opportunities and experiences, while those low on this factor prefer to keep things the same and consistent.

Conscientiousness—orientation toward hard work, dependability, follow through. Those high on this factor tend to be highly motivated and work toward goals, while those who are low tend to be lazy, disorganized, and unreliable.

Neuroticism—reflects on the person's emotional stability. People low on this factor tend to be more calm, confident, and in control, while those high on it tend to be emotionally reactive and prone to and reactive to psychological distress.

Agreeableness—relates to the quality of interpersonal relationships. Those high on this factor tend to be flexible, good-natured, and cooperative, while those who are low on it tend to be cold, distant, and in the extreme, antagonistic and unpleasant.

United States. Unfortunately, given the way that it is typically used, it is less effective than it could be. A structured interview has the following characteristics:

- The interview is limited to measuring factors that have been identified in a job analysis.
- Questions are written ahead of time.
- Scoring standards are identified for each question; that is, the characteristics of a good answer and a bad answer, at a minimum, are written down. This alleviates the problem of interviewers writing "great" questions, only to learn later that even they can't determine what constitutes a good or a poor response!
- All applicants are asked the same questions in the same order, thereby giving everyone a "level playing field."
- Applicant answers then are compared to the scoring standards to evaluate how well they performed.

Unfortunately, most interviewers don't use these structural elements and to the extent that they don't the accuracy of their inter-

view decisions decreases. There are several reasons for this state of affairs. Many employers view the hiring process as a test of their own personal intuition. They don't view the interview as a distinct tool. Instead, they believe that their personal intuition is the tool and that the interview simply provides a time, a place, and a process in which to utilize their intuition. If in fact the interview is really nothing more than an opportunity to apply intuition and perspicacity, then it requires no prior preparation. In addition, many employers, physicians, and their business managers included, don't want to take the time to prepare a proper interview. As a result, the interview is often a morass of questions that are either "pets" (posed to all applicants irrespective of the job) or created on the spot with little or no thought regarding what is being measured or how to evaluate the applicant's response.

Irrespective of the research evidence, interviewers usually are convinced that they make good employment decisions. Two factors usually operate to create this fallacious belief in success. First, many tend to selectively

**Exhibit 4–5** Candidate Potential Report

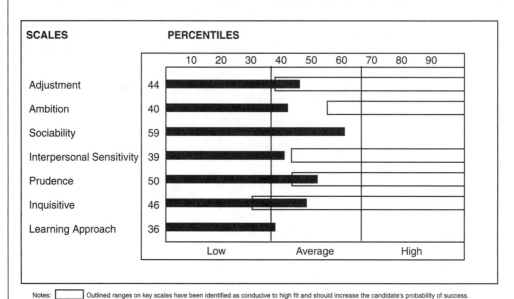

## SECTION II – GRAPHIC REPORT – HOGAN PERSONALITY INVENTORY

Notes: Outlined ranges on key scales have been identified as conducive to high fit and should increase the candidate's probability of success.

| Scales | Scale Descriptions |
|---|---|
| Adjustment | Concerns composure, optimism, and stable moods. |
| Ambition | Concerns taking initiative, being competitive, and seeking leadership roles. |
| Sociability | Concerns seeming talkative, socially bold, and entertaining. |
| Interpersonal Sensitivity | Concerns being agreeable, considerate, and skilled at maintaining relationships. |
| Prudence | Concerns being conscientious, dependable, and rule-abiding. |
| Inquisitive | Concerns being curious, imaginative, visionary, and easily bored. |
| Learning Approach | Concerns enjoying formal education and actively staying up-to-date on business and technical matters. |

## SECTION III – OVERALL EVALUATION OF CANDIDATE

Based on the assessment results, and in comparison to the job specific profile for your company, the overall fit for the position is:

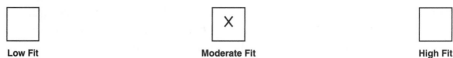

**Low Fit**                    **Moderate Fit**                    **High Fit**

*Source:* Hogan Assessment Systems © 2005. All rights reserved, used with permission.

remember the past. Good employment decisions tend to be remembered, and bad ones tend to be forgotten or explained away. Second, there will always be a natural incidence of success. Even if you make hiring decisions by tossing a coin, some of those chosen will be successful employees. If a job is minimally demanding or if your recruiting is effective, some proportion of the applicants might well have the appropriate skills because those who are unable or uninterested will tend to self-select out. As a consequence, even poor interviewing will likely result in some hiring success, and the interviewer will be led to overestimate his or her contribution to this success. The interviewer then will continue to use the interview in ways that contribute little or nothing to obtaining better employees.

Many review studies have consistently pointed to the superiority of structured interviews over the unstructured anecdotal interviews conducted by most healthcare organizations.[11–13] For example, Weisner and Cronshaw noted that the average correlation between interviewers' predictions of job performance and actual job performance was 0.20, but when interviewers used a structured interview method, the correlation increased to 0.63. Because of the nature of the number scale for these values, the degree of predictability for the structured interview was actually almost *10 times higher* than for the unstructured interview.[14]

Now, let's turn to the issue of *what* to measure with a structured interview. Schmidt and Hunter noted that the employment method that added the second highest level (24%) of incremental to GMA was called a work sample. In a work sample, applicants perform aspects or simulated aspects of critical job elements. For example, you might have clerical applicants do word processing of typical documents that appear on the job. As a result, you get a sample of their performance during the application process that shows you how they would probably perform on the job. As with integrity tests, I will have a separate section later in this chapter discussing work samples in greater detail. For now, however, let's think about how the structured interview could also be used as a work sample. Consider what you are asking applicants to do during an interview: *communicate* and *interact* in a social situation. A successful structured interview strategy, therefore, will utilize the interview to assess those things for which an interview is a natural work sample and will do this in a structured manner. It will focus, therefore, on interpersonal skills and communication skills. Applied examples could include ability to use conversational medical terminology, negotiate a fee agreement or payment plan, communicate policy accurately to front office staff, supervise front office staff, and so forth. You would probably unconsciously abide by the work sample rule for interviewing in extreme cases. Few employers, for example, would ask an applicant whether he or she is a good typist! Obviously, applicants could say whatever they please, whereas a simple typing (word-processing) test would provide much more accurate information. Beyond simplistic examples, however, employers are inclined to misuse the interview in other absurd, if less-obvious, ways. For example, if you use the interview to assess technical skills, reliability, learning ability, intelligence, work attitudes, honesty, or personality traits, you are misusing it. It's not that these issues are unimportant, it's just that the interview isn't the best way to assess them.

**Exhibit 4–6** contains some examples of structured interview questions and response categories for a supervisory skills factor. Notice that the scoring categories are not specific answers but instead delineate the

**Exhibit 4–6** Structured Interview Questions and Response Categories

---

*Supervisory Skills for Business Manager Position:* Exhibiting patience and tactfulness when dealing with fellow employees, remaining open to new ideas and suggestions, and listening to and understanding employee needs.

1.  How would you handle a situation in which there is a deterioration in a subordinate's performance?
    A.  *Good:* Answer refers to attempts to determine the cause and to institute corrective actions.
    B.  *Fair:* Answer refers to confrontation with and warning of subordinate.
    C.  *Poor:* Answer refers to dismissal of subordinate, or no attempt at corrective action, or to corrective actions that does not directly address the performance problem.

2.  Lori is a secretary who collects patient fees and does word processing and other clerical tasks. She comes to you with an idea for improving the negotiation of patient fees. Negotiation of patient fees is your job, not hers. How would you respond?
    A.  *Good:* Answer refers to sincere evaluation of the subordinate's suggestion and to attempt to understand the reasons why it was suggested.
    B.  *Poor:* Answer refers to superficial acceptance without evaluation, or to outright rejection of the idea of a subordinate making such a suggestion.

3.  An employee comes to you to discuss a personal problem. How would you respond to this situation?
    A.  *Good:* Answer characterized by setting aside time to examine with the employee the problem's possible job-related consequences, as well as the personal consequences.
    B.  *Fair:* Answer characterized by a discussion of the job-related consequences only.
    C.  *Poor:* Answer characterized by discussion of the personal consequences only.
    D.  *Very poor:* Answer characterized by refusal to discuss the problem and telling the employee, implicitly or explicitly, to leave personal problems at home.

---

*characteristics* of what constitutes better versus worse response. People are very creative, and you will never anticipate all the unique answers that applicants will produce. Generally, however, there will be three or four themes that run through answers, which intuitively characterize their quality. This is what you are trying to build your scoring categories around. *If you can't write good scoring categories, then you probably have a poorly worded or ill-conceived question! Remember, if you can't specify characteristics of what you are looking for, then don't expect applicants to, or expect that you will be able to after you've interviewed several applicants!*

It is usually sufficient to anticipate three levels of response to a question, such as "outstanding," "acceptable," and "not acceptable." The number of evaluation categories is arbitrary, and should depend on what you find to be useful. Some questions might generate five easily separated categories, whereas other questions could be evaluated with only two categories.

When you conduct the interview, you should concentrate on what the applicant is saying and take notes for later evaluation. After the interview, you can rewrite your notes into a more complete narrative evaluation, so you can more easily recall the applicant's responses. You can also then classify the responses into scoring categories. If the applicant says something that you want to pursue during the interview, feel free to pursue it. Be certain, however, to come back to the point of departure and proceed from there.

It is very important to understand that your evaluation criteria express a value system.

For example, look at question 3 in Exhibit 4–6. Some physicians might consider category "D" (the lowest category) to be desirable, and they personally would evaluate applicants who would discuss the personal and business implications of a personal problem (category A) with a subordinate as having poor supervisory skills. Scoring categories often represent a value system that should reflect *your* preferences. There is nothing wrong with this, as long as you understand your preferences and *consciously* build them into the applicant-evaluation process. Problems arise when you select employees on one basis, but then ask them to perform in a contrary manner. To achieve consistency between your preferences and employee characteristics, you may have to engage in some serious introspection. If you feel that the best strategy for running a practice is to refuse to discuss personal problems, then don't hire applicants whose natural inclination is to do the contrary.

Keep in mind that the interview will best assess applicants' abilities when they are using their skills as they would use them on the job. For example, if you are trying to assess medical terminology skills, then develop questions around discussions that require the understanding and correct utilization of medical language. On the other hand, if you are trying to assess general language skills and good grammar, then get the applicant to talk on any topic familiar to them, such as hobbies, career goals, or previous jobs. Concentrate on *how* applicants communicate as opposed to the *content* of their communication.

If you are familiar with the job and have developed a clear list of selection factors, then it should take an hour or so to develop questions and evaluation criteria for the relevant interview factors. Keep in mind that the questions and evaluation criteria for each factor may be used again for this job in the future and for other jobs that require the same factor, so think of this as reusable instrument rather than a throw-away tool. If, for example, you have several clerical jobs that require good verbal skills, then you can most likely use the same questions and criteria for all these jobs going forward.

## WHO SHOULD DESIGN AND CONDUCT YOUR TESTING?

Testing is truly a double-edged sword. It provides considerable power, but specific knowledge about this subject is necessary if this power is to be effectively used. As was pointed out, it is possible for your staff to identify employment factors, select tests, and put the process into operation without any outside help. This is especially the case if you have a staff person who is interested in the subject and is willing to do some reading and self-education. Generally, however, physician leaders working in private practices and smaller healthcare organizations that don't employ a human resources specialist should consider using a consultant to help guide the introduction of testing. One cost-effective way to find a knowledgeable consultant is to contact the business or psychology department at a local college or university. Another approach is to contact major testing companies, such as Hogan Assessment Systems or E.F. Wonderlic, as two examples. They provide selection design services to ensure that the selection procedures are appropriate for jobs and comply with federal equal employment opportunity laws (see Chapter 10). This extra level of assurance is especially important if your staff is new to this approach to employment.

A consultant can work with your staff to develop accurate job descriptions, write structured interview questions, identify and obtain testing materials, develop work samples, train your staff to correctly administer the employment methods, provide your staff with an effective model of how to combine the information to make hiring decisions, and give them confidence. Remember, once you find a method (test, work sample, etc.) that satisfactorily measures a job-related factor, it can be used for any other job that requires that same performance factor. Ideally, the employment tests that a consultant recommends should be scorable by your staff or the test publisher online so you can get immediate results. Be suspicious if a consultant recommends tests, other than work samples, that are "self-developed" or only scorable by the consultant. Locking yourself into this kind of arrangement may limit your future flexibility, as well as result in inflated consulting fees. Your staff should be able to do a creditable job of constructing work samples, especially if the initial efforts are supervised by a knowledgeable consultant.

Structured interviewing is a task that business managers and office managers should be able to perform themselves. If they have no experience doing structured interviewing, then some initial training is desirable. In general, interviewing should not be totally contracted out to a consultant. The personal involvement of your staff in selecting their colleagues will more than compensate for their initial lack of structured interviewing experience. Generally, an employee will be more knowledgeable than a consultant about the position. Finally, using employees to conduct structured interviews will develop their interview skills, thereby giving you the flexibility to respond to unexpected employment needs and to keep your consulting costs down.

Whether physicians should get personally involved depends on the position, and how you value your time. If you will be working closely with whomever is selected, you will probably want some involvement. Obviously, you will only want to use your time to inter-

view the best applicants—those who have already cleared other selection hurdles. Positions more removed from the focus of your personal activities might not require your personal attention. This is, however, a matter of personal preference. Some practice-based physician leaders insist on personally interviewing all their employees, even if only to have the final selection approval.

Physician leaders in larger healthcare organizations should expect the human resources (HR) staff to be thoroughly competent in the use of tests, structured interviews, work samples, and other modern employment methods. If this is not the case, then the appropriate role for the physician leader is to set goals for the HR staff to obtain these skills. This may include hiring someone with the appropriate expertise, or having a current staff member obtain formal training in testing, work sampling, and structured interviewing.

## THE RÉSUMÉ

Résumés are valuable sources of information for two reasons. First, résumés are samples of applicants' behaviors. They are statements that applicants prepare by themselves or at least approve of the final product! They do this at their own pace, stating what they feel is important about themselves, and what qualifies them for a job. Look at a résumé first, therefore, as a work sample. Second, each résumé is a statement of what the applicant has been doing with his or her life.

When examining a résumé as a work sample, consider its orderliness, neatness, and organization. How clearly and concisely does it convey information? If the applicant takes two pages to express what could be presented in one page, this may indicate that the applicant will not be able to construct concise documents or arguments or "get to the point" on the job. This would be an hypothesis to evaluate during the employment process, if you feel the applicant otherwise is qualified for the position. Does it appear that some thought has gone toward organizing information in a logical manner? If the résumé is confusing or illogically organized, this is an indication that the applicant may not be able to present information in a logical, understandable manner to you, your employees, patients, and so forth. Are spelling, punctuation, and grammar correct? If you find mistakes, then it may mean that the applicant does not have basic language skills, is a lazy or sloppy worker, or tends to be rushed and make mistakes. Irrespective of the causal hypothesis, focusing on the behavior is sufficient to exclude the applicant.

After you have evaluated the résumé as a work sample, evaluate its content. First, examine the applicant's previous experience and education to determine whether he or she has the skills required for the job. This does not mean that the applicant must have performed a job with the same job title or previously worked for a medical organization. For example, bookkeeping in a medical practice is little different from bookkeeping in any other type of professional or service organization. An applicant who has worked for an accounting firm, a lawyer, or an architect should have little difficulty making the transition to a medical practice.

Examine how frequently the applicant has changed jobs. Eliminate applicants who have a history of frequent job changes. They are job hoppers who will be dissatisfied in any situation, and their dissatisfaction will cause disruption and dissension. Look for a logical order or progression to the job changes. Good applicants will show a history of increased skills and responsibilities. A bookkeeper who then became a secretary, and then the receivables administrator for a 15-physician practice, and who now is applying to become the manager of a 5-physician

practice is moving in the right direction. The manager of a 5-physician practice who is now willing to take a secretarial position is going in the wrong direction. The associated pay and status reductions can create all sorts of acting out and displaced anger. Going back to our betting analogy, this latter applicant is a bad bet.

Examine the résumé for unexplained gaps in employment. If you find any, the applicant must account for them—*all of them*. An employment gap sometimes indicates failure at a job, perhaps even time in jail. Discuss any gaps with the applicant during the interview. You will have to make a judgment concerning the reasonableness of the applicant's explanation.

For many jobs, education and experience are to some degree interchangeable. An applicant for a bookkeeping position who has no previous experience but has received appropriate, documented education might well be able to perform the job. Jobs requiring skills that normally are not obtained through formal education, such as insurance billing, are best performed by people who have had previous experience. This, of course, creates a problem for the inexperienced applicant: how to obtain experience if the only people who are hired are people with experience. This is a problem, but it is not *your* problem.

Generally, the person screening the résumés for a position should be the one to whom the incumbent will report. Managers (physician and nonphysician) may be tempted to delegate initial résumé screening to others. Your ability to judge with whom you can work, however, can rarely be matched, and never exceeded, by the judgment of others.

## THE APPLICATION FORM

Generally, the initial screening of applicants will be based on résumés, followed by short telephone interviews. Survivors then will be invited in for additional interviewing, testing, and so on. It is desirable at this point to have all applicants complete an application form. This will make it easier to compare applicants on education, previous experience, and the like. The alternative is to dig this information out of the résumés, which is a frustrating, time-consuming job. Another important reason for using an application form is that it can provide legal justification for immediately dismissing an employee who lied about qualifications, credentials, previous experience, and so on. The application form should state that supplying false or misleading information may result in the immediate termination of employment.[15]

Application forms should only request job-relevant information. Do not ask applicants about their race, religion, sex, national origin, age, or disability, because these are not relevant to evaluating applicant performance. **Exhibit 4–7** contains a sample application form. State laws vary considerably regarding what questions are permissible, and you should contact your attorney before using any application form. Refer to Chapter 10 for a more complete discussion of equal employment opportunity and how to utilize your attorney.

Finally, if the employee will be working without a written contract, the application form should contain a strong at-will employment provision, as does the form in Exhibit 4–7. At-will employment gives you flexibility to terminate an unsatisfactory employee. Once again, refer to Chapter 10 for a discussion of at-will employment and written contract employment arrangements.

## ADDITIONAL TESTING

### Performance and Skills Tests

As noted previously, GMA should be the core of your selection process for most of the jobs in your practice or healthcare organization. There may be other critical job skills where testing is appropriate. Often, this will be the case with clerical and technical positions. For example, imagine having to put a check mark next to the pairs of numbers that are the same in **Exhibit 4–8**. The task on its face is easy. Imagine, however, that you now had to scan 200 such pairs and do it in 4 minutes! Obviously, some people are much better at this task, which assesses underlying skills of speed, attention to detail, eye-hand coordination, and working under pressure. The average score on this test is 112 correct identifications, yet some people can get 180 or more correct, while others only 50. In the busy front end of a medical practice, these are relevant clerical skills. In addition, these skills are uncorrelated with GMA and personality. The test just described is called the Hay Aptitude Test Battery: Number Perception.[16] Now, imagine that you have two clerical applicants to choose from who are roughly equal on the other aspects of the employment process, and one scores 100 on this test and another scores 150. It's clear where you should place your bet.

This test, as an example, raises the question of how you find out about tests that could be useful to you. There are several ways you can do this. One is to hire a consultant to help you develop selection processes for jobs. If you don't want to do this, then I suggest contacting major test publishers. **Exhibit 4–9** contains a limited list of test publishers. Once you are familiar with your jobs through job analysis, you can knowledgably talk with publishers about the skills you are trying to assess, and determine if their tests may be appropriate. In addition to the short list in Exhibit 4–9, you can do Google searches to find additional test publishers. When talking with test publishers always ask about their validity studies.

**Exhibit 4–7** Application Form with At-Will Statement

APPLICATION FOR EMPLOYMENT WITH GREENWICH MEDICAL ASSOCIATES, P.C.

| Last Name | First Name | | Middle Name | |

| Present Address (Street, City, State, Zip Code) | Telephone Number | Social Security Number |

| Position Applying for | Date Available |

| Names and Addresses of Schools Attended | Dates From | To | Degree | Major or Subject Area | Grade Point Average |
|---|---|---|---|---|---|
| | | | | | |
| | | | | | |
| | | | | | |
| | | | | | |
| | | | | | |

| Licenses or Certificates | Granting Agency | Expiration Date |
|---|---|---|
| | | |
| | | |
| | | |
| | | |

Honor Societies, Professional Societies, Etc.:

List all previous work experience. Begin with most recent position held. Use additional Application Forms if Necessary.

| Employer's Name and Address | Supervisor's Name and Title | Job Title and Work Description | Salary | Employed From | To |
|---|---|---|---|---|---|
| | | | | | |
| | | | | | |
| | | | | | |
| | | | | | |
| | | | | | |
| | | | | | |

| Work or Educational references Name of reference | Name of organization | This Reference Was Your: |
|---|---|---|
| | | |
| | | |
| | | |

I acknowledge that I am seeking employment with Greenwich Medical Associates, P.C. I further state that all of the information that I have provided is true. By signing this application form, I acknowledge that employment may be denied or terminated if I have supplied false or misleading information. I also understand that the position that I am applying for is an at-will position, and that if I am hired my employment can be terminated a the sole discretion of the employer.

Job Applicant's Signature: _____   Date _____

Reputable publishers don't sell a test unless they have scientifically validated it on samples of applicants, and can statistically demonstrate that their test really measures what it purports to measure. Just because a test is named "Clerical Speed Test" doesn't tell you how well it measures this construct or in fact whether it measures it at all. The proof is in the data, so always ask to see validation data.

**Exhibit 4–8** Number Comparison Task

| Place a check mark next to the items that are the same. | | |
| --- | --- | --- |
| 6767 | 6767 | ____ |
| 25334 | 25334 | ____ |
| 845 | 854 | ____ |
| 6798 | 6798 | ____ |
| 29423 | 29423 | ____ |
| 38995 | 38959 | ____ |
| 7402 | 7402 | ____ |
| 87994 | 87994 | ____ |
| 2492 | 2492 | ____ |
| 10772 | 10772 | ____ |

**Exhibit 4–9** Selected Test Publishers and Potentially Useful Tests for Practice Selection

Wonderlic, Inc.
1795 N. Butterfield Rd.
Libertyville, IL 60048
(800) 323-3742
www.wonderlic.com/default.asp
Test Types: GMA, Integrity, Personality

Hogan Assessment Systems
P.O. Box 521176
Tulsa, OK 74152
(918) 749-0632
(800) 756-0632
www.hoganassessments.com/
Test Types: Personality, Integrity, Organizational Fit

Personnel Decisions, Inc.
2000 Plaza VII Tower
45 South Seventh Street
Minneapolis, MN 55402-1608
(800) 633-4410
www.personneldecisions.com/
Test Types: GMA, Personality, Integrity

Psychological Assessment Resources, Inc. (PAR)
16204 North Florida Avenue
Lutz, FL 33549
(800) 331-8378
www3.parinc.com/default.aspx
Test Types: GMA, Personality

Although most tests are available and usable by anyone, distribution of some psychological tests is restricted to those with appropriate qualifications. If you or your staff don't meet the publisher's qualifications, don't try to circumvent these restrictions because this indicates that the test requires a sophisticated understanding of testing theory or specific training in the test to use it effectively. Remember, if you use a test improperly, you may deceive yourself regarding the quality of applicants whom you hire. Either make the investment and get the necessary training, or continue looking for another test that assesses the same factor. There are thousands of tests available, and usually any given factor can be assessed using literally dozens of unrestricted, published tests. The difference between restricted and unrestricted tests is often analogous to the difference between the prescription and nonprescription strengths of some medications. The "nonprescription" test may be more than adequate for your purpose, as well as easier to score and less expensive. Finally, some test publishers are hesitant to sell their tests unless you contract with them for a job-analysis study, which they can do by questionnaire. In some instances, this may be an effective way for you to do a job analysis and ensure that the selection instruments are appropriate for the job. In other instances, this is simply a testing company's attempt to extract extra revenue from a potential client who already knows what needs to be assessed.

## Honesty/Integrity Tests

As noted, Schmidt and Hunter found that integrity tests added the largest amount (27%) of incremental validity to GMA. Also as suggested, personality testing, which looks at a combination of conscientiousness and other Big 5 personality variables correlates highly with integrity tests, so if you are doing personality assessment, then integrity assessment certainly is not necessary. That aside, however, there may be some specific reasons why you might want to consider integrity testing. All of us have heard stories about the trusted employee who embezzles funds.[17] Theft of cash, supplies, and inventory is an important business problem, with annual estimates of financial losses running between $15 billion and $25 billion. One attempt to reduce losses due to theft was to use a polygraph or lie detector test to screen applicants. Research strongly indicated that the polygraph was not effective at screening applicants.[18] In addition, the Employee Polygraph Protection Act of 1988 makes the use of polygraphs illegal for screening applicants for virtually all organizations.[19]

Generally, organizations try to reduce theft through cash control methods, such as separating the collection of cash from the accounting for it, and regular monitoring and reconciling of financial reports, such as revenue, receipts, and write-off reports. Although these tactics are important, they are essentially defensive and reactive in nature. *Integrity tests*, sometimes called *honesty tests*, are easily administered and scored paper-and-pencil tests that can be used to screen job applicants for "organizationally delinquent" behaviors, including likelihood to steal or commit sabotage, alcohol and drug abuse, absenteeism, lying, unreliability, immaturity, insubordination, and the like.

Conceptually, integrity tests assess deviance from accepted socialization standards.

Socialization appears to be normally distributed, with a few individuals being overly conscientious, most being generally rule compliant, and a few being rule resistant, which in extreme cases results in law violations. Hogan and Hogan, who have conducted extensive research on identifying organizational delinquents, concluded:

> ". . . there are people who, although hostile to rules, manage to avoid becoming involved with the legal system, and, therefore, are not identified as delinquent. We believe that they are the people who cause most of the problems in organizations."[20]

How well do integrity tests work? In order to answer this question, please recall the concepts of true-positive and false-positive errors, and that selecting applicants with higher test scores increases the chance of a true positive but also increases the chances of false negatives. Now, let's look at the results of one study to illustrate the potential strengths and weaknesses of integrity testing.[21] An integrity test was given to 482 grocery store applicants before employment. Because this was an experiment, the test results were not used, and all 482 applicants were hired. After 8 months, 17 had been identified as thieves and of these, 94 percent (16 of 17) had failed the integrity test. This certainly sounds like a success. Of the remaining employees, however, 48 percent also had failed the test! Some of these may have been thieves who had not been caught or who hadn't yet stolen, but many were undoubtedly false positives.

From a decision-making perspective, if we had used the test to make hiring decisions and rejected all applicants who failed the test, we would have eliminated 94 percent of the theft, but we also would have had to identify an additional 225 applicants to fill all 482 positions because of the incidence of false positives. Recruiting and screening an additional 225 applicants is obviously an expensive and time-consuming process. Scaling this down to selection ratios more typical of a healthcare organization, this would suggest that if your current employment methods require you to evaluate 10 applicants for a receptionist position, you might have to evaluate on average 15 to find an applicant who both is qualified on your other tests, interviews, and so forth *and* passes the integrity test.

What about legal issues? There is a substantial body of data indicating that professionally developed integrity tests do not discriminate unfairly on the basis of race, gender, or age.[22] Privacy law generally has focused on the invasiveness of the information collection process, such as blood, urine, and polygraph testing. There are virtually no privacy cases that challenge the content of integrity tests. The Employee Polygraph Protection Act of 1988, which essentially outlawed polygraph testing by private employers, specifically excludes oral and written tests. As with most aspects of life these days, however, you may want to consult your attorney for any recent cases or statutes in your state.

Integrity testing is controversial, and there is still some disagreement in the field about whether it really provides a useful indication of counterproductive behavior. There have been some allegations, for example, that the tests can be easily faked and that coaching can affect scores.[23] Few applicants, however, will have access to coaching help, and many integrity tests contain scales that effectively detect faking. If integrity testing sounds like it might be helpful, and if you feel ethically comfortable using this type of instrument, then contact several test publishers including those listed in Exhibit 4–9. Have your business manager or personnel/human re-

sources department consider the specific delinquency issues assessed, cost, administration time, validation data demonstrating that the test really works, and convenience of scoring when deciding whether to use a particular test. Integrity testing, as with personality testing, will be more expensive than GMA or performance and skills tests, so if you decide to use one, use it only on finalists who otherwise are fully qualified. This will keep your evaluation costs down.

## Drug Testing

Drug testing of applicants may be appropriate under certain circumstances. Bear in mind, however, that a recent national survey indicates that the overall presence of workplace impairment due to illict drugs is less than 3 percent of the workforce.[24] Drug testing is a relatively expensive procedure, so you should give careful consideration to when and how you use it. There are a number of different drug tests. The least expensive, at a cost of about $15 to $20, is thin-layer chromatography (TLC). Its interpretation is also the most subjective. Enzyme immunoassay (EIA) and radioimmunoassay (RIA) are slightly more expensive but provide more definitive results. These tests can detect the eight major abused drugs or drug classes: amphetamines, barbiturates, benzodiazepines, cannabinoids, cocaine, methaqualone, opiates, and phencyclidine. EIA and RIA are the most commonly used employment drug tests and cost between $30 and $50. Finally, gas chromatography and mass spectroscopy offer much greater sensitivity than EIA, RIA, and TLC. Because they are significantly more expensive, they are generally reserved for situations in which extreme accuracy is essential, such as a follow-up to an initially positive finding.

All the tests discussed are susceptible to various degrees of cross-reaction. A *cross-reaction* is when a legal substance, such as poppy seeds, falsely indicates the presence of an illegal substance, such as heroin. With these facts in mind, you may want to consider testing an applicant in the following instances:

- The applicant, once hired, would have ready access to prescription drugs or large sums of cash.
- Other information indicates that the applicant may have a history of illicit drug abuse, but because of other qualities the applicant is at the top of your hiring list.
- The drug screen is the final employment hurdle.

In such situations, employers will generally use an EIA or RIA. If a positive finding is returned, the possibility of a false positive is evaluated using either gas chromatography or mass spectroscopy. Obviously, it is essential for the testing laboratory to retain all samples so that retesting is feasible.

## WORK SAMPLES

Let's use some common sense. One obvious way to know whether a person can perform a job is to put the applicant on the job for a period of time, observe performance, and determine whether it is both minimally adequate and superior to that of other competing applicants. In an ideal world, this is how we would select employees. Unfortunately, there are obvious problems with this approach, the first of which is that it would take excessive time and would be organizationally disruptive to staff, patients, and others to have new applicants cycling through a position. Work sampling, however, uses this principle of obtaining a sample of work, by

reducing its size and length, and isolating applicants from the rest of the organization and patients, so it becomes feasible. If we do this effectively, then we may get a good indication of the applicant's skills. Schmidt and Hunter noted that work samples added 24 percent incremental validity to GMA. More recent meta-analyses also support the validity of work samples.[25]

A commonly used example of this strategy is a word-processing test. This is especially the case if the work sample is constructed from existing practice files and charts, so it is typical of the daily tasks the employee will perform. *A work sample is only appropriate when you do not intend to train the new employee in the particular skill.* For example, word-processing ability is a good work sample candidate, because you certainly wouldn't intend to train a new employee to use Microsoft Office (Word, Excel, Outlook, etc.) when there are many trained applicants looking for jobs. A work sample using your proprietary scheduling software would not be appropriate, because it's not reasonable to expect that applicants will be familiar with it. Another limiting factor for work samples is the complexity of the simulation that you will have to devise, and the amount of time that it will take to assess an applicant. For example, you may be able to devise a work sample for word processing that would take 5 hours to administer and would be very indicative of applicants' abilities, but it would take so much time and be so expensive that it would be impractical.

Here is how to construct a work sample, using word-processing skills as an example. The same basic procedures can be used to design other work sample measures, such as collection actions, and taking BP and other physiological measures. First, review the job description to get a good idea of the nature of documents typed and the word-processing programs used. If you have any doubt, talk to an incumbent and also review documents from current office files. The work sample should contain typical word-processing tasks normally performed, such as a letters, lab reports, patient notes, and the like. Because your goal is to make the work sample representative of office word processing, the range of skills, such as commands, macros, formatting, printing, merging addresses into form letters, exporting to other programs, and so forth also should be represented in your work sample. This may be achieved by pulling together parts from several different documents. It may also require you to construct an item or document that is typical in character and gives applicants a good opportunity to exhibit their skills in a particular area, such as developing style sheets.

Generally, it is best to make the work sample long enough so that even the very best applicants won't be able to finish. This will ensure that you get plenty of range in the scores. It is very important to standardize the work sample testing conditions, so that everyone is tested under similar conditions. Avoid testing in noisy rooms or where applicants may get interrupted by current employees or patients.

Give the applicants plenty of time to learn the "feel" of your word-processing equipment. The test should provide enough time for applicants to fully exhibit their word-processing ability, including speed and accuracy. Use your common sense to develop reasonable scoring criteria. Set reasonable minimum standards in obvious knowledge areas, such as speed, errors, and ability to format, use tables, macros, and style sheets. The particular scoring criteria that you adopt are not as crucial as the consistency with which you apply them. As long as the rules are generally reasonable, the scoring criteria relate

to actual job performance, and the criteria are consistently applied across applicants, the resulting rank ordering of applicants should reflect their relative skill levels.

There are many other opportunities to develop work samples. For example, telephone skills can be assessed by staging a work sample during an interview. Play the role of a caller and have the applicant turn away so as not to react to your facial expressions or body language. Then develop a conversation to assess the applicant's abilities to use language, respond appropriately to questions, and so on. Keep the evaluation criteria simple; this will increase reliability. Develop two or three evaluation criteria, such as these:

- *Adequate:* Handled all questions and situations using appropriate language or tact.
- *Minimal:* Had some problems with appropriate language or tact.
- *Inadequate:* Had substantial problems with appropriate language or tact.

It is important not to confuse personal style preferences with skill. For example, if there is a particular way you like the telephone answered, it is *not* appropriate to expect your preference to be anticipated by applicants. The new employee can be trained in these stylistic matters. Instead, you should be looking for fundamental telephone answering skills, such as tact, appropriate language and grammar, appropriate voice level, and cordiality. In addition, keep your notes to support your conclusions. Later, you may want to review your evaluation of an applicant, and your original notes will allow you to reevaluate and weight the test conclusions.

Collection is another candidate for work sampling. You can construct a work sample around an aging analysis. See whether applicants can determine the highest-priority cases to work, then have simulated case folders available for typical problem accounts. Have applicants draft letters, determine action follow-up dates, recommend actions, and so forth. This process can be much more effective than asking applicants during an interview "How good are you at collection?" Other factors amenable to work sample assessment include writing, filing, checkbook balancing, interacting with patients (using a simulated patient), negotiating patient payment plans or fees (using a simulated patient), problem solving, and responding to insurance claim denials.

## REFERENCES AND RECOMMENDATIONS

References and recommendations are very difficult tools to use, because you can never be certain what motivates those who provide them.[26] Schmidt and Hunter noted that they added only 12 percent incremental validity to GMA. Past employers can have many reasons for giving former employees a good reference, including keeping their own unemployment insurance rates down and fear of legal action on the part of the former employee. Remember, everyone can find someone who will provide a good reference. Even Al Capone had his friends and beneficiaries.

It is very important to limit references to those people who had an employment relationship with the applicant. A personal reference is generally worthless, because the reference has not observed the applicant's actual work performance. In addition, the motivation of the person giving a personal reference is highly suspect. You may be talking to the applicant's brother-in-law. You may be doing this even with an employer reference!

The best way to use a reference is as a means to verify or validate information that you have obtained elsewhere in the employ-

ment process. Personally, I find that it is best to talk on the telephone with whomever is providing a reference. Sometimes, you can obtain more information than the person is willing to commit to writing, and on occasion the person will inadvertently reveal some unintended information by their voice inflection, pauses, and so on.

One of the best ways to use references is as a way of verifying information obtained in another part of the employment process. For example, if psychological testing indicates that an applicant is highly conscientious and strives to deliver the best quality, attempt to verify this by asking "Could you describe some of John's most outstanding qualities?" If the reference doesn't mention anecdotes related to conscientiousness, then you might then state, "Give me an example of an incident that is typical of John's focus on getting the job done." Similarly, if an applicant has indicated that a significant part of his or her job involved insurance collection, you could ask the reference "What were some of the major duties that Sally had?" The answer should verify whether insurance collection was a primary or secondary responsibility.

Asking good questions and designing a strategy by which to use the reference to confirm or disconfirm hypotheses generated in previous employment steps takes time and thought. As a result, obtaining references should be the *final* step in the selection process. Ideally, it should only be used for the top one or two applicants as determined by your other employment methods.

## SELECTION STRATEGY

After reviewing all the selection tools that are available, you may feel that doing a good job of hiring employees is a time-consuming and complicated process. It doesn't have to be. The key to hiring good employees, and doing it in a timely, cost-effective manner, is understanding how to *organize* the process.

The first step in implementing a successful selection strategy is to create a large applicant pool as quickly as possible. The applicant pool is the set of applicants who apply for the job. It is a waste of time and effort to identify and sequentially evaluate a few applicants and then repeat the whole process time and time again. First, there is always a time delay between recruiting efforts and the receipt of résumés. Obviously, if you have to repeat the whole process even once, you will waste considerable time simply waiting for the arrival of additional résumés.

A second and perhaps more important consideration is that a sequential recruiting process may not identify the most qualified applicant. For example, suppose you only use a limited recruiting method, such as word of mouth, that generates a selection pool of three or four applicants. One of these applicants may appear to be an adequate, although not outstanding, prospect. As a result, you find yourself in the difficult position of having to decide between offering this applicant the job or resuming your recruiting efforts. There will be a strong temptation to hire the "bird in hand," because this will relieve your anxiety and allow you to move on to other, more pressing matters, such as practicing medicine. It may be, however, that a far more qualified applicant is out there and that a broader initial search, simultaneously using a newspaper ad, online recruitment, and recruiting at a local university or technical school would have identified this applicant.

Also necessary for developing a successful selection strategy is understanding how to sequence the events and how to process all the applicant information. Generally, the best way of sequencing is to use "multiple hurdles." This means that you order the se-

lection process into sequential stages, so that subsequent employment methods are only applied to the survivors of previous stages. An effective sequencing uses the least expensive and least time-consuming procedures early in the employment process, and reserves the more expensive and more time-consuming procedures for those applicants who have survived the initial hurdles. For example, a reasonable order of events for a clerical position might be as follows:

1. résumé review
2. telephone interview of applicants
3. face-to-face interview and testing of applicants including GMA and any relevant performance and skill testing
4. work sample, personality test
5. telephone reference check

Ideally, you would only conduct the telephone reference check for your top candidate.

An example of a selection sequence for processing 26 applicants is illustrated in **Exhibit 4–10**. In step 1, the 26 résumés are classified as good or bad. Only the 14 good applicants pass on to step 2 and are interviewed by telephone. Of these survivors, six pass the telephone interview, and one self-selects out of the process. Following this step and all subsequent steps, those who are "survivors" are asked if they are still interested in the position, so those who are uninterested can easily self-select out. Six move on to step 3, which involves testing and initial face-to-face interviewing. Based on the testing and interviewing, applicants A, D, and E stand out. They are invited back for a second interview and personality testing. Applicant A is evaluated as superior and continues to express interest in the job, so his or her references are checked. The references' comments are consistent with the previous testing and interviewing, so A is offered the position. If

**Exhibit 4–10** Sequence of Employment Steps

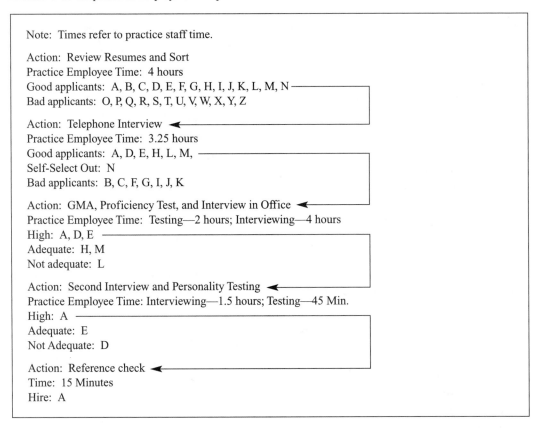

Note: Times refer to practice staff time.

Action: Review Resumes and Sort
Practice Employee Time: 4 hours
Good applicants: A, B, C, D, E, F, G, H, I, J, K, L, M, N
Bad applicants: O, P, Q, R, S, T, U, V, W, X, Y, Z

Action: Telephone Interview
Practice Employee Time: 3.25 hours
Good applicants: A, D, E, H, L, M,
Self-Select Out: N
Bad applicants: B, C, F, G, I, J, K

Action: GMA, Proficiency Test, and Interview in Office
Practice Employee Time: Testing—2 hours; Interviewing—4 hours
High: A, D, E
Adequate: H, M
Not adequate: L

Action: Second Interview and Personality Testing
Practice Employee Time: Interviewing—1.5 hours; Testing—45 Min.
High: A
Adequate: E
Not Adequate: D

Action: Reference check
Time: 15 Minutes
Hire: A

A's references had not checked out, then E would move to the reference check, and if they checked out, then E would be offered the job. If E failed, then the process would begin again. Exhibit 4–10 indicates that 26 applicants could be evaluated and a job offer realistically made with the expenditure of about 15½ hours of practice employee time.

You also will benefit from providing applicants with detailed, realistic information about the job early in the selection process. This is called a *realistic job preview*. Realistic job previews enable uninterested applicants to drop out of the process, saving you the trouble of evaluating their qualifications. For example, always indicate the salary range early in the evaluation process, such as in the initial telephone contact or perhaps even in

the advertising. Similarly, you should describe the job in some detail in the telephone interview, so uninterested applicants can drop out at that point. During the first face-to-face interview, review the position's duties and responsibilities, and, if possible, show the applicant where he or she would work. Fill in any gaps left by the job description and provide a fair statement of the work, warts and all. Applicants who have unrealistic job expectations and would be likely to quit after a short time on the job tend to self-select out when told the truth.

The selection strategy used for a job is critical to filling the position successfully and economically. This is especially the case the first time or two that you apply these methods to jobs in your practice. It is very important, therefore, to devote your best thinking to the design of the selection strategy. This is an appropriate place for your personal involvement. Subsequently, as your staff becomes more experienced and they can look to past examples, your personal supervision becomes less critical. If you don't have the time or inclination to supervise the early implementations of these methods, then consider retaining a consultant.

Once a selection strategy has been designed for a job, it can be used again for that job. In this way, over time, selection strategies will be acquired for all jobs. These strategies need not change unless the content of jobs change or there is some indication that the selection methods are not working properly, such as dissatisfaction with the quality of hired employee.

Finally, an effective selection strategy is one that is put into practice with *patience*. It is disruptive and perhaps frightening to have an important position vacant. It is far worse, however, to fill the position with the wrong person. Your employment methods may give you answers you don't like. They may indicate that many applicants who initially appeared to be well qualified are not good employment risks. Be persistent, and don't easily take a less-than-adequate applicant simply to fill the position and move on to other issues.

## SELECTING PHYSICIANS AND OTHER PROFESSIONAL EMPLOYEES

Hiring a physician is one of the biggest challenges faced by physician leaders in group practices and large healthcare systems.[27] The right decision can enhance the practice's professional reputation, the quality of services provided, control costs, and increase profitability. A wrong decision can

lead to frustrating interpersonal problems, difficulty in recruiting other physicians, and financial catastrophe. When the stakes are this high, you need to ask yourself "Are the evaluation methods that I'm using simply giving me an excuse to select one applicant over another, or are they *really* able to identify the better candidate?"

As noted, using GMA should be a standard part of the employment process for virtually all jobs in a medical practice. Hiring physicians, however, is the exception. Physicians have gone through an extensive, highly selective educational process, which will result in little useful GMA range. If physicians didn't have adequate GMA to handle the job, they would have been screened out as an undergraduate, in medical school, internship, residency, or licensing. GMA, therefore, has been very adequately assessed, and by definition if a physician is applying for a position in your practice this is not an issue. This brings us back to the questions of *what* to assess; or stated another way, why do physicians fail? After talking with many physicians over the years, the most commonly mentioned theme is "interpersonal stuff"; the ability to work with colleagues and staff, get along well with patients, be flexible, adaptable, and motivated to do a good job.

Considering these issues, unfortunately, résumés, references, and unstructured interviews don't work any more effectively with physicians and other professionals than they do for the administrative and technical positions just described. If your evaluation is limited to interviewing physician applicants and perhaps talking with their references, then you are overlooking several important sources of information that could help you to make a better decision. Certainly, very few *Fortune* 100 companies would fill an equivalently important management or technical position on the basis of an unstructured interview and references. Why? Because there are important job performance issues that can be better measured using the other assessment methods that were discussed previously, including structured interviews, work samples, and, in some cases, psychological testing.

Just as with any job, it is unlikely that unstructured interviews will reveal much information that will allow you to separate physician applicants based on their abilities on the skills just noted. Structured interviews, as we have seen, are more promising. Here, for example, is a sample structured interview question that assesses physician teamwork and respecting collegial boundaries:

While covering for Dr. Jones, you notice that Mrs. Smith is receiving a drug that in your opinion is inferior to the drug that you routinely prescribe. How would you handle this situation?

A. *Characteristics of an effective answer:* Review patient history and response to drug. Change medication only if clinical outcome has been less than satisfactory. If clinical outcome is satisfactory, don't change drug.

B. *Characteristics of an ineffective answer:* Any expression of passive-aggressive tendencies toward colleague, such as comments that might subtly undermine the patient's confidence in the colleague. Failure to take into account prior clinical outcome when making prescription decision.

You may personally disagree with these two scoring categories. If this is the case, then I'm willing to bet that you can write better ones, and it is exactly these better ones that you would use to evaluate applicants' responses. The point here is that you have probably encountered or know of a number of these interpersonal and work issues that *have* created all sorts of intrapractice conflict. These are all potentially structured questions to ask applicants. It is also appropriate to ask applicants who give low-scoring responses an opportunity to reply to higher categories. For example, if an applicant gives a B category response to the Dr. Jones question, then you might ask, "What do you think of (action consistent with category A)?" Note their response. An applicant who expresses consideration of category A actions will be more likely to fit in than one who rejects it out of hand in a condescending manner.

Work samples and other procedures that mirror the complexity of the job have great potential. Perhaps one of the best "work samples," if it can be arranged, is a visit to the applicant at his or her current location. A cardiac surgery practice used this approach as a final screen before making a selection, when this was feasible given the applicant's current work setting. One retired partner commented that generally it had been the interpersonal issues that created problems. He noted that it was possible for someone to create a facade for a short period of time, a few hours or a day. He commented that when you have been in the operating room with someone for several days, however, you see indicators of how he or she will really interact with others and how they will perform. Roughly quoting one of the physicians who conducted this work sampling: "You really learn how a surgeon feels about quality when you see him put in a stitch that isn't *quite* right. What does he do? Does he take it out and replace it correctly?"

If this process isn't feasible, it may be possible to have an applicant pair with a physician. In a family practice, for example, this could involve doing several joint patient consultations, with the evaluating physician retaining ultimate responsibility for all clinical decisions. During this process, the evaluating physician can observe the quality of the clinical decisions and the nature of the patient-physician and physician-physician interactions.

A locum tenens arrangement is another possibility. Working with someone for 6 months to 1 year is certainly an extended work sample. Would it be inconvenient or expensive then to part ways? Certainly. But what are the financial and interpersonal costs of a faulty hire? Many practices in fact use this approach with a longer trial period, when they hire a new physician and contract to an "up-or-out" partnership decision to be made in X years.

Finally, you may want to consider obtaining a psychological test profile on finalists. This can provide information about issues such as Big 5 personality characteristics, work attitudes, values, and ethics. The profile can highlight areas to be investigated further with interviews, references, and work sample observations. A psychological profile then would be one additional piece of information to utilize in combination with the other data to reach a decision. An additional use of a psychological report would be to help guide the entry of a new physician who is hired into the practice. Understanding the new physician's potential interpersonal strengths and areas that could become contentious, make it possible for the new physician's mentor to begin developing the physician so he or she becomes a more effective colleague and team member. **Figure 4–3** contains part of a report from the Personal Characteristics Inventory. This figure shows an evaluation on the Big 5 factor of Neuroticism, which in this report is called Stability, as well as two subfactors or parts of stability that are named Self-Confidence and Even-Temperment. Notice that the information provided on this factor could be very useful in placing information obtained in the selection process into context. If this applicant is hired, it also provides some helpful information on potential problem areas, so

the physician's awareness can be increased and skills developed. This type of testing should be performed by a testing professional, such as an industrial or clinical psychologist with experience in personnel selection. The testing firms noted in Exhibit 4–9 can provide this type of testing.

Might some good physician applicants resist these "unorthodox" methods? Perhaps. These ideas, however, are not unorthodox in most other industries and are in fact the norm for critical positions at *Fortune* 100 companies. As healthcare organizations grow in size and increasingly rely on proven business methods to improve quality and reduce costs, we will see more of them adopting these methods. Are the costs in terms of dollars and time worth it? Only you can answer that question. As you are considering your answer, however, you might also ask yourself: "What would General Electric do?"

## EQUAL EMPLOYMENT OPPORTUNITY

You should use all your selection methods without regard to the race, religion, sex, national origin, age, or disability. In addition, you cannot allow applicants' medical conditions or medical histories to affect your employment decisions, unless this directly affects the applicant's ability to perform the job, and you cannot make any reasonable accommodation to their condition. The employment methods described in this chapter provide healthcare organizations with greater legal defensibility than traditional unstructured interviews. This is a consequence of basing employment decisions on job-relevant issues that have been assessed through demonstrably valid methods. Specific guidelines for complying with federal equal employment opportunity requirements are discussed in Chapter 10.

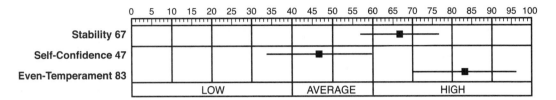

**Facilitating Characteristics:** Those scoring in the high percentile range are even-tempered, calm, and secure. They are often described as being in control of their emotions and do not become easily excitable so they can concentrate on matters of importance. They do not worry about unimportant things. They set aside their own personal wishes to be better able to meet their responsibilities. They cope well in novel or difficult situations and perceive themselves as being capable of handling difficult situations. Their demeanor is usually easy going and they have a steadying influence on others. They tend to maintain their poise and appear relaxed at work. They are generally free of dramatic swings in mood and negative emotions like guilt, sadness, hopelessness, or despair. They seldom get depressed, jealous, apprehensive, fearful, tense, anxious, nervous, emotional, or angry. They tolerate stress well and are seen by others as patient, well-adjusted, stable, and durable. They tend to be seen as controlled rather than casual or spontaneous. They do not get frustrated easily and are able to accept constructive criticism as they feel very secure about themselves. They are comfortable in social situations and do not dwell on negative or embarrassing situations as they are able to get over these situations quickly and do not feel vulnerable or insecure. They appear unshakable, self-reliant, self-sufficient, and adaptable in most situations where they can take stressful events in stride.

**Inhibiting Characteristics:** They may need to balance emotional control with appropriate expression of empathy. They may tend to display too much emotional control and appear to lack of interest, compassion, or interpersonal sensitivity. They may tend to minimize personal discomfort and not openly share their emotions. At times they may not be aware of their own developmental needs. They may lack understanding of others in securities and be a little overbearing or obnoxious. They may tend toward over-confidence and overlook minor issues that could potentially become problems.

### Even-Temperament

Those scoring in the high percentile range are very calm and relaxed. They are even-tempered, secure, and are very steady emotionally. They do not have dramatic swings in mood and their demeanor is usually easy going. They are often described as being in control of their emotions and do not become easily excitable. They tend to maintain their poise, appear relaxed, and seldom get jealous, tense, anxious, nervous, emotional, or angry. They typically will not become depressed, fearful, or apprehensive. They tolerate stress well and are seen by others as patient, well-adjusted, stable, and durable. They typically tolerate others' idiosyncratic behaviors and do not get frustrated easily. They generally keep their cool, take things as they come, and have a steadying influence on others. However, they may tend to minimize difficulties and not be open in their emotional expressions.

### Self-Confidence

Those scoring in the middle percentile range tend to feel secure about themselves. When faced with crisis situations, they usually remain calm. They usually cope adequately in stressful situations. Occasionally, they may experience negative emotions like guilt or sadness. They do not tend to dwell on things that might go wrong. They may be somewhat sensitive to criticism.

**Figure 4–3** Factor Report Sample Report.
*Source:* © 2000, E.F. Wonderlic, Inc. 1795 North Butterfield, Libertyville, IL, 60048. Used with permission.

## CASE APPLICATION: HIRING A BUSINESS MANAGER

The purpose of this case description is to provide you with an example of how selection methods and strategy can be applied in a real employment situation. It illustrates how to use the general guidelines presented earlier in a realistic and practical manner. The case also illustrates how to adjust your employment procedures to take advantage of the changing reality of the selection process.

A family practice employing six physicians was seeking a new business manager. The current business manager had fallen behind in collection and did not have the organizational skills, efficiency, or motivation to fix the problem. The job description for the position was organized into five technical skill factors, two interpersonal skill factors, and one personal trait (**Table 4–2**). The evaluation methods were résumé, structured interviews, work samples, psychological tests, and reference check. The sequence of selection methods was as follows:

1. résumé review
2. telephone interview
3. face-to-face interview and psychological testing
4. second face-to-face interview and work samples
5. reference check

Recruiting methods included word of mouth and two newspaper advertisements spaced 1 week apart. These generated 18 résumés. **Exhibit 4–11** shows the résumé (disguised) of the applicant who was eventually selected for the position. This résumé shows experience on most, if not all, of the selection factors. Ms. Johnson's résumé was well organized and contained appropriate language with correct spelling and grammar. The information was presented in a neat, logical, and concise manner. Her résumé made an acceptable initial impression. It indicated that she was experienced in the following areas: revenue collection, developing systems to deal with business problems, efficiency, and interpersonal relations on the job. Their importance to her, however, did not guarantee that she did these things well. The time break between the last two jobs was acceptably accounted for in the initial telephone contact.

Next, Ms. Johnson was interviewed on the telephone by Dr. Frederick, the practice's physician leader. Dr. Frederick took on this task because the position reported directly to him, and he considered this worth his

---

**Table 4–2**  Business Manager Job Description Factors, Selection Factors, and Selection Procedures

| Job Description Factor | Selection Factor | Selection Procedure |
|---|---|---|
| Collections | Technical Skill | Resume, Work Sample, Structured Interview |
| Insurance Billing | Technical Skill | Resume, Work Sample, Structured Interview |
| Payroll | Technical Skill | Resume, Work Sample |
| Taxes | Technical Skill | Resume, Work Sample |
| Fee Negotiation | Interpersonal Skill | Work Sample |
| Management Reports | Technical Skill | Work Sample |
| Problem Identification | Trait | Psychological Test |
| Teamwork | Interpersonal Skill | Psychological Test, Structured Interview |

**Exhibit 4–11**  Resume (Disguised) of Business Manager Applicant

Ann Johnson
342 Main Street
Virginia Beach, Virginia 23456
(757) 555-1212

*Experience*
Andrew Carey, M.D., Surgeon
1867 Oats Road
Eastville, Connecticut 06387
Position: Business Manager (November 2003 to August 2007)
My objective, as an effective business manager, was to achieve a consistent income for the practice by utilizing proven, effective means of collection. With this end in mind, I initiated a turnover system so that within 12 hours after a patient's visit the insurance had been processed. By thoroughly understanding the mechanisms of different insurers, we were able to achieve a 100 percent collection rate month after month. By streamlining different tasks and implementing time management principles, much of the loose paperwork was eliminated, and fewer errors were made. Consistent with this objective was my desire to create a satisfying environment for all employees. All employees had their own sphere of importance and expertise, which afforded them some control over their work and resulted in higher productivity.

John Blanchard, M.D.
Professor and Chair
New England Medical School
Westville, Connecticut 06774
Position: Practice Manager–Executive Secretary (March 2002 to July 2003)
The position encompassed two areas: private practice manager and secretary to the chair of OB-GYN. As practice manager, I was responsible for patient records, transcription, coding, charges, and patient scheduling. As secretary to the chair, I was involved with the residency program for obstetrics and gynecology.

Nutmeg Roofing
87 Westover Street
Westville, Connecticut 06774
Position: Office Manager (September 1998 to June 2000)
I ordered supplies, maintained inventory, payroll, and accounts receivable and payable, and did the preliminary figures for the quarterly taxes.

*Education*
New England Business College: Eastville, Connecticut (2005)
Principles of Accounting, Business Management, English, Principles of Information Processing
Connecticut Community College: Eastville, Connecticut (2004)
Biology, English, English Literature, American Literature
Smith Business School: Westville, Connecticut, 2000
Medical Terminology I, II, Physiology I, II, Medical Transcription I, II, Insurance I, II, Psychology, English, Typing I, II, Shorthand I, II

time. His objectives were to acquire more detailed information about Ms. Johnson's previous work experience, assess her verbal skills, familiarize her with the job description to clarify whether the job interested her, and determine whether the salary range for the job was acceptable. The telephone interview was organized with the most fundamental qualification issues discussed first, so it could be quickly ended if the applicant was not appropriate for the job.

The telephone interview began by verifying that Ms. Johnson was still in the job market. Next, the job was described to her in considerable detail. She was encouraged to ask questions at any point during the interview. After the job description had been reviewed, she was once again asked whether she was interested in the position. Salary range and benefits (vacation time, sick leave, retirement plan, and health insurance) were then described, and once again, she was asked whether she was still interested in the position. Finally, she was told that the next step would include a face-to-face interview and testing. She was informed that testing was included in the next step, so she could drop out if this was a problem for her. An evaluation of her performance in the telephone interview is included in **Exhibit 4–12**.

Dr. Frederick decided that Ms. Johnson was a very promising candidate, so he scheduled her for an interview. He stated his reasons for immediately scheduling interviews with promising candidates as follows:

> When I conclude during the telephone interview that the applicant is a very good candidate, I schedule the next step in the employment process before I end the call, so I don't waste time recontacting the applicant. This can be advantageous for three reasons. First, we can easily lose a day or two trying to recontact and schedule an applicant who is in demand. Second, the selection process works two ways. The applicant also is making decisions. I am in competition with other employers, and if the appli-

---

**Exhibit 4–12** Structured Telephone Interview Format and Evaluation

1. Ask the applicant to identify him- or herself.

2. Ask the applicant whether he or she is still in the job market.

3. Describe the position to applicant, and tell the applicant to ask questions at any point during this interview.

4. Ask what the applicant is looking for in a position.
(*Ms. Johnson:* Position with responsibility, enjoys getting the money in, place where she fits in, long-term relationship)

5. Ask the applicant to describe their previous work experience.
(*Ms. Johnson:* Handled accounts to $650,000; stressed her ability to organize, look for efficient ways of working; has done insurance billing, posting, collections; no experience with local TRICARE, some with state BC/BS)

6. Discuss salary and benefits.
(*Ms. Johnson:* No problem)

7. Next step is interview and testing.
*Evaluation of skills*
Language was always appropriate. No observable mistakes in grammar or syntax. Asked relevant questions at several points, possibly indicates good problem-solving ability. Technical skills appear to be appropriate. Overall, she appears to be intelligent, qualified, and interested.

cant is tied down interviewing with me, then she *can't* be interviewing with my competition! Similarly, if she's scheduled to interview with me and finds a job she likes, she might delay accepting that job until she's had my interview. Finally, scheduling the next step will shake out the serious from the nonserious applicants. The danger in scheduling the applicant at the end of the telephone interview is that she may not be as good as the next two or three that I will assess on the telephone, but I can always call back and cancel. In reality, deciding whether to immediately offer the second step or postponing that decision is usually not difficult. Those applicants who are really good stand out.

The next step in the selection procedure consisted of a structured interview and administration of a personality test. The interview focused on technical questions related to insurance billing and collection. The goal was to explore the depth of the applicant's knowledge and assess her ability to make the shift into another medical field. **Exhibit 4–13** presents selected interview questions and the interviewer's notes, although not the scoring categories into which he subsequently classified her answers. The first five questions were used with all applicants. The sixth question was specific to this applicant because her last job had been in another state and her previous experience had been in another medical field.

The most important consideration on this job was collection, so the interview questions focused on this factor. Obviously, it was impossible for Dr. Frederick to assess every facet of Ms. Johnson's collection knowledge, so he identified particularly important areas that would give an indication of the depth and degree of her knowledge. In addition, he used the structured questions as points of de-

parture. If the applicant said something that raised another question or made a comment that didn't seem quite right, Dr. Frederick followed up until he felt confident that he had satisfactorily resolved any uncertainties.

The personality test used in this instance was the California Psychological Inventory (CPI). In my opinion, there are tests available now that provide better more easily understandable applicant information than the CPI provides. Examination of Ms. Johnson's profile indicated that she had many traits that would contribute to success on the job. **Exhibit 4–14** shows Ms. Johnson's CPI interpretive report.

The interview took 45 minutes to complete, and the CPI took 65 minutes. Dr. Frederick, however, was only present during the interview. The test was then sent off for scoring and interpretation. As a result of Ms. Johnson's superior performance in the interview, her CPI results, and her stated interest in the position, it was decided to suspend assessment of other applicants until a decision could be made about her. It made sense, therefore, to change the ordering of assessment procedures and to proceed immediately with the telephone reference checks because these would consume less time than the second interview. The reference's comments were positive and Ms. Johnson was asked back for a second interview and work sample testing.

The work sample was designed to end any remaining doubts regarding Ann's knowledge of revenue collection and insurance. The applicant was presented with a real account (name disguised) that had a large outstanding balance. She was told to analyze the account and identify any problems with it. She analyzed the account by identifying copayments, insurance payments, and write-offs for each procedure, and she then assembled personal and insurance balances. When asked what

**Exhibit 4–13** Structured Interview Questions and Responses

1. What is the procedure that you use when a patient has more than one insurance carrier?

   Answer indicated that she would identify the primary, hold billing on the secondary until the primary had paid. Addressed some of the difficulties of identifying the primary. Overall, an informed answer, quickly given.

2. How do you handle a delinquent account? (Follow with role play)

   Answers indicated the necessity to act quickly but with reason. If patient is in office, meet face to face. First, ask if there are any personal circumstances to account for not paying. Depending on the situation, use humor, sternness, and the like to achieve the goal. Obtain a partial payment on credit card if necessary. If patient is not present, use telephone call first, then short series of letters. Indicated that she did not like to use form letters. This was then role played. I stated, "OK, I'm the patient. Talk to me." She was direct and courteous and asked me to make behavioral commitments. Overall, appropriate answers given quickly. Answer stressed reason, control, logic, the need to be systematic.

3. How do you handle a delinquent insurance company?

   Answer given with humor. Stated that she really "liked to go after them." When pushed on how you identify outstanding insurance claims, she stated that she assumed that there would be some aging reports available. Also indicated that she has simply looked through patient files. When pressed about how she would identify slow payers, she indicated that the key was systematic review of accounts, ideally on a weekly basis. When asked how she would review 800 accounts in a week, she stated that she would separate out the bad ones based on an aging report and review them regularly. Overall, her answers were adequate. She seemed somewhat hampered or frustrated by not knowing our procedures.

4. What do you consider an acceptable standard for accounts receivable?

   Previously indicated a standard of two times current as the upper end of what would be acceptable, implying that this was marginally not acceptable. Body language and verbalizations indicated that she thought our accounts were out of control.

5. How would you go about reducing this practice's accounts receivable?

   She didn't have a particular strategy and seemed somewhat confused or surprised by the question. Her first response was that it would take long, hard work. She then asked if there was anyone else in the practice who could assist. This indicated to me a standard thought process of looking for available tools that could be utilized on a project. She then asked how long she would have to get the "AR plug" fixed. I indicated that it should all be gone, as well as current accounts properly handled, in 6 months. She stated and/or indicated through expressions that this was a reasonable if not generous time period.

6. Your background is in working in a surgical practice in Connecticut. What problems do you anticipate in doing billing in a family practice in Virginia?

   She indicated that there were differences between fields but that they were not major—related to knowing what codes to use, what diagnoses would be paid for, etc. In regard to the insurance companies, she stated that it was just a matter of getting on the phone, calling, and asking a lot of questions. She didn't minimize the shift across medical fields or in having to deal with new insurers, but she clearly was not intimidated by it, nor did she express overconfidence. A very appropriate and reasonable answer.

**Exhibit 4–14** CPI Outcomes and Interpretation

**CPI Overall Conclusions**

A dominant theme is a strong sense of obligation and a need to meet the expectations of others. She wants to fit in and meet the needs of those whom she values. There is a strong need to be needed, but there is also evidence of assertiveness and perhaps aloofness and detachment. She is perceptive of others' needs and abilities, likes to be with other people and work with them, and is competent in interpersonal situations, but ultimately trusts her own ability to get things done more than she is willing to delegate to others.

She is serious, proper, stable, competent, rational, able to accept constructive criticism, disciplined, and concerned about her performance. There is a desire for structure and predictability and to stick to plans, which probably results in an aversion to risk taking.

Her behaviors are always appropriate, she strives for competence, and ascribes to the Protestant work ethic. She works hard, intelligently, and efficiently, and this effort is characterized by planning, setting of priorities, and anticipation of consequences. Overall, her personality and work are characterized by optimism and a positive attitude. Her pattern is opposite to that of a passive-aggressive behavior pattern.

**Response Set Evaluation**

Fake Good Scale was within normal limits. No indication of an attempt to fake good.

**Class Evaluation**

The high degree of consistency within classes indicated that class interpretation was appropriate. Class I scales indicate a self-confident person who is outgoing, competent in interpersonal situations, and interpersonally oriented. The relatively low self-acceptance score may indicate that she tries to put her evaluation of her own capabilities into a reasonable perspective, if not consciously minimize them, so as not to appear self-aggrandizing.

Class II scales suggest a person who has a sense of duty, behavioral control, and a dislike of taking risks.

Class III scales indicate that she is achievement oriented and uses an intellectual strategy as opposed to a brute force strategy to approach problems.

Class IV scales are mixed and cannot be interpreted as a set.

**Structure Evaluation**

Structural scale characteristics indicate that she is a weak Alpha, which is an ambitious, action-oriented, productive type of person, a doer who does socially acceptable things and feels comfortable in interpersonal relationships. At their worst, Alphas can be self-centered, opportunistic, and manipulative. She has an exceedingly high v.3 score. This indicates that she has a superior development of the positive aspects of the type. This indicates a high degree of self-reflection and optimism regarding the future.

**Selected Individual Scale Interpretations**

Responsible level of dominance (Do), indicating that she is not overbearing but can be assertive when necessary.

Capacity for status (Cs) indicates that she aspires upward, should be sensitive to management's perspective, and can handle stress and pressure.

Sociability (So) indicates an ability to relate to people in an appropriate manner, enjoys interpersonal reactions, but is not a "backslapper" or inappropriately boisterous.

Social presence (Sp) indicates enthusiasm and ties in well with So, indicating a comfort with social situations.

Self-acceptance (Sa) is inconsistent with the previous two scales. This may indicate a conscious attempt to keep her own self-impression under control, to be modest, and to be socially appropriate regarding her own skills.

*continues*

**Exhibit 4–14** continued

Independence (In) is at levels indicating appropriate goal-oriented behavior and an appropriate level of assertiveness.

Empathy (Em) indicates insight regarding her interpersonal behavior. As a result, her behaviors are viewed as reasonable by others.

Responsibility level suggests a sense of responsibility and a desire to follow through on obligations.

Sociability (So) is at levels associated with sincerity, honesty, and compliance with social norms.

Self-Control (Sc) indicates a preoccupation with detail, a tendency toward compulsiveness, and a reliance on facts as opposed to her intuition. She plans ahead and is good at developing systems and procedures for getting things done. She thinks before she acts but may also repress feelings and occasionally explode.

Tolerance (To) indicates a nonjudgmental, tolerant appreciation for differences and a trust of others.

The achievement scales suggest that she is comfortable working in organized structured situations, but at the same time she can act independently and still need a minimum of supervision.

Intellectual efficiency (Ie) indicates that planning, anticipation of events, and establishing priorities are very important to her. She does not act impulsively.

Psychological Mindedness (Py) suggests that she is more comfortable in dealing with concepts and abstracts than in delegating responsibility. She is perceptive of others' needs and empathic. She would rather do something herself than delegate it.

Flexibility (Fx) level is consistent with someone who is deliberate and determined. She is not afraid of change but probably has a realistic concern with and skepticism of it.

Femininity/Masculinity (F/M) level indicates a balance between being tough minded and sensitive to the needs of others.

**Special Scales**
Her level of work orientation is very high. This is consistent with a person who is reliable, disciplined, and dependable. Similarly, managerial potential is well above average. This indicates that she creates a good impression and is confident, socially effective, emotionally stable, mature, realistic, optimistic, and well-organized; shows foresight; and gets things done.

she would do regarding the personal balance, she stated, "I'd call the patient on the telephone because the balance is large and long overdue." Because that type of conversation had already been role-played in the first interview (question 2, Exhibit 4–13), there was no need to role-play it again. Her ability to bill insurance companies successfully was assessed by presenting her with several insurance forms containing errors, such as missing diagnosis codes and undercoding that would have resulted in the practice re-

ceiving lower payment than merited, along with insurance company EOBs.

This was followed by a simulated fee negotiation in which a secretary played the part of the patient. Finally, she was presented with sample payroll reports from which to determine when and to whom to make tax payments.

The second interview focused on specifying the needs of the practice's medical director, Dr. Frederick, and providing Ms. Johnson with a realistic preview of the job and the personnel with whom she would work. Salary and benefits were discussed in detail, and a job offer was made. This second interview and the work sample testing took 2 hours. The telephone reference checks took 15 minutes. The time expended by practice personnel for Ms. Johnson's selection is shown in **Table 4–3**.

In this instance, the entire selection process was directed by Dr. Frederick, the practice's managing physician. Dr. Frederick described his job as 80 percent clinical work and 20 percent administration. He felt that the business manager position was so important that he should personally assume the responsibility for filling it. In this regard, this case is not typical.

This case illustrates how a small medical practice can fill a critical position in a timely, cost-effective manner and at the same time obtain an employee with an excellent chance of success. The same principles can be applied to selection in a larger practice, hospital, or any other medical setting.

## CASE APPLICATION: A SELECTION FAILURE—A PERSONAL PERSPECTIVE

In retrospect, one of the biggest employment mistakes I made occurred when an applicant pool wore me down. As a result of

---

**Table 4–3** Time Consumed to Select an Applicant

| Procedure | Time (hours) |
| --- | --- |
| Resume Review | 0.10 |
| Telephone Interview | 0.50 |
| Interview & Testing | 0.75 |
| Reference Check | 0.25 |
| Second Interview & Work Sample | 2.00 |
| Total | 3.60 |

---

bad luck, poor applicants, ineffective recruiting, or whatever, applicant after applicant failed to survive some critical part of the employment process. One particular problem was that many applicants were scoring at high levels on the Fake Good Scale of a personality test. A high Fake Good score may mean that the applicant is trying to present a false impression on the test.

Unfortunately, the high Fake Good applicants generally performed better than others in the interview and on the various ability tests. In effect, the Fake Good Scale was the only thing keeping the medical practice to whom I was consulting from hiring a business manager. The physician was growing more anxious as applicant after applicant was rejected. I explained the problem to the physician, and we jointly chose to "take a chance" and ignore the Fake Good warnings. With the Fake Good Scale no longer an impediment, I recommended an applicant who, although well into the questionable range on that scale, otherwise had excellent testing and interviewing results. Needless to say, the employee's subsequent job performance was marked by covering up problems, deception, manipulation of employees, and outright mendacity. The personal and financial costs of searching for a few more days or weeks would have been far-less burdensome than the problems caused by hiring this applicant. This experience proved to me that there are times when one must "tough it out." Hire a temporary employee, use a contractor to cover, or do whatever is necessary, but don't easily compromise your hiring standards.

## CONCLUSION

You should now understand that there are many tools, procedures, and methods for selecting and hiring employees. **Exhibit 4–15** provides a summary of different employment

**Exhibit 4–15** Employment Methods and Their Uses

| Method | Performance Factors |
| --- | --- |
| Resume | A Work Sample<br>Experience<br>Education<br>Work History<br>Practicalities |
| Application Form | Same as Resume |
| Interview | Interpersonal Skills<br>Verbal Skills<br>Communication Skills<br>Motivation/Career<br>  Aspirations<br>Sell Applicant on Job |
| Testing | Technical Job Knowledge<br>Technical Proficiency<br>Aptitiude (Ability to<br>  Learn)<br>Personality<br>Honesty |
| Work Samples<br>  & Simulations | Technical Job Knowledge<br>Technical Proficiency<br>Decision Making<br>Problem Solving<br>Setting Priorities |
| In Basket | Decision Making<br>Problem Solving<br>Setting Priorities |
| References | Verification of<br>  Information (?) |

methods and their uses. By beginning with a good understanding of job content and using the methods discussed in this chapter, you will be able to develop and implement selection methods that will assess job-related skills in a timely, cost-effective manner for all jobs, including physician positions. This approach to employment will greatly increase your chance of hiring successful employees. You also should now have a better understanding of your role as a physician leader in this process as well as the roles of staff and consultants.

## NOTES

1. Warehan, J. (1981). *Secrets of a Corporate Headhunter*. Playboy Press, Chicago: 213–225.
2. If you live in an area where a number of people move in and out, then online provides a unique advantage, because it provides easy exposure from and to people who will be moving to the area. Tidewater Virginia, for example, has a significant transient population due to the large local military population.

3. Validities can also be negative. A validity of -.50 would mean that there is an inverse relationship between performance on the test or interview and job performance. In this case, you would be hiring applicants who performed low on the test or interview in order to get high-job performance. The statistic used to calculate these correlations is usually the Pearson Correlation Coefficient.

4. Standard deviation (SD) is a measure of variance from the mean. One SD above the mean includes approximately 34 percent of the total distribution. The next SD includes approximately another 14 percent. Therefore, two SDs above and below the mean encompass approximately 95 percent of the population.

5. Some large companies will randomly hire applicants to test new employment methods. As a result, they will be able to observe how applicants perform; whom the selection procedure predicts will fail. This strategy for evaluating the predictiveness of employment methods is called *predictive validity*.

6. Few medical practices would hire the number of applicants as in this example. The same phenomenon could be observed, however, by plotting the performance of applicants hired over a long period of time. Even though a practice may only be filling one position at a given time, the same forces illustrated in this example will be at work.

7. This could be due to several reasons, such as better recruiting sources, improved wages, better working conditions, location, and so forth.

8. Schmidt, F. and J. Hunter. (1988). The Validity and Utility of Selection Methods in Personnel Psychology: Practical and Theoretical Implications of 85 Years of Research Findings. *Psychological Bulletin*, 124(2): 262–274.

9. Cortina, J., N. Goldstein, S. Payne, H. Davison, H., & S. Gilliland. (2000). The incremental validity of interview scores over and above cognitive ability and conscientiousness scores. *Personnel Psychology*, 53: 325–351.

10. The HPI is one company's proprietary implementation of the Big 5, which includes renaming some of the factors and breaking others into smaller components. Openness is broken into Inquisitive and Learning Approach, Conscientiousness is defined as Prudence, Agreeableness is defined as Interpersonal Sensitivity, Extroversion is broken into Ambition and Sociability, and Neuroticism is defined as Adjustment. Think of this as the equivalent of proprietary names for drug compounds and proprietary combinations of drug compounds.

11. Weisner, W. H., & S. F. Cronshaw. (1988). The moderating impact of interview formate and degree of structure on interview validity. *Journal of Occupational and Organizational Psychology*, 61: 275–290.

12. Huffcutt, A. I., & W. Arthur. (1994). Hunter and Hunter (1984) revisited: Interview validity for entry-level jobs. *Journal of Applied Psychology*, 79: 184–190.

13. Schmidt, F., & R. Zimmerman. (2004). A counterintuitive hypothesis about employment interview validity and some supporting evidence. *Journal of Applied Psychology*, 89(3): 553–561.

14. The coefficient of determination is the square of the correlation. In this instance for the unstructured interview, it is $.20 \times .20 = .04$; and for the structured interview $.63 \times .63 = .397$.

15. Courts have held that inadvertent or minor misstatements may not be reason for termination. For example, misspelling an address or transposing a telephone number would be very questionable reasons for dismissal.

16. The test publisher is Wonderlic Personnel Tests, Inc.

17. Parts of this section first appeared in: Solomon, R. (1993). Integrity testing can help you avoid hiring a thief. *American Medical News*, 26.

18. Saxe, L., D. Dougherty, & T. Cross. (1985). The validity of polygraph testing. *American Psychologist*, 40: 355–366.

19. Some employers are still permitted to use polygraphs to screen applicants. These include employers with national defense contracts, parts of the nuclear power industry, businesses with access to highly classified U.S. government information, and city, state, and the federal governments.

20. Hogan, J., & R. Hogan. (1989). How to measure employee reliability. *Journal of Applied Psychology*, 72(2): 273–279.

21. Lillienfeld, S. O., G. Alliger, & K. Mitchell. (1995). Why integrity testing remains controversial. *American Psychologist*, 50(6): 457.

22. Ones, D., & C. Viswesvaran. (1998). Gender, age, and race differences on overt integrity tests: results across four large-scale job applicant data sets. *Journal of Applied Psychology*, 83(1): 35–42.

23. Ones, D., C. Viswesvaran, & F. Schmidt. (1995). Integrity tests: Overlooked facts, resolved issues, and remaining questions. *American Psychologist*, 50(6): 456–457.

24. Frone, M. (2006). Prevalence and distribution of illicit drug use in the workforce and in the workplace: Findings and implications from a U.S. national survey. *Journal of Applied Psychology*, 91(4): 856–869.

25. Roth, P. (2005). A meta-analysis of work sample test validity: updating and integrating some classic literature. *Personnel Psychology*, 58: 1009–1037.

26. For an examination of the legal issues involved in *providing* references, see the discussion of the tort of defamation in Chapter 10.

27. Parts of this section first appeared in: Solomon, R. (1994). There are ways to check skills before hiring a doctor. *American Medical News*, 41.

# CHAPTER 5

# Compensating Employees

## Chapter Objectives

An effective compensation plan will help you to hire, retain, and motivate good employers, while keeping your payroll costs under control. The objective of this chapter is to provide you with a strategy and procedures for determining how much to pay each of your employees. Although compensation is largely dispensed in the form of direct wages, most medical practices also provide some benefits, which can include life insurance, health insurance, a retirement plan, vacation time, sick leave, educational benefits, and for physicians, profit sharing. Benefits will be discussed as a means of fine-tuning your compensation plan to best meet your needs and those of your employees.

The methods that are presented in this chapter are most directly relevant to larger healthcare organizations that deal with many more positions and compensation decisions than smaller organizations, such as small group practices. Nevertheless, the same compensation concepts that are used by larger organizations are applicable to physician leaders working in smaller private practice settings.

Physician leaders in practices and larger healthcare organizations will find that basing a compensation plan solely on intuitive judgments of appropriate salaries for positions will create personnel and compensation problems. In particular, employees might become dissatisfied with their pay, which can manifest itself in such symptoms as absenteeism, tardiness, productivity problems, and turnover. Alternatively, the size of your payroll might become excessive. If you notice either of these conditions, you should take a closer look at your compensation plan.

Physician leaders working in large practices or healthcare organizations, such as hospitals and healthcare systems, will want to use either a consultant or their professional human resources staff to build a compensation plan. The information contained in this chapter will help you more effectively utilize these compensation professionals and apply the results of their work.

Physician leaders in smaller practices may conclude that use of the methods described in this chapter for determining salaries for their limited number of positions is overkill. If that is the case, you can improve the results you obtain from an intuitive approach to compensation by considering the compensation concepts discussed in this chapter. Seeing how these concepts translate into procedure in larger organizations will give you a model around which to build your intuitive compensation strategy. If you understand what compensation should be based on and the goals that any compensation plan—either large or small—should achieve, you will be able to make better intuitive judgments and arrive at more equitable salaries. Physician leaders in smaller practices will find that they can determine salary rates for front office personnel without the use of a consultant, although whether this is a cost-effective use of their time is problematic.

## WHO SHOULD CONSTRUCT YOUR COMPENSATION PLAN?

If you are a physician manager in a private practice who wishes to develop a compensation plan, you will either have to do most of the work yourself, or delegate it to a consultant. With the exception of some data collecting tasks, such as obtaining published wage and salary surveys, the tasks should not be delegated to subordinates in the practice. The need for judgment, having a practice as opposed to an employee perspective, as well as the potential for influencing their own salaries, makes these decisions inappropriate for your subordinates.

Hiring a consultant to construct a practice compensation plan is the preferred strategy for three reasons. First, and perhaps most importantly, contracting this work to a consultant gets you out of the compensation business and back into practicing medicine. Generally, physicians in private practice are more successful if they leave technical personnel issues to those with expertise. Using a consultant puts the physician leader in the more appropriate role of knowing enough about compensation to be able to communicate with, evaluate, and implement the consultant's work. Second, hiring an experienced consultant will give you the benefit of knowledge and perspective in a task where these commodities are very important. Finally, the objectivity that a consultant can provide will give your plan greater credibility with and acceptance from your employees and your partners.

Compensation plans in larger healthcare organizations should be developed either by experienced consultants or by HR staff with compensation expertise. The goal of this chapter in this circumstance is to give you an understanding of compensation process, so you can work more effectively with your HR staff or consultants.

Some consulting firms have their own proprietary compensation plans that they utilize, with minor adaptations, for all clients. Large national compensation firms, such as Hay Associates, use plans that have been developed and refined over many years. Generally, these plans do a very good job of achieving equity. In addition, these firms maintain large databases that can be very helpful when establishing benchmark job rates and making comparisons between your compensation rates and those of other hospitals and large practices.

## EQUITY: A THEORY AND STRATEGY FOR DETERMINING COMPENSATION

The goal of any compensation plan is to achieve equity in the minds of employees. *Equity* is a judgment made by the employee regarding the fairness of compensation. Equity judgments are comparative, not absolute. An employee judges the equity of compensation by making a comparison of his or her rewards and the work he or she performed to the rewards of and work performed by others. Equity is therefore a personal, cognitive ratio of rewards to performance compared with the ratio of rewards to performance for significant others. Three equity conditions can be expressed conceptually as:

$$R_e/I_e = R_o/I_o \text{ Equity}$$

$$R_e/I_e < R_o/I_o \text{ Inequity due to underreward}$$

$$R_e/I_e > R_o/I_o \text{ Inequity due to overreward}$$

where $R_e$ represents the rewards received by the employee, $I_e$ is the inputs made by the employee, $R_o$ is the rewards received by the other person, and $I_o$ is the inputs made by the other person.

The reward component in these equations includes all rewards associated with the job. In addition to salary, retirement plan, vacation leave, and health insurance, this would include nonmonetary considerations such as friendships, status, working conditions, and the like. The work inputs, similarly, would include all items that the employee perceives him- or herself as contributing, including items that may not be mentioned in the job description. These could include loyalty and willingness to adapt to the employer's needs (e.g., overtime, adjusting work hours, changing projects, etc.). Generally, however, the largest single reward element is salary, and the largest single input element is the sum total of the job description.

An important point to remember throughout this discussion is that equity is ultimately judged by the *employee,* and the employee's judgment regarding what is equitable may differ substantially from the conclusions of an independent, unbiased observer. This is significant because the equity of your compensation plan ultimately will be judged through your *employees'* eyes, not yours.

Employees do not consciously calculate mathematical equity ratios for themselves and others. Although some equity judgments may result from conscious comparisons, most equity judgments are based on semiconscious or unconscious evaluations. In addition, many of the data that the employee uses to form an equity judgment are "messy." For example, although John, your business manager, has good data regarding the rewards you provide, he may somewhat distort his input by overevaluating the importance of his job or how well he is performing his job. Also, suppose John compares his rewards and inputs to those of Jane, a business manager at another practice. His data regarding Jane's rewards may or may not be accurate. He may be drawing his conclusions, for example, based partly on the clothes Jane wears, the car she drives, the neighborhood in which she lives, "hints" she has dropped during conversations indicating satisfaction with her compensation, and so on. The data regarding Jane's inputs also might be questionable. These might include self-serving remarks made by Jane, a halo effect based on the reputation of the other practice, comments made by a Blue Cross claims representative regarding the ease or difficulty of working with Jane, and so on. John then combines all these data at a semiconscious or unconscious level and forms an impression of the equity of his compensation.

Given these circumstances, there is a real possibility that what you perceive to be fair, just, and equitable may not be similarly perceived by your employees. The degree to which your employees will perceive their compensation as equitable will be affected by a number of issues besides salary, including:

- the general climate of employee relations in your practice
- the quality of your performance-appraisal feedback

- the "reasonableness" of employees in choosing peers for comparison
- other characteristics of your compensation plan

The employee relations climate will have a pervasive impact on many aspects of your practice. If there is disharmony and unpleasantness, employees will add them to the $I_e$ component. For example, suppose that, in your heart of hearts, you know that on occasion you can be overbearing when working with Dolores, your nurse. When Dolores calculates her equity ratio, she adds "working with an overbearing . . . . " to the $I_e$ component. To some degree, this will offset the value that you will be adding to the $R_e$ component through your compensation package. The offset may be even greater if Dolores has a friend who works for a physician who is always calm and reasonable, and whom she uses to make her equity comparison. On the other hand, if you have very good employee relations with Dolores and she prizes this, it can add value to the $R_e$ component.

Performance-appraisal feedback sets the stage for your employees' equity judgments. The quality and truthfulness of your performance appraisals will also have a profound impact on your employees' perceptions of equity. Suppose that you have a laboratory director with some serious performance problems that you choose not to address in the performance review. Given the lack of criticism, the laboratory director will assume that his or her performance is at least adequate. If you then give the director a small pay raise based on your recognition of the inadequate performance, he or she probably will perceive this reward as inequitably low. Similarly, providing a glowing appraisal for an employee who is competent but certainly not outstanding may result in an average pay raise being viewed as inequitably low.

An employee's perception of equity is partly based on comparisons with peers. The peers whom your employees choose will certainly have an impact on the evaluation of your compensation plan. Unfortunately, this matter is largely out of your control. If you have an employee who makes unreasonable comparisons, there is little that you can do about this. Generally, employees do not discuss these comparisons with their employer, and, as you have seen, they may only be vaguely aware of the comparison process.

This brings us to your compensation plan, something over which you do have considerable control. By using the methods discussed in this chapter, you will be able to determine equitable compensation rates based on your market and develop a compensation plan that creates equitable compensation differences corresponding to the various jobs and employees in your organization. You can also increase the fairness of the plan by talking with your employees to better understand the types of compensation that they desire.

## USING EQUITY TO CONSTRUCT A COMPENSATION PLAN

To use equity concepts effectively, it is important to make a distinction between compensating jobs and compensating people. Jobs have value to your organization irrespective of the job incumbent. For example, no matter how well a secretary performs, the value of the job has an upper limit. This is why secretaries are not paid $75,000 per year. No matter how well the incumbent performs, and regardless of the employee's years of service, dedication, and commitment, *the work itself* simply does not merit this level of compensation. Similarly, the value of each job has a lower limit. Assuming that the incumbent is competent enough to retain in the position, the duties dictate that the incumbent be paid at least a minimum amount. There is a pay range, therefore, that exists for each job irrespective of the characteristics or performance level of the incumbent.

To establish an effective compensation plan, therefore, you first must think of the pay for each job as being composed of an equitable pay range that is associated with the *position*, independent of the job incumbent. For example, you may determine that the pay range for a billing specialist is $25,000 to $34,500, for a level I secretary from $14,000 to $17,000, for a marketing director from $80,000 to $95,000, and for a family practice physician from $120,000 to $150,000.[1] Next, you determine a specific employee's pay level from within this range based on job performance, seniority, experience, and so on. Perhaps, as a result, Tim Singh's pay as a training specialist will be $30,800, and Dale Yee's salary as a secretary will be $15,000.

Determining a reasonable salary for an employee requires consideration of three distinct types of equity: internal, external, and individual. These are summarized in **Exhibit 5–1**. *Internal equity* comparisons are comparisons among jobs within the practice or healthcare organization. The director of the

physical therapy department, for example, might compare inputs and rewards associated with his or her job with the inputs and rewards associated with the department heads of nursing, radiology, various hospital laboratories, and so forth. He or she will also probably compare their salary with subordinates' salaries in the department and with the boss's salary. Once again, the data regarding the contributions and rewards of each of these positions and the people who occupy them may vary in accuracy and will certainly have a subjective aspect to it. Nevertheless, each employee will make internal equity comparisons. To achieve internal equity, jobs that are generally recognized as having lower value, being less demanding, or requiring less training should, all other things being equal, be paid less, whereas the opposite should be true for more difficult, higher-value jobs. Your compensation plan, therefore, must have a mechanism to ensure logic and consistency between and among jobs in your organization.

This can be a particular problem for healthcare systems that have been acquiring physicians and putting them on salaries. These physicians' initial salaries are generally related to their productivity prior to ac-

---

**Exhibit 5–1** Internal, External, and Individual Equity

| Concepts | Tools for Assessing | Outcomes |
|---|---|---|
| Internal Equity–<br>Relationships Between and Among<br>Jobs in the Organization | Job Descriptions<br>Job Analysis<br>Job Evaluation | Cost Control |
| Individual Equity–<br>Relationships Between and Among<br>Individuals Within Jobs | Performance Appraisal<br>Merit<br>Seniority | Attract Competent<br>Employees<br><br>Retain Competent<br>Employees |
| External Equity–<br>Relationships Between and Among<br>Jobs in the Labor Market | Wage and Salary Surveys<br>Anecdotal "Going Rate" Data | Motivate High<br>Performance |

quisition. As a result, the healthcare system may have a wide range of salaries within a specialty, such as family practice or cardiology. At some later point in time, however, this could become a problem as performance differences between physicians change and as the relative market value of various specialties adjusts to the marketplace changes. One effect, for example, is that the value of primary care physicians may increase relative to specialists. As a result, the healthcare system needs a mechanism to adjust for the changing relative value (internal equity) across specialties.

*External equity* comparisons are made between the jobs in your organization and jobs in other organizations. External equity is the perception of the so-called going rate or market rate for a job. A compensation plan with external equity allows you to attract and retain qualified employees. The positions in other organizations that employees use as the "comparison other" can be medical, non-medical, or both. For example, practice-based employees may evaluate the equity of compensation for clerical, business, and management positions by making comparisons, in addition to other medical practices, with banks, law firms, construction companies, and so on because these are other viable employment alternatives. Physician employees will make comparisons with peers in other healthcare organizations, such as other healthcare systems, HMOs, medical schools, and private practices. Once again, the accuracy of the perceptions of the rewards and inputs of the "comparison others" may be questionable. The process will vary from fully conscious investigation by collecting wage and salary data to semiconscious and unconscious ruminations. Nevertheless, employees make these comparisons and in part act on them.

Both internal and external equity comparisons are essentially comparisons among *jobs. Individual equity* comparisons are comparisons among *employees*. In its simplest form, individual equity relates to the differences in pay received by different incumbents on the same job. For example, if you employ several family practice physicians, then pay differences between them will be subject to individual equity judgments. Once again, one or all physicians may be operating on the basis of poor or inaccurate information. Nevertheless, they will make inferences and take actions based on their assessments. Each, individually, will subjectively discount experience, training, seniority, job performance differences, and so forth, and form a conclusion about whether his or her pay is equitable. Sometimes, employees will make individual equity comparisons across jobs. For example, a nurse might compare him- or herself with a secretary by discounting job and performance differences. Similarly, a physician may do the same with a top-level administrator. If they can account for all the perceived salary differences as being due to job and performance differences, then they will conclude that their pay is equitable. If there is a discrepancy, they will perceive themselves as either underpaid or overpaid.

Employees combine their internal, external, and individual equity data to form conclusions about the fairness of their compensation. For example, a secretary might go through the following cognitive exercise (not necessarily consciously):

I'm making $17,000 per year. I think that is pretty good. I saw an ad in the newspaper last month that offered $15,000 for a medical secretary over at Dr. Li's practice. I know that Dr. Li doesn't have automated scheduling, so you don't have to be as computer capable as I am. On the other hand, that probably means that his secretaries have to work harder to do the same amount of work.

I prefer to work in a more automated office anyway. (external equity comparisons)

Badra, our business manager, is probably paid about $10,000 more than I am. I've been here almost 2 years. She just bought a new Toyota Prius with all the options—those cars cost about $30,000! Her being single and all, why she must be making $29,000 or $30,000. Also, she always dresses very well. Not terribly expensive, but stylish and up to date. Yeah, she's probably making about $29,000 or $30,000. She's responsible for collecting all the money, making certain that all the bills are paid, and supervising the rest of us. She also has to train us on all the computer programs used in the office, and she knows them all really well. (internal equity comparisons)

I've heard, however, that she's not a superstar; she issued six incorrect W-2s a few months ago. Also, insurance collections have been slow, and I know that Dr. Simpson is not happy about that. He also knows that sometimes she has problems getting along with some of the rest of us. (individual equity comparisons)

Dr. Simpson always tells me that I am doing a super job and in my last performance review, Badra gave me the highest evaluation possible in four of the five evaluation factors. My super performance should make up for some of the difference in the importance of our jobs. It would be fair if Badra made $6,000 or $7,000 more than me, but not $13,000. She does have a more important job, but I am better at what I do than she is at what she does. (individual equity comparison)

I really think that she is being paid at least $30,000. That's not really fair. If she gets that much, then I should be making another $5,000 or $6,000. She just isn't worth that much more than me. I know that secretaries at some of the local offices of big companies like TRW and DuPont have salaries in the middle to upper twenties. Steve works for DuPont, and he as much as told me that. (external equity comparisons)

Maybe I really put too much into this job. When I switched schedules to cover when Jacob was sick, I didn't get anything for it other than a "thanks" from Dr. Simpson. If he really wanted to thank me, he would pay me more. He obviously has the money—look at what he's paying Badra! I guess I should stop putting myself out. I should do a good, competent job, but not anything extra. (overall equity decision)

This example illustrates how an employee can integrate several sources of information and combine external, internal, and individual equity data to reach an overall judgment regarding the fairness of compensation. It also illustrates one other very important point: Employees *always* achieve equity *one way or another*! When employees feel that their rewards are inequitably low, they will achieve equity by reducing inputs. When employees cannot reduce inputs enough to achieve equity, then they will take more extreme measures, including passive-aggressive behavior, noncompliance, open disobedience, sabotage, and ultimately leaving.

Employees who perceive that they are overpaid also will achieve equity. They will increase the quality or quantity of their work or will psychologically adjust their perceptions of their input or the rewards they receive, until they perceive equity. Some physician leaders may be tempted to increase the compensation of valued employees to inequitably high levels to "freeze" them and thereby deter turnover. This strategy is dangerous, because it creates internal inequities relative to *other* employees, thereby causing dissatisfaction and motivating other employees to act out or to leave. Of course, the compensation of all employees could be raised to inequitably high levels, but this would inflate the size of the organization's payroll to unnecessary levels.

Generally, employees are relatively less concerned about external equity than about internal and individual equity. This is because it is easier to rationalize working for somewhat lower compensation compared with someone across town than it is to rationalize differences compared with someone at the next desk. For example, "the work atmosphere is nicer here," "parking is easier," "this healthcare system is the dominant one in the area and I like that prestige," "Dr. Fisk is a pleasure to work for," and so on are all justifications for working for somewhat lower compensation. If, however, the pay is less than that of another employee in the same organization, it is much more difficult to produce convincing rationalizations, because the comparison is with someone working under the same circumstances.

Because of internal and individual equity considerations, it is not sufficient simply to pay the going market rate to each employee. First, it is simply too time consuming and difficult to identify the market rate for all jobs, with the possible exception being the smallest practices. Second, using the average rates for jobs in your local labor market will not necessarily produce a pay plan that is internally equitable. The market rate for a job is based on an amalgam of below-average, average, and above-average performers in organizations with varying mixes of job content for a given job title. In effect, not all positions labeled insurance billing specialist perform the same tasks. Some insurance billing specialist positions are more demanding and require more skills and abilities than other positions with the same job title. Adopting the average or market rate across all positions in your organization won't take into account real performance differences between your employees or the mix of tasks as they exist in your organization. As a result, you need ways to build internal, individual, and external eq-

uities into your compensation plan based on the mix of jobs and performance levels *as they exist in your practice or healthcare system*. Column two in Exhibit 5-1 lists the methods that are used to achieve each of these equity goals. Finally, column three in this exhibit describes the outcomes when you develop a compensation system that achieves adequate levels of internal, individual, and external equity.

## JOB EVALUATION METHODS FOR ACHIEVING INTERNAL AND EXTERNAL EQUITY

Job evaluation is the process that compensation professionals use to build internal and external equity into their compensation plans. There are three major job evaluation methods and many variations on these themes. These methods do two things. First, they order jobs based on their internal content and worth to the organization. This achieves the internal equity goal. Next, they identify the market rate for some of the jobs. These jobs are called *benchmark jobs*, because they will be used to benchmark or anchor the internal ordering of jobs to outside market rates.

Generally, you will want to identify some benchmark jobs toward the top, middle, and bottom of the internal equity order. Once benchmark pay levels have been determined, then pay levels for jobs between the benchmark jobs can be resolved. These rates will be derived subjectively, through interpolation, or by calculation, depending on the particular job evaluation method that is used.

We will examine two job evaluation methods. The ranking method is the simplest and easiest to use. Simplicity and ease can be real advantages for a small practice. Its disadvantage is that it becomes cumbersome to use when there are many jobs to be evaluated or when the jobs are highly technical or complex. Smaller private practices and healthcare organizations will find that the ranking method may be sufficient to develop compensation plans for front office, technical, and professional positions.

The other method that we will cover is called a *point plan*. Point plans require more time, effort, and skill to create. They can, however, cover large numbers of jobs and jobs that are complex in their work content. Point plans are the most common job evaluation method used in the United States. Large group practices and healthcare organizations, such as hospitals and hospital systems, will generally find the point system to be appropriate.

Before looking at how to use job evaluation methods, we must discuss who will do this. Because equity is the eventual goal, two considerations to remember are that the eventual plan must be understandable by those whom it covers, and that these employees must accept the results as valid. As a result, larger organizations often use a committee to develop their compensation plans. Often, these committees span several employee groups, such as administrative, technical, professional, and medical. Using broader representation gives additional perspective to job content and provides more "real-world" data on what employees really do on a job. In addition, participation often improves acceptance. If nurses know, for example, that they had representation on the team that developed the compensation plan covering their positions, then they are more likely to accept the results.

## USING A RANKING METHOD OF JOB EVALUATION

The object of a ranking method is to rank jobs on the basis of their overall value to the organization. The procedure works as follows:

1. Assemble all the job descriptions to be covered in the compensation plan. Generally, a practice will have several compensation plans. For example, all clerical positions might be in one plan, nursing and technical positions in another, physicians in yet another, and so forth.
2. Read all the job descriptions so you are fully familiar with their contents. Validate that the descriptions are current, and resolve any questions regarding what employees really do on a job.
3. Considering all issues covered by the descriptions, identify the job that is most important to the organization.
4. Next, identify the job that is least important to the organization.
5. Of the jobs remaining, identify the one that is most important, then the one that is least important. Repeat this process until all jobs have been ranked.

The first two columns in **Table 5–1** illustrate the outcome of this ranking process. This ranking expresses the internal equity ordering of jobs in this practice. Because we

**Table 5–1** Rank Ordering of Nursing/Technology Line of Positions

| Rank | Job Title | Benchmark Rate |
|---|---|---|
| 1 | Nursing Supervisor | |
| 2 | Nurse Practitioner | $55,000 |
| 3 | Nuclear Medicine Technologist | $51,500 |
| 4 | Ultrasound Technician | |
| 5 | RN-Physician Assistant | $40,800 |
| 6 | Medical Assistant II | $24,600 |
| 7 | Medical Assistant I | |

are using ordinal measurement, however, the "distances" between jobs are not meaningful; that is, the "importance difference" between nurse practitioner and nuclear medicine technologist (NMT) probably isn't the same as between medical assistant I and medical assistant II.

Using the ranking process obviously requires an ability to subjectively evaluate the composite of compensable factors possessed by each job. For example, the nursing supervisor position may require more experience and supervisory skills than the NMT, yet the NMT may require more formal education and have greater responsibility. Nevertheless, when there are a fairly small number of jobs and the evaluator or evaluating team really understands the jobs, the relative worth or value of the positions to the organization can be captured with the ranking process.

Next, benchmark jobs must be identified. Benchmark jobs are jobs for which you know the fair salary level. The standard way of obtaining benchmark information is with a wage and salary survey. **Table 5–2** is from an online wage and salary survey published by the U.S. Department of Labor Bureau of Labor Statistics (BLS).[2] Wage and salary surveys can be obtained several ways. First, you can conduct a survey yourself. Some large companies conduct their own surveys. Larger healthcare systems, may have personnel staff who are capable of conducting a local wage and salary survey. This approach is not a cost-effective alternative, however, for most healthcare organizations. A second alternative is to commission a consultant to conduct a wage-and-salary survey. This option provides accurate, current data for jobs that are comparable to the ones in your organization. Larger healthcare organizations that have a continuing need for current data may find this to be a cost-effective alternative. This is not the case, however, for most

private medical practices. A variation of the second theme is to use a consultant who conducts ongoing wage-and-salary surveys in the medical field. Generally, these consultants provide survey data for a subscription fee. This approach often provides the most feasible source of wage-and-salary survey data for healthcare providers that are looking for market rates for jobs specific to healthcare, such as medical secretaries, nurses, radiation technologists, and respiratory therapists.

Another source of wage-and-salary data may be your local or state medical association,[3] which might conduct wage-and-salary surveys for the use of its members. Generally, each organization that wants a copy of the survey pays a nominal fee and also completes a survey questionnaire. A consultant hired by the association collects, analyzes, and interprets the data, and the association then provides the wage-and-salary survey to participating members. Survey reporting formats vary. An example of one is found in **Exhibit 5–2**. Each reporting practice in this example is reported by a code number. In this way, physician leaders at each practice can examine the data to see how their organization compares with others and with group statistics, yet complete anonymity is maintained for everyone.

Other possible sources of published wage-and-salary data include your state employment commission or department of labor, local chamber of commerce, and local trade and professional associations. Generally these sources won't provide surveys containing medical jobs. Nevertheless, you may be able to get some good data on selected other jobs, such as clerical and business-related positions, that are not unique to medicine.

Irrespective of the source of your survey, remember that the data it contains will be approximate because of the data collection

**Table 5–2** Bureau of Labor Statistics Wage and Salary Survey for Office and Administrative Occupations—Virginia May, 2005

| Occupation Code | Occupation Title | Employment (1) | Median Hourly | Mean Hourly | Mean Annual (2) |
|---|---|---|---|---|---|
| 43-0000 | Office and Administrative Support Occupations | 588,770 | $13.39 | $14.89 | $30,970 |
| 43-1011 | First-Line Supervisors/Managers of Office and Administrative Support Workers | 35,790 | $21.61 | $24.49 | $50,940 |
| 43-2011 | Switchboard Operators, Including Answering Service | 4,420 | $10.17 | $10.67 | $22,190 |
| 43-2021 | Telephone Operators | 820 | $18.40 | $17.09 | $35,560 |
| 43-2099 | Communications Equipment Operators, All Other | 160 | $18.90 | $19.44 | $40,430 |
| 43-3011 | Bill and Account Collectors | 12,290 | $13.44 | $14.54 | $30,250 |
| 43-3021 | Billing and Posting Clerks and Machine Operators | 12,780 | $13.91 | $14.26 | $29,660 |
| 43-3031 | Bookkeeping, Accounting, and Auditing Clerks | 45,680 | $14.69 | $15.41 | $32,040 |
| 43-3051 | Payroll and Timekeeping Clerks | 6,220 | $15.60 | $15.94 | $33,160 |
| 43-3061 | Procurement Clerks | 2,940 | $17.42 | $17.21 | $35,800 |
| 43-3071 | Tellers | 16,120 | $10.30 | $10.65 | $22,140 |
| 43-4011 | Brokerage Clerks | 1,360 | $15.57 | $15.97 | $33,220 |
| 43-4021 | Correspondence Clerks | 370 | $16.20 | $18.15 | $37,760 |
| 43-4031 | Court, Municipal, and License Clerks | 1,930 | $14.14 | $15.04 | $31,270 |
| 43-4041 | Credit Authorizers, Checkers, and Clerks | 2,020 | $14.56 | $14.84 | $30,870 |
| 43-4051 | Customer Service Representatives | 53,670 | $13.13 | $14.24 | $29,610 |
| 43-4061 | Eligibility Interviewers, Government Programs | 3,380 | $15.05 | $15.76 | $32,780 |
| 43-4071 | File Clerks | 4,930 | $10.65 | $11.50 | $23,930 |
| 43-4081 | Hotel, Motel, and Resort Desk Clerks | 7,200 | $8.30 | $8.75 | $18,200 |
| 43-4111 | Interviewers, Except Eligibility and Loan | 4,810 | $12.12 | $12.69 | $26,390 |
| 43-4121 | Library Assistants, Clerical | 2,130 | $10.87 | $11.47 | $23,850 |
| 43-4131 | Loan Interviewers and Clerks | 6,740 | $15.64 | $16.25 | $33,800 |
| 43-4141 | New Accounts Clerks | 2,140 | $12.67 | $13.11 | $27,270 |
| 43-4151 | Order Clerks | 7,520 | $11.64 | $13.12 | $27,280 |
| 43-4161 | Human Resources Assistants, Except Payroll and Timekeeping | 4,750 | $16.37 | $16.68 | $34,690 |
| 43-4171 | Receptionists and Information Clerks | 28,140 | $10.35 | $10.90 | $22,670 |
| 43-4181 | Reservation and Transportation Ticket Agents and Travel Clerks | 4,440 | $15.66 | $15.49 | $32,230 |
| 43-4199 | Information and Record Clerks, All Other | 15,440 | $20.86 | $25.41 | $52,860 |
| 43-5011 | Cargo and Freight Agents | 1,120 | $17.16 | $18.70 | $38,900 |

*continues*

**Table 5–2** continued

| Occupation Code | Occupation Title | Employment (1) | Median Hourly | Mean Hourly | Mean Annual (2) |
|---|---|---|---|---|---|
| 43-5021 | Couriers and Messengers | 3,000 | $10.97 | $11.89 | $24,730 |
| 43-5031 | Police, Fire, and Ambulance Dispatchers | 2,490 | $13.79 | $14.46 | $30,080 |
| 43-5032 | Dispatchers, Except Police, Fire, and Ambulance | 4,200 | $14.22 | $15.20 | $31,620 |
| 43-5041 | Meter Readers, Utilities | 1,240 | $14.01 | $14.59 | $30,350 |
| 43-5051 | Postal Service Clerks | 2,160 | $23.27 | $22.52 | $46,840 |
| 43-5052 | Postal Service Mail Carriers | 8,730 | $21.94 | $21.02 | $43,720 |
| 43-5053 | Postal Service Mail Sorters, Processors, and Processing Machine Operators | 4,630 | $21.76 | $20.70 | $43,050 |
| 43-5061 | Production, Planning, and Expediting Clerks | 9,300 | $19.12 | $19.81 | $41,200 |
| 43-5071 | Shipping, Receiving, and Traffic Clerks | 18,080 | $12.49 | $12.96 | $26,970 |
| 43-5081 | Stock Clerks and Order Fillers | 43,280 | $9.79 | $10.69 | $22,230 |
| 43-5111 | Weighers, Measurers, Checkers, and Samplers, Recordkeeping | 2,070 | $12.36 | $13.12 | $27,280 |
| 43-6011 | Executive Secretaries and Administrative Assistants | 18,870 | $18.78 | $19.59 | $40,740 |
| 43-6012 | Legal Secretaries | 3,120 | $19.08 | $19.22 | $39,980 |
| 43-6013 | Medical Secretaries | 4,370 | $12.76 | $13.52 | $28,130 |
| 43-6014 | Secretaries, Except Legal, Medical, and Executive | 24,390 | $14.86 | $15.42 | $32,070 |
| 43-9011 | Computer Operators | 3,340 | $15.90 | $16.85 | $35,060 |
| 43-9021 | Data Entry Keyers | 7,300 | $10.85 | $11.89 | $24,720 |
| 43-9022 | Word Processors and Typists | 2,520 | $12.87 | $14.05 | $29,230 |
| 43-9031 | Desktop Publishers | 1,280 | $15.10 | $15.89 | $33,060 |
| 43-9041 | Insurance Claims and Policy Processing Clerks | 5,160 | $14.67 | $15.11 | $31,430 |
| 43-9051 | Mail Clerks and Mail Machine Operators, Except Postal Service | 5,710 | $11.32 | $11.87 | $24,690 |
| 43-9061 | Office Clerks, General | 114,920 | $12.26 | $13.03 | $27,100 |
| 43-9071 | Office Machine Operators, Except Computer | 2,750 | $11.79 | $12.16 | $25,300 |
| 43-9081 | Proofreaders and Copy Markers | 260 | $11.81 | $13.73 | $28,560 |
| 43-9111 | Statistical Assistants | 270 | $19.26 | $19.24 | $40,010 |
| 43-9199 | Office and Administrative Support Workers, All Other | 6,020 | $14.20 | $14.59 | $30,340 |

*Source:* Adapted from Bureau of Labor Statistics: http://www.bls.gov/oes/current/oessrcst.htm.

**Exhibit 5–2**  Coded Wage and Salary Survey for Practice Manager Position (Direct Wages Only)

Job  Description: The practice manager is responsible for the major day-to-day financial and supervisory functions in the practice. Typically, this involves supervising all clerical staff and business operations, responsible for the effective design and operation of all business systems. Typically reports directly to the managing physician.

| Rank | Code | Annual Salary ($k) | Rank | Code | Annual Salary ($k) |
|------|------|--------------------|------|------|--------------------|
| 1  | XO37 | 68.9 | 25 | ER77 | 56.3 |
| 2  | EK94 | 65.2 | 26 | LL49 | 54 |
| 3  | JK23 | 64.9 | 27 | KK34 | 52 |
| 4  | OI38 | 64.9 | 28 | IO38 | 51.5 |
| 5  | FI34 | 63   | 29 | UT44 | 50.5 |
| 6  | KL99 | 62.5 | 30 | RR67 | 50 |
| 7  | OF39 | 62.5 | 31 | TW78 | 50 |
| 8  | HL81 | 62.1 | 32 | IQ37 | 50 |
| 9  | JG88 | 62   | 33 | OO99 | 48 |
| 10 | BBl2 | 62   | 34 | PU38 | 47.3 |
| 11 | CM31 | 61.7 | 35 | HH78 | 46 |
| 12 | XM44 | 61.5 | 36 | RQ56 | 46 |
| 13 | VM55 | 61.5 | 37 | UT48 | 44.1 |
| 14 | MM21 | 61   | 38 | OW60 | 42 |
| 15 | NN39 | 60.5 | 39 | UW29 | 41 |
| 16 | ZX94 | 60.5 | 40 | NV39 | 40 |
| 17 | AQ51 | 60.3 |    |      |    |
| 18 | PL81 | 60   |    |      |    |
| 19 | PP79 | 60   |    |      |    |
| 20 | PU42 | 59.7 |    |      |    |
| 21 | YT30 | 59.3 |    |      |    |
| 22 | TT28 | 59   |    |      |    |
| 23 | YT23 | 58.8 |    |      |    |
| 24 | UZ39 | 58.5 |    |      |    |

| | |
|---|---|
| Mean Salary ($k) | 56.23 |
| Standard Deviation ($k) | 7.58 |
| 75th %–25th % ($k) | 50–62 |

method. When employers receive a request for data from the BLS or any other surveying organization, they also receive a set of job descriptions. Each employer selects the jobs in his or her organization that most closely match the job descriptions provided by the surveyor, and then reports the salary and benefits data for those jobs. The salary data reported across a number of employers will be a blend of data for jobs that vary in their de-

gree of closeness to the survey job descriptions. *It is important, therefore, to use the wage-and-salary survey figures as a starting point.* You may conclude that it is best to establish benchmark job rates at levels somewhat above or below the survey rates, based on your judgment of how similar the survey job descriptions are to your jobs.

A final method of obtaining external equity data that would be appropriate for a smaller practice is to contact a few major hospitals and colleagues in your area to obtain salary information about selected jobs. *This is not the same as conducting a scientifically valid survey, so your data have none of the precision of data collected from a representative sample of employers.* Nevertheless, if you have a small practice, need data on only a few jobs, understand the concept of external equity, and can make some good intuitive inferences, this method can provide useful "starting point" information. It certainly can be a cost- and time-effective way of collecting information. Finally, many hospitals conduct or purchase wage-and-salary surveys. Some hospitals may be willing to provide affiliated physicians and practices with these data, especially if you routinely hospitalize there, while others may consider these data privileged, and will not share them. You have nothing to lose, however, by asking.

As a result of using one or several of the methods discussed, you may be confident that you have good market rate data on some of your jobs, less confident about the market rates of other jobs, and perhaps no data at all on a few of your jobs. That is fine. Even large organizations do not try to obtain market data for all jobs. As noted, given the mechanics of conducting a survey, this would be an impossible task. Those jobs where you have obtained good market data will be used as your benchmark jobs. In Table 5-1, benchmark rates are listed in the third column for those jobs where the organization felt confident about the data. These jobs then will be used to anchor the compensation plan.

Next, base compensation rates are determined for the nonbenchmark jobs through interpolation. For example, we know (Table 5–1) that the rate for ultrasound technician must be somewhere between the NMT and the RN–physician assistant. Similarly, we know that the medical assistant I should be below $24,600, and the nursing supervisor should be above $55,000. If the evaluators are knowledgeable about the content of the jobs, they generally can make valid interpolation decisions. Is it possible for evaluators to make bad interpolation decisions that result in the perception of inequity? Certainly! But that is the disadvantage of this method and the other side of the ranking method's ease and simplicity.

Job evaluation methods, such as the ranking system, provide a systematic way of handling *most but not all* of the jobs in a practice. Every now and then there will be jobs that are exceptions. For example, there may be some quirks in the marketplace such that a job's compensation level is out of line. Local or national undersupply can lead to higher salaries than the job evaluation plan suggests is equitable. For example, perhaps certified opthalmic technicians (COT) are in short supply in your area and as a result the salary has escalated beyond what the job would normally merit. If you price the job according to your ranking analysis, the salary that you will be offering will be below market. If you proceed to do this, you would have difficulty hiring or would probably hire low-quality employees, and have high COT turnover. In this circumstance, you would have to offer the salary that is consistent with the market level. This is called *red circling* a job. It's an outlier, you know it's an outlier, and this is the only thing you can do with this job. You don't, however, allow it to distort the other jobs in your ranking. You don't, for example use COT as a benchmark job. In addition, you keep a close eye on this job. Usually, jobs with out-of-line salaries fall back into line after the high salaries attract more people into the field. Outliers must be dealt with idiosyncratically and paid either what you can get away with, as in the case of a low outlier, or what is necessary, as in the case of a high outlier. Don't allow these few exceptions, however, to corrupt the remainder of your compensation plan. Deal with the outliers for what they are: exceptions.

## GOING BEYOND A RANKING METHOD

The ranking job evaluation method just described is feasible for private practices to use. It's better than simply trying to guess at equitable market rates, or using no method at all to manage internal equity considerations. That said, it has some real limitations:

1. It places great reliance on being able to effectively interpolate between benchmark jobs.
2. Ranking treats jobs as wholes, because they are evaluated based on their overall worth. Jobs, as was discussed in Chapters 3 and 4, are composed of factors, such as education, responsibility for money, supervision, and so forth. For example, if one job is high in responsibility and moderate in supervision, and another is high in supervision and low in responsibility, then these relative differences should have an effect on each job's relative compensation.

A more sophisticated job evaluation method will take this complexity into account and provide a better way to determine compensable distances between jobs. The point system of job evaluation is capable of handling this complexity. It is the most widely used job evaluation method in the United States. Unfortunately, the point system's complexity and the technical human resources skills required to develop one are generally not possessed by medical practices, even large ones. Some large healthcare systems are capable of developing point systems, but even they typically implement point systems through consultants or perhaps as part of a consortium of hospitals, which cooperate to develop the basic plan. Some "off-the-shelf"[4] point systems, or one developed by a consultant specifically for your practice, nevertheless can be an effective choice for practices. In addition, some of the concepts and thinking associated with point systems provide useful ideas for physician leaders who are responsible for compensation issues.

### Point System Description

A point system is based on identifying compensable factors that apply to all of the jobs covered in the compensation plan. A compensable factor is an issue for which you or the labor market is willing to pay. Generally, for example, organizations are willing to pay for supervision, responsibility, education required, and so forth. Factors then are weighted to reflect their relative compensability, and broken into levels, which are called *degrees*. Finally, points are assigned to each degree level within each factor. An example of a point system is found in **Appendix 5A**. Next, the point chart is used to evaluate benchmark jobs based on their job descriptions. Once again, benchmark jobs are those for which you are confident that you know the fair market rate. **Table 5–3** contains an analysis of two jobs using the point system in Appendix 5A.

It is important to remember that you are evaluating *what is required by the job*, not the characteristics of a particular incumbent. Many incumbents possess skills, education, or experience not required by their jobs. Because these are characteristics of the person and not job requirements, you should not pay for them, and they should not enter into the evaluation of the job. For example, look at the education levels (1–9) for the knowledge (**Table 5A–1**) in Appendix 5A. Now, suppose that you have a clerical position in which the demands of the job require a high school education and some specialized courses. The incumbent happens to have a bachelor's degree. Because the job only requires a high school education and some spe-

**Table 5–3**  Point Evaluation of Two Benchmark Jobs

| Factor | Computer Operator/Secretary | | Business Manager | |
| --- | --- | --- | --- | --- |
| | Degree | Points | Degree | Points |
| Knowledge | 1A | 110 | 3D | 200 |
| Nonsupervisory Responsibility | 3C | 185 | 4D | 270 |
| Ingenuity | 2B | 170 | 4B | 400 |
| Personnel Management Responsibility | 1A | 120 | 6C | 225 |
| Outside/Patient Relations | 2B | 120 | 3B | 240 |
| Total Points | | 705 | | 1,335 |

cialized courses, it would be evaluated at degree 2 and would receive 135 to 255 points, depending on the number of years of experience required to perform the job adequately. The important thing to remember is that you are evaluating the worth of *jobs*, not people. Paying for irrelevant skill or experience that contributes nothing to job performance is simply a waste of money and ultimately will reduce perceived equity.

Table 5–3 contains an evaluation for the job of computer operator/secretary (see Exhibit 4–1 in Chapter 4 for the job description). The job requires a high school education with experience of less than one year, so it receives 110 points for the knowledge factor. The amount and nature of the job's nonsupervisory responsibility is best described by degree 3C, so the job receives 185

points for this factor. Given the evaluations on the other three factors, the job receives a total of 705 points. A similar evaluation of the business manager position produces a total of 1,335 points. *The point totals represent the relative worth of the jobs in terms of the compensable factors.* This is the internal equity determination process.

The next step is to convert points into dollars. This is accomplished once again by identifying benchmark jobs as described for the ranking job evaluation method. **Table 5–4** contains data for the benchmark jobs of computer operator/secretary, collection administrator, and business manager. You can now derive the point–pay relationship in two ways:

1. Use regression analysis to derive the straight-line formula for the relationship

**Table 5–4**  Determining Base Pay Using a Point System

| Benchmark Job Title | Points | Benchmark Salary | Projected Salary |
| --- | --- | --- | --- |
| Computer Operator/Secretary | 705 | $23,700.00 | |
| Insurance Biller I | 847 | | $27,461.40 |
| Collection Administrator | 950 | $30,100.00 | |
| Business Manager | 1335 | $40,800.00 | |
| Practice Administrator | 2010 | | $59,095.00 |

Benchmark Regression: Salary = $4,423 + (27.2 × Points)

between points and pay.[5] This results in a *y* intercept of $4,423, with each point (slope) worth $27.20. *Warning:* Regression analysis is only appropriate if the data essentially are linear. If the data are graphed and there is a clear bend or curve in the plot, do not use regression analysis. In this event;

2. Plot the relationship,[6] and eyeball a line that fits the data (see **Figure 5–1**). If you decide to eyeball a line, remember that measurement errors may cause your benchmark jobs not to perfectly line up. Sometimes, also, the point-pay relationship is best described by a smoothly curving line. Once again, use your judgment. If you can eyeball a line that appears to do a reasonable job of describing the data, that will be sufficient.

Because the line (expressed either as a formula or on paper) is based on benchmark jobs, *which by definition represent the equitable relationship between points and pay,* any point on the line should represent equity. The line can be used, therefore, to calculate an equitable salary for other jobs. Table 5–4 illustrates this by showing projected salaries for Insurance Biller I and Practice Administrator.

## PAY RANGES

Having one pay rate for a job could create a number of problems. For example, if $35,000 represents equity for a job, you will want the flexibility to pay somewhat above or below this amount to take into account individual equity differences between employees, such as merit and seniority. Developing pay ranges will give you this flexibility. A *pay range* treats the equity level of a job as the midpoint of a range. Pay ranges can be applied to compensation rates derived

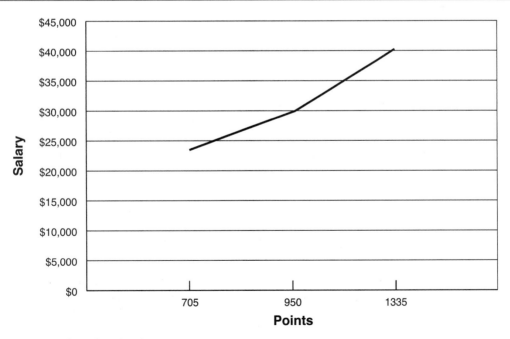

**Figure 5–1** Point-Salary Graph.

through either ranking or point job evaluation methods.

There are no incontestable ways of determining the correct size of a pay range. Generally, rules of thumb are applied. At the low end of a pay scale, spreads may vary from 10 percent to 20 percent of the pay grade midpoint. At higher pay levels, spreads may vary from 20 percent to 40 percent. Judiciously applying these rules of thumb to the positions listed in Table 5–4 might result in the salary structure found in **Table 5–5**. Obviously, this can result in some overlap between ranges. That is, a high performer or very senior employee occupying a lower position may actually make somewhat more money than a low performer or junior employee occupying a higher position. Generally, these overlaps are perceived by employees as equitable. It is generally advisable, however, to develop pay ranges so that salaries for supervisors and subordinates don't overlap, or will do so only in extreme and rare cases.

Realistically, pay levels substantially below equity will not be used very often because of the difficulty of recruiting at these levels. Labor markets, however, are not perfect, and the combination of job evaluation and wage-and-salary survey data only provide you with an estimate of equity. Employees and applicants will form their own equity judgments. As a result, you probably can hire some applicants at below-midpoint salary levels. If you find resistance to these lower levels, then you will have to raise your salary offer.

Once you have a pay range associated with a job, the next task is to decide where an employee fits within that range. This decision should be based on job performance, seniority, or some combination of the two. It is essentially a subjective decision, and in making it, you will have to rely on your evaluation of the employee's performance and the employee's value to the practice. The discussion of performance appraisal in Chapter 3 gives a number of ideas about how to obtain the performance data needed to make salary decisions on the basis of merit. Some organizations use a salary matrix that is based on the outcome of the performance appraisal (**Table 5–6**). This matrix expresses the interaction between job performance and current pay level in the pay grade.

Pay ranges can be a very effective control for excessive payroll expenses. When employees hit the top of a pay range, they cannot receive any additional increases, *because of the compensability of their jobs*. When employees start to approach the top of the range for their job, it is time to do one of the following:

• Increase the employee's duties and responsibilities to justify a higher salary. This option may be limited by the ability or

**Table 5–5**  Pay Ranges

| Benchmark Job Title | Points | Salary Midpoint | Pay Range % | Low | High |
|---|---|---|---|---|---|
| Computer Operator/Secretary | 705 | $23,700.00 | 10 | $21,330.00 | $26,070.00 |
| Insurance Biller I | 847 | $27,461.40 | 10 | $24,715.26 | $30,207.54 |
| Collection Administrator | 950 | $30,100.00 | 10 | $27,090.00 | $33,110.00 |
| Business Manager | 1,335 | $40,800.00 | 15 | $34,680.00 | $46,920.00 |
| Practice Administrator | 2,010 | $59,095.00 | 20 | $47,276.00 | $70,914.00 |

**Table 5–6** Performance Appraisal–Salary Matrix

| Current Salary Level % of Grade Midpoint | Greatly Exceeds Performance Standards % | Exceeds Performance Standards % | Meets Performance Standards % | Below Performance Standards % | Significantly Below Performance Standards % |
|---|---|---|---|---|---|
| 110 | 6 | 4 | 2 | 0 | 0 |
| 100 | 8 | 6 | 4 | 0 | 0 |
| 90 | 10 | 8 | 6 | 0 | 0 |
| 85 | 12 | 10 | 8 | 4 | 0 |

willingness of the job incumbent to take on different duties, or by the degree to which these changes would make sense given other jobs in your organization.

- Prepare the employee for a shift into another position. This option may be limited, once again, by employee ability, interest, and practice need. In a larger organization, such as a hospital or hospital system, this career path approach to staff development can be a powerful selling point to job applicants, and a real incentive.
- Tell the employee that with the exception of cost-of-living adjustments to the whole salary structure, he or she will not be able to make more money in this job. If you do this, the employee may leave. Depending on other considerations, such as staff morale and the employee's job performance, it may be reasonable to risk the employee's resignation because it could provide an opportunity to hire an acceptable replacement at a significantly lower pay level.
- Continue to give the employee pay raises, fully recognizing that you are overpaying for the job. You may be able to justify this on the basis of staff morale or simply because it makes your life easier. Overpayment, however, should be the result of a conscious, informed decision; be aware of

the probable effects on the payroll and the potential for creating internal equity problems. At some point, the overpaid employee will become costly enough in terms of payroll expenditures and equity problems that the inconvenience associated with turnover becomes greater than the benefit achieved by continuing to grant pay increases.

If you decide that you want to give merit pay increases, it is important to have wide enough pay ranges to make meaningful distinctions among employees. A merit system will be counterproductive if employees perceive that meaningful differences in performance result in trivial compensation differences. This can be a particular problem at the low end of the compensation plan, where the spread between low and high for a job might only be 20 percent. The problem is compounded by the fact that most people expect an annual salary increase. You probably will find that it is best to base pay raises on a combination of seniority and merit. The seniority component might account for 1 percent to 3 percent. The merit component might account for an additional 1 percent to 10 percent. For example, a healthcare system decides that each department will get a 7.5 percent increase in wages based on total salaries of all positions below executive level, to be distributed as follows: 2.5 percent based on seniority, and 5.0 percent based on merit. If the physician manager of the physician services office wishes to give one employee a 10 percent raise on the merit component, he or she will on average have to give other employees merit component raises of less than 5 percent to achieve the 5 percent merit average.

## INFLATION

For the past several decades, the inflation rate in the United States has been low and stable. Contrast that with the early 1980s when the annual inflation rate was over 18 percent. As an employer, the inflation rate has a lot to do with how you deal with it. When inflation is low and stable, it makes no sense to expressly incorporate inflation as a compensation component. Instead, focus on merit and seniority. Cost of living (COLA) has nothing at all to do with how well an employee is performing or their long-term commitment to you (seniority). COLA should not be confused with seniority, which is really an expression of the mutual commitment between the employee and the employer. Nevertheless, over several years, even low inflation may become a significant issue. If it does, then address it through a new job evaluation study, which looks at then-current relationships between *all* practice benchmark jobs and compensation. It should not be addressed by automatically giving everyone X percent more each year.

If inflation should become rampant again, then it would be impractical to be running job evaluation studies every year or two. Utilizing a COLA adjustment is an unrefined but effective way to keep the compensation plan somewhat equitable for several years. One way to think about a COLA increase is that you are uniformly increasing the whole compensation line in Figure 5–1 by a fixed percentage. Don't, however, raise the salary line by the full cost-of-living increase, because you want to maintain equity in total compensation through including some compensation for merit and or seniority. Cost-of-living adjustments, therefore, should lag cost of living increases by several points.

## COMPENSATION PLAN COVERAGE

Generally, organizations have several different compensation plans. One plan may cover administrative positions, a second might cover professional nonphysician positions, and the third might be for physicians. This is because the underlying job factors relevant to the different compensation plans will vary. For example, the job factors that medical and other healthcare professional positions load on would be different from those that would be appropriate for administrative positions.

## PRACTICAL CONSIDERATIONS

The compensation process discussed in this chapter may sound like overkill for a small private medical practice. For most small practices, using a ranking method with limited investigation of benchmark rates is feasible. For example, a cost- and time-effective strategy for a small practice might include using the free regional BLS *Area Wage and Salary Survey* to acquire data on some generic jobs, such as secretary and computer operator positions. Phone calls to a few hospitals and colleagues might provide ideas about the going rate for medical jobs. A ranking system then could be used to determine base rates for those positions for which you were not able to obtain market data. A "devil's advocate" pay line could be eyeballed. Salary spreads could be created and then adjusted based on your judgment of what makes sense for your practice.

At a minimum, this approach will cause you to ask yourself penetrating questions as you make compensation-related decisions. It almost certainly will give you a better outcome than using no system at all. It will provide an answer when employees ask how their pay was determined. Finally, it will probably save you money by controlling payroll costs.

Larger healthcare organizations may find it advantageous to form alliances to jointly develop a point plan. For example, several regional hospitals may use a joint task force to identify compensable factors, weight factors, and write degree definitions. Each individual hospital then can take the jointly developed point plan and use its own benchmark job data to create its own compensation plan. In this way, competitors can share common expenses to develop the point plan, but go their own separate ways as they use it. Regional and state medical societies similarly can share these infrastructure costs for its members. In effect, they develop the point system as colleagues, but then each individual practice determines how it wants to price a point.

Irrespective of whether you run a small practice or a large healthcare organization, the compensation methods discussed in this chapter are best used as a means of forming hypotheses. Formal methods should never replace good, sound management judgment. If a wage-and-salary survey gives answers that you don't like, then ask yourself why you don't like them. Is it because you really don't want to hear that a fair salary for a position is $3,000 higher than you want to pay? Or is it because the survey was inaccurate or inconsistent with anecdotal information? By forcing yourself to ask questions and investigate, formal compensation methods can help you make better compensation decisions.

## INCENTIVE PLANS

In an incentive plan, an employee receives compensation as a direct result of a change in some performance indicator. For example, a business manager who receives a percentage of the gross receipts as part of his or her compensation is receiving an incentive. A physician executive who receives a bonus as a result of an increase in the healthcare system's net income also is receiving an incentive.

Incentive plans are appealing. After all, who can argue with the logic that employees will perform better if they directly benefit from their own performance? In addition, because the incentive payment is based on an objective index, both the employer and the employee have unambiguous commitments. There are no uncertainties, such as those that characterize linking performance appraisals to merit compensation decisions.

Incentive plans can be highly motivating, but unfortunately they also can be very dangerous. Employees will direct their performance toward maximizing their incentive payments. This can be detrimental to other job-performance areas. For example, the business manager who receives a percentage of the gross receipts may neglect those duties that do not immediately affect the bottom line. Responding inadequately to patient inquiries, neglecting accounts payable duties, working on "easy money" accounts while avoiding more difficult accounts, and neglecting cost-control responsibilities all could be dysfunctional outcomes of such an incentive plan.

It is important, therefore, to anticipate dysfunctional reward contingencies. Some organizations attempt to counteract dysfunctional behavior by creating several incentives, so that employees cannot neglect a major aspect of the job. This quickly can become a cumbersome arrangement in which crafty employees may meet the letter of the incentive agreement but still manage to avoid doing all that the job requires. Generally, front-line positions in medical practices, such as collection clerks, receptionists, and business managers, should not be on incentive plans. There simply are too many possibilities to "game" behavior, which may adversely affect patients and other employees in ways that are not obvious to management.

It also is important to remember that most performance indexes can vary for many reasons. It may be very difficult to say with certainty that one person has made any contribution to an increase or decrease in a performance index, such as gross receipts, insurance collections, reduced accounts receivable, or net income. Additional capital investment, effective employee selection, good marketing, an increase in the quality of services, local demographic changes and hiring of additional physicians and employees all can contribute to raising objective indexes. As a result, employees may benefit even when their performance has not affected the outcome. Under these circumstances, an incentive arrangement will be unfair to the organization because employees will receive pay increases as a result of factors neither due to their efforts nor under their control.

It is critical, therefore, to thoroughly think through the possible consequence of an incentive plan. If you still feel that an incentive is valuable, then try to build an incentive plan that will protect you from possible dysfunctional consequences. For example, limit incentive payments to only those employees whose individual performance as noted on their performance appraisal exceeds some threshold level, such as adequate perfor-

mance on *all* factors. Another alternative is to require that the organization achieve some productivity increase, such as an increase in net income of at least 10 percent, before any incentives are payable. Employees would then share in any increase over the 10 percent level.

Incentives can be particularly important to large healthcare systems that are trying to achieve organization integration (Chapter 9). Organization integration refers to getting the parts of the healthcare system to act in a coordinated manner that furthers the total organization's objectives. Sometimes, parts of a healthcare system will excel at its own objectives to the detriment of the whole organization. Incentive plans can be used to penalize this suboptimal behavior.

For example, **Figure 5–2** illustrates a few of the divisions in a healthcare system with a matrix organization structure. (Matrix structures are discussed in Chapter 9.) The goal of this structure is to concentrate the focus of executives on critical success factors. The executive in charge of Hospital A has the job of integrating all services within the hospital to maximize quality and productivity for that facility. The director of information systems has charge of information systems across the complete healthcare system. His or her responsibility is to develop and operate information technology in the most effective manner across all system locations. The goal is to get both the product division and business division directors to work cooperatively. The danger is that if each is measured and rewarded only on the success of their own component, then each may optimize at the expense of the whole healthcare system.

For example, suppose that this health system will be implementing a new electronic medical record (EMR). These systems are very expensive and intrusive. Doing it "right"

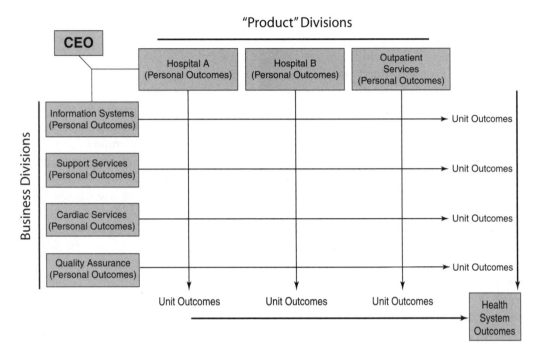

"Product" Divisions

CEO

Hospital A (Personal Outcomes) | Hospital B (Personal Outcomes) | Outpatient Services (Personal Outcomes)

Business Divisions

Information Systems (Personal Outcomes) → Unit Outcomes

Support Services (Personal Outcomes) → Unit Outcomes

Cardiac Services (Personal Outcomes) → Unit Outcomes

Quality Assurance (Personal Outcomes) → Unit Outcomes

Unit Outcomes | Unit Outcomes | Unit Outcomes | Health System Outcomes

**Figure 5–2** Matrix Organization Structure and Comprehension Incentives.

is crucial. Information Systems may favor an EMR that is relatively inexpensive and easy to maintain. This keeps acquisition and maintenance costs down, and makes the Information Systems division look good. If, however, the EMR lacks decision support capabilities, situation sensitive support menus, and other user focused characteristics, then it may waste physician time, be frustrating for them to use, and not produce other quality of care improvements that are advantageous from the healthcare system's perspective. Similarly, if Hospital A's "cash cow" service is cardiac surgery and Hospital B's is orthopedic surgery, then each may want to have an EMR with screens and characteristics desired by their surgeons, and Outpatient Services may favor a primary care focused EMR. Incentives may help us to gain the cooperation that will be needed to make an expensive, controversial, and intrusive project such as this succeed.

The first component is based on individual performance against personal goals. For example, one goal set by the health system CEO for the director of information systems might be to successfully bring a new EMR online. A second component of the IS executive's incentive plan is based on the performance of the information system division. Did they meet their cost budget? How do users, such as physicians, rate the quality of information system services? Is the automated pharmaceutical-dispensing process in the hospitals actually resulting in cost savings and reduced errors? The final component of this executive's bonus is based on a healthcare system's performance, such as net income, the system meeting quality improvement goals, and return on total assets.

Usually, these three components are linked, so that the incentives received for succeeding personally and divisionally are greatly reduced unless the whole healthcare system meets or exceeds its goals. For example, the director of information systems' incentive plan may be apportioned with 30 percent of the bonus based on individual performance, 40 percent based on the performance of the information systems division, and 30 percent based on overall healthcare system success. If, however, the healthcare system's net income is not 110 percent of last year's net income, then there is no system-based bonus; if it is less than 105 percent of last year's net income, the personal and divisional incentives are reduced by 50 percent; if it is less than 100 percent of last year's net income, the divisional bonus is eliminated; and if system net income is less than 95 percent of last year's net income, the personal component is eliminated. Plans of this nature create an incentive for division heads to be concerned about how their unit's actions affect other parts of the healthcare system, and total organization performance.

Physicians who have sold their practices to hospitals and healthcare systems often find themselves working for the first time in their lives without productivity incentives. Previously, the more these physicians worked, the more they earned, whereas now they are receiving straight salaries with annual percentage increases. Many healthcare organizations are finding that these physicians, who previously were working 50 and 60 hours per week, have turned into "clock punchers." They put in their 40 hours or so each week and go home. Profit and productivity estimates that were based on physician work habits and production levels before purchase have proven to be wildly optimistic. As a result, many healthcare organizations are rethinking how they compensate employed physicians. A consensus is developing that physician salaries need to be supplemented by bonuses or rewards based on performance. Once again, carefully specifying performance, so that perverse incentives are not created, is critical if the healthcare organization is going to achieve the type of performance it desires.

In summary, incentive payments can motivate behavior, but the behavior that is motivated may not be in the best interest of the organization. If you determine that you want to use incentives, do so with caution, and examine the arrangement from the employee's perspective to determine possible unintended consequences.

## BENEFITS

Benefits are an important part of any compensation package. As with direct wages, the benefits provided will affect the attractiveness of the organization to job applicants and will influence employee satisfaction and job performance. Some benefits, such as vacation time, are simple and generally available, whereas others, such as retirement plans, are complex and require the consultation of a specialist. Data on many benefits can be found in wage-and-salary surveys. These benefits include vacation time, sick leave, holidays, and insurance (health, life, disability, and dental).

When considering the selection of benefits, look closely at the operation of the organization. In a private practice, for example, is the day before Christmas normally a slow day? If it is, consider making this a holiday, thereby providing a benefit to employees at little cost to yourself. Do you really want to work the day after Thanksgiving? If you don't intend to work, close the office. Once again, it will be a relatively inexpensive benefit. Do you want to keep employees for a longer time, or do you prefer some turnover so as to keep salaries down? If the former, then consider offering better retirement and education benefits. If the latter, then offering these benefits would be counterproductive.

Health insurance and sick leave are benefits that can have an important effect on your employees' productivity. Employees who delay medical treatment don't take the time to get well. Those who are worried about their medical expenses will be less-than-fully productive. Good health insurance can also contribute to lower employee turnover because it will tend to tie employees to your organization.

When you are considering which benefits to provide, it is important to determine the needs of your employees. At a minimum, both large and small healthcare organizations should consider surveying their employees to find out what benefits they most desire. You are simply wasting money if you spend it on unwanted benefits. A survey can be as simple as a listing of potential benefits accompanied by a rating scale (e.g., extremely desirable, very desirable, somewhat desirable, slightly desirable, not desirable).

Some companies use a cafeteria benefits plan in order to offer benefits that are most useful and valued to their employees. A cafeteria-benefits plan allows employees some flexibility in choosing a set of benefits to meet their needs. In a cafeteria-benefits plan, each employee receives a basic package of benefits, such as health insurance, minimum number of vacation days, minimum life insurance, and minimum vacation time. They also get a number of benefit points, which is based on their salary. For example, Ramon earns $30,000 in base salary and gets the base benefits plan plus 1,000 points to use however he wishes. Perhaps moving from an HMO to a PPO costs 800 points. If so, then Ramon could upgrade his health insurance and have 200 points left over to upgrade some other benefits option, such as vacation time, tuition reimbursement, etc. Larry, on the other hand earns $50,000 in base salary. He gets the same base benefits package as

Ramon, but the higher salary also has associated with it 1,800 points, thereby providing him with an additional degree of benefit quality and flexibility. By allowing employees to select benefits based on their personal need, the value of the benefits is increased to the employee, since you allow them to spend the benefits where each derives the most value.

The concept of a cafeteria compensation plan ties in nicely with the discussion of the expectancy theory of employee motivation in Chapter 6. There are some disadvantages to cafeteria plans. Employees can make bad choices and find themselves exposed to predictable emergencies. Obviously, this is not your personal responsibility, but to the extent that an employee is distracted, his or her performance may suffer. Cafeteria plans may cost a bit more because of the extra management burden. Finally, employees will tend to select those benefits that they will use. For example, those with health problems may tend to select higher quality and therefore more expensive health options, while healthy employees remain with the HMO. This adverse self-selection may increase the overall cost of benefits to the organization.

Retirement plans have a number of advantages for employers and employees. Not only do they provide a means of accumulating retirement funds, but they can also be used to defer taxation and allow accumulation of funds at tax-deferred rates. For most physicians, the retirement plan is one of the cornerstones of their personal financial plan. Because of tax and pension reform legislation, the provisions that govern contributions to physicians' retirement plans are inextricably tied to the benefits offered to other employees. This can make a retirement plan a very complex and expensive benefit.

Retirement plans can take on a number of different forms. A pension plan becomes a fixed obligation. Contractually, your organization is committed to making certain contributions to the plan. If you have agreed to a defined contribution plan, then you are obligated to make these contributions for all qualified employees, irrespective of the organization's profits, in good years and in bad. If you have a defined benefits plan, then you are obligated to make contributions that will support the benefits promised to employees upon retirement, once again in good years and in bad. The pension plan approach to retirement planning can be burdensome for a young private practice, where income may vary from year to year and substantial funds may have to be reserved for capital investment to support growth.

Profit-sharing plans provide some of the same retirement and tax advantages as pension plans. Contributions, however, are made out of profits. If there is no profit, then there is no obligation to fund the plan. This is advantageous for young practices, for example, because it provides greater discretion in the use of corporate funds. Currently, however, the amount of funds that can be sheltered in a profit-sharing plan is less than in a pension plan. Physicians in a private practice setting should carefully analyze their practice's financial needs before making a commitment to a retirement plan. In addition, personal introspection regarding your need for predictability and flexibility is necessary before you can determine whether your retirement needs are best met by a pension or profit-sharing strategy.

Another option is a 401K plan. A 401K plan can be used to amend a profit-sharing plan to allow employees to contribute part of their salary to the plan. These contributions are deducted from the employee's taxable income and at the same time constitute a corporate expense. This can be advantageous because employees, including you, can make contributions even if there is little or no profit

available to fund a profit-sharing plan. This flexibility is limited, however, by Internal Revenue Service (IRS) rules that govern the size of contributions and the ratio of contributions that can be made by high-salaried and low-salaried employees.

The taxation issues and the IRS rules that govern whether a plan qualifies for preferential tax treatment are very complex and change on an annual basis. It is *essential,* therefore, for smaller healthcare organizations to consult an advisor who specializes in retirement planning. In addition, you should remember that creating a retirement plan is like having a baby. It is going to be with you for the remainder of your corporate life. It will be constantly consuming time and resources. There are annual IRS statements and financial reports that must be assembled and filed in a timely manner. The plan will have to be updated from time to time to comply with current law. In addition, someone will have to administer the plan and make investment decisions. Larger healthcare organizations should have a position, perhaps even a department, devoted to retirement planning and management. Physicians in closely held organizations, such as private practices, should obtain the advice of a professional who understands both their personal financial objectives and their organization's objectives.

## CASE APPLICATION: MRS. WILSON'S EQUITY

Dr. Early was an owner and the managing physician of a group family practice. He received a résumé from Mrs. Wilson for his vacant business manager position. Mrs. Wilson had previously worked for Dr. Johnson's group radiology practice at a salary of $75,000, directing the group's billing functions. When Dr. Johnson retired, the remaining partners eliminated Mrs. Wilson's position and her entire staff, with the justification that it would be more economical to "outsource" the function to a billing service. Mrs. Wilson's experience appeared to be excellent, and at the interview she gave the impression of being a calm, mature 50-year-old woman who knew that she could do the job.

Dr. Early had some reservations about hiring Mrs. Wilson. The salary for his business manager position was $50,000, which he knew was a fair salary, perhaps even somewhat above the median salary for this type of position. Dr. Early sensed that Mrs. Wilson's real job at Dr. Johnson's practice had been to supervise an overstaffed office, and that she hadn't been in the trenches actually running a fast-paced office for many years. He knew that in his practice the business manager was in the front line and personally had to follow up on problem claims, negotiate payment plans with delinquent patients, and manage other front office employees, among other things. Dr. Early was concerned that the combination of more demanding work and substantially lower pay would result in perceptions of inequity, irrespective of the fact that he had given Mrs. Wilson a realistic job preview, and that she was voluntarily taking a job at a much lower salary than in her previous job.

Mrs. Wilson, however, insisted that she knew that she would have to take a pay cut wherever she went, and that it was important to her to work for people with whom she felt comfortable. After two interviews with Dr. Early and his staff, she said that she would enjoy working at his practice. Mrs. Wilson was the most qualified applicant in Dr. Early's selection pool, and he needed to fill the position as soon as possible, so he hired her in spite of his reservations.

Mrs. Wilson's tenure turned out to be unsettling to all involved. She quickly grew frustrated with the demands of the job. Her frustration manifested itself in temper tantrums and insubordinate comments and actions toward Dr. Early and the other associates. She resigned after 4 months of employment. Dr. Early had these comments:

It started to go wrong right from the start. She was used to a country club atmosphere in which she was also overpaid. She quickly grew to resent realistic job demands at a realistic salary. She treated me like it was *my* fault that she was in this situation, that she was no longer employed by a sugar daddy practice! Toward the end, she even tried to manipulate me into firing her, so that she wouldn't have to take the responsibility for her circumstances!

She never did get her equity equation readjusted to reality. Her "comparison other" was this image of herself at the previous practice, which had no grounding in the real world. How could I fight that? The answer is that I couldn't, and I should have realized this, despite her assurances to the contrary.

Dr. Johnson's largess made Mrs. Wilson largely unemployable. It would be a rare individual who has the self-awareness to be able to take a career step backward of this magnitude. Mrs. Wilson couldn't do it, and I suppose that I shouldn't hold that too much against her. At the same time, however, I've learned that you can't fight unrealistic equity perceptions. In her mind her previous employment situation was equitable, and only she can change that perception. If she doesn't find another sugar daddy practice, she will eventually have to adjust her expectations. I have sympathy for any practice that she encounters between now and then. I'll never hire a person under these circumstances again. I've learned my lesson.

## PHYSICIAN COMPENSATION

During the mid-1990s Meridia Health Care in Cleveland, Ohio, began purchasing primary care practices as part of an effort to build an integrated delivery system.[7] Compensation was based on physicians' salaries at the time of acquisition. Benefits were based on those provided to Meridia's executives. Billing, collection, and practice management were contracted out to a management company. After these acquisitions, physician productivity precipitously declined, with losses on average exceeding $100,000 per physician. The moral of this story is that physicians' incentives and their performance are linked. Physicians, who previously were performing at higher levels, changed their behavior once their compensation was no longer related to their financial productivity.[8]

Physician compensation is potentially the most contentious business issue that physicians face in group practice. In order to effectively manage this it is necessary to focus first on *what* is to be compensated. If you don't identify the "what" first, then developing a compensation plan will be rooted in personally directed self-interest characterized by a confrontational zero-sum-game atmosphere.[9] This is a situation in which the distinctions between integrative and distributive negotiations and positions and interests (see Chapter 8) are particularly relevant. Group practices create integrative opportunities for their members that they otherwise would not have access to: clinical, marketing, staffing, and managerial resources; contracting opportunities; and collegial opportunities including clinical coverage and personal time. The practice can provide value that is more than the sum of its individual parts if the physicians are motivated to work in integrative ways. Always begin the compensation development process with a discussion of *practice*, meaning *mutual* strategic goals. Focus the discussion toward mutual underlying interests and away from specific positions. If interests are not identified, then developing the compensation plan will become a zero-sum-game negotiation in which each stakeholder simply becomes positional

by arguing for a formula that he or she believes will maximize personal gain.

At a minimum, a physician compensation plan should determine how to allocate collections based on physicians' billings including an equitable distribution to cover common expenses, such as rent, telephones, and managerial and front office personnel, etc., and personally identifiable expenses, such as an assistant, personal equipment, and the like. In addition, the compensation plan can support integrative practice opportunities by rewarding physicians for achieving *practice* goals, such as specific quality improvement objectives, which have been identified through a participative process involving the practice's physicians.

In order to determine what will be compensated for, and then develop a compensation plan that will make this happen, we will rely on concepts discussed in earlier chapters, specifically:

1. Identifying critical physician performance factors
2. Goal Setting and Performance Planning

In addition, we will do these things within the context of:

1. Achieving equity as defined earlier in this chapter.
2. Distinguishing between positions and interests—Interests are fundamental objectives that you are trying to achieve. Positions are tactics or ways of achieving an interest. For example, achieving equity and insuring long-term financial success may be two interests that you want to achieve when developing a practice's physician compensation plan. The characteristics of the specific plan per se, such as what is compensated for and the compensation formulae, etc. are positions.

Often, there is more than one position that will more or less achieve an interest. Understanding this creates the opportunity for negotiation. This is discussed in more detail in Chapter 8 (Negotiation).

3. Aligning specific compensation objectives with the practice's marketing plan and the strategic goals that have been identified to achieve practice success. Developing a marketing plan is discussed in detail in Chapter 7.

The physician compensation plan will be the outcome of a well-considered analysis of these five points. "Well-considered" means that you must immediately and completely explore all of the possible options on each of these five points. If time and cost are not considerations, then a thorough job on these points must be done. Develop a level of comfort that is mutually satisfactory to the partners today. Next month or next year the partners may mutually decide that additional exploration on one or more of these points is desirable.

## Practice Business Strategy and Critical Physician Performance Goals

Physicians will be the leaders for achieving practice goals. Creating personal incentives for achieving practice goals is one way to ensure that all are working toward these common goals. **Table 5–7** provides an illustration for a cardiology practice. The first column identifies some long-term practice objectives that the physicians have identified as central to their business strategy, which is an outcome from the practice's marketing plan. The second column identifies some physician performance factors that are consistent with or help to achieve some of the strategic initiatives. The goal of the practice compensation plan will be to create incentives for physicians to excel on these physician performance factors, and through them achieve practice objectives. Column three contains some operational measures, which are available today and included in the practice's compensation plan. Notice that many of the physician performance factors have not been developed into physician compensation factors. In this instance, the practice recognizes what is important to assess (physician performance factors), but either because of time, difficulty, or failure to achieve a consensus yet, it has not developed operational measures (physician compensation factors) for all of them. Nevertheless, it's clear that the practice has a plan of where it needs to go in refining it's compensation plan.

Let's assume for the moment that the practice has not formally identified strategic objectives. This might be the time to begin discussing these issues. Even if you don't comprehensively identify practice strategic objectives, the discussion will provide information going forward. For example, everyone may agree that working on primary care physician satisfaction is an important practice issue, and that to some degree physicians who are outliers on this factor should be affected by their performance on it. It would be too soon to begin doing this, because no one has determined yet how to measure PCP satisfaction. The consensus that it is an important and potentially compensable issue begins the process of identifying how to do this, so it will appear in a future development of the compensation plan.

## Evaluating Performance, Setting Goals, and Performance Planning

If your compensation plan is going to provide incentives for "doing the right thing," then somehow, you have to be able to assess performance. Ideally, physician compensation

**Table 5–7** Cardiology Practice Compensation Issues

| Selected Practice Strategic Objectives | Physician Performance Factors | Physician Compensation Factors |
|---|---|---|
| *Clinical Programs* | | |
| Lipid Management Protocol Program | Quality of Care | |
| Congestive Heart Failure Study | Protocol Compliance | Not Assessed |
| Angina Management Program | Charting Compliance | Not Assessed |
| Women's Health Initiative | Satisfaction | |
| | Patient Wait Times | Not Assessed |
| | Patient Satisfaction | Patient Satisfaction Survey |
| | PCP Satisfaction | PCP Satisfaction Survey |
| | Clincial Outcomes | Not Assessed |
| | Clinical Productivity | |
| | FFS Productivity | FFS Net Income |
| | MC Productivity | MC Net Income |
| *Administration* | | |
| EMR Intensification | Clinical Program Leadership/Participation | 360° Colleague Evaluation |
| Cost Management Task Force | Clinical Program Leadership/Participation | 360° Colleague Evaluation |
| Internal Practice Committees | Clinical Program Leadership/Participation | 360° Colleague Evaluation |
| *Practice Development* | | |
| Alliances—Health Systems, Med School, MDs | Teaching | Not Assessed |
| | Committee Service | Not Assessed |
| Reputation Enhancement | Research Publications/Conf. Presentations | Not Assessed |
| | Community Service | Not Assessed |

factors should be quantitative, with the numbers coming directly from physician performance. Examples include Relative Value Units (RVUs), gross revenue, net revenue, managed care revenue, percent treatment protocol compliance, patient satisfaction survey data, and the like.

The basis for goal setting and performance planning was discussed in Chapter 3. In Chapter 3 the basis for doing physician goal setting and performance planning is collegiality. For example, a physician who is well recognized for her or his successful relations with referral sources works with a colleague who seeks to improve in this area. The link now to compensation simply places additional emphasis on setting reasonable goals and developing the skills and motivation to do it. In short, motivation is not only based on satisfying a personal need for achievement, but also on financial consequences.

### Developing a Physician Compensation Plan

A compensation plan that results in wild compensation fluctuations based on relatively short-term annual performance on limited but important variables will not be perceived as equitable. Therefore, a successful compensation plan will balance the "pay-for-performance" aspect with a dependable, predictable, equitable component based on simply doing your job. If a physician isn't doing the basic job at a minimally acceptable level, then this is a performance appraisal issue and should be handled accordingly. There are two basic physician compensation strategies. One is internally focused and the other is externally focused.

Internally focused strategies focus solely on the within practice distribution of rewards. For example, a physician's compensation is based on collections (cash basis) or net revenue (accrual basis). Deductions from collections are made to cover the physician's share of practice fixed and variable costs, budgeted future practice capitalization and cost items, and individually identifiable fixed and variable costs. If there is a pay-for-performance component, then an additional increment is withheld, which will be divided based on performance.

Externally focused strategies first use external wage-and-salary data to anchor physician compensation. For example, each physician in a cardiology practice may receive a base pay equal to the 50th percentile in the Medical Group Management Association's (MGMA) wage-and-salary survey. This approach assumes that the physicians as a group are as productive as those in the wage-and-salary survey, and that practice costs also are in line with those in the survey. Physician salaries then are treated as a practice expenses, and this expense along with all other expenses then are subtracted from practice net collections (cash basis) or net revenue (accrual basis). As with internal models, any fixed or variables costs that can be allocated to a particular physician are subtracted from his or her net collections or revenues. After budgeting for any future practice expense and capitalization needs, any residual goes into a bonus pool, which is allocated to physicians based on their performance. The base and bonus components can be adjusted, so that next year, for example, the base component might be set at the 60th percentile or the 45th percentile of the wage and salary survey, thereby reflecting practice performance, or the degree to which the partners wish to incentivize physician performance.

The specific details of how to arrange internally focused and externally focused plans are limitless. The objective for any practice should be to develop a plan that addresses its physicians' own strategic objectives as just discussed, and do this in a way that the partners see as equitable. As a way of illustrating this, let's take a look at a few compensation plan examples.

### Straight Salary

Using this internally focused approach, all partners are paid an equal salary. Generally, this is set at some large percentage of expected revenues or actual past cash collections based on past history so that there is no annual deficit. At the end of the year, any practice net income is equally distributed to the physicians. The advantage of this approach is that it is simple. If everyone is producing at about the same level on all important issues to the practice, and everyone likes this approach, then this may be an easy and successful plan. As a colleague of mine says, "If you have a tree growing in the middle of your living room, and you like the tree, and you think it adds ambiance to your living room, and you decorate it for Christmas, it's not my place to be critical." There are, however, many potential disadvantages. If there is physician productivity or cost variance, then higher producers will be subsidizing lower producers. It also doesn't create any incentive to excel, because there is no reward for seeing additional patients, reducing costs, improving quality, or developing new referral sources.

### Salary + Incentive Bonus

This is the same as straight salary, but salary is targeted at a level, which is based on past and current performance and ensures that there will be a residual at the end of the year. The residual is then allocated based on performance. Once again, there is a potential subsidization problem if there is physician productivity or cost variance. High produc-

ers may get some of this back from the bonus pool, but low producers may still be collecting more than their productivity merits.

### Salary + Market-Based Incentive

In this approach a wage-and-salary survey is used to identify a relationship between a salary driver and salary, such as gross revenue and salary level. In **Figure 5–3**, the salary curve reflects the salary-productivity relationship at the 50th percentile in this market based on a wage-and-salary survey. The base salary for each physician is set at a level that everyone is expected to exceed, such as the 35th percentile in the market, which in this case is $200,000. The net effect of this is that everyone is guaranteed a salary floor. Once the physician exceeds $550,000 in gross revenue, then compensation is based on the wage-and-salary survey data curve, so generating $700,000 in gross revenue would result in salary of $340,000.[10] It is unlikely that high performers will have to subsidize low performers, because the guaranteed salary is set at a less than expected level. Once again, if a physician performs below this floor, then this may be a performance appraisal and goal-setting issue. Why would a practice wish to risk subsidizing *any* salary? Perhaps, to control for illness, a new physician whose productivity is uncertain, or as a general safety net should the practice's market position change in unforeseen ways.

In this example, the driver for allocating the incentive is gross revenue, however, as long as the practice is exceeding the market productivity level, it can also reward other incentives, such as those described in Table 5–7. For example, suppose that the practice is actually performing at the 60th percentile productivity level. After salary based on gross receipts is distributed, there will still be a residual, which now could be awarded based

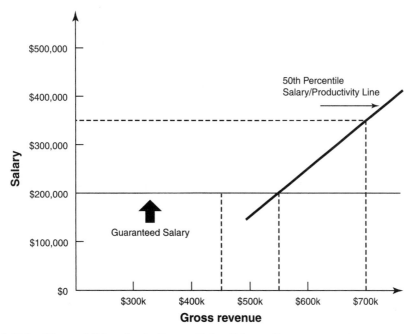

**Figure 5–3** Using Wage and Salary Survey Data to Relate Salary to Revenue.

on clinical outcomes, protocol compliance, or patient or primary care physician satisfaction.

There are an infinite number of specific compensation plans that medical compensation advisors can construct. They all, however, reduce to the objective of achieving equity. Focusing the discussion first on practice strategic interests will allow the partners to work with the consultant to develop a practice plan, with a relative degree of objectivity and civility.

## CONCLUSION

Making good compensation decisions has both artistic and technological components. The technological parts are the compensation processes that you use, while the artistic parts are the choices that you make to effectively recognize stakeholders' interests, so they perceive equity. The most significant message of this chapter is the importance of achieving equity. The tools described are essentially aids for achieving equity. Some smaller practices may find that understanding the objectives of individual, internal, and external equity at the conceptual level will allow them to make good compensation decisions. Larger practices and other healthcare organizations will find it necessary to use empirical compensation tools, such as wage-and-salary surveys, point job evaluation plans, pay ranges, and structured physician compensation plans to achieve these objectives. Consultants can be particularly useful in designing compensation plans, because experience is important for making good compensation design decisions. In addition, an effective consultant can dispationately explore the interests of the practice stakeholders, identify alternative positions, and facilitate an effective discussion of these issues, so the eventual compensation plan achieves practice and stakeholder objectives.

## NOTES

1. This assumes that the physician position is salaried, such as it might be in some larger healthcare systems. Generally, in practices, physician compensation is based on collections.
2. BLS has many wage and salary surveys, some of which contain medical occupations. See www.bls.gov/home.htm.
3. See, for example, the Santa Barbara County Medical Society at www.sbmed.org/webpages/pm .asp and the Michigan State Medical Society at www.rehmann.com/default.cfm?t=service_ industry.cfm&L2=HEACAR&L3=HCSURV& regionId=6.
4. These are proprietary, but semigeneric systems. The consulting firm starts with its standard point system factors and charts, but may modify them, or how they are used based on internal practice issues. They then use their own internal databases to identify benchmark jobs and develop a compensation plan that is internally and externally equitable.
5. Regression analysis requires a large enough sample size so that the resulting statistical conclusions are meaningful. This case has only three observations so errors in using the point chart or identifying true benchmark rates could easily change the regression formula.

6. It's also not advisable to project the line much beyond your data points, because the real point/pay relationships may be above or below your projected line. Because you don't have data in these regions, your projections are speculative.
7. Davis, A., & Hardy, T. (1999). New compensation model improves physician productivity. *Healthcare Financial Management,* 53(7): 46–50.
8. It should be noted that financial productivity is only one aspect of productivity. It is possible, therefore, that physicians increased the quality of their work while decreasing the quantity or at least the revenue associated with their work.
9. A zero-sum-game occurs when the size of the pie is fixed and the negotiation is over how to divide it. If I win $50, you lose $50, and the sum of the two is $0.00.
10. Actual compensation is calculated with a regression formula that describes the relationship between the salary driver, in this case gross revenue, and the dependent variable of salary. The Salary/Productivity line in Table 5–8 displays the regression line for the underlying statistical formula.

# Point System of Job Evaluation

*This point plan is provided for illustrative purposes only. The factors that it contains, their weighting, and the degree definitions may not be relevant to your practice. If you wish to use a point system, contact a qualified compensation professional.*

## KNOWLEDGE (TABLE 5A–1)

*Knowledge* is the combination of education and experience that is required by the job. *Education* refers to knowledge that is normally acquired through formal schooling; *experience* is knowledge that is normally acquired through on-the-job training or work experience.

## NONSUPERVISORY RESPONSIBILITY (TABLE 5A–2)

This factor considers the degree of analytical ability, judgment, discretion, and timeliness involved in making decisions. It is concerned with how education and experience are applied to the job, but it does not cover responsibility for personnel administration, which is covered elsewhere.

Consider the following issues when evaluating degree of review and impact:

- What decisions are made?
- What are the most difficult decisions and actions?
- Is independent judgment required, or are decisions based on precedent?
- How frequently are decisions made?

- Consider all the responsibilities for the position, even if some of them are delegated to a subordinate. For example, an office manager may be responsible for collection even if some specific collection tasks are delegated to a billing clerk.
- Remember, making decisions is more important than making recommendations.

Consider the following issues when evaluating degree of independence:

- To what extent are decisions reviewed by superiors?
- What is the potential cost or seriousness of errors, and how often does the position require making decisions for which there is a chance of serious cost or consequences?
- What is the time span that could occur before an error is detected?
- Evaluate the job under normal day-to-day conditions. Don't place disproportionate weight on unusual or unlikely circumstances.

If a subordinate position merits more points than the position being evaluated on either the degree of review and impact or degree of independence scales, then assign the number of points associated with the subordinate position.

## INGENUITY (TABLE 5A–3)

This factor is concerned with the creativeness and resourcefulness required by the position. This can occur as a result of creative

**Table 5A–1** Factor: Knowledge

| Education | A Under 1 Yr. | B 1 Yr.–2 Yr. | C 2 Yr.–3 Yr. | D 3 Yr.–4 Yr. | E 4 Yr.–5 Yr. | F 5 Yr.–6 Yr. | G > 6 Yrs. |
|---|---|---|---|---|---|---|---|
| 1. High school degree | 110 | 120 | 135 | 150 | 170 | 195 | 230 |
| 2. High school degree plus some specialized courses | 135 | 145 | 160 | 175 | 195 | 220 | 255 |
| 3. High school plus many additional courses; up to 1 year of college | 160 | 170 | 185 | 200 | 220 | 245 | 300 |
| 4. Extensive courses beyond high school, 1 or 2 years of college, business school, or technical training. | 210 | 220 | 235 | 250 | 270 | 295 | 350 |
| 5. Courses equivalent to 2 or 3 years of college | 265 | 275 | 290 | 305 | 325 | 350 | 405 |
| 6. Bachelor's degree | 325 | 335 | 350 | 365 | 385 | 410 | 465 |
| 7. Master's or equivalent graduate degree. | 385 | 395 | 410 | 425 | 445 | 470 | 525 |
| 8. Master's degree or equivalent plus other graduate degree or certification | 445 | 455 | 470 | 485 | 505 | 530 | 585 |
| 9. Doctorate | 510 | 520 | 535 | 550 | 570 | 595 | 650 |

**Table 5A–2** Nonsupervisory Responsibility

Degree of Review and Impact: Column Definitions

A. Decisions and actions reviewed regularly. Limited effect on operations.
B. Decisions/actions reviewed regularly. Inadequacies would only result in minor problems.
C. Decisions/actions usually reviewed. Inadequacies could cause moderate problems or expense.
D. Decisions/actions occasionally reviewed. Inadequacies could cause considerable problems or expense.
E. Decisions/actions occasionally reviewed. Inadequacies would cause extensive problems or expense.
F. Decisions/actions rarely reviewed. Inadequacies could cause extensive problems or expense.
G. Decisions/actions rarely reviewed. Inadequacies may affect long-range practice plans and strategies.
H. Decisions/actions usually final. Inadequacies may affect long-range practice plans and strategies.
I. Decisions/actions usually final, and inadequacies will seriously affect long-range plans.
J. Decisions/action are final and inadequacies will seriously affect long-range plans.

|  | | | | | Degree of Review and Impact | | | | | |
| *Degree of Independence* | A | B | C | D | E | F | G | H | I | J |
| --- | --- | --- | --- | --- | --- | --- | --- | --- | --- | --- |
| 1. Operating procedures are well defined, and independent activity is limited. | 120 | 140 | 165 | 195 | 245 | 315 | 415 | 560 | 765 | 1060 |
| 2. Operating procedures are generally coverd by clear rules, regulations, instructions, etc. Decisions/actions required are not complex. | 140 | 160 | 185 | 215 | 265 | 335 | 435 | 580 | 785 | 1080 |
| 3. Makes operating decisions and takes some actions of importance. Occasionally, decisions are of considerable complexity. | 165 | 185 | 210 | 240 | 290 | 360 | 460 | 605 | 810 | 1105 |
| 4. Make operating decisions, and takes actions of moderate difficulty. Occasionally, actions/ decisions are of considerable complexity. | 195 | 215 | 240 | 270 | 320 | 390 | 490 | 635 | 840 | 1135 |

*continues*

**Table 5A–2** continued

| Degree of Independence | Degree of Review and Impact | | | | | | | | | |
|---|---|---|---|---|---|---|---|---|---|---|
| | A | B | C | D | E | F | G | H | I | J |
| 5. Makes frequent operating decisions and takes actions of considerable difficulty. Assists in the formulation of recommendations on difficult and important issues. | 245 | 265 | 290 | 320 | 370 | 440 | 540 | 685 | 890 | 1185 |
| 6. Assist in the formulation of and on occasion independently formulates recommendations on difficult and important matters. | 315 | 335 | 360 | 390 | 440 | 510 | 610 | 755 | 960 | 1255 |
| 7. In addition to the above, makes some independent decisions and takes independent action on important matters. | 415 | 435 | 460 | 490 | 540 | 610 | 710 | 855 | 1060 | 1355 |
| 8. Frequently makes independent decisions and takes independent action on important operating matters. | 560 | 580 | 605 | 635 | 685 | 755 | 855 | 1000 | 1205 | 1500 |
| 9. Continually makes independent decisions, and takes independent action on very important operating matters. | 765 | 785 | 810 | 840 | 890 | 960 | 1060 | 1205 | 1410 | 1705 |
| 10. Continually makes independent decisions and takes independent action on matters of the greatest importance. | 1060 | 1080 | 1105 | 1135 | 1185 | 1255 | 1355 | 1500 | 1705 | 2000 |

**Table 5A–3** Factor: Ingenuity

| Degree Definition | A | B | C |
|---|---|---|---|
| 1. Requires little original or independent thinking. | 100 | 115 | 130 |
| 2. Requires occasional ingenuity in the refinement of ideas by others. | 150 | 170 | 195 |
| 3. Ingenuity is definitely required, but usually involves the refinement of established ideas, procedures, methods, etc. | 225 | 260 | 300 |
| 4. Some original and independent thinking in originating and developing new or improved ideas. | 350 | 400 | 475 |
| 5. Frequent application of a high degree of original and independent thinking and developing complex ideas in new undefined areas. | 550 | 625 | 700 |
| 6. Continuous application of a high degree of creativeness, resourcefulness, and inventiveness. Originates very complex creative ideas in new and undefined areas. Creativity has major effect on the practice. | 800 | 900 | 1000 |

The "B" point values should be used when the definition closely matches the job. The "A" or "C" columns can be used for jobs that are somewhat above or below the definition, but not to a significant enough extent to warrant selection of a higher or lower Degree Definition.

thinking, or developing new ideas, plans, or methods. Evaluate the job based on how much ingenuity is normally required, as opposed to overweighting unusual circumstances. The key issue is whether the job requires ingenuity, not whether a particular incumbent happens to be personally creative.

## PERSONNEL MANAGEMENT RESPONSIBILITY (TABLE 5A–4)

This factor assesses the job requirements for organizing, leading, coordinating, training, and controlling employees. This factor assesses both line and functional responsibilities. *Line responsibilities* are defined as organizing, selecting, training, promoting, dismissing, setting performance objectives, evaluating, and directing the actions of others. An example of a line relationship would be a business manager who directly controls the actions of a subordinate secretary.

Functional responsibilities are concerned with implementing programs and policies through employees, but the position does not have direct line authority over the implementing positions. An example of a functional relationship would be a business manager who develops collection policies, which are used by secretaries who report to the collection administrator. The following issues should be considered when evaluating jobs on this factor:

- Only consider responsibility for managing people.
- It is important to determine whether the position has line responsibility, functional responsibility, or both.
- When evaluating line responsibility, consider the diversity of supervisory activities involved, the type of people being supervised, and any extenuating or complicating issues.

**Table 5A–4**  Factor: Personnel Management Responsibility

| Degree of Line/Functional Responsibilty | Number of Line Employees Supervised | | | | |
|---|---|---|---|---|---|
| | *A* *None* | *B* *1–5* | *C* *6–10* | *D* *11–15* | *E* *16 or More* |
| 1. Little or no line or functional responsibility. | 120 | 130 | 140 | 155 | 170 |
| 2. Line responsibilities are primarily simple and routine, or functional responsibility is limited to advice or guidance with no responsibility for control or follow-up. | 130 | 140 | 150 | 165 | 180 |
| 3. Line responsibilities are generally routine involving the same or similar activities, or some functional advice and guidance usually without responsibility for control or follow-up. | 145 | 155 | 165 | 180 | 195 |
| 4. Line responsibilities are somewhat complex and occasionally difficult, involving the same or similar activities, or frequent functional advice and guidance usually without responsibility for control or follow-up. | 160 | 170 | 180 | 195 | 210 |
| 5. Line responsibilities are moderately complex and occasionally difficult, involving varied activities or work groups, or frequent functional advice and guidance with some control responsibilities or limited complexity. | 180 | 190 | 200 | 215 | 230 |
| 6. Line responsibilities are generally complex and difficult involving varied, moderately complex activities, or moderately complex functional control responsibilities. | 205 | 215 | 225 | 240 | 255 |
| 7. Line responsibilities are complex and difficult and involving diverse complex activities or work groups, or complex functional control responsibilities for upholding practice standards. | 235 | 245 | 255 | 270 | 285 |
| 8. Line responsibilities are highly complex and diversified involving highly complex activities or work groups, or highly complex functional control responsibilities for upholding practice standards. | 275 | 285 | 295 | 310 | 325 |
| 9. Line responsibilities are of extreme complexity involving activities and work groups of extreme importance, or functional control responsibilities of extreme complexity and importance. | 420 | 430 | 440 | 455 | 470 |
| 10. Line responsibilities are of maximum complexity, or functional control responsibilities of maximum complexity and importance in the practice. | 790 | 800 | 810 | 830 | 860 |

- When evaluating functional responsibility, consider the diversity of activities, the types of employees with whom the incumbent must work, and any extenuating or complicating issues.
- It is often more difficult to get things done through people in a functional relationship than in a line relationship.
- If a subordinate position merits more points than the position being evaluated, assign the number of points associated with the subordinate position.

## OUTSIDE RELATIONSHIPS (TABLE 5A–5)

Outside relationships assess the extent to which the position must interact with others outside the healthcare organization. This could include insurance companies, patients, physicians, and the like. It is important to determine whether these outside contacts involve simply exchanging information or whether something more significant occurs, such as influencing the decisions of others. Consider the level of people being contacted, the frequency of contact, and whether the nature of the communication is to elicit or provide information.

**Table 5A–5** Factor: Outside Relationships

|  | *Point Values* | | |
| *Degrees* | *A* | *B* | *C* |
|---|---|---|---|
| 1. Outside contacts limited to the exchange of information with employees in other organizations who do not make decisions. Little tact or few negotiation skills required. | 50 | 65 | 80 |
| 2. Outside contacts are required, which involve some tact, and diplomacy, and on occasion they may influence decisions, or contacts may occur frequently, but they only involve the exchange of information. Alternatively or additionally, patient contact to provide information or make simple transactions. | 100 | 120 | 150 |
| 3. Outside contacts are a central requirement of the position. They necessitate tact and diplomacy and frequently influence decisions that are of moderate importance. They could involve discussions with relatively high levels of management. Alternatively or additionally, patient contact regarding significant financial or business issues. | 190 | 240 | 300 |
| 4. Outside contacts are a major job responsibility. They involve important decisions, require negotiation and tactical skills, and occur at high organizational levels. | 360 | 430 | 500 |

The "B" point values should be used when the definition closely matches the job. The "A" or "C" columns can be used for jobs that are somewhat above or below the definition, but not to a significant enough extent to warrant selection of a higher or lower degree definition.

## CHAPTER 6

# Leading Your Employees and Colleagues

---

**Chapter Objectives**

This chapter will help you to:

1. Effectively lead colleagues and subordinates using a variety of leadership styles based on relevant situational issues.
2. Introduce significant change into your practice or healthcare organization, and manage the change process to benefit from and overcome opposition to new ideas and ways of doing things.
3. Motivate others so they will work toward organizational goals.

---

## INTRODUCTION

The glue that holds a practice or health system together is the management skills of its leaders and managers. The effectiveness of a physician leader's financial, marketing, and strategic skills is greatly diminished if he or she cannot successfully bring them to bear through the actions of subordinates, peers, and superiors. As a physician leader, much of your work will be performed through the actions of others. Some of your ability to do this is based on your reputation and the network of associations and relationships that you bring to the job. Much of your success at marshalling the efforts of others, however, will be based on your leadership skills, your ability to manage change in the face of resistance, and your ability to motivate others to follow through on the direction that you have set or caused to be set.

For example, you have been given the job of evaluating the feasibility of starting an obstetrics triage center for your hospital, which your practice would help to staff. You are aware of the importance of constructing a financial model to evaluate the costs and profitability of the center (see Chapter 1). You also know that you need to determine how it will improve acute obstetrical care outcomes, and how it will affect resident staff, who formerly provided treatment in the emergency department. After you identify the information and data that you want to examine, others will collect and assemble them into spreadsheets and reports. Next, you will probably discuss the financial and medical implications with those who will be affected by this change, including emergency department staff, obstetrics staff, residents, administration, and so forth. The success of this project will be due in no small measure to your ability to understand the incentives of the individuals involved, so you can:

1. create a vision of how the change will be beneficial and galvanize others to help make the change a success

2. incorporate good ideas suggested by others
3. overcome resistance on the part of some stakeholders

Leading and managing the process with subordinates, peers, and superiors and anticipating potential sources of resistance and overcoming this resistance will be as much a determinant of the project's success as properly evaluating the financial and clinical considerations.

Two terms that capture the essence of the skills necessary for success are *leadership* and *motivation*. Both skills are concerned with getting employees to work toward organizational goals. Leadership is the process of how you interact with other critical players. Often, leadership is concerned with influencing behavior through inspiration, personal example, words, and actions. Leaders lead in a variety of ways, which include delegating, consulting, and on occasion being directive. Motivation is the process of causing employees, peers, partners, and others to work toward the organization's goals by providing rewards that they desire. Sometimes, these rewards are monetary, but often they are less tangible such as recognition, a sense of achievement, and the opportunity for personal/professional growth. When personally valuable rewards are contingent upon reaching organizational goals, then employees are motivated to attain them.

## LEADERSHIP

Leadership methods and principles are best understood in the context of real problems. When I'm conducting physician leadership programs, I always discuss these ideas in the context of real physician leadership situations. Often, I will ask the participating physicians to describe leadership issues that they have confronted in their practices or in their hospital roles. In addition, I have the physicians read a practice-based case, so they can discuss and apply the leadership ideas discussed in the program to a shared situation. The case I will use in this book is called United Family Practices Ltd. and you will find it in the appendix at the end of this chapter. Please read this case before continuing with this chapter.

Effective leadership has at least three aspects to it. *Vision* involves an intuitive ability to see where the practice, organization, or group needs to go. The visionary physician leader has ideas about what the practice needs to be doing and how to do it. At United Family Practices, both Mr. Reynolds and Dr. Anderson are visionary. They see the need to change and they have some ideas regarding what the practice needs to do to achieve this vision. *Inspiration* is the ability to get others to convert this vision into actions. It is a way to motivate others to act. The inspirational physician leader can translate the OB triage center project discussed previously into a compelling story that will motivate specific actions by critical stakeholders. Often, these visionary and inspirational aspects appear together in great leaders. For example, Martin Luther King, Winston Churchill, and Cesar Chavez are often identified as great leaders. Each was able to formulate a vision of what could be, and then inspire others to act in ways to achieve the vision. Mr. Reynolds and Dr. Anderson both need to think about how they could inspire the changes that they are proposing. Unfortunately, a leader's visionary and inspirational skills are to a large degree the baggage that they are or are not carrying. It's very difficult to teach someone how to be creative or how to enthuse others, although certainly leaders need to try.

These aspects of vision and inspiration separate the issue of *leadership* from *management*. Leadership results in something *changing*, and leaders create *change*. Management is the process of effectively using *current* methods, procedures, and rules. Physicians need to be involved in both the *leadership* and *management* of their organizations. Stated another way, healthcare organizations need both physician leaders and physician managers. Often, this is the same physician in the same job, who simply is being faced with a different (leadership or management) challenge. Healthcare organizations need physicians who can create new ways of doing things and make current ways of doing things work effectively, and the fact that they are physicians allows them to utilize their medical knowledge to achieve results that are sensitive to both clinical and business considerations.

A third aspect of leadership is critically important and it is learnable. This part is *how to involve others in the decision-making process*. By knowing how to effectively involve others, the leader can improve the quality of outcomes, its acceptance by those in the organization, and get the problem solved or the change implemented in a timely manner. The issues of who, when, and how to involve the other physicians is the immediate leadership challenge that is facing Dr. Anderson.

Leadership is the process of getting subordinates, peers, and others to work toward organizational goals. Sometimes, effective leaders simply make decisions without consulting others. Effective leaders, however, also recognize that under the right conditions the best way to achieve the organization's goals is to transfer decision making to others. Effective leaders understand, for example, that when others have goals that are aligned with the organization's goals, and that others possess sufficient technical knowledge relevant to the problem, that the best way to lead is to involve these other motivated,

knowledgeable stakeholders in the process. Effective leaders, then, use a range of leader behaviors that vary from delegating the work to others, to working with others in a participative style, to consulting with them to get their input, and on occasion simply making a directive, autocratic decision themselves, with no one else's input.

Sometimes, it is easier to identify a successful leader than it is to understand what he or she does to be a successful leader. Successful leaders seem to have the following four characteristics in common:[1]

1. They use exceptional communication skills to make ideas and visions tangible to others.
2. They generate trust through clear, consistent behavior.
3. They have a realistic sense of their limitations.
4. They reject the notion of failure.

As broad guiding principles, these four points are interesting and may even be helpful to Dr. Anderson, but it's difficult to apply them to obtain specific operational guidance at UFP. Originally, management scientists thought that leadership was a combination of personal or personality characteristics. Effective leaders were expected to have more or less of some combination of personal traits and characteristics, such as intelligence, charisma, integrity, strength, bravery, self-confidence, extroversion, height, attractiveness, and so forth.[2] When research studies found too many exceptions to this approach, it then was proposed that leadership was a set of behaviors. For example, researchers at Ohio State University concluded that leaders exhibit varying amounts of concern for employees' welfare, which they called "consideration," and concern for getting the task accomplished, which they called "initiating structure."[3] Using this approach, a leader is less concerned with who you *are* (personal characteristics: charismatic extrovert with above average height), than how you *act* (behaviors: develop strong personal bonds with subordinates, and give them project schedules and goals). This approach to understanding what made leaders effective was more successful, but once again too many exceptions were found to conclude that particular behaviors or behavioral strategies per se, such as being high on both consideration and initiating structure, are the essence of successful leadership.

A more recent approach to understanding leadership focuses on examining leader attributes and behaviors *in the context of specific situations.*[4] Successful leaders seem to be able to choose certain behaviors or decision-making styles that are appropriate given the situation at the time. This is called a *situational approach to leadership*. Sometimes, a leader has to make autocratic decisions, whereas at other times delegating decisions to others will produce the best results; it all depends on the circumstances. There also are many situations in which a leader will be most effective if he or she uses methods somewhere between these two extremes.

There is considerable research and applied case evidence supporting the validity of this situational approach to leadership.[5] Imagine, for example, the behaviors of the model Marine Corps drill instructor: autocratic, strict, loud, organized, and highly structured. He or she certainly would typify the directive leader. Imagine, however, that it's 7 PM and this very directive Marine Corps drill instructor is now in charge of leading a voluntary church organization, and uses the *same behaviors* as with his or her day job! It is obvious that the result would be a disaster, and that soon there would be a leader with no followers. Conversely, leadership behaviors characterized by flexibility, participation, and

consensus building that would bring success to the volunteer church organization would be equally inappropriate for leading Marine recruits. The key to leadership, therefore, is to *match the leadership style to the situation*. There are very few organizations in which a leader can be successful using only one leadership style. The truly successful Marine Corps sergeant will recognize that if the nature of the work changes, delegating decisions and involving others in a participative decision-making process are necessary for success. Once again, the skill is to know *when* to choose a particular decision-making style. Applying this approach to the situation faced by Dr. Anderson at United Family Practices indicates that he has a conscious choice to make about how to involve the other physicians, and that this choice should be dependent upon his assessment of key situational issues.

The challenge that leaders have, therefore, is to be sensitive to the right situational issues, and to know how to match their leader behaviors to those circumstances. Obviously, some leaders intuitively do this. They have a sense of when to delegate to others, when to bring everyone together and reach a joint consensus, when to ask for information before making a decision themselves, and when to simply make a decision without consultation *now*. Think of effective leaders whom you personally know. Almost certainly this ability to vary how they interact with others in their organizations characterizes how they lead. Similarly, this leadership flexibility characterizes well-known business leaders, such as Jack Welch who led GE to great success and Louis Gerstner who revived IBM. Certainly, you have some of this ability also. The question is how *much*—and given whatever your leadership ability is at this point—could it be *improved* by a thoughtful strategy of situational assessment followed by conscious leadership-style choices? The answer to this question is yes, and what I will present is a way to do this.

The following discussion presents a way of thinking about leadership. It is based on a line of research begun by Victor Vroom[6] at Yale University and followed by many others.[7] Vroom's approach to understanding leadership was based on observing successful leaders. He reached several conclusions about the strategies that successful leaders use. This approach, called the *Leader Participation Model*, integrates three issues: leadership style, situation, and the goals that successful leaders try to achieve. Let's begin with this latter issue, because how you act as a leader is focused on achieving goals. Vroom found that successful leaders make decisions that:

- *Protect the Quality of the Decision*— Effective leaders are concerned with achieving successful outcomes. If the decision involves developing a critical care pathway for pneumonia, then producing a pathway that provides effective clinical care, controls costs, and coordinates personnel and facilities is of primary concern and an effective leader will ensure that these goals are achieved.
- *Protect the Acceptance of the Decision*— Effective leaders understand that a high-quality decision that others will resist, will fail to implement, or don't understand will not produce an effective outcome. Effective leaders, therefore, use a leader style that will result in others accepting the decision.
- *Are Timely*—Effective leaders understand that late decisions may be irrelevant. Sometimes, time is of the essence.
- *Develop the Skills and Abilities of Their Subordinates*—Effective leaders understand that subordinates and peers make many daily decisions that they don't even know about. As a result, effective leaders develop, *when feasible*, others' leadership

and decision-making abilities, so the overall level of organizational decision making improves.

All of these outcomes are relevant to United Family Practices. The quality of the decisions is certainly critical. If, for example, they institute a new performance appraisal and compensation plan that is roundly viewed as inequitable, they will have a personnel disaster on their hands. Similarly, the financial implications of these decisions will be large enough so if they implement them poorly they will jeopardize the existence of the practice. Imagine, for example, the consequences of investing in EMR hardware and software that is disliked by users and doesn't provide timely information. They won't have the financial reserves to redo this decision. Similarly, if they fail to implement some version or subset of the initiatives, they also will have a low-quality outcome and most likely will jeopardize the practice's survival.

Acceptance is obviously a critical issue. The case stated that the practice was structured as it was in order to keep the physicians' lives as similar to the past as possible. When they learn that their professional lives will need to radically change in order to capture some benefit from this large-group practice model that they have created, many may resist. Timeliness is also an important consideration for Dr. Anderson. It is unlikely that failure to institute these changes in the next few months, or maybe even for a year or longer would be fatal to the practice. If, however, they don't make these changes for 5 years, then they may not survive. At some point, therefore, there is a cliff out there and they will fall off of it, but it's probably further off than proximate. Understanding that time is *not* of the essence is important, because it gives Dr. Anderson the time to identify how to achieve quality and the time to build acceptance. Think of leaders whom you may have experienced who have rushed to decisions, and as a result had less-than-successful outcomes, when in fact there was no real need for haste.

Development, on the other hand, is arguably a critical issue. Imagine, for example, involving physicians in this decision who don't have the business background to understand *why* the changes that are being proposed are essential for the success of a large-group practice. The consequences would be that they would make uninformed decisions. Similarly, imagine if physicians who are not directly involved in the decision-making process also don't understand why these costly and unpopular decisions are being made. Resistance, opposition, and perhaps even civil war within the practice might result. Having business-savvy physicians both directly and indirectly involved in these decisions is critical for United Family Practices.

Vroom found that quality and acceptance are the most important goals for effective leaders. Timeliness and employee development also are very important, but are lower priority than quality and acceptance. This order of priorities is important to appreciate. It means that leaders should not sacrifice quality and acceptance to make a decision "on time." Instead, effective leaders emphasize quality and acceptance, and then *manage* the time issue as a secondary, although still important, consideration. Similarly, effective leaders may involve others as a way of developing their decision-making skills, such as by delegating a project to them or significantly involving them in a joint decision, but they don't do this if it sacrifices quality or acceptance.

Vroom also found that effective leaders use a range of leader behaviors or decision-making styles (**Exhibit 6–1**). As you can see, the level and type of involvement by others

---

**Exhibit 6–1** Leadership Styles

Decide—You make the decision alone and either announce or "sell" it to the group. You may use your expertise to collect information from the group or others that you deem relevant to the problem.

Consult Individually—You present the problem to the group members individually, get their suggestions, and then make the decision yourself.

Consult Group—You present the problem to the group members in a group meeting, get their suggestions, and then make the decision yourself.

Facilitate—You present the problem to the group in a meeting. You act as a facilitator, defining the problem to be solved and the boundaries within which the decision must be made. You strive to reach a mutually satisfactory solution in an atmosphere of free and open exchange of information and ideas. Your objective is to reach consensus on a decision. Above all, you take care to ensure that your ideas are not given any greater weight than those of others simply because of your position.

Delegate—You permit the group to make the decision within prescribed limits. The group undertakes the identification and diagnosis of the problem, develops alternative procedures for solving it, and decides on one or more alternative solutions. Although you play no direct role in the group's deliberations unless explicitly asked, your role is an important one behind the scenes, providing needed resources and encouragement.

*Source:* Adapted from Vroom, V. (2000). Leadership and the decision-making process. *Organizational Dynamics*, 28(4): 82–94.

varies across these styles in this exhibit. Using Decide involves no one else. The leader collections any necessary information him- or herself, and then makes the decision. Consulting means acquiring information from others. The difference between Consult Individually and Consult Group is where the leader does the consultation. Consulting individually provides privacy for others as they give their views or provide information. Sometimes, people say things in private that they won't say before team members or colleagues. Consult Group filters the information that each person provides through a group process. This back-and-forth dialogue, the testing of ideas that others can critique and build upon, can result in the ideas and perspectives that come from a Consult Group process being significantly different from or refined from those that individuals might offer in a Consult Individually process. The downside of Consult Group is that groups at times are subject to a process called *Group Think*.[8] This occurs when group members become so concerned with achieving consensus and concurrence that it becomes extremely difficult for members to offer minority opinions or deflect the direction in which the group is going. Examples of this include the Bay of Pigs decision in which several of President Kennedy's cabinet members did not express their concerns about the plan. Similarly, engineers who opposed launching the space shuttle *Challenger* felt that NASA management considered their minority opinions to be a problem, so some didn't express them. A related phenomenon is Group Shift in which the camaraderie of the group leads to riskier recommendations than group members as individuals would recommend. Considering these issues indicates, once again, that *when* to use a particular leader style is important.

If you use Facilitation, then team members are empowered to contribute on an equal footing with the leader. There is a lot implied, however, in the definition of Facilitation by the words, "You strive to reach a mutually satisfactory solution in an atmosphere of free and open exchange of information and ideas." Suppose, for example, that the way in which you normally lead is that you come up with the ideas, and you expect others to put them into action with little or no comment. Your view is that if others offer ideas, it's your role to quickly point out everything that is wrong with them. You do this not out of disrespect for your colleagues and others, but because you firmly believe that the best way to get *good* solutions is to quickly point out everything that is *wrong* with a proposal. Finally, you don't "suffer fools kindly," and you quickly put them in their place. Now, suppose that in spite of this history you come to the realization that there may be times when leading through Facilitation would in fact be beneficial. A situationally appropriate opportunity arises, so you turn to your colleagues and subordinates and say in effect, "Let's work on this together, and I'll just be another team member of equal rank with equal say." Most likely, no one will believe you. They will wonder when the sandbag will fall, and they will be very hesitant to behave in an *effective* facilitative manner. Availability of these leader styles, therefore, is not a given. It may take you 6 months or a year to bring some of the less-directive leader styles into the feasible set depending on your past leadership actions.

Vroom's research also identified several situational variables that effective leaders consider either consciously, semiconsciously, or unconsciously when selecting a leadership style (**Exhibit 6–2**). As you examine these, you can see their obvious relevance for deciding how to lead. For example, if Leader Expertise is low, then common sense tells you that you don't make autocratic (Decide) decisions. It's obvious when you say this out

**Exhibit 6–2**  Situational Issues for Leaders to Consider when Selecting a Leader Style

---

**SITUATIONAL ISSUES**

Decision Significance—The significance of the decision to the success of the project or organization. Focus on whether this is externally important to the organization rather than its impact on the group.

Importance of Commitment—The importance to the success of the decision of team members' commitment to the decision. Having the "right" answer may not be enough if Importance of Commitment is high and you don't get it.

Leader's Expertise—Your knowledge or expertise in relation to this problem.

Likelihood of Commitment—The likelihood that the team would commit itself to a decision that you make on your own. This is the degree to which the group is likely to support your solution to the problem. Consider your personal relationship to members, and their trust and confidence in you. Do they view you as an expert? Do they *think* you should make the decision?

Group Support for Objectives (Goal Alignment)—The degree to which the team or its members supports the organization's objectives at stake in the problem.

Group Expertise—Team members' knowledge or expertise in relation to this problem.

Competence Working as a Team (Team Competence)—The ability of team members to work together in solving problems. Do they have the social skills and teamwork capabilities necessary to collaboratively work together? A group may possess the relevant knowledge and expertise, but lack the qualities identified in this issue. Both social skills and technical knowledge are integral to effective group problem solving.

*Source:* Adapted from Vroom, V. (2000). Leadership and the decision-making process. *Organizational Dynamics*, 28(4); 82–94 , and Expert System CD.

---

loud, but how many times have you seen leaders violate this rule? If Group Expertise is low, then don't delegate to others for similar reasons. Generally, in life, we work to achieve our own goals and objectives. If you determine that Goal Alignment is low, then don't delegate or facilitate, because the group will make decisions to satisfy their own needs and not those of the organization. We could proceed by going through the situational issues and logically relating them to leadership styles and their likely impact on Quality and Acceptance, but **Tables 6–1** and **6–2** express these relationships based on many years of research on leaders in real organizations. Leader styles identified in these tables produce the highest levels of quality and acceptance given the situational circumstances. Notice that there are separate tables

for Timeliness and Development. They are treated as mutually exclusive outcomes in this version of the Leader Participation Model. If time is of the essence, then you don't have time to develop others. On the other hand if time is not critical, then you do have time for development. Later versions of the model use a computer-based expert system, and Time and Development are scaled in their importance. You can say, for example, that Time and Development are both important, or that both are important but one is more important than the other.[9]

Tables 6–1 and 6–2 are useful as a devil's advocate to ensure that you think about the critical situational issues before making a leadership decision about how to involve others. They will help you to explore the situation, and point out where you may need to

**Table 6–1** Leader Participation Model: Development Driven Model

| | Situational Factors | | | | | | Leadership Style |
|---|---|---|---|---|---|---|---|
| Decision Significance? | Importance of Commitment? | Leader's Expertise? | Likelihood of Commitment? | Goal Alignment? | Group Expertise? | Team Competence? → | |
| H | H | | H | H | H | H | Delegate |
| | | | | | | L | Facilitate |
| | | | | | L | — | Consult (Group) |
| | | | L | L | H | H | Delegate |
| | | | | | | L | Facilitate |
| | | | | | L | — | Consult (Group) |
| | L | — | — | H | H | H | Delegate |
| | | | | | | L | Facilitate |
| | | | | | L | — | Consult (Group) |
| L | H | — | H | — | | — | Decide |
| | | — | L | — | | — | Delegate |
| | L | — | — | — | | — | Decide |

*(Rows 1–9 labeled vertically "Problem"; rows 10–12 labeled vertically "Statement.")*

*Source:* Adapted From Vroom, V.H. (2000). Leadership and the decision making process. *Organizational Dynamics,* 28(4):82–94.

**Table 6–2** Leader Participation Model: Time-Driven Model

| | | | | *Situational Factors* | | | | |
|---|---|---|---|---|---|---|---|---|
| | *Decision Significance?* | *Importance of Commitment?* | *Leader's Expertise?* | *Likelihood of Commitment?* | *Goal Alignment?* | *Group Expertise?* | *Team Competence?* | → *Leadership Style* |
| Problem Statement | H | H | H | H | — | — | — | Decide |
| | | | | L | H | H | H | Delegate |
| | | | | | | | L | Consult (Group) |
| | | | | | | L | — | |
| | | | | | L | — | — | |
| | | | L | H | H | H | H | Facilitate |
| | | | | | | | L | Consult (Individually) |
| | | | | | | L | — | |
| | | | | | L | — | — | |
| | | | | L | H | H | H | Facilitate |
| | | | | | | | L | Consult (Group) |
| | | | | | | L | — | |
| | | | | | L | — | — | |
| | | L | H | — | — | — | — | Decide |
| | | | L | — | H | H | H | Facilitate |
| | | | | | | | L | Consult (Individually) |
| | | | | | | L | — | |
| | | | | | L | — | — | |
| | L | H | — | H | — | — | — | Decide |
| | | | | L | — | — | H | Delegate |
| | | | | | | | L | Facilitate |
| | | L | — | — | — | — | — | Decide |

*Source:* Adapted From Vroom, V.H. (2000). Leadership and the decision making process. *Organizational Dynamics,* 28(4):82–94.

acquire additional information about a situational issue before making a decision. They should not be used in a mechanical, uncritical manner. Instead, use them as a guide. After using them for a while, you will find that you incorporate their logic into your leadership thinking.

Now, let's use them to help guide Dr. Anderson at United Family Practices. First, he needs to decide on the relative importance of Time and Development. As noted, time is not of the essence, although eventually these are issues that the practice needs to address. Development, on the other hand, in the form of UFP's physicians acquiring business skills (marketing, finance, strategy, etc.) could be critical for them to reach high-quality decisions on the Anderson/Reynolds proposals. The first contribution, therefore, of the Leader Participation Model is that is prompts Dr. Anderson to consciously consider the relevance and implications of Development and Time. Therefore, we will use the Development Driven Model in Table 6–1. The first situational issue to consider is Decision Significance. As noted, these are critical issues to UFP, so Decision Significance is high. Importance of Commitment is also high. If the physicians aren't committed to following through, and they are constantly sabotaging the initiatives, then the practice will fall into chaos. Note also, that having high commitment doesn't necessarily mean that the physicians need to *like* the outcome. It simply means that irrespective of whether they like it or not, they are *committed* to implementation. Table 6–1 then directs us to evaluate the Likelihood of Commitment. This is low for many of the UFP physicians. They are unlikely to commit to decisions handed down from above that will in many cases radically change their professional lives, as well as impact their bank statement.

The Goal Alignment issues are complex. All of the physicians probably have some common goals. They all want to make money, and hopefully they all want to provide quality medical care, act ethically and legally, and so forth. Where they may diverge is how they see the proposed changes relating to the additional organizational goals of better utilizing fixed costs and reducing variable costs, better utilizing staff, acquiring new staff capabilities, making large investments in infrastructure (information systems, EMR, etc.), and all of the implications that these changes have for changing practice patterns of care. Those who see these changes as inconsistent with personal needs or their vision of how to practice medicine will have low Goal Alignment, while those who embrace new practice patterns and agree with or at least acquiesce to managing the practice as a business will have high Goal Alignment.

The model now indicates that those with low Goal Alignment should be brought together as a group (consult group), the new proposals discussed, their thoughts and ideas listened to, but that they should not be involved in the final decisions. For those with high Goal Alignment, we consider their Group Expertise. In this instance Group Expertise relates to their business skills. Do they have the financial, marketing, and strategy skills to make high-quality decisions on the proposals, or will they simply defer to naïve and uninformed information and assumptions? If their Group Expertise is low, then work with them using a Facilitative process. If it is high, then consider their Team Competence. Team Competence is low in this case. The physicians have recently formed into this group and prior to this experience they were competitors. Once again, the leadership prescription is Facilitate.

This analysis probably leaves you feeling uncomfortable. After all, we've split the physicians into two groups, and in effect said that some will have more say than others.

This could be a formula for disaster! However, consider what would happen if the low-Goal Alignment physicians are in the middle of the decision-making process; chaos, deadlock, and rejection of any significant change. Neither one of these situations is desirable, *but given a choice of the former and the latter, the former is the least bad choice*. Now, remember that the Leader Participation Model is focusing *on the situation as it currently exists*. It is not saying this is an ideal decision-making situation, or that if you follow the model's recommendations that it will produce great decisions or high-quality outcomes, simply the *best* ones given the *current* circumstances. It's saying that if you are stuck in these unfortunate circumstances, then the best that you can do is to minimize the disruptive opportunities of those with low Goal Alignment, and use Facilitate with high Goal Alignment physicians. The Leader Participation Model is prescriptive *given the defined situation*.

The Leader Participation Model also has identified the Goal Alignment issue as critically important. Under these circumstances Dr. Anderson could take this information and conclude that time is not of the essence, but development is. He could change the basis on which *all of* the physicians are looking at these proposals by using the time available to develop the physicians' understanding of the finance, marketing, strategy, and other relevant contextual business issues, so the stakeholders will understand *why* these changes are essential to United Family Practice's survival, and will be able to more effectively participate in their development. One consequence of this might be that those who wish for a simpler more medically focused life may realize that they made a mistake by joining UFP. Many of these physicians will realize that that they should have considered these issues before joining the practice, because the financial situation will make it extremely costly for them

to leave now, or for them to continue with a UFP that doesn't change. So Dr. Anderson comes out of this analysis realizing that he has time on his side and that he needs to use this time to increase the business literacy of his physicians, so they can effectively contribute as partners to reach high-quality consensus decisions on these issues.

Developing the physician's appreciation for the business issues that UFP must address can also have another beneficial effect. Although it would be desirable to have all of the physicians involved in these decisions to some degree, the logistics of a 25-physician deliberating team would be cumbersome. Increasing the physicians' average business literacy may also result in increasing Likelihood of Commitment, with the result that the final decision making could be done by a smaller group of well-chosen physicians whom all or most trusted to represent their interests to build a more effective practice. Similarly, breaking physicians into committees each charged with considering one part of the Anderson/Reynolds plan becomes also a viable option.

The end result of this analysis is that Dr. Anderson takes a much more sophisticated look at the decisions to be made, and identifies a more effective process, really a plan, for how to evaluate Mr. Reynolds' proposals, improve them through effective physician participation, and gain widespread acceptance by the physicians.

When I discuss this case with practicing physicians they often comment: "But I knew that all the physicians would have to be involved. That's just how we are, and how we do things. It would never fly to have an autocratic decision handed down from the top." The critical element here, however, is *when* the physicians are involved and the *skills* that they bring to the table. Participation without relevant skills results in bad decisions. Dr.

Anderson and UFP will do much better if they slow down, make an investment in developing physicians' business skills, and then involve them in facilitative ways with developing plans that build on the Anderson/Reynolds plan. The Leader Participation Model's value here is that it focuses Dr. Anderson's thinking onto the critical issues. It does more than prescribe, "be facilitative." It helps Dr. Anderson identify critical situational issues, so he can consider how to change the situation to improve the outcome.

## LEADING THE CHANGE PROCESS

Change has always been a difficult issue for both people and organizations to respond to and to accept. Take the example of scurvy. The disease was documented in ancient times, but did not become a pressing issue for western civilization until the trade routes to the Orient were cut with the fall of Constantinople in 1453. European countries responded with technological innovation by developing larger sailing ships and navigation instruments and methods that enabled sailing for long periods of time out of sight of land. Infrequent reprovisioning exacerbated the always-present threat of scurvy to epidemic proportions due to the inadequate naval diet. For example, in 1497 Vasco de Gama sailed from Portugal to India returning 2 years later having lost 100 of his 160 sailors, most of whom perished from scurvy. There were many urban legends regarding scurvy treatment options, one of which was citrus. In 1601 James Lancaster commanded one ship in a fleet of four sailing to India. He brought bottles of boiled lemon juice, which he gave to the sailors on his ship. His sailors remained healthy until he ran out of the juice, while the other ships in the fleet were wracked with scurvy. Upon returning to England he published his findings. In 1617

John Woodall published the first comprehensive naval medical text in which he unequivocally stated that citrus prevented and cured scurvy. He even provided dosage recommendations. Woodall's widely distributed medical text had very little influence. The prevailing theory of disease attributed scurvy to an imbalance in the humors. Citrus was the wrong cure for the affected humor given the theory, so most physicians rejected citrus out of hand. In 1747 James Lind, a Royal Navy surgeon, conducted one of the first recorded medical clinical trails, when he placed scorbutic sailors on *HMS Salisbury* on a citrus regimen along with six control groups.[10] The sailors given citrus responded so well that they nursed their shipmates in the other groups. He published his results in 1753 and they were roundly ignored. Lind, being a surgeon, had a low rank in the Royal Navy's medical hierarchy. As a result, during the Seven Years War, which concluded in 1763, the Royal Navy reported that it conscripted 184,899 sailors, of whom 1,512 were killed in action while 133,708 died of disease, which was mostly due to scurvy. It took the persistence of James Lind, the power and reputation of Capt. James Cook and others of high status, and increased recognition of the link between nutrition and health before the British Admiralty required the daily issue of lime juice to its sailors in 1795. The British Board of Trade adopted a similar measure for the British Merchant Marine in 1867. It is estimated that between the time John Woodall published his naval medical text in 1617 and the uniform adoption of citrus by the Royal Navy in 1795 over 1 million British sailors died from scurvy, this in the presence of both anecdotal evidence of a simple and effective preventative and cure.

The message is clear. Good ideas, even good ideas supported by data, don't necessarily sell themselves. They often fall to ignorance, misunderstanding, self-interest, fear, pride, and habit. Implementing many of the ideas in this book will require significant change in practice procedures, how physicians and staff view their roles, and in some instances, physician and staff personal skills. Utilizing financial analysis methods, developing and using strategic plans, employing marketing methods, implementing effective performance appraisal procedures, leading in unfamiliar ways, utilizing new technology, implementing clinical best practices, assessing outcomes—the list goes on. All are good ideas. All can be supported by data, and all invariably will encounter resistance of one form or another. One of your roles as a physician leader, therefore, is to manage the change process to anticipate this resistance, to benefit from the good ideas of others, and to successfully overcome it when it is counterproductive. Returning to United Family Practices, it's clear that Dr. Anderson will need to consider resistance. The changes that Dr. Anderson and Mr. Reynolds are considering are controversial, and their success in this endeavor will be as much a function of Dr. Anderson's ability to address this resistance, as it will be the quality of his proposal.

Given this warning about the problem of resistance to change, note that not all resistance is bad. Consider what the consequence would be if the organizational level of resistance to change is too low. Changes would be put into effect that are not fully considered. The result would be chaos due to frequent course changes, and disaster due to low quality. Resistance that is grounded in truly improving ideas is beneficial. Utilizing the concepts of interests and positions defined in Chapter 5, consider the resistor's interests. If their interests and your interests are aligned, then listen carefully to their position. This will give you clues on how to proceed. If an adversary has the same interest that you do, but the resistance is arising over a positional issue, then consider how you can change your position.

Many successful leaders intuitively know how to facilitate change, just as many intuitively know how to lead or identify evolving marketing opportunities. Distilling this intuitive approach to change into a systematic conscious process that you can utilize is the goal of this discussion. **Exhibit 6–3** contains a six-step change implementation plan.[11] Once again, let's use the United Family Prac-

Exhibit 6–3  A Change Implementation Plan

1. Create Urgency—This provides motivation.

2. Build a Change Implementation Team—Generally, broad-based changes are more successful and more difficult to defeat.

3. Develop a Vision—Inspire others to think about the ultimate outcome. Show them how the immediate change leads to the ultimate objective.

4. Act Assertively—Use effective implementation methods to communicate with stakeholders and decisively address resistance.

5. Obtain Short-Term Wins —Show that there are immediate benefits and that the plan has merit. Create momentum by doing something now!

6. Make Change Stick—Anchor it in the organization's culture, so it becomes an intrinsic part of how the practice operates.

tices case to illustrate the parts of this change plan. Consider possible actions that Dr. Anderson and Mr. Reynolds could take that fit into the Change Implementation plan. What follows is conjectural, because the case doesn't say how Dr. Anderson will implement the change. In addition, we need to make some reasonable assumptions about the practice, which in real life leaders would have better information about.

**Create Urgency.** Dr. Anderson and Mr. Reynolds have concerns about the current situation. Sharing these concerns with their colleagues should be the basis for creating urgency. Examine the financial implications of the current course of action and do pro forma ("What if") projections of likely practice and physician financial outcomes for a few years into the future (see Exhibits 1–6, 1–7, 1–22 and for examples of pro forma analyses). Projecting current trends forward, such as declining revenues, flat referrals, stagnant or declining salaries, and increasing costs can present a compelling picture. Similarly, discuss what the competition is doing and how more highly integrated practices are competing in the marketplace for employer contracts, patients, specialist access, health system alliances and support, and so forth. The key to creating urgency is to visualize the problem to others. Stories and cases are often more powerful than financial data in isolation. You want to achieve both rational buy-in and emotional buy-in. The goal of creating urgency is to make the status quo seem more dangerous than change to some large percentage of those affected.

**Build a Change-Implementation Team.** Big changes are often too much work for any one person. In addition, broad-based change teams are more likely to be successful, because ownership is infiltrated through the practice, and ownership and acceptance often go together. Team member selection is criti-

cal. Members need sufficient interest, influence, and respect to be effective change agents. It's important to draw from various constituencies and across organizational levels and avoid organizational silos. If a change will affect professional management as well as physicians, then include them in the process. In a multispecialty practice, be certain that all specialties are adequately involved. The change team's task is to develop a vision of the changes needed, and a realistic plan for putting them into place. A critical concern when selecting team members is to realize that technical skills don't necessarily translate into good teamwork skills.[12]

Applying these points to United Family Practices, Dr. Anderson should be looking for a broad-based team of physicians and managers to develop the details of the change process. Based on the previous leadership discussion, the initial change objective will be to develop an adequate level of physician business skill, so those who participate can be effective, and so those physicians who won't be directly participating will understand the need for change and be more willing to accept the proposals. A particularly important constituency on the change team is those physicians who are not particularly business savvy, but who nevertheless understand that the large practice model that they have created depends on effective business operations. These physicians should be prime targets for inclusion along with those physicians who already have these skills.

**Develop a Vision.** Develop a statement of long-term objectives and express it in ways that are understandable, easy to communicate, and that will appeal to stakeholders. The UFP change team might say:

> We want the practice to implement operational changes in how we run this practice, so that staff compensation and evaluation is equitable across locations, personnel and

operating costs can be reduced, and the practice can support physician compensation averaging the 65th percentile. We know that many who helped found this practice did so to achieve the benefits of both traditional practice patterns and the economies of scale associated with a large group practice. Therefore, the processes that we will develop and recommend to the board will focus on improving financial and clinical performance, but will be sensitive to how we achieve this. Our initial efforts and recommendations will be to provide UFP physicians and managers with information and skills so they can most effectively participate in our future.

**Act Assertively.** Specific content for the last three aspects of the change management plan in Exhibit 6–3 depend on the change team's vision, so discussion at this point becomes more generic. Act assertively by communicating the vision in the most effective ways possible. Physician-to-physician, nurse-to-nurse, and manager-to-manager marketing are examples of customized stakeholder communication. At UFP, the initial change efforts will be to raise the overall level of business literacy, so broad-based participation in developing the details of and implementing the Anderson/Reynolds plan will be effective. One challenge will be from those physicians who resent devoting time to learning new skills. They should be engaged by appealing to their collegiality, intellectual stamina, and ability to continue to be part of the process. Converts can be particularly effective proselytizers to resistors. Wrap converts into the change process, and give them roles that utilize their unique access to others.

**Engage Resistors.** Be on the lookout for resistance and actively engage it quickly and decisively. Don't assume that it will go away.

**Exhibit 6–4** summarizes some methods to do this. Several of these methods may be appropriate for the UFP change team to use. Certainly, Education/Communication is the cornerstone. Educating UFP personnel on why change is necessary defuses resistance on the part of those who will rationally evaluate the situation from a business perspective. Selective use of Participation can achieve buy-in and can improve the final iterations of the Anderson/Reynolds plan by bringing new ideas and additional perspectives to the proposals. Facilitation and Support is essential to overcome the fear, much of which may be realistic; that the world will be changing and particular individuals may be stretched to adapt. Particular individuals may be susceptible to Negotiation and Cooptation. For example, if a physician in one of UFP's seven locations is particularly influential there, then coopting this individual by perhaps giving him or her leadership of the IT committee that will take the lead on EMR implementation may be effective. Manipulation and Coercion are listed in Exhibit 6–4, because we all recognize that organizations use them. However, these methods are not endorsed and they would be particularly inappropriate at UFP. At best they achieve short-term compliance, but the cost in collegiality and long-term resentment and retribution make them inappropriate to any but the most desperate situations. Their use should be limited to when you see only one way to success: Organizational *survival* depends on it, and if the change is not implemented *now* then there won't be a practice in 6 months within which to suffer the inevitable retribution. Note, however, that the described circumstance makes organizational survival unlikely anyway, so you may also want to consider your reputation and legacy following its very likely demise.

**Exhibit 6–4** Methods for Engaging Resistors and Overcoming Resistance

| Tactic | Definition | Best for | Advantages | Disadvantages |
|---|---|---|---|---|
| Education/Communication | Familiarizing resistors with the reasons behind the change. | Resistance based on lack of information, inaccurate information, or analysis about the nature or need for change. | Once educated, people will often help with implementation because they accept the reason behind it. | Possibly time consuming. Educated resistors are more difficult to deal with. |
| Participation | Resistors participate in the design of the change. | When initiators don't have all of the necessary information needed to design the change, and others have considerable power to resist. | Participants become committed to avoid cognitive dissonance. Relevant information resistors will be integrated into the change. | Potentially time consuming. Resistors could sabotage change from inside. |
| Facilitation & Support | Operational training. Provides skills to operate in the new situation. | Adjustment problems. When people don't have technical skills and fear they can't learn them. | Best tactic for addressing fear due to lack of knowledge or skill. | Potentially time consuming and expensive, and may still fail. |
| Negotiation | Buying out resistors by giving them something for cooperation. See Chapter 8. | When a resistor will lose something as a result of the change, and he/she has considerable power to resist. | Relatively easy if you have something to offer. | May be expensive. Sets negotiation precedent for others. |
| Cooptation | Make a resistor an integral part of the change through a desirable or visible role. | Situations where a few individuals are influential with many other resistors or potential resistors. | Aligns self-interests. Variation on negotiation. | Can create equity problems for those not coopted. |
| Manipulation | Covertly, selectively providing information. Half-truths, deception, lies. | When other tactics won't work or speed is critical. | Quick and inexpensive. | Costs future credibility. Leads to future retribution. |
| Coercion | Using brute force or threats of force. | When speed is critical and initiators have considerable power. | Quick and inexpensive. Overcomes all kinds of resistance. | Risky. Leaves people angry with motivation to seek retribution. |

*Source:* Adapted with permission from P. F. Schlesinger, et al. *Organization: Text, Cases, and Readings on the Management of Organizational Design and Change.* Burr Ridge, IL: Richard D. Irwin, 1992, p. 352.

**Obtain Short-Term Wins.** Complex changes that attempt to be all encompassing and therefore take a long time often fail because participants become exhausted and demoralized. You need short-term wins to retain momentum. Rapid Cycle Improvement is one example of this approach to creating change. **Figure 6–1** illustrates this approach with the PDSA cycle for planning and conducting low-impact projects. UFP's initial change effort is to improve physician business literacy. A PDSA example would be a 1-day program for physicians and managers on cost-volume-profit (CVP) financial issues, which were discussed in Chapter 1. At the end of the program, the participants are broken into several small teams, each of which is to look for one way to utilize CVP concepts to implement measurable change at UFP (PDSA step 1). The teams follow the PDSA steps, and the outcomes from these focused studies are then assembled by the change team and distributed throughout the practice (PDSA step 6).

**Make Change Stick.** It's important to maintain the sense of urgency at UFP after the initial PDSA projects and to publicize the results. This should quickly be followed by another development initiative, such as a discussion session on the application of the

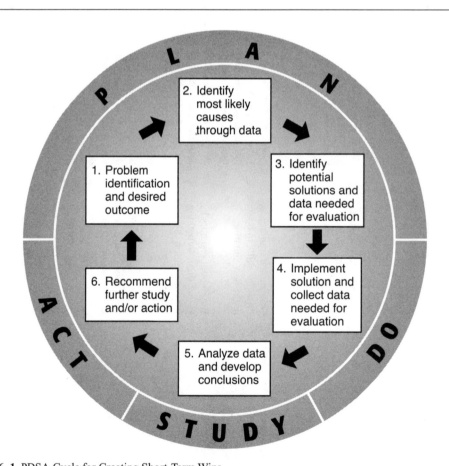

**Figure 6–1** PDSA Cycle for Creating Short-Term Wins.
*Source:* Adapted from 02_CQIEducationalWorkshop_CCE.ppt slide #10. Loyola University Health System. Used with Permission.

CVP program to UFP's current situation. This then might be quickly followed by another program to provide the basic skills on performance evaluation or strategic marketing, both critical to understanding why the Anderson/Reynolds plan is critical, and, which once again could be followed by PDSA projects and working sessions to discuss applying concepts to UFP's situation. Remember, also, that people come and go in practices. It's important that as new physicians and managers join the practice that they are brought up to speed on both the acquired skills and the organizational history. Change sticks when it becomes part of the organizational culture. At UFP, this means that the accepted culture needs to become that as business systems and clinical solutions evolve, becomes the practice sensitive to the larger business and medical environments.

## Leading Meetings

Leading meetings is a common situation. Utilizing some leadership concepts discussed earlier in this chapter, along with common wisdom from experienced executives provide some useful direction on how to lead a meeting. First, have a clear idea of some of the qualities of the outcomes that you want from the meeting. The four objectives that characterize successful leaders—Quality, Acceptance, Timeliness, and Development—also provide useful touchstones for any meeting. The challenge is how to conduct meetings that achieve these outcomes. Generally, there are two reasons for having a meeting; decision making and information evaluation. The preceding leadership discussion indicates that meetings are appropriate when the situation calls for using Consult Group (information collection) and Facilitation (decision making). Delegation may require meetings, but these will be meetings that others will manage. Some meetings are held to convey information, but this is often a very inefficient way to achieve this objective. Consider memos, e-mails, phone calls, and the like as more efficient ways to communicate *simple* content.

Considering *when* to call a meeting is the first key to success. Consider calling a meeting when at least one of the following applies:[13]

- Information needs to be shared, but no single person has all of the information. A meeting may be an efficient way to reciprocally share information.
- When it's not clear what information is needed.
- To create commitment in situations where commitment is necessary for success. Stated another way Importance of Commitment is high and Likelihood of Commitment is low.
- When it's important to gauge the *reaction* of many people to information.
- When the problem is complex, and you believe that a group process will bring out nuances and result in new and better ideas.

There are several methods that you can use to enhance the group's process during a meeting:

1. Brainstorming—rules are used to both promote the generation of ideas and reduce inhibitions to expressing them. These include the following:

    - No idea is ridiculous. Members are encouraged to state extreme "outlandish" ideas. On occasion, outlandish ideas, once refined, achieve breakthroughs.
    - All ideas belong to the *group*. As a result, the group builds on ideas without the concern of trampling on others' turf.
    - No criticism. The purpose of the meeting is to generate ideas, not to evaluate

or criticize them. Evaluation should be done in a separate meeting. If you try to do both in the same meeting, this may cut off the generation of new ideas, because team members may prematurely seek closure on an issue.

2. Nominal Group Technique—this process is composed of three phases, which separate idea generation from evaluation.

- Phase 1—Members sit around a table, but do not speak to each other. Each person writes an idea on paper. After a fixed time, say 5 minutes, each person presents his or her idea. A recorder writes ideas on a flip chart for all to see. Several rounds of writing and recording may take place, until everyone agrees they have no more ideas. Throughout this process, there is no discussion.
- Phase 2—There is structured discussion of each idea including necessary clarification from the idea generator. The leader manages the process so that evaluation is focused on the ideas, not the idea generators.
- Phase 3—Evaluation. Each person privately rank orders the ideas. The group decision is the result of the pooled rankings.

In a Facilitate situation, the leader would implement the team's decision. In a Consult Group situation, the team's decision would be the information that the leader would then use as data to reach his or her own conclusion about what to do. In both instances, it is critical for the leader to let the team know the "operating rules." If this is a Consult Group situation, then don't let the team think that their decision will be directly implemented. Similarly, if this is a Facilitate situation, then let the team know this so they understand the significance of their decision.

Next, consider *who* to invite. Inviting too many people, too few, or the wrong people all can lead to failure. The Goal Alignment situational issue discussed earlier is important to consider. Generally, you want those in the meeting to have aligned *outcome* goals, but this does *not* mean that everyone agrees on *how* to get there. If you call a meeting in which the members seek to achieve totally different outcomes, then you may have so little basis for discussion that the group discussion degenerates into nonproductive arguments. At the same time, you need to avoid the problem of groupthink. Groupthink occurs in highly cohesive and close-knit groups. Irving Janis,[14] who did much of the original research on this subject in political organizations, defines it as "deterioration of mental efficiency, reality testing, and moral judgment."[15] Groupthink tends to occur when:

- Members feel invincible.
- Members Moralize; opposition to group views is considered weak, evil, stupid, etc.
- Feelings of Unanimity and Group Conformity—Members don't share their reservations with others, so they won't appear to be weak (see previous bullet). Both active and informal norms are present that discourages divergent views. The group exerts pressure to conform.
- Dismissing Opposition—Outside dissenting views are dismissed out of hand or receive little or no serious consideration. The group shows strong favoritism for its own ideas and seeks out confirmatory information or data, while simultaneously rationalizing away, dismissing, minimizing, or failing to collect conflicting data.

Balancing the need for some degree of cohesiveness, and avoiding the problem of groupthink is an art that effective leaders manage to achieve. At United Family Practices, for example, the overall goal of business effectiveness might be a reasonable meeting inclusion standard for a meeting on how to achieve this outcome. There would still be many different opinions about how to achieve this, but that would be the focus of the meeting. Inviting physicians who believe that attending to *any* and all business issues would probably lower meeting productivity, because these physicians would simply act as obstructionists to those who were trying to develop some effective business ideas. Keep in mind that as a UFP physician leader you may have another objective, which is to change these other physicians' minds about the importance of business issues, but this should be addressed in another setting.

Next, plan and manage the meeting. Have an agenda and give the agenda to meeting participants well ahead of time. This will greatly help introverts. Introverts like to process their ideas and fully consider them before acting in an extroverted way, such as talking about them. Extroverts, on the other hand, often think out loud, sometimes not even knowing what they will say until they say it. When you mix the two together in a meeting, as is typically the case,[16] the danger is that the extroverts will drown out the introverts. By the time the introverts get around to talking, the extroverts have moved the conversation along. By publishing an agenda, you level the playing field for the introverts. In addition, one of your roles as meeting leader is to actively manage the meeting. You might, for example, ensure that everyone has a chance to talk by establishing a rule for at least part of the meeting, that no one talks twice until everyone has had a chance to talk once. Similarly, you can call on those who haven't actively participated to be certain that their ideas get heard. Let meeting members know the ground rules. Will they as a team be providing advice or actually making a decision? How will conclusions be reached? For example, will there be a majority rule vote, will alternatives be rank ordered, or is the objective to reach a consensus that all can accept?

As you run the meeting, strive for participation. Ask open-ended questions instead of phrasing them so they can be answered with a simple "yes" or "no." Ask for reactions to comments made, and consciously try to include those who are not volunteering comments. At the same time, avoid disrupting the natural flow of ideas across members and personally dominating the discussion. Try to use team member's terminology. The business concepts in this book will be particularly helpful when you are leading a nonphysician business meeting. In this regard, don't be afraid to acknowledge when you are a little shaky on some of these business concepts. Illustrate issues with concrete examples. This is analogous to the cases in this book. Real-life examples make issues more real and often provide others with a more accurate picture of what you are trying to say.

Finally, close the meeting with a summary of what has transpired and any decisions made. If there are specific "to-do's" and personally identified actions that came from the meeting, be certain to review these so those who are responsible will follow through on the right items, and with the right delivery dates. Recording meeting minutes is problematic. Some meetings by organizational rules require minutes. Most meetings do not. Minutes may stifle open discussion, and create more paper that few will probably read.

## MOTIVATION

Motivation is another tool that leaders can use to put plans into operation and to direct the actions of others. Your practice's compensation plan is one very important element in motivating employees, but there is more to motivation than monetary compensation.

Think about the things that motivate you. If you are typical of many physicians, other likely motivational issues include a sense of career achievement, clinical accomplishment, achieving patient satisfaction, the recognition of others, providing for your family, and self-actualization, which was defined in the old Army recruiting theme, "be all that you can be." Others, to varying degrees, will also be motivated by these and other nonmonetary issues. Note, however, you cannot replace equitable monetary compensation with these other nonmonetary issues. We've all heard of examples of people including physicians who are happily working on a job for less money than they could make elsewhere, because of some aspect that brings significant additional satisfaction. It may be a desirable part of the country, the opportunity to work with an outstanding mentor, being close to family and friends, or in some cases, a job that is very undemanding. A situation in which an employee actively seeks out a job that accentuates these nonmonetary characteristics is very different, however, from one that you as a physician leader try to manufacture within the walls of your practice. The motivation strategy discussed, therefore, is predicated on a fair and equitable compensation plan (Chapter 5). If, in addition, you then can provide other elements that are particularly motivating to an employee, you will be more likely to see the benefits of motivated employees. These include more concern for job performance, higher satisfaction, and a greater retention rate across employees. Keep in mind, also, that not all employees want a more challenging job, or one that requires taking on responsibility, or has the potential to instill a sense of achievement. Recognize that some people, including physicians, may simply want to work a set schedule, contribute nothing out of the ordinary, go home at 5:00 PM, and leave their job behind them. People vary in what they desire in life and on a job, and any effective motivational strategy will need to take this variance into account.

The key to motivating employees and colleagues is to understand their long-term goals in life, and then to manage the rewards that the practice provides, so they relate as best as possible to these long-term life objectives. This statement is derived from expectancy theory, which is arguably the most comprehensive behavioral motivation theory. Expectancy theory is supported by a significant body of research,[17] as well as practical application. It states that rewards obtained from a job are intermediary benefits that will be used to satisfy other more fundamental personal needs. For example, a nurse ostensibly works for a salary, which he or she then uses to buy a car, go on vacation, continue education, contribute to a personal sense of worth, or provide for family. The nurse's motivation or force to perform is ultimately a function of the long-term personal life goals, which salary just happens to lead toward. This also implies that there may be other and better ways that the nurse could achieve some of these ultimate personal outcomes, and there may be other nonmonetary things that the practice could do to facilitate her or his achieving these personal goals, such as flexible schedules, or educational benefits. Note also you may conclude that given an employee's or colleague's long-term personal objectives, that what he or she seeks is not consistent with what you can provide. Expectancy theory, therefore, can help you to know when you *can't* motivate someone.

Expectancy theory has a number of components, which will help you as a leader to understand the particular motivational opportunities and limitations available to use with each of your employees and colleagues. As you read about each of these components think about how they are expressed in your practice and their relevance to particular employees:

- *Actions* (*i*) are things an employee does on the job. In the case of the nurse, it might be those things that he or she would do to develop new cost control procedures for disposable items (e.g., gowns, syringes, etc.) or delivering clinical services on a daily basis. This also could imply some rather remote activities, such as taking a statistics course to better implement total quality management, or receiving training to monitor new pain management medications. There are lots of *i*'s that everyone performs on a daily basis, and in sum they constitute everyday job performance and accumulate into a level of overall success.
- *First-level outcomes* (*j*) are outcomes that are directly related to the job. These often are rewards that the company provides, such as compensation or benefits. They may also be positive or negative comments made by colleagues and patients, and include any other immediate consequence of job performance.
- *Second-level outcomes* (*k*) are outcomes of larger significance in someone's life. Generally, they are long-term life goals. They vary in importance, but by definition they are things that we are striving to achieve in life. Examples might include a personal sense of satisfaction and accomplishment, financial security, buying a new house, or providing education and a comfortable life for one's children. We all have lot's of *k*'s or things that we strive for in life.[18]
- *Valence* ($V_j$ and $V_k$) is the expected value or anticipated satisfaction that one expects from achieving a certain outcome. $V_j$ indicates the satisfaction anticipated from a first-level outcome. $V_k$ indicates the satis-

faction anticipated from a second-level outcome.
- *Expectancy* ($E_{ij}$) is the likelihood that an action (those things an employee does on a daily basis) on the employee's part will result in receiving or achieving a given first-level outcome. It can be expressed as a probability, and therefore it is measured on a scale of 0.00 to 1.00. The subscripts (*i*) and (*j*) indicate that Expectancy links Actions to First-Level Outcomes.
- *Instrumentality* ($I_{jk}$) is the relationship between first- and second-level outcomes. It can be conceptualized as a correlation, and therefore it is measured on a scale ranging from $-1.00$ through 0.00 to $+1.00$. For example, if a particular employee always associates a first-level outcome of a $5,000 pay raise with his personally determined second-level outcome of financial security, then $I_{jk} = 1.00$. If a first-level outcome is never associated with obtaining the second-level outcome, then $I_{jk} = -1.00$. If a first-level outcome is perceived to be unrelated to a second-level outcome, then $I_{jk} = 0.00$. In this specific example, the outcome of a $5,000 raise would probably be "somewhat" related to financial security, because it leads in that direction. Many employees might perceive an $I_{jk}$ of .20, .25, .31, or so forth. Ultimately, perception is reality, so whatever the employee perceives the instrumentality to be will influence their actions. For some employees, for example, who have very significant financial needs, or who are in significant debt, this $5,000 raise would have little meaningful impact on the second-level outcome, and $I_{jk}$ may be perceived as close to .00.
- *Force* ($F_i$) is the desire, predisposition, or motivation to act.

The following equations describe how these components relate to each other:

$$V_j = f(V_k \times I_{jk}) \qquad (6\text{--}1)$$

$$F_i = f(V_j \times E_{ij}) \qquad (6\text{--}2)$$

Expectancy theory recognizes the reality that we are all motivated by different objectives, and by commonly offered rewards to varying degrees. As a leader, therefore, the first important implication to derive from the expectancy theory is that if you are going to effectively motivate people in your practice, *then you must get to know them as individuals.* You may be able to make some fairly reasonable assumptions that the standard rewards of pay and benefits will tie in with virtually everyone's second-level outcomes, and that more is better than less, but to go beyond this, you will need to know what your employees and colleagues seek as individuals. Obviously, this takes time. For physician leaders who also practice clinical medicine, time is what you sell to generate revenue. You won't want to make the same time investment with all employees. Employees in less-critical positions may merit little or no time investment on your part. Employees in distant positions may be more effectively motivated by others in your practice, such as your business manager or nursing supervisor. Employees in critical positions who report to you may merit substantial personal time investment.

Let's examine the motivational implications of the equations in greater detail, and discuss how you can use them in your practice. As noted, we all have lots of $k$'s or second-level outcomes. In addition, second-level outcomes vary in their importance to each of us, which is expressed by the term $V_k$. The first equation says each person considers how each second-level outcome ($k$) that he or she desires in life is related to first-level outcomes ($I_{jk}$) provided by the employer, and that we sum across all of our $V_k \times I_{jk}$ prod-

ucts to get the anticipated satisfaction ($V_j$) with the first-level outcomes provided by the employer, such as compensation and verbal recognition. Stated another way, this is how satisfied we expect to be with the rewards the employer is providing.[19] One important implication is that if you are offering rewards with low instrumentality, then $V_j$ will be low, even though the employee has lots of things he or she is seeking in life and is *potentially* very "motivatable." Notice that the person's anticipated satisfaction ($V_j$) coming out of the first equation becomes an *input* in the second equation.

In the second equation, the employee adjusts the anticipated satisfaction ($V_j$) by the probability ($E_{ij}$) that if he or she acts in appropriate ways to achieve the first-level outcome, that he or she will in fact achieve it. The second equation, therefore, indicates the amount of *effort of motivation* that a person puts forth. We have all experienced at one time or another the implication of this adjustment of anticipated satisfaction by the probability that we will succeed. We consider that if we get the reward, it would be wonderful (high $V_j$), but when we look at the chance of success, we conclude that it is so small that there is no point working toward the objective. Notice that no matter how large $V_j$ is, that if multiplied by a small ($E_{ij}$), the Force or predisposition to act becomes small. When we perceive that there is *no* chance of success ($E_{ij} = 0$) irrespective of how tempting the reward, we will not act on it at all ($F_i = 0$).[20]

The implications for a leader trying to motivate practice employees and colleagues include the following:

• Get to know your employees personally, so you can determine some of their second-level outcomes. This is sometimes difficult to do. Employees often are wary of telling supervisors their true life goals, because they are uncertain how this information will be used. Some goals may be obviously incompatible with the practice, such as moving to a different part of the country, or changing career. Nevertheless, as a leader trying to motivate employees, the most critical thing you can do is to build enough trust over time so that employees will communicate their second-level outcomes. Obviously, this is a long-term process that is best achieved in a climate of trust in which you've proven in the past that you are trying to make the practice a personally rewarding place to work. Sometimes, you can get some idea of a person's second-level outcomes in subtle ways, such as the photos on their desk, or a comment made over lunch.

- Consider likely instrumentalities for specific employees when you set first-level outcomes (rewards) that result from the job. Think about the first-level outcomes that you provide, and consider how you can customize them so they just fit more naturally into the employee's second-level outcomes. One way of doing this is through a cafeteria-benefits plan as discussed in Chapter 5. Consider also, the power of positive feedback for employees who seek recognition and self-actualization. This is easily supplied on a daily basis and should be an important consideration when doing performance appraisal and goal setting for employees with these second-level outcomes (Chapter 3).

- Influence expectancy by really changing the probabilities of success; provide training, resources, inspiration. As a leader, you can influence the probability that an employee can succeed. This closely relates to your goal-setting responsibilities, because you have a responsibility to go beyond noting substandard performance to help the employee develop a plan that leads toward success. If a nurse is receiving poor patient satisfaction evaluations, then ensuring that he or she mentors with one who is good on this factor really *does* change the probability of success. If formal statistical training is needed to successfully implement quality improvement methods (to which you are being pushed by insurers and employers), then making certain that effective training is provided really *does* change the probability of success. Finally, don't underestimate the power of the Knute Rockne half-time pep-talk. It is not a replacement for real solutions for impediments to success, but it can inspire employees who have the skill to attack the problem. If you are a respected leader and you truthfully tell an employee or colleague that you believe they can succeed, then they most likely will succeed.

- You can guide an employee's actions ($i$) through performance appraisal, training, and goal setting. Sometimes, employees fail because they don't know what to do and are afraid to ask, or because they incorrectly define the task. The business manager who doesn't understand the appropriate reports to scan or the databases to construct in order to prevent new collection problems and reduce receivables falls into this category. The employee's direct supervisor, who may be you or another practice manager, can redirect his or her actions. These actions really *do* change the expectancy or chance of success.

- You may conclude that you cannot motivate some employees. For example, an employee who is seeking second-level outcomes that you cannot satisfy, and whose performance is low, is not salvageable. This is a losing proposition, because there is no way that you can effectively increase instrumentality. Under these circumstances, provide clear goals, choices, and known conse-quences regarding job performance. You may say, for example, "George, I know that the overall level of reward that you get from the collection administrator position doesn't fit well with what you are looking for in life. We pay an equitable wage, but there's more that you are looking for that we can't seem to provide. Nevertheless, we need a better level of patient interaction, paperwork compliance, and aggressive ac-tion. If there are things we can do to help you where you don't understand the job, then we need to explore this. The current level of job performance, however, is not adequate and we need this to improve. If you can't do this, then we may need to part ways." Then, follow this with any relevant goal setting that is feasible, hold George to standards that you set, and terminate him if there is no improvement.

Expectancy theory has significant impli-cations for Dr. Anderson at United Family Practices. Understanding the physicians' second-level outcomes will be critical in order to most effectively use Participation, Negotiation, and Cooptation. Another way to think about the proposal to develop physi-cians' understanding of the underlying busi-ness issues is that it provides the knowledge so that physicians will be able to more accu-rately determine how the changes (first-level outcomes) relate to their own personal second-level outcomes. Some of the physi-cians will conclude on balance that when they net out all of the $(V_k \times I_{jk})$ products that the final proposals will produce greater an-ticipated satisfaction than the current situa-tion or the projected situation a year or two from now. Others will see a loss. Understand-ing the expectancy theory components can help Dr. Anderson clarify these issues to his colleagues, so they can make more rational decisions about their futures.

## CONCLUSION

This chapter focuses on three aspects of leadership: how to make decisions and involve others in those decisions, how to lead the change process, and how to motivate others in your practice. Leadership involves convey-ing a vision of what you want, and then in-spiring, motivating, or managing others to work toward that vision. Effective leaders are sensitive to relevant situational issues, and ad-just how they lead to achieve their objectives.

Effective leaders know that identifying the best path is not enough. Resistance in or-ganizations is natural, so effective leaders are on the lookout for it, try to prevent it, and ef-fectively address it when it occurs. Some leaders intuitively know how to adjust to re-sistance. For the rest, being familiar with some strategies for addressing resistance and consciously applying them will result in more successful change.

Finally, considering the life goals of oth-ers, as well as their expectancies and in-strumentalities, can help you to motivate colleagues and employees to perform at higher levels. This chapter has outlined a mo-tivation strategy that is supported by signif-icant research and is eminently practical. It focuses on structuring monetary and non-monetary incentives, so that employees achieve their own personal goals in the process of working toward achieving the or-ganization's goals.

The popular business literature is replete with universally applicable leadership tru-isms. The approach presented in this chapter is quite different, proposing that effective leaders adjust their actions based on attend-ing to relevant situational variables. Some-times, being directive will lead to success, while at other times, delegating will be the key. Sometimes, focusing on increasing a key player's expectancy that he or she can suc-ceed will be the critical element, while at other times facilitating PDSA projects that others create will inspire the practice to continue on a difficult but essential path. Leadership, therefore, is a process and not a set of personal characteristics or mechanically applied tools. The effective leader looks around, sees the challenges and opportunities, and adjusts accordingly. There are, un-

fortunately, no magic leadership bullets, as much of the popular literature suggests. The methods presented in this chapter are grounded in the organizational behavior, psychology, and management research literatures, but a leader who is sensitive to internal practice issues and personalities will best implement them.

---

## NOTES

1. Bennis, W. (1984). The four competencies of leadership. *Training and Development Journal*, 15: 15–19.
2. See, for example: Zaccaro, S. (2007) Trait-based perspectives on leadership. *American Psychologist*, 62(1): 6–16. Also: Zaccaro, S., R. Foti, D. Kenny. (1991). Self-monitoring and trait-based variance in leadership: An investigation of leader flexibility across multiple group situations. *Journal of Applied Psychology*, 76: 308–315.
3. Stogdill, R., & A. Coons. (Eds.). (1951). *Leader Behavior: Its Description and Measurement*. Research Monograph #88, Columbus, OH: The Ohio State University Bureau of Business Research.
4. Vroom, V., & A. Jago. (2007). The role of the situation in leadership. *American Psychologist*, 62(1): 17–24.
5. See for example: Robbins, S. (2005). *Essentials of Organizational Behavior*. Princeton, NJ: Prentice Hall, pp. 161–165.
6. Vroom, V. (2003). Educating leaders for decision making and leadership. *Management Decisions*, 10: 968–978.
7. See, for example: Yun, S., S. Faraj, & H. Sims. (2005). Contingent leadership effectiveness of trauma resuscitation teams. *Journal of Applied Psychology*, 90(6): 1288–1296. This study was conducted on trauma teams composed of attending physicians, trauma resuscitation nurses, surgery fellows, residents, and trauma resuscitation technicians. Results indicated that directive trauma team leaders (attending physicians) provided better care than did empowering leaders when patients were severely injured, or when the trauma team was inexperienced, but that empowering leaders provided better care when time was not of the essence or team experience was high. Empowering also provided more learning opportunities than did being directive.
8. Eisenhardt, K., J. Kahwajy, & L. Bourgeois. (1997). Conflict and strategic choice: How top management teams disagree. *California Management Review*, 39(2): 42–62.
9. Contact Victor H. Vroom, Ph.D., at: victor. vroom@yale.edu. The expert system is available on CD.
10. Bown, Stephen H. (2003). *Scurvy: How a Surgeon, a Mariner, and a Gentleman Solved the Greatest Medical Mystery of the Age of Sail*. NY: St. Martin's Press, pp. 95–97. The six control groups were: cider; elixir of vitriol; vinegar; sea water; a paste of nutmeg, garlic, mustard seed, dried radish root, balsam of Peru, and gum myrrh; and a no treatment group. All were common treatments at the time.
11. This is based on an eight-step process described in Kotter, J. (1996). *Leading Change*. Boston: Harvard Business School Press.
12. Note that the same issue is addressed in the leader participation model by the situational variable team competence.
13. Whetten, D., & K. Cameron. (2007). *Developing Management Skills*, (7th ed.). Princeton, NJ: Prentice Hall, p. 657.
14. Janis, I. (1973). *Victims of Groupthink: A Psychological Study of Foreign Policy Decisions and Fiascos*. Boston: Houghton Mifflin.
15. A classic example of groupthink is President Kennedy's cabinet's recommendations regarding the Bay of Pigs invasion. Arguably, a more recent example is President Bush's 2003 invasion of Iraq as described in Woodward, B. (2006). *State of Denial: Bush at War, Part III*. NY: Simon and Schuster.
16. In a sample of 1,234 physicians assessed using the Myers Briggs Type Indicator colleague William Geary and I found that 36 percent were introverts and 64 percent were extroverts. The percentage varied with specialty. For example, emergency

medicine (I = 47%; E = 53%) and oncology (I = 21%; E = 79%). In contrast a sample of 167 nonphysician administrators attending a physician leadership program were 51 percent E and 49 percent I.

17. Van Eerde, W., & H. Thierry. (1996). Vroom's expectancy models and work-related criteria: A meta-analysis. *Journal of Applied Psychology,* 81(5): 575–586.

18. It is possible to think of 3rd, 4th, nth levels of outcomes. For motivational purposes, this added complexity adds no explanatory value. It is sufficient to collapse everything down to what an employee receives from the job (first-level outcomes), and everything that these outcomes lead to (second-level outcomes).

19. This process is almost always an ongoing unconscious or semiconscious process. Nevertheless, many who have a rational approach to life recognize in these equations how they consider these issues. Expectancy theory isn't indicating that we literally calculate these products, simply that the equations describe how we act. Research studies designed to evaluate expectancy theory's validity often do have subjects assign numbers to the components, thereby translating a semiconscious or unconscious process into a conscious activity.

20. A personal example is betting in the state lottery. For some, $V_j$ is very high, but $E_{ij}$ is zero, so there is no motivation to do those things $i$'s that are necessary to bet in the lottery.

# United Family Practices, Ltd.

When Fred Anderson, MD, signed the final document creating United Family Practices, Ltd., he wondered whether he and his colleagues really knew what they were getting into. The financial logic behind the joining of 7 previously independent practices and 25 family practice physicians was compelling.

As a group, they would constitute a significant percentage of local family practice physicians, and would have to be reckoned with by insurers, smaller practices, and employers. Their purchasing power should result in obtaining the best possible prices for medical and business supplies and capital items. Over time they planned to consolidate their locations, thereby reducing fixed costs for rent, personnel, and capital equipment. By controlling these costs, they would be both more profitable and have the resources to invest in the best technology and personnel, and thereby provide the highest quality care.

No, Dr. Anderson wasn't worried about the finances. After all an assemblage of CPAs and consultants had assured everyone that this was a sound financial and strategic decision. What Anderson was worried about was how to *manage* 25 physicians, and an initial support staff of 94 others.

The plan that Dr. Anderson, the other physicians, and consultants developed to organize United Family Practices, Ltd. (UFP), seemed to make sense. One physician from each of the seven founding practices would serve on a board of directors. The board would elect from its members a managing physician, or chief executive officer (CEO),

who would be appropriately compensated for this work. In addition to his or her clinical practice, the CEO would make most daily decisions needing physician concurrence, such as final approval of advertising and promotions, and "operational" purchases within the constraints of the budget. The CEO would seek board involvement and concurrence for decisions with major financial or long-term implications, such as making a job offer to a physician, major system changes such as the introduction of an electronic medical record, and developing a practice strategic plan.

The CEO and the board hired an administrator, Pete Reynolds, who had an MBA and 4 years of experience working with hospital-owned primary care practices. His job at UFP would be to handle day-to-day practice management. His duties included developing internal practice policies and personnel procedures, assisting the CEO, making sure that costs in all parts of the practice were being controlled, and coordinating all aspects of daily practice operation. This included supervising department heads such as office managers, billing, collection, and the like. Dr. Anderson was somewhat concerned about Reynolds' lack of independent practice-based experience. Dr. Anderson and the rest of the selection committee felt, however, that Reynolds' strong financial and managerial skills would more than compensate for this limitation.

The seven founding practices were spread across the local region. In order to keep things simple and retain some semblance of normalcy for the physicians, the new practice retained most of the old physician-staff reporting relationships. The former office managers of each practice were still responsible for the operation of their locations, and they reported to Reynolds. Billing remained decentralized, but each office manager sent Reynolds daily reports, such as work completed, cash receipts, insurance billings, insurance collections, and aging analyses. In addition, physicians retained their previous staffing relationships with nurses and secretaries. Purchasing of supplies was centralized through Reynolds. Physician compensation was based on personal collections, adjusted for local practice (location) costs, and the location's share of "corporate costs," such as Reynolds' salary and Dr. Anderson's administrative salary.

Dr. Anderson and most of the other physicians strongly supported this organization structure, because they retained significant local control, which made the whole experience less frightening. For example, if a secretary or a nurse had performance problems, the affected physician and local manager could quickly handle it. Hiring would be handled locally also, with the needs of the local physicians being paramount.

A feeling of local control was especially important for Location A, which primarily had an inner city Medicaid patient base, and Location F, which was positioned in an affluent suburban county, and still had a high proportion of traditional insurance patients. Physicians in these locations felt that their needs and their patient's needs were somewhat different from the group's other locations, and it was important to them to be able to practice accordingly.

A minority of physicians had some reservations about the practice's structure. Dr. Early commented:

> One reason for forming a large group practice was to operate more efficiently. The

way we have organized, however, doesn't do much to help us act as *one* practice. We need to encourage interdependent, coordinated behavior, but our organization structure appears to work against this. The days of 25 or even 7 Lone Rangers, each charging off in their own direction are over, or will be over soon. But how do we integrate the parts of United Family Practices, Ltd., so that as a group we are better than we were as seven competing practices?

Reynolds has a plan to address these issues. Reynolds and Dr. Anderson are at one of their regularly scheduled weekly meetings. They often have discussed the need to improve practice integration during these meetings. Reynolds has been considering this issue of integration—how to get the parts of the practice to work more effectively as a coordinated whole, and he has some ideas. After 3 months of observation and focusing on daily practice operations, Reynolds assembles a plan to move the practice forward toward this goal in several critical areas. He proposes to implement the following changes over the next 3 months:

1. Centralize the recruiting and hiring of front office and staff positions.
2. Develop practice-wide front office and staff (not physician) performance appraisal and compensation plans to ensure equal treatment across the practice locations, as well as create some control over the compensation process.
3. Eliminate the positions of the former business managers, retrain and reposition these personnel as best as possible, but offer those who cannot fit into the new structure "outplacement" assistance.
4. Create a new position to develop and manage integrated practice-wide management information systems related to patient care, patient records, and financial information.

5. Create new positions to coordinate and manage practice-wide business functions, such as scheduling, billing, human resources, and quality improvement.

Dr. Anderson looked at the list and commented, "Pete, you've done a very good job developing this proposal. This gets us moving toward an integrated practice. We need to start someplace and personnel issues, information systems, and quality improvement are critical places to begin. I'm going to distribute this to the board, and we will begin working on it at the next board meeting. These certainly are board-level issues."

Reynolds looked up from his notes, hesitated, and then stated, "Fred, I'm not sure that the board is really where we need to go with this. I know that you need to go there next, but maybe we need to involve all 25 physicians in this."

"So you're recommending, Pete, that I go to the board and ask them to involve all 25 physicians in deciding about this plan? And if I do, what do I specifically ask the board to authorize? That we consult with all the physicians? That we allow *them* the final say—delegate to them? I'm pretty certain that most of the physicians won't grasp the business reasons for doing these things. All they may see is the pain and disruption to their accustomed ways of practicing. And then there's the issue of cost—they won't like that aspect very much. Do they replace the board as the decision makers on this? Somehow we need to achieve economic and operational improvements if United Family Practices is going to survive, but we need to do this without sacrificing what makes us happy to come to work every morning!"

"I'm not sure, Fred. It's going to be contentious however you and the board decide to proceed."

# CHAPTER 7

# Marketing

---

## Chapter Objectives

The primary objective of this chapter is to get you to think about the medical services that you deliver through the eyes of someone with a marketing perspective. As a physician, you can then select those aspects that help you to effectively deliver your services, while knowledgeably rejecting those aspects of marketing that you feel uncomfortable with, or view as unethical. In order to make these decisions, you will need to know your practice's strengths and weakness and external market opportunities and threats. This chapter gives you ways to evaluate these issues. You also learn that marketing is really analogous to taking a strategic look at your practice, because you systematically will evaluate the products and services that you offer (Product), where and when you offer them (Place), the value that you offer (Price relative to quality), and finally, how to inform people (Promotion) about all of these issues. After considering these issues, you will learn how to develop a marketing plan, which is your strategy for addressing these issues. Generic market strategies are presented as a way to generate some brainstorming on your part about how to develop your own specific marketing plan. Finally, specific applied promotion suggestions are offered, once again with the objective of generating some brainstorming on your part on how to best promote your practice.

---

## INTRODUCTION

This chapter differentiates marketing from selling. Marketing is based on evaluating your organization's internal competitive strengths and weaknesses, and identifying and analyzing potential threats and opportunities in your environment. Physicians who market their services first identify their customers' needs. Customers can include patients, patients' families, other physicians, and employers. Physicians who consciously utilize marketing provide products and services that their customers want, at a price, and in a location that is attractive to them. Marketing, therefore, affects the quality and characteristics of the products or services you offer. An alternative to marketing is *selling*. Physicians who use a selling philosophy begin with the products and services that they wish to offer. Subsequent communication efforts, such as advertising, are aimed at convincing patients and customers why they should acquire what the physician wants to sell. When an organization markets its services, it recognizes that no matter how excellent they are, they are incomplete if customers fail to use them because they are:

- Less useful than some other provider's services
- Unaware of them
- Offered at an inconvenient time, or place, or in an inconvenient manner
- Not affordable or viewed as unfairly priced

Marketing professionals have traditionally talked about four types of decisions that must be made regarding the marketing of any product or service. Often referred to as the Four Ps, these decisions concern:

1. *Product* or service characteristics
2. *Place* or distribution of the product or service
3. *Promotion* of the product or service so that customers will be aware of it, one form of which is advertising
4. *Price* of the product or service

The *marketing mix* is the specific combination of the Four Ps that you develop for your practice as a whole, or for particular services, such as a coronary artery bypass graft (CABG) or colonoscopy.

Product decisions concern the specific products and services you intend to offer. To make these decisions, you need to identify groups of potential customers (patients, patients' families, employers, referring physicians, insurers, etc.), learn how they can be best served, and determine which products and services will attract them. The service that you offer might well include more than clinical outcomes. For example, it might include satisfaction, a sense of respect, patient choice, quick scheduling, and patient involvement. Patient-focused units and maternity centers are examples of how medical services can be modified to better encompass patient (customer) desires. Similarly, CABG critical paths that can discharge some patients from the hospital sooner and reduce costs represent an expanded product definition that better satisfies

employer and insurer needs. Colonoscopies offered in an office offer patients lower co-payments coupled with a more personalized practice experience. Concierge practices offer high-service levels and personalized attention.

Place or distribution decisions concern where and when to offer services. Location and office hours are choices that can contribute to success. Using satellite, storefront, and shopping center locations, and offering staggered and extended office hours are distribution options. Offering e-mail consultation to answer current patient questions is a distribution option. Convenient parking, easy access, and proximity to existing or desired patient bases (neighborhoods) are place considerations.

Promotion can include various forms of paid advertising, such as newspaper ads, TV infomercials, and Web sites. It also can include speeches at professional conferences, seminars to probable patient-referral sources, free or low-cost blood pressure or cholesterol checks, and any number of activities that will familiarize the public or referral sources with the organization, its physicians, and its services.

Pricing decisions concern the cost of services to customers. This includes decisions related to participating with an insurance company and accepting its fee structure, participating with preferred provider organizations (PPOs) and HMOs, and agreeing to capitated contracts. Physicians and other healthcare providers can adopt conscious pricing strategies to undercut, match, or lead the market. Each pricing strategy can be appropriate if it fits into a coherent strategy to attract market segments. For example, undercutting the market with a low price is a strategy to use in mature markets to gain market share. If you are a *low-cost* practice or healthcare system, it can be an effective approach. Matching the market generally makes pricing a nonissue, so you can compete on other issues such as quality, location, or unique services. Leading the market can be effective if your services are in great demand. Generally, consumers perceive higher-priced services and products to be of superior quality, so a price leader position can be consistent with introducing state-of-the-art procedures.

## DEVELOPING A MARKETING PLAN

Because marketing is composed of decisions that affect the Four Ps, a comprehensive *marketing plan* will contain a product plan, a place plan, a promotion plan, and a pricing plan. These four component plans must fit together as an integrated whole, so in combination they provide a competitive advantage. The specific combination of product, place, promotion, and pricing that you implement is sometimes called the *marketing mix*. Marketing plans are developed as a result of a thorough analysis of *internal* organizational strengths and weaknesses and *external* opportunities and threats in the environment. This process is referred to as SWOT (strengths, weaknesses, opportunities, and threats) analysis. For example, internal factors, such as your practice's or hospital's financial resources, the medical and professional skills of physicians and others, equipment and facilities, and the organization's mission must all be assessed in terms of strengths and weaknesses, so the marketing plan can build on your strengths and compensate for your weaknesses. Similarly, healthcare organizations do not operate in a vacuum. Important external factors include the opportunities and threats associated with the number, quality, characteristics and pricing of competitors, local geography, local and national economies, changes in medical technology, standards of care, government regulation, and local ethics regarding acceptable forms of promotion, services, and places of service delivery. The process of acquiring the data necessary to conduct the SWOT Analysis is called *situational analysis*. **Exhibit 7–1** shows the relationship between situational analysis, SWOT analysis, and the marketing plan. Now, let's look at each of these components in more detail. Remember, the ultimate goal is to develop a

---

**Exhibit 7–1** Situational Analysis, SWOT Analysis, and Marketing Plan

| Situational Analysis | SWOT Analysis | Marketing Plan |
|---|---|---|
| *External Factors* | | *Product Plan* |
| Competition | | Services |
| Environment | Threats | Procedures |
| Life Cycle | | Etc. |
| Demand | Opportunities | *Place Plan* |
| Distribution | | Location(s) |
| | | Hours, Days |
| . . . . | | Internet Access |
| | | *Promotion Plan* |
| *Internal Factors* | | To Patients |
| Professional Skills | Weaknesses | Media: TV, Print, Internet |
| Business Skills | | To Referring Sources |
| Financial Resources | Strengths | *Pricing* |
| Personal Goals | | Fee Schedules |
| . . . . | | Participation/Insurer |

marketing plan, but the process begins with the situational analysis.

## Situational Analysis

The goal is to assess issues that pertain specifically to *your* practice or healthcare organization. The list of situational analysis issues in Exhibit 7–1 is generic, but it is a good starting point.

## External Factors

### The Competition

To compete effectively, you must know who your competitors are and will be. Consider sources of new competition, such as specialists or primary care physicians who are broadening their sphere of practice. Are there any relevant nonmedical providers, such as psychologists, nurse practitioners, massage therapists, or chiropractors? If you are a practice, are hospitals, emergency departments, or emergency care centers competitors? What are their competitive advantages and disadvantages? For example, do they have unique training, skills, cost structures, management skills, or equipment that set them apart? Do some have inside ties with hospitals and other potential referral sources? Do they have better or inferior locations? If you can understand the competitive advantages of your competition, then you may be able to:

1. Use similar strategies to your advantage.
2. Avoid head-to-head competition that you cannot win.
3. Devise tactics to circumvent your colleagues' competitive advantages.

### The Environment

Environmental issues provide the scientific, professional, ethical, and social context for your market strategy and plans. Some en-

vironmental issues come and go, whereas others are more or less permanent. For example, the "war on drugs" has been enduring since the 1970s. Our social, legal, and political environments are saturated with this issue. A marketing plan that takes into account the public's enduring interest in the drug problem may benefit your organization as well as lead you to provide a needed public service.

In contrast, eating disorders, such as anorexia and bulimia, are no less real now than they were a decade ago, but they no longer occupy the public spotlight. Does this mean that a healthcare system shouldn't develop programs to treat these disorders? Certainly not. The resources devoted to the problem and other marketing mix decisions, however, should take into account the current relative disinterest in the topic and the large number of medical and nonmedical providers that are now competing for this market. As a result of the changing social environment, a marketing plan that you would design today for an anorexia or bulimia treatment program probably would look very different from one that you would have designed in the past.

It also is important to take into account local environmental issues. For example, the Hampton Roads area in Virginia has a very large military population. This population is such a significant part of the local market that it should be considered in the marketing plan of any local physician, hospital, or healthcare system. The implications of this market segment include the following:

• Directing product/service decisions at young, low-income, temporary residents and providing services that might be highly utilized by this segment, such as obstetrics and children's disease.
• Taking into account insurance coverage for military families and associated usual and

customary rates, and the difficulties of working with the Tricare system (pricing)

- Accessing the military system and other referral sources to selectively reach this market segment (promotion)
- Selecting a location that coincides with areas of heavy military housing and commuter routes to the three major area bases and providing practice hours to harmonize with military base commuting schedules and routes (distribution)

Another environmental issue in the Hampton Roads area is the road system. The local highway system was poorly designed and does not have sufficient capacity. As a result, some parts of this area become virtually inaccessible between 7:00 AM and 9:00 AM and between 3:30 PM and 6:30 PM. This means that at any given time a trip that normally takes a few minutes can take an hour or longer. These transportation problems result in residents seeking services in their immediate locality, avoiding certain areas and roads except during midday, and planning commitments, such as medical appointments, to avoid the high-traffic times whenever possible. These considerations affect customer choices including the physicians and hospitals they will use.

Another important environmental issue to consider is local ethical standards regarding the use of promotion by healthcare organizations. For example, physicians in most parts of the country now feel comfortable placing a display ad in the daily newspaper describing their services. In addition, many physicians think that appearing on a local television talk show is an appropriate public service/promotional activity. What is the reaction to a 30-second paid commercial extolling your skills and services? Many physicians feel this goes beyond the bounds of good taste or is even unethical, yet in-

creasingly we are seeing physicians using advertising such as this. What would the consequences be if you were one of the first in your area to use this promotional approach? How would your peers react to you, and might there be some form of subtle or not-so-subtle retaliation?

Another area of environmental concern is changing medical technology. This issue, which obviously has educational, technical, and financial implications, also has significant marketing implications. How would new equipment or new surgical methods allow you to provide new or better services to your patients? How can you let patients or referring professionals know about your capability to provide new services? To what extent will your colleagues follow suit, thereby limiting your competitive advantage to a window in time? Similarly, a technological change could be a major threat, if it eventually renders one of your services obsolete.

### *Life Cycle*

Another external consideration is the life cycle of each service or procedure you offer. It is easy to understand that a product such as a computer or a car can have a life cycle. It is introduced into the market, demand for it grows, the market eventually becomes mature and stabilizes, then the demand for the product declines as tastes change or as competing products enter the market, and finally there is little or no need for it. Many medical services and procedures also go through a life cycle of birth, growth, maturity, decline, and death. In most cases, the underlying disease continues, but the services, procedures, and medications that physicians use to treat the disease go through a life cycle. The change from one life cycle stage to another can be due to changing technology, such as new equipment or drugs, or to changing public awareness and acceptance of treatment options.

Marketing professionals have noted that products or services in a particular life cycle stage have characteristic attributes. For example, the introductory phase is characterized by low sales, technical and marketing problems, and high costs in relation to revenues. These characteristics are due to the start-up costs and the costs of initial marketing. Physicians who decide to provide a service or procedure that is in the introductory stage should be future oriented and willing to assume some risk. The eICU[1] is in this stage. The eICU is an advanced monitoring technology that allows specially trained intensivists to monitor critically ill patients in the ICU, or for that matter simultaneously in several ICUs. Monitoring takes place 24 hours a day, 7 days a week from a remote location. Utilizing an elaborate network of cameras, high-speed data transmission, and two-way communication links, doctors and critical care nurses in the eICU command center can make "virtual rounds" on patients. The eICU technology potentially offers higher-quality clinical outcomes and reduced cost.

The growth phase is characterized by rapidly increasing demand for services. Generally, the physicians who benefit most from the growth stage of a new service or procedure are those who first introduce it to an area. In the growth stage, it is not unusual for demand to exceed the ability to supply the service. The high revenues associated with the growth phase can also lead to a failure to control costs and may create the temptation to overextend. Overextension can be manifested as risky growth, such as buying new equipment or acquiring new facilities that will only pay for themselves if the growth continues. It also can be manifested as overwork. In short, the euphoria associated with the growth phase has inherent dangers. Laparoscopic gastric bypass surgery is currently in this phase.

The beginning of the mature phase is characterized by slowing growth. Eventually patient demand relative to the number of providers flattens and may begin to decline. Most medical services and procedures will be in the mature stage, and some will remain there for many years. Healthcare organizations that are well entrenched and well managed will prosper even when providing mainly mature services and procedures. Because growth is no longer occurring as a result of increased demand from patients, growth only can be achieved by increasing market share. This means taking business away from competitors. Generally, this results in price competition. Therefore, controlling costs and differentiating yourself from your peers are particularly important in this stage. For instance when the last edition of this book was written, vision correction surgery was in the growth phase. Now it is in the mature phase. Predictably, price competition now is rampant with TV ads and direct mail advertising featuring low prices and financing options.

The decline stage of a procedure or service is characterized by a decreased usage or patient demand. This can be a slow and steady decline, such as would be characterized by changing social factors that might affect, for example, specific elective plastic surgery procedures. Declines resulting from technological change, on the other hand, can be precipitous. Much lip augmentation surgery has been replaced with injectables.

### Demand

*Demand* is the extent to which current consumers seek the services or procedures you offer or intend to offer. To understand the demand for a given service or procedure, you must understand how potential patients currently buy similar services or procedures. Scott and associates[2] lists a number of considerations related to the nature of patient demand for medical services to consider:

- Number of physicians whom patients consider when seeking medical care
- Extent to which patients seek information before selecting a physician
- Loyalty that patients have to physicians used in the past or to referral sources, such as hospitals and other healthcare professionals
- Sources of information used by patients, such as the Yellow Pages, Internet, physician referral services, other healthcare professionals, and friends
- Who makes the physician selection decision, and who influences the decision (e.g., the husband, wife, father, or mother)
- Degree of patient interest in the physician selection process (Is the decision more like a decision to purchase hairpins or an automobile?)
- Perceived risk involved in making a bad physician selection decision
- Attitudes regarding whether the illness or procedure is viewed as a necessity or a luxury (Is the purchase of the medical service more like the purchase of food or a cocktail dress?)
- Length of the anticipated time involvement with the physician (Is the time involvement analogous to that of buying gum or dining room furniture?)

The objective of asking these and other questions is to uncover implications for your services and procedures. By determining the answers, you may be able to design more effective services or communicate them more effectively.

Another issue related to demand is the concept of market segmentation. *Market segments* are groups of people who will respond in a similar manner to the marketing mix. By understanding the different demands associated with the segments of your market, you can more precisely direct your marketing efforts. If, for example, a plastic surgeon determines that a significant number of his or her rhinoplasty patients are women between the ages of 25 and 35 years, and reside disproportionately in two of the seven local counties, then this information can be used to design a more effective marketing plan. Similarly, if the decision about where to take a child with a cold for treatment is made by the mother in 75 percent of families, then this should influence promotion decisions. Segmentation will be discussed in greater detail later in this chapter.

### *Distribution*

Consider where and when competing services are offered. Are there some new opportunities available to distribute your services? For example, some large retailers, such as Wal-Mart, are providing health clinics in their stores. Often, nurse practitioners and other nonphysicians staff them. Nevertheless, they could be a market niche, as an additional service that you provide, and as a new source of patients who come to your practice after a positive emergency care experience.

## Internal Factors

### *Professional and Business Skills*

To develop an effective marketing plan, it is important to assess your organization's professional and business skills. It makes no sense to market a service that cannot be delivered either clinically or managerially, to undersell a valuable or rare service, or to take on a well-entrenched competitor with little hope for success. Self-deception is self-defeating; you are obviously dependent on a realistic determination of the relative quality of your professional and business skills.

The business end of your organization provides the support necessary for the delivery of professional services. If your business operations have weaknesses or strengths, then these must be understood, compensated for, taken advantage of, or changed. An assessment of your organization's business strengths and weaknesses is very important because an effective marketing plan will put additional pressures on business operations. First, the marketing plan will, one hopes, result in an increase in patients treated, procedures performed, revenue, and so on. This, of course, will result in an increase in associated support work, such as laboratory testing, insurance filing, chart management, report writing, and so forth. At the practice level, for example, marketing activities may include writing press releases and speeches and arranging appointments with referral sources, all of which take time and energy. Do you have an employee with enough skills to write a press release? Are your secretaries going to be able to take the additional load if you decide to produce a training and nutrition manual for the local Little League?

A thorough and honest assessment of your clinical skills is arguably the most fundamental internal analysis that you can perform, and perhaps only second in importance to your personal goals. Consider both the breadth of your skills and your professional interests. If, for example, you are a psychiatrist who is much more interested in medication than psychotherapy, then it is important to understand this and to build this choice into your marketing plan.

### Financial Resources

Any marketing plan will have financial implications. Developing new services and locations as well as promoting them cost money. Developing a pro forma budget can be a helpful exercise. Some promotional methods may cost little or nothing; many others can be quite expensive. It is important to be realistic about the funds that are available for product and service development, as well as the cost of promoting them.

### Personal Goals

For physicians in private practice, this is arguably the single most important internal environmental issue. What do you and your partners *want* to do? What do you want your practice to be like? What kinds of patients (defined any way you like) do you want to treat, and what type of clinical work do you really want to undertake? There is nothing so frustrating as working hard to achieve success, only to realize that what you accomplished was not what you really wanted.

Consider more than just your clinical work when defining your goals. If, for example, it is important for you to have significant amounts of time with your family, then this should be taken into account in your marketing plan. For example, a plan, which if successful would result in your conducting 50 clinical hours per week, not to mention marketing and administration duties, is obviously inconsistent with a significant home life. Other issues, such as your status in the community, or your ability to help ameliorate social problems, may be important to you. So might the personal satisfaction that you derive from your office-based practice versus ICU coverage. You will be happier and certainly more successful if your personal goals are reflected in the marketing plan that you develop.

Healthcare organizations similarly should pay attention to life goals, but in this context we usually use the term organizational mission. A for-profit healthcare system should develop a marketing strategy and specific plans that are consistent with its for-profit mission. Similarly, not-for-profit healthcare systems often have significant parts of their missions defined in terms of returning value to the community. Once again, the strategy and plans should derive from these goals.

### SWOT Analysis

A SWOT analysis utilizes the situation analysis data to determine an organization's strengths, weaknesses, opportunities, and threats. Threats are external factors that result in an organization performing at lower levels than it would otherwise. Threats might include the following:

- Numerous competitors in your specialty
- Insurance carriers that have adopted lower compensation rates and require more burdensome authorizations, preauthorizations, and documentation as prerequisites for payment
- A new emergency care facility that has opened two blocks from the hospital, skimming "cream" cases and revenue from the emergency department
- A downturn in the local economy that makes preventive healthcare generally less affordable
- Physicians who are major referral sources to the hospital forming an outpatient surgery center

Opportunities are openings in the external environment of which you might be able to take advantage. Some examples include:

- The local school system decides to contract with a physician to provide medical examinations for all students in its athletic programs.
- An older physician with a successful practice is retiring and is interested in working out an arrangement for the care of her patients.

- A major commuting route passes your office, which allows you to provide treatment during commuting hours.
- Physicians, who aren't part of the forming outpatient surgery center feel vulnerable, and may be willing to work more closely with the hospital to develop new service lines.
- Both healthcare systems and physicians underserve a rapidly growing suburb.

Weaknesses are internal factors that limit your ability to compete for patients or to provide services. Weaknesses might include:

- A patient reception area that is too small to support practice growth.
- Front office staff who are having difficulty coping with the current volume of patients.
- A dislike on your part of talking before large groups.
- Undeveloped management information systems, so that the hospital or practice has poor cost data and, as a result, has difficulty making knowledgeable bids on contracts.
- Your location is in an older part of town with demographics that include declining income and increasing crime.
- Your AR is out of control and you don't have a process in place to fix this problem.

Strengths are internal factors that provide you with a competitive advantage over other organizations. The following are some hospital- and practice-level examples:

- Physicians in hospital-affiliated practices have been educated in business issues. They understand the need for hospital cost control, and actively pursue total quality management thinking to improve quality and reduce costs.

- An artificial hip critical path is integrated with financial and medical management information systems.
- Financial reserves allow you to deal with growth, or any unforeseen circumstances expeditiously.
- Both you and your staff are fluent in Spanish, and there is a significant local Spanish-speaking population.

## GENERIC MARKETING STRATEGIES

Once you have conducted a situational analysis to collect critical information on environmental and internal issues, you then recast this information into a SWOT analysis. This will provide you with a picture of how your practice or hospital fits into a competitive context. Next, filter the SWOT analysis through some generic marketing strategies. These are common marketing themes that organizations in all types of industries have used to consider their approach to the market. Use them as templates to stimulate your thinking. They may give you some ideas for an overall organizational (practice, hospital, or health system) approach to the market, but just as likely you may see them as a way of structuring your marketing of a particular procedure, service, or service line.

### The Low-Cost Provider

This strategy may be relevant when you are trying to attract groups of patients from a large employer, a group of employers, or a managed healthcare system, or when you are targeting certain types of patients.[3] The strategy is to cut costs to the bone, so you can offer lower prices and thereby gain market share. High volume is leveraged to create low costs by getting the best prices from suppliers and more efficiently utilizing fixed costs (see Chapter 1). Offering low prices relative to competitors means that the organization must be cost conscious in every aspect of business. Tight budgeting, elimination of waste, frugal design of office space, and thin personnel staffing are intrinsic to this strategy. Often, this strategy is adopted when there are many providers, growth is flat, and providers are trying to steal market share from each other by lowering prices. Currently, this characterizes vision correction surgery, so it is not surprising that we see ads for $100 procedures.

### Differentiation

A differentiation strategy is based on identifying purchasers or patients with different sets of needs. One or more of these needs form the basis for a strategy. Medical services can be differentiated on each of the Four Ps. For example, the orthopedic surgeon who can offer hip replacement patients a complete in-house package of radiographic examination, surgery, and physical therapy has a different product than the one who only offers the surgery component. Shouldice Hospital utilized a differentiation strategy built around the Shouldice hernia procedure. It offered patients unique advantages, including lower cost, faster recovery time, and perhaps most importantly, a sense of personal control and participation. By exclusively focusing on this procedure and only taking patients for whom it was appropriate, Shouldice successfully executed a differentiation strategy. Similarly, centers with reputations for excellence, such as the Texas Heart Institute, the Jones Reproductive Clinic, and the Cleveland Clinic have managed to differentiate themselves on perceived, if not actual, quality. Interestingly, this can also allow them to be the low-cost provider. The perceived high quality allows many centers of excellence to compete for regional and national contracts, which results in higher volume. This, in turn, results in better utilization of fixed costs, and allows them to negotiate lower costs on variable cost items, both of which result in a lower cost structure, which permits lower pricing. High quality and low price is obviously a very powerful combination. Differentiation, however, can also fail when the price is too high or if the patient does not perceive the value even if it is real.

## Attacking

Generally, it is not acceptable in medicine to openly attack your competitors through direct criticism. You can, however, attack your competitors' strengths and weaknesses. Opening satellite locations "across the street," using image advertising to kill a competitor's fledgling program, and using price reductions to take advantage of your high volume and the adversary's low volume are all forms of attack. For example, a healthcare system in eastern Virginia, has a national reputation for its heart surgery program. A smaller system recently opened a heart program. The larger system has run full-page print and TV image ads focusing on its outcomes data, size, and reputation. None of the ads mention the much smaller new competitor, but the target of the ads was obvious. Similarly, Wal-Mart and other retailers are attacking primary care and emergency care practices by opening no-appointment care centers staffed by nurse practitioners.

## Guerrilla Warfare

Guerrilla warfare is a variation of an attack strategy. It is characterized by attacks directed at specific weak points of carefully selected competitors who often are much more powerful. It can be a very effective strategy for a smaller healthcare organization in a market with mature, larger, well-entrenched competitors. This strategy also can be useful for new practitioners in a no-growth or slow-growth market.

Guerrilla attacks focus on a market segment or service that is weakly defended. For example, hospital systems may be vulnerable to attacks on selected surgical procedures that can be performed in physicians' offices. Surgeons who selectively seek contracts by offering insurers better rates for practice-based procedures that formerly were hospital based are conducting guerrilla warfare. See, for example, the use of an activity-based costing approach by a gastroenterology practice in Chapter 1 (Exhibit 1–19) to move work that was formerly hospital based into the practice.

## Fortifying and Protecting

This is a defensive strategy designed to block the advances of adversaries. Generally, service businesses use a fortifying and defending strategy to protect referral sources. Obtaining written contracts, wining and dining, acknowledging referrals, and providing quality service make it difficult for challengers to divert referrals. Some healthcare systems have been purchasing primary care practices as a defense against the entry of outsiders into a local market. By buying up the available sources of primary care, they make it very difficult or very expensive for outside players to enter the market.

## Harvesting

*Harvesting* is a strategy for orderly withdrawal from a market while at the same time collecting a harvest of cash. Harvesting is accomplished by cutting budgets to a minimum, reducing advertising expenses, reducing quality in those areas where it will not show, eliminating nonessential services, reducing or eliminating equipment maintenance, subletting or selling excess office space, and so on.

Harvesting is appropriate when an organization is in an undesirable position and the goal is to restructure the organization or kill it off. Harvesting also is appropriate for services where demand is flat or declining *and* you have a small market share. Harvesting can create the capital necessary to finance a turnaround, or it can precede liquidation. In any event, it is a strategy that can buy time for a final decision.

Consider the following case example. Dr. Singh did not enjoy his solo private practice. He found the experience to be lonely, he did not enjoy cultivating referral sources, and he did not find managing the day-to-day affairs of a small practice to be rewarding. In addition, his financial position had been in a long steady decline, because the economics of solo practice were no longer favorable. His lease expired in 6 months, and he decided that he would prefer working for a large hospital doing clinical, educational, and administrative work. While negotiating

an agreement to work for the hospital, Dr. Singh began a harvesting strategy. He eliminated a part-time clerical position, a nursing position, and a telephone line and reduced his supply inventory to a minimum. He also accelerated into his remaining months of private practice any legally appropriate personal expenses that he thought his future employer might not compensate him for, such as buying a new cell phone and laptop computer. Finally, he limited the time each day that his business manager would take patient calls so that she could work back accounts and maximize account collection.

## Boston Consulting Group Strategies

The Boston Consulting Group developed generic strategies that integrate the issues of relative market share and market growth rate. Dichotomizing both growth rate and market share results in a 2-by-2 table (**Exhibit 7–2**). Begin in the northeast cell. Low share of a

**Exhibit 7–2** Boston Consulting Group Generic Strategies

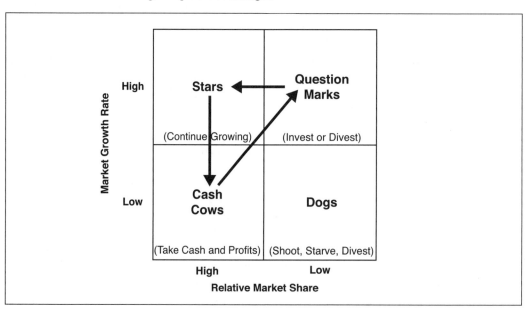

high-growth market often characterizes the introductory life-cycle phase of products and services including those that are medical. Generic strategies in this cell are either to invest to gain market share while the competition is fragmented and margins are large, or get out (harvest), and reinvest capital, effort, time, etc. in other products/services/procedures. Growing market share generally results in both negative cash flow and income statement net income, because of the need to reinvest gains to continue gaining market share. This phase is called the Question Mark, because of the uncertainty of a procedure's or service's future.

Over time, demand for the procedure or service hopefully increases. If you are successful, then your devotion to growing this procedure or service as it is "catching on" should result in attaining a high-market share of a high-growth market (northwest cell). High-market share creates economies of scale and lower costs, and results in a very competitive market position. The generic strategy in this cell is to grow at the maximum digestible rate. As Satchel Paige said, "Don't look back because someone may be gaining on you!" This phase is called the Star. The goal in this cell is to obtain the largest possible market share. Reinvestment of net income continues, and Stars often are cash and net income neutral. A danger in this phase is that it is hard to tell when it ends and demand starts to flatten out. During this phase of rapid growth, exuberance abounds. There is the tendency to make linear growth predictions and to take on fixed costs based on projected growth. If you miscalculate the inflection point of the growth curve, then serious problems can occur.

As with all markets, products, and services, eventually the growth rate declines, and you move to the southwest cell. Here, we often see price competition as competitors try to increase volume in a flat market by stealing it from their competitors. If you have been successful to this point, meaning that you have attained high-market share, then you can choose to undercut the competition on price, or match them on price and gain substantial net income and cash. This is the Cash Cow phase. Here, the generic strategy is to milk the cow, take cash and profits, but not kill it. Simultaneously, you should reinvest some net income in new question marks, because they will be your future.

The final cell (southeast) is a low share of a low growth market. It is referred to as a Dog. Generally, you get into this cell by never gaining market share during the growth phase. You simply drop from a low share of a high-growth market to a low share of a low-growth market. You can also get yourself a Dog by defining what you do as a *procedure* when a new procedure to solve the same medical *problem* comes along. There is low or no growth for your procedure of choice, and you have a low share of the *market* that your obsolete procedure addresses, because competitors are using a more attractive alternative. The generic strategy here is to shoot the dog, starve the dog, harvest the dog, or divest the dog. The problem is that Dogs are often pets; a pet hospital, clinic, program, procedure, or service, and it is often difficult to kill off a pet.

Thinking of your practice as a portfolio of different medical products and services, you would like to see a distribution across all of the cells except the Dog. The Question Marks are your future. The Stars represent what you do well now. The Cash Cows are your reward for doing things well in the past.

This approach may be helpful if market share and growth convey competitive advantages. Some products and services, however, are not sensitive to these issues. For example, Lexus, Mercedes-Benz, the iPhone and healthcare organizations that cater to overseas cash patients and patients desiring upscale or personalized service are examples that run counter to this model. In these cases, market share and market growth are less important than various quality image and attentiveness attributes.

## Turnaround

A turnaround strategy is appropriate when an organization is in crisis and is worth saving, but the current strategy has led to very serious financial or management problems. The first task in a turnaround strategy is diagnosis. A misdiagnosis can be fatal, because the organization by definition is already in a weakened state. It is essential at this point to determine whether the crisis has been caused by poor implementation of an effective strategy or an ineffective strategy. Common problems that can precipitate the need for a turnaround strategy include the following:

- Buying market share with low fees while underestimating the actual cost of delivering the services; this can be a real danger of capitation, HMO, and PPO arrangements
- Excessive fixed costs associated with underutilized office space, equipment, or personnel
- Insufficient market share, either as a result of internal incompetence or competitors' actions
- Overreliance on a new procedure or technological innovation that does not generate the expected revenues

Attempting a turnaround can be very risky. Hall studied 64 companies that had attempted a turnaround and none of them succeeded.[4] The turnaround attempts failed, because the firms either waited too long to begin or had insufficient cash or managerial talent to recover in slow-growth markets. Here are five generic approaches to undertaking a turnaround:[5]

1. *Revamp the existing strategy.* If the cause of the problem is strategic as opposed to operational, then this approach is appropriate. Strategic problems are essentially flaws in the approach to the market. Operational problems usually result from incompetent execution of the strategy. Revamping can be undertaken with any of the strategies just noted.
2. *Increase revenues.* This approach is necessary when there is no way to cut expenses. The strategy for approaching the market remains the same, but operational changes are made to increase revenues. Revenues can be increased through better utilization of physician time, using more physician extenders, offering additional services, adding office hours, coding more thoroughly, and so on. If demand is inelastic and you are a nonparticipating physician with an insurance plan, you can raise your fees. If demand is elastic, raising your fees may result in driving patients to your competition, thereby reducing your revenues. This is a difficult strategy to implement.
3. *Reduce costs.* Once again, the strategy for approaching the market remains the same. Operational plans, however, stress cost reductions in all organizational aspects. Reducing costs will only work if the items associated with the costs do not generate revenue, or if their associated costs can be reduced at a greater rate than their associated revenues. To use this tactic, cost inefficiencies must be identifiable, and the cost-volume-profit relationship must be understood (see Chapter 1). Costs can be reduced by eliminating unneeded or underemployed positions, eliminating underutilized services, making better utilization of automation (e.g., electronic claims), using flexible budgets to manage expenditures, and undertaking a general belt tightening.

4. *Sell assets.* Big-ticket capital items (e.g., radiology equipment, computers, and laboratory equipment) that are not being efficiently utilized can be sold. The cash generated then can be used to finance other revenue-generating programs and services.

5. *Use a combination of approaches.* A turnaround need not be elegant. Use any and all of the approaches that seem relevant. A change of strategy can be coupled with the other approaches, or these approaches can be used with the current strategy. Generally, the more serious the problem, the more likely it is that you will have to consider a broad, rapid attack on the problem.

## OUTCOME: THE MARKETING PLAN

The marketing plan is analogous to saying, "We will open a second front in France in June 1944," then indicating which divisions will land where, what their objectives are, determining the equipment and supplies they will need, and developing a plan to get troops, the equipment and supplies to the right places in a timely manner. The four elements of the marketing plan (product, place, price, and promotion) must fit together into a synergistic whole, and there must be a logical tie back to your SWOT analysis. **Exhibit 7–3** provides an example of a marketing plan for a psychiatrist.

---

**Exhibit 7–3** Marketing Plan for a Psychiatrist

---

### PRODUCT PLAN

My objective is to spend 60 percent of my time doing medication work and hospital rounds. I do not want to be involved in much short-term psychotherapy, so I will select my psychotherapy cases to be longer-term, more chronic cases. I will refer out short-term psychotherapy cases to my psychologist, while retaining the medical component of the case.

I want to develop an eating disorders program. My primary interest, however, is in the medication and hospitalization components. I will try to find a psychology practice to jointly develop and market this program. The psychology practice will handle the psychotherapy, and I will handle the medical component.

### DISTRIBUTION PLAN (Place Plan)

My practice is currently well situated to serve my patients. I will not expand my hours. The eating disorders program will have to be based in the "allied" practice. This practice must be in the eastern part of town, no more than 5 minutes or so from an expressway exit and no more than 15 minutes from my practice.

### PROMOTION PLAN

#### Paid Display Advertising

$13,500 over the next 12 months in paid print advertising. This will be divided: $6,500 on display ads in the local entertainment newspaper two times per month, and $7,000 on a smaller weekly display ad in the science section of the daily newspaper. The ads will stress the personalized nature of my services and the comprehensiveness of psychiatry as opposed to the more limited skills of competitors, such as psychologists.

When the new eating disorders program comes online, I am planning $5,000 in some form of advertising. The specific nature of these ads will be determined with the partnering practice, but the ads will reflect a high-quality, scientific (as opposed to "pop psychology") professional image.

*continues*

**Exhibit 7–3** continued

---

### Referral Source Development

1. I will refer out a significant proportion of psychotherapy patients to well-qualified and professionally competent allied providers, such as psychologists and clinical social workers, with the objective of receiving medication referrals.
2. I will provide six evening seminars over the next 12 months in my office for psychology and clinical social work practices on medication issues.
3. I will hold a 1-day training program for family practice physicians to acquaint them with ways of determining when child behavior problems should be referred to a psychiatrist.

### Television and Radio

I will have my secretary obtain a list of the names and addresses of all local talk show hosts. I will write each one a letter describing timely topics that I can talk about on his or her show. In addition, I will mail each one a press release on a specific issue at least once every 2 months.

### Free Media

1. I will write at least one news release each month. These will be on the latest developments in mental health based on information obtained from my professional journals. The news releases will be mailed to reporters and to local television and radio news departments. My secretary will follow up on these to see if interview appearances can be scheduled.
2. I will conduct four free 1½-hour workshops/seminars each year, which will be held in a nearby church auditorium. These will cover such issues as smoking, eating disorders, phobias, problem children, etc. The workshops will emphasize the unique role of psychiatry in treating these disorders.
3. Six weeks before each free workshop, I will distribute a press release about it to all local newspapers and other media for inclusion in community announcements as well as to local churches and civic groups for inclusion in their newsletters.
4. I will try to find some source of free, recurring media exposure, such as a weekly mental health segment on a television news program or a weekly or monthly newspaper column.

### Internet

I will develop a Web site for the practice. Based on discussions with a Web site design consultant I am budgeting $5,000 for Web site design and will budget for ongoing Web expenses after they are determined.

### PRICING PLAN

I will participate with Blue Cross/Blue Shield and other major insurers in the area. I will set my fees for uncovered services at about what my peers charge, but if I am off, I will be on the high side.

---

A marketing plan is subject to constant revision. For example, suppose that the first of the quarterly workshops referred to in Exhibit 7–3 is a great success. Many people attend, and within a week several become patients. Investigating why the workshop was so successful through the patient intake process, and as a consequence revising the number and timing of workshops would be justified. Similarly, if the newspaper display ads are producing no noticeable results after 2 months, then the ad content should be reexamined, and ultimately the budget for display ads may need to be reduced or eliminated.

## FOCUSING ON PROMOTION

Promotion is probably what first comes to most people's minds whenever they hear the term marketing. As you can see from the preceding discussion, promotion is only one part of the entire marketing process. Promotional activities, however, are often the most visible part of an organization's marketing activities, because they are focused toward the outside. The goal of this section is to acquaint you with a number of specific promotional activities, and to suggest how and when to use them.

### Personal Contact

Personal contact is one of the most effective ways of promoting a healthcare organization. Personal contact means talking to large or small groups of people, or individuals. The target of personal contact can be potential patients or referral sources. One reason that this form of promotion can be so effective is that it is often not perceived as promotion. Another reason is that potential patients and referral sources get to know you and begin to see you as a person, not merely as a name or a title.

Let's first discuss how to promote yourself to groups of potential patients or referral sources. It is important to draw a distinction between making one or two presentations to groups and developing an ongoing personal contact strategy. The former is dabbling, the latter is promotion, and the distinction between the two is important. A real promotional effort requires commitment. In particular, it requires time and energy spent developing good presentations and a willingness to make presentations over an extended period of time. Hospital systems, for example, often have speaker series that are designed to familiarize potential patients with affiliated physicians and hospital facilities through the means of education.

Any form of promotion, to be effective, requires repetition, and personal contact is no exception. Physicians using this approach need ways to consistently develop interesting presentation materials. How do you do this? You create a special niche for yourself. Think about your specialty and interests. Select two or three treatment or disorder areas about which you are particularly knowledgeable or would like to be. Don't necessarily limit yourself to areas of current expertise. Be willing to expand your knowledge base when that is necessary or personally desirable. For example, if an employee assistance program will be conducting a seminar on drug testing, give it a shot even if you aren't an expert on the subject. A few hours of paid library work on the part of a student, coupled with a computer search, will give you the specialized knowledge, which in combination with your medical experience and education, will allow you to make an informative and effective presentation. Remember, you don't have to present yourself as an expert on a subject or procedure to make an interesting and useful presentation. You do have to present yourself, however, as one who knows what is current regarding a subject or procedure.

Remember also that the value of the personal contact lies largely in the quality of communication between you and your audience. The very fact that you are there has promotional value. Develop your presentation so that, whenever possible, it involves your audience. Asking your audience questions and giving them plenty of opportunities to ask you questions will help you establish a two-way dialogue. The presentation should allow your audience to sample your behavior. If your objective is to let the audience know that you are competent, concerned, and approachable, then conduct your presentation in this way. Give them facts, but also show them the type of person you are. Conduct the presentation so they understand that you care about their problems and are willing to listen to them. "But I don't have the time to do all that preparation," you say. If you really don't have the time, then you probably don't need the referrals in the first place, or you should seek other means to promote to patients and referral sources. Once you have defined a few presentation subjects, the next problem is finding someone who will listen. Begin by asking yourself "Who else works in these areas?" For example, suppose that you feel that you could make an effective presentation on sexual abuse. You might want to contact family service agencies, rape hotlines, churches, women's groups, police departments, and others that come into contact with sexually abused individuals.

Personal contact also can take place at the individual level. One of the most effective ways to conduct one-on-one promotion is over lunch. Meeting a referral source over lunch is advantageous in that neither of you "wastes" an hour (unless, of course, you normally don't eat during the day). Also, it allows you to develop a series of similar time-limited promotional opportunities that can be easily arranged by you or your secretary. If you make it a point to hold three luncheon meetings a week for a month, you will have captured approximately 12 hours of referral development time at virtually no cost in clinical hours.

### Paid Ads

**Exhibit 7–4** contains an evaluation of the strengths and weaknesses of various major media. Many physicians use newspaper display ads in which they state their names and the services that they offer. If newspaper ads are to work, they require repetition. Given the high cost of space in daily newspapers, this will invariably result in a large initial cost before results are likely to be seen. If you are considering placing a display ad in a newspaper, be certain to ask yourself what will differentiate you from other physicians running similar display ads.

You also should consider the geographical area from which you draw patients. Although a newspaper may be read by hundreds of thousands of readers, most of this exposure may be of little value if your patients largely come from within a few miles of your practice. For example, a family practice located near residential neighborhoods may draw 90 percent of its patients from within a 10-mile radius. An advertisement in a widely distributed daily newspaper may be largely a waste of money, because most readers will not travel long distances because there will be many competitors located between you and them. On the other hand, a specialist in cosmetic plastic surgery or a cardiologist may have a regional clientele, in which case the wide circulation of the daily newspaper could be useful for reaching potential patients.

An alternative to advertising in the daily newspaper is to use smaller newspapers and newsletters. These especially can be effective if the publication targets an audience that is more likely to want your services than the general population. In addition, the lower advertising rates will allow you to achieve greater repetition. For example, a display ad in a Norfolk, Virginia gay and lesbian newspaper which publishes monthly can be run for a year for a lower cost than a single display ad in the daily newspaper. The gay newspaper could be a very good place for a practice to advertise, if the gay and lesbian population would be particularly interested in the practice's services. If gays and lesbians would not be more interested than the general population, then it would in fact be a very expensive advertising outlet, because its circulation is much smaller than that of the daily newspaper.

**Exhibit 7–4** Media Strengths and Weaknesses

| Source | Advantages | Disadvantages |
| --- | --- | --- |
| Newspapers | Good coverage in local markets<br>Short time commitment<br>Easy availability<br>Tangible and believable | Low demographic selectivity<br>Relatively short life<br>Low reproduction quality<br>Declining market share with young adults |
| Television | Combines sight and sound<br>High attention<br>Conveys "Big League" image<br>Entertaining, energetic, and forceful | Low demographic selectivity<br>Very short message life<br>High production and presentation costs<br>Commercial clutter |
| Radio | Low production and presentation costs<br>High demographic selectivity<br>Reaches mass markets | Less attention getting than visual messages<br>Very short message life<br>Commercial clutter |
| Billboards | High repetition<br>Low cost<br>Visual | No demographic selectivity<br>Very limited message<br>"Low class" image |
| Magazines | High message permanence<br>High demographic selectivity<br>High reproduction quality | Long purchase lead time<br>No guarantee of position |
| Direct Mail | Demographic selectivity<br>Personalized<br>No competition surrounding your message | High cost per number of exposures<br>Junk mail image |
| Internet Web Page | High message permanence<br>High reproduction qualilty<br>Low cost<br>"Big League", "With It" image<br>Attractice to young adults | Being found<br>Initial design costs |

*Source:* Adapted from: Fajen, S. "More for your money from the media." *Harvard Business Review,*1978, Sept.–Oct.

For example, if an ad in the daily newspaper costs $400 and is seen by 500,000 readers, then each dollar of advertising translates into 1,250 readers. By placing a similarly sized ad costing $30 in the 10,000-circulation gay and lesbian newspaper, each dollar reaches 333.33 readers. Advertising in the gay newspaper would be reasonable if you had a service or a message that would result in a response rate from gays that is 3.75 times greater than the general population newspaper.[6] Promoting AIDS services or advertising the fact that you have special interest in helping gay and lesbian patients might produce a favorable return. Whenever you advertise in a specialty newspaper or bulletin, you should consider designing your ad to speak *directly* to the publication's audience. Customizing the ad may cost a little more, but it will allow you to convey your message in a manner that might be particularly attractive to that market. Another benefit of utilizing smaller newspapers and newsletters is that some organization within the specialty audience may ask you to present a workshop or give a presentation, thereby providing additional exposure.

Another place to advertise is the Yellow Pages. An ad in the Yellow Pages is a passive form of advertising because it does not increase demand for your services. A newspaper or television commercial can educate potential patients regarding the symptoms of a problem or the need for preventive care, thereby increasing demand. In addition, it intrudes upon them so you are creating exposure. Yellow Page browsers, on the other hand, must already know that they need your services in order to find you. Many Yellow Pages referrals are price shopping. The Yellow Pages also represent one of the last places that people look for healthcare services. Yellow Pages shoppers often have exhausted other potential referral sources, such as friends and healthcare professionals. As a result, Yellow Pages referrals are less likely to show up for the initial appointment. One practice reported an overall first appointment show rate of 74 percent, whereas the rate for Yellow Pages show rate was 51 percent.[7]

Yellow Pages ad copy should be designed for the consumer who does not know you. The top line should stress the services that you provide, not your name (an exception is when the practice name is descriptive of the services provided, such as "Liver Specialists, P.C."). Listing the most common symptoms you work with and a few of the most common disorders you encounter will also help Yellow Pages readers determine whether you can help. Other Yellow Pages ad design pointers are as follows:

- Use a large black border around your ad. A ¼-inch border will set your ad off from others.

- Color is not cost effective. In addition, as more advertisers resort to color, the color ad's ability to catch the eye is lost. Finally, many color ads look gaudy and do not promote a quality image.
- Strive to get the ad placed near the alphabetical listing. This will result in increased readership. The "dollar bill"–size ad has a greater chance of being placed near the alphabetical listing. Alternatively, create a small display ad in the alphabetical listing by purchasing several lines.
- Being toward the beginning of the listing is not that important. Many readers will fan through the book from back to front and will therefore search the listing in reverse order.
- Copy should use upper- and lower-case letters to increase legibility. Put your name near the telephone number. Don't use a map. It will waste space, and your ad may be torn out of the book. A short quotation in parentheses will attract attention.
- If you have been practicing for a while, note that in your ad. A group practice may be able to state, for example, "Over 40 Years of Professional Experience."

Finally, Yellow Pages spending should be a carefully assessed part of your overall advertising budget. By tracking how referrals are generated, you can determine the cost per referral, and comparisons can be made with other forms of promotion. The Yellow Pages budget then can be increased or decreased depending on the relative effectiveness of your Yellow Pages advertising.

Television and radio both present messages that are very transitory but can have high impact. A daily newspaper may sit on a table for a day, and a monthly newspaper or magazine may have exposure for several weeks (or years, if in a physician's office!). A 30-second television or radio ad is gone in 30 seconds. These media, however, can be exceedingly effective. The question is whether they are appropriate for you. Radio and television ads require significant repetition if they are to have an impact. A rule of thumb is that the ad has to be seen or heard at least three times before the viewer or listener will fully comprehend the message, and be able to recall the advertiser's name. In addition, the development, design, and production of the ad are critical, because you have such a short time to make your point, and of course this costs money.

Production and air time costs will vary greatly depending on the market. In the Norfolk–Virginia Beach market (ranked 31st nationally), a simple 30-second television commercial can be produced and taped for about $2,000. The cost of air time will vary based on the ratings of programs on which the ad appears. For example, the local 6:00 PM news in this market costs about $1,000 for a 30-second ad. On the other hand, 30 seconds on David Letterman is currently selling for $400 in this local market. If you have a $10,000 ad budget, the 6:00 PM news may not provide the repetition you need to have a good chance of success, but Letterman might. This would especially be the case if the demographics of your patients better aligns with Letterman's demographics. Production costs for radio are substantially lower than for television. Some radio stations will produce ads at no cost in return for purchasing advertising time.

Larger healthcare providers can use television effectively. With their greater financial resources, they can achieve the needed repetition. In addition, they can use alternative formats. Large healthcare systems have developed public service programming that includes several half-hour or hour-long infomercials that appear in prime time spread over the course of a year. This is supplemented by 30-second spot commercials and print ads promoting the longer infomercials.

The focus of the programming is to create public awareness of healthcare problems, such as stroke, heart disease, prenatal care, and so forth, that can be addressed at the system's facilities or by its physicians. Often commercials within the infomercials promote talks given by its physicians and others.

An understanding of patient characteristics is critical to effectively use electronic media. For example, suppose that you are promoting a service that will be used primarily by women, such as cosmetic surgery. There are specific hours and programs that attract a disproportionate number of female viewers. Sometimes, the rates will be lower for hours or programs that are most attractive to a particular market segment because *overall* viewership may be lower. A well-designed media plan for running an ad during hours and on programs where lower viewership is coupled with disproportionate viewing by your target market segment can make the cost-effectiveness formula for television and radio very favorable.

Television and radio stations have considerable amounts of data on ratings and demographics for various programs and time periods. Radio can be a particularly effective medium for targeting specific market segments, because each station has a well-defined format that appeals to a different segment of the population. For example, talk radio stations tend to attract higher-income, better educated listeners, and rock stations have a high proportion of teenage and young adult listeners.

When talking to a station's advertising personnel, you should remember that their job is to sell advertising. Advertising that works is in their long-term interest, because you will continue to run ads if they generate patients. As with any purchase, however, be aware of the unscrupulous salesperson or the salesperson with a short-term profit orientation.

According to one television executive,[8] "A ratings book is like the Bible. You can find whatever you are looking for in it. An ad salesman will know what to show you to tell his story."

Given the 30- to 60-second length of electronic media ads, your ad must be well designed if it is going to be effective. This is one area in which you should heavily rely on professional advice. Television and radio professionals know how to take your ideas and convert them into visual and audio content that will attract viewer attention and communicate your message. You should be involved in the ad development process, but you also should recognize your limitations. Focus on communicating to the media professionals the visual and audio message that you want to convey, along with some thoughts on advertisement characteristics. For example, you might outline the message content, and ask whether the message should be presented by actors in dialogue, by one actor, or by you talking directly into the camera. When media professionals suggest an approach and can give you a reasonable case for proceeding as they suggest, then defer to their judgment. That said, these are your ads and you need to feel comfortable with content and format. You also should be involved in the selection of actors, graphic displays, and other decisions that will affect the appearance and placement of the message. Defer to professional judgment regarding specific use of language and technical production considerations, such as lighting, background, music, camera angles, dress, and make-up.

An alternative to this level of personal involvement is to hire a media consultant to act as an intermediary between you, the advertisement production personnel, and the television or radio station. The media consultant will also be able to tell you which local market programs will provide the best mix of viewers and listeners to meet your marketing objectives. If you use a media consultant, it is critical to spend enough time together so you can make known your objectives and the image you wish to present.

If you decide to use paid advertising, you must be especially cognizant of the local ethics regarding this issue. If you get too far out in front of your colleagues, you may be subject to retribution ranging in form from mild ostracism, to loss of referrals, and perhaps official censure. On the other hand, being out in front of your colleagues can be a very valuable competitive advantage.

Finally, if you determine that your practice might benefit from paid advertising, it might be worthwhile to read about some of the approaches used by successful advertising executives. This may give you some ideas for developing your own ads and ad copy, and also may help you judge the ideas proposed by marketing and media consultants. For example, David Ogilvy, who developed a number of successful advertising campaigns, described his formula for print layout as follows:[9]

- Place an illustration at the top of the page with a caption below it.
- Print the copy in a serif typeface.
- Set the copy in three columns 35–45 characters wide.
- Start the copy with drop initials.
- Print the copy in black ink on white paper.

One particularly effective modification of Ogilvy's formula was used by Washington Hospital Center (**Figure 7–1**). This display ad uses color and paradox (luxury and cuisine in the context of a hospital ad) to attract the reader. The ad clearly is targeted at a market segment. In addition, the ad was run in *Washingtonian Magazine,* whose readership demographics are consistent with the ad's

Gourmet food prepared to order. A waiter in bow tie and tails. Definitely not what you're used to in a hospital.

*Luxurious. Comforting. Tranquil. Warm. If these are the last four adjectives you'd ever associate with the word "hospital," you'll know why we're announcing The Pavilion at Washington Hospital Center. An entire wing of deluxe, private hospital suites doing its very best impersonation of a luxury hotel. There's soft, incandescent light that flows from delicate, crystal fixtures. Carpeting so thick it makes your shoes feel more expensive. And a complete, gourmet menu prepared by The Pavilion's own chef, in The Pavilion's own kitchen.*

*In your suite there's fine art, fine furniture and fine linens. A spacious, tiled bathroom with marble vanities and heated towel racks. There are complete concierge and business services. And perhaps the best feature of all, utter quiet. In other words, the list of amenities goes on and on.*

*Even after you leave, your VIP treatment can continue, thanks to the personalized attention offered by the VNA Integrated Home Care System.*

*To determine if your doctor is affiliated with Washington Hospital Center, or to receive more information about deluxe suites at The Pavilion, call 202-877-DOCS. Washington Hospital Center. The area's most experienced hospital.*

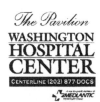

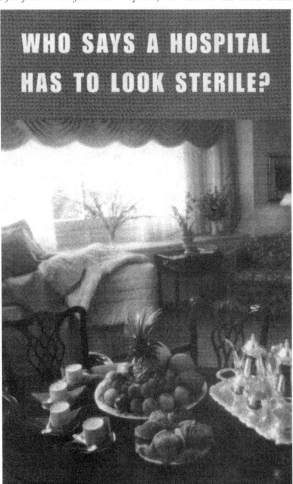

**WHO SAYS A HOSPITAL HAS TO LOOK STERILE?**

**Figure 7–1**  Segment Directed Display Ad Using Modified Ogilfy Format.
*Source:* Courtesy of Washington Hospital Center.

message. Of additional interest is the contrarian market strategy that the ad implies. At a time when everyone was trying to obtain managed care contracts, this organization targeted the "self-pay" segment as part of its customer mix. Ads of this type for a hospital hardly raise an eyebrow these days. The physician who is first in a market with aggressive ad copy may obtain a real competitive advantage, as well as the envy and criticism of peers.

**Unpaid Ads**

Some of the most effective promotions come in the form of free advertising. There are countless ways of getting free advertising, including the following:

- Writing letters to the editor
- Placing announcements in community bulletins about new services that you offer or workshops that you can or will conduct
- Sending announcements to the local newspaper of honors that you have received, or new associates who have joined your practice, open houses, talks, blood pressure clinics, cholesterol clinics, etc.
- Volunteering to write a column for a local newspaper or newsletter
- Distributing a press release on a newsworthy subject
- Appearing on a local television or radio program or obtaining your own program[10]

A few of these strategies deserve particular comment, because of the exposure they can provide. Press releases are a particular favorite in the free ad category. As you might imagine, television ads during prime time can be very expensive. Writing effective press releases can get you the equivalent of several 2-minute television ads per year, as well as newspaper coverage that is equivalent to a large display ad. But these are *better* than ads, because they have the appearance of unbiased news. The key to writing an effective press release is to remember your audience. Your target is a reporter who needs a story. A press release must tell the reporter that he or she can get an interesting, timely story by calling you. The format of a press release is important. It should cover the five Ws of newspaper reporting (who, when, what, where, and why), and do this in a concise, clearly worded manner.

**Exhibit 7–5** contains a press release. The *who,* of course is you. Indicate this in a clear visually exciting way. Next, you want to indicate the *when,* or the date of release. The *what* should be summarized in your headline. The headline needs to be enticing, but it should not be sensationalistic. Reporters are bombarded with press releases, and if they sense that you are trying to overstate your case, you will be quickly filed in the wastepaper basket. The *why* should be in the body of the press release. Here, you must *succinctly* demonstrate the significance of your release. Why should the reporter care? Why should his or her readers, listeners, or viewers care? Generally, a good tactic is to point out the personal importance of the information to the reporter's audience. Another tactic is to tie your message to some compelling statistic. Finally, you want to end the press release with a clear statement of *where* the reporter can go to get additional information. This can be a paper or workshop that you will be presenting, your name and office telephone number, e-mail address, and so forth. You don't have to be a national expert to distribute a press release. The only requirements are that you be knowledgeable about the subject and possess a minimal amount of audacity.

**Exhibit 7–5** Sample News Release

---

NEWS RELEASE FROM THE OFFICE OF
DR. ROBERT BROWN

JULY 18, 20XX

***FOR IMMEDIATE RELEASE***

*Driver Training Students Tour Bayview Hospital Emergency Room*

Students in Riverside High School's Driver Education Program are being given a tour of Bayview's emergency room in an effort to educate them on the perils of reckless and drunk driving. Emergency room personnel familiarize the students with the typical injuries suffered by accident victims and the necessary medical procedures.

Dr. Robert Brown, who initiated the program, stated, "Teens makes up 7 percent of licensed drivers, but suffer 14 percent of fatalities and 20 percent of all reported accidents. I hope that seeing the possible consequences of reckless behavior will act as a deterrent."

The program has been in effect for 3 weeks, and 47 students have toured the emergency room.

FOR ADDITIONAL INFORMATION CONTACT:
Robert Brown, M.D.
(555) 555-7639

5673 Anderson Dr., Virginia Beach, VA 23456

robert.brownMD@mac.com

---

Once you have developed a press release, the next task is to get it to the right people. Look in the local newspaper for reporters who are writing local articles. Do not limit yourself to the health, fitness, and science reporters. Your objective should be to assemble a mailing list of local newspaper, television, and radio reporters. By reading the newspaper each day and by noting television and radio talk show hosts, you can establish a mailing list with virtually no effort. The same task can be given to your secretary or another employee.

Another tactic is to target a media outlet for concentrated attention. Because newspaper, television, and radio reporters receive dozens of press releases each day, 95 percent of them are thrown out immediately after or even before they are read. To be effective, you have to get enough distribution of your press release within the newspaper or station to overcome the natural propensity to throw it out. This can be accomplished by targeting a cross-section of the organization. For example, you might target a television station by mailing releases to several reporters, the program director, the assignment director, and the public affairs director as well as the hosts and producers of any locally produced programs. A reporter may throw the release out, but perhaps it will appeal to the assignment director, who then may instruct a reporter to see whether there is an interesting story there.

In television, early morning news crews, noon news crews, and especially weekend news crews are often looking for program material. Be certain that your press releases get to these personnel. How do you obtain all these names? Have your secretary call your targeted media outlets and ask for names and job titles. It is that simple.

Getting a mention in a newspaper article or television story is often a function of timing. If you want to develop this aspect of marketing your practice, then you must be responsive to the needs of reporters. When a reporter calls, you must talk to him or her *then* or call back *very shortly* thereafter. Remember, reporters work under tight deadlines, and they need answers quickly. A print reporter probably will be in the process of writing the story at the time he or she telephones you. If you are not immediately available, the reporter will call the next physician down the list. The reporter will pass you by even if it was *your* press release that provided the initial idea for the story!

Another advantage of consistently responding quickly to reporters is that they will come to rely on you for medical information. Reporters will begin to call you and quote you in stories that they generate. For example, if there is testimony in a trial regarding a prescription drug, a reporter may contact you for information regarding the possible side effects of the drug. You then may be mentioned in the story: "Dr. Maria Martinez noted that the drug could cause the side effects claimed by the defense but that these side effects are rare." Another example of this type of promotion is presented in **Figure 7–2**. In this article, several local physicians give their opinions about a national news item.

Do not overlook distributing press releases to appropriate church, community, and specialty newsletters. Although their readership may be small, your chances of scoring a hit may be significantly greater. Also, a church or community newsletter may give you exposure to a relatively high proportion of potential patients. Once again, sending your press release to multiple targets within each organization will increase your chances of scoring a hit.

A personal appearance on a local radio or television program is another favorite in the free media ad category. You need a "hook" to get on a program, and a press release is a good start. Another alternative is to call a local talk show host and explain what you would like to talk about on the program. The reaction you will get to this approach will vary, with the probability of success being greater in smaller markets.

How should you conduct yourself when you appear on a local television or radio talk program? It is important to remember that effectively communicating with the typical television audience is best achieved with simple, direct language. If you use a technical term, you should immediately define it or explain it. Being very specific and using examples also will increase your communication effectiveness. Keep your discussion at the level of greatest general interest. Viewers will be less interested in your topic than your patients would be. Patients care about their bodies, so they tend to be interested in what you have to say. If a viewer does not feel that your discussion is directly pertinent, he or she will probably not care, and with a remote control and 200 cable alternatives readily available, you may be quickly "deselected."

Finally, a word of caution. No matter what you say or how clearly you state it, reporters will make mistakes. You will be frustrated because they will miss a major point you were trying to make, misquote you, or present only part of the total picture. All this "goes with the territory." As an example, take the story of a physician who was trying to persuade the city council in a rural Virginia community to allocate more money for emergency mental health services. She told a local newspaper that the cost of 24-hour-a-day emergency services was about $1.50 per year

# Henson's pneumonia treatable if diagnosed

## Antibiotics could have saved him

**By April Witt**
*Staff writer*

The virulent strain of pneumonia that reportedly killed Muppets creator Jim Henson is common and usually curable if treated quickly with antibiotics, local doctors say.

"The streptococcus pneumonia is the most common kind of pneumonia to occur at home," Dr. William Edmondson, a Norfolk internist, said Thursday.

"It hits hard and once you have it you usually get sick enough to get help," he said. "It's something that drives you to the doctor quickly. It is the rare patient that toughs it out and does not get help."

Dr. Oscar E. Edwards, a Norfolk internist said: "Streptococcus pneumonia is tragic to die of. It is the most eminently treatable of them all. If he'd have just come in sooner, with a little bit of penicillin, and he'd probably have been well."

Henson, the creator of Kermit the Frog, Miss Piggy and a host of other beloved Muppets, died Wednesday in a New York Hospital of what his doctor said was "a massive bacterial infection, more specifically known as streptococcus pneumonia."

Dr. David M. Gelmont, director of intensive care at New York Hospital-Cornell Medical Center in New York, said the 53-year-old was healthy until coming down with flu-like symptoms Friday.

Asked why Henson failed to seek more aggressive treatment for his illness, Susan Berry, a spokeswoman for Jim Henson Productions, said: "My guess is he's totally absorbed. He couldn't be bothered. He was very cavalier with his health."

Henson worsened, returned to New York on Monday and checked into the hospital the next day. But by then the infection had spread through his body, damaging vital organs so severely that it could not be controlled by antibiotics, the usual treatment, Gelmont said.

Pneumonia, which strikes about 2 million Americans annually, is an inflammation of the lungs. Although a variety of bacteria and vi-ruses can cause pneumonia, it is most commonly caused by streptococcus, the bacteria that reportedly killed Henson.

Once known as the "captain of the men of death," pneumonia has been much more easily treatable since the invention of antibiotics.

But pneumonia still kills more than 40,000 Americans annually. Most of those who do not survive pneumonia are either very young, elderly or debilitated by a serious disease such as cancer.

Among those at especially high risk of dying are people whose immune systems have been weakened by diseases such as AIDS or who are taking immune-suppressing medicines.

Asked Thursday whether Henson had AIDS, his doctor said: "Categorically, he did not have AIDS."

Dr. Scott A. Miller of Norfolk said no one needs to invoke AIDS to explain a pneumonia death in 1990. "If you get someone who comes in too late with this, you can't save them," said Miller, a Norfolk internist who specializes in infectious diseases. "It's upsetting, but it's the way of the world.

"A few years ago I took care of a 24-year-old woman — healthy, no AIDS — who came in with a little pneumonia and was dead in 24 hours. We don't have to invoke AIDS and we don't have to invoke alternative lifestyles to explain it. Mother Nature can do all of those things."

Streptococcal pneumonia is caused by a common bacteria. "Some people carry it in their mouths and are not affected by it," said Dr. Ignacia Ripoll of Norfolk, a specialist in pulmonary medicine.

People typically contract streptococcal pneumonia when "they have a little cold or a little virus," Ripoll said. "Then their body becomes more susceptible to this infection.

"Once they have this infection, they get sick very fast. Within a matter of hours, people are having chills and a fever and they feel quite ill."

Given a small dose of penicillin or another antibiotic, patients typically improve within 24 hours, Ripoll said.

Untreated, the infection can spread into the blood and damage vital organs, he said.

"We can still reverse it, but these people typically spend weeks in intensive care," he said. "When people develop multi-organ failure, 70 percent of them will die regardless of what you do."

**Figure 7–2** News Story with Local Physicians.
*Source:* Reprinted with permission from The Virginia Pilot, May 18, 1990, 2.

for each county resident. In an attempt to put the cost of these services in perspective, she lightly dropped the comment that these services would be cheaper than a six-pack of beer. The next day the local newspaper headline proclaimed "Crossroads Emergency Services—Cheaper than a Six-Pack!" To top it off, Crossroads at the time was a dry county.

Finally, writing a letter to the editor is another effective type of unpaid ad. A good strategy for getting a letter published is to expand on an issue or topic already covered by an article printed in the newspaper. An example is shown in **Exhibit 7–6**.

### So What Promotions Work Best?

At this point, you may well be asking "But what works? What will give me the most promotional effect for my time and money?" All the ideas discussed can and do work *if you use them effectively and if you use them long enough.* A cornerstone of most successful medical promotion is personal contact with potential referral sources and patients, including one-on-one meetings, lunches, community services, and community presentations. Paid media can be useful if you can adequately finance the projects. The expression "It takes money to make money" is particularly apt when it comes to advertising. Paid advertising, irrespective of the media, is most effective with repetition, and that costs money.

In general, the best way to generate referrals through the media is to get something to appear in print. People tend to cut out your name or announcement or an article that you wrote or in which you are quoted. They often will keep the clipping for weeks or months, and when they finally do need medical services, they will seek you out. In many ways, the ad, announcement, or article is like a business card with your name on it.

Television gives you outstanding visibility and name recognition. The fleeting nature of the medium, however, is a limitation, and you should not have great expectations based on a single appearance on a talk program. The cost of radio is substantially less than the cost of television. Once again, however, a few

---

**Exhibit 7–6**  Letter to the Editor

Solid as a Seatbelt

The arguments against the HPV vaccine on Tuesday's letters page were really an attempt to provide an alternative view laced with anecdotal hearsay and a belittling of 3,700 deaths.

The use of a vaccine to protect against cervical cancer that can be given in the tween years provides a veritable slam-dunk argument in favor of approval.

Dr. Hugh McPhee's letter last Sunday made a perfect analogy of protecting children with the HPV vaccine as one would use a seat belt to protect a child from an unforeseen traffic accident. When states initially started mandating the use of passenger seat belts, the opposition would cite unverifiable reports of a friend or relative who was saved by being thrown clear of a fatal injury because they were not belted in. But logic ultimately triumphed, and seat belt laws were passed, with a precipitous drop in subsequent injuries and deaths from auto accidents.

Arguments against vaccines were alive and well over the last 100 years with smallpox, polio, mumps, rubella, measles and hepatitis B. Yet a whole generation and beyond will never have to experience these illnesses in their unfettered state. My two daughters (ages 9 and 13) have always been advised to wear a seat belt and now can be counseled to roll up their sleeve for another lifesaving intervention.

John Harrington, M.D.
General pediatrician, CHKD
Norfolk

*Source:* © *The Virginia–Pilot.* February 11, 2007, pg. J4. Used with permission.

sporadic appearances will not constitute an effective radio campaign. Unless you devote substantial funds to advertising, the importance of these media lies in the part that they can play in your overall promotional effort, and this part should not be underestimated.

The final selection of a physician is often the result of many events that occurred over an extended period of time. It may result from name recognition gained over months or years of published letters to the editor, appearances on radio and television programs, quotations in the newspaper, and a few personal encounters. Slowly, a prospective patient or referral source becomes familiar with you, and comes to believe that you are someone who may be able to help. When the prospective patient finally needs medical services, he or she is likely to call you because, in a sense, he or she has "known" you for an extended period of time. It should be clear from this that promotion is a long-term activity that must never cease but may change in nature as your practice develops and matures.

Patients can come from anywhere, and virtually anyone can become a referral source. If you are cognizant of this essential truth, then any interpersonal contact has promotional potential. Whether you are visiting your dentist or lawyer, getting your car repaired or your plumbing fixed, or simply mingling at a party, you should always be open to the possibility that you are talking to a potential patient or referral source. When appropriate, manage to work a few comments into the discussion about your profession. The key word here is *appropriate.* Remember, if you do this in a clumsy manner or in a way that is inappropriate given the context of the conversation, you may be doing more harm than good. It is far better to unobtrusively state your profession, and then illustrate your good qualities by being an attentive listener and making appropriate additions to the conversation.

Finally, your own patients can be among your best referral sources. John Ernhardt, MD, has offered several excellent suggestions for marketing to your own patients, including these:[11]

- Show regard for patients' time. This involves being punctual for your appointments and devoting sufficient time to each patient.
- Provide extra time for each patient who is hospitalized, and also make it a quality visit. Try to reduce the patient's anxiety.
- Be available to talk on the telephone. In nonemergency situations, this could include having a staff person tell patients that you will return calls during a specified time period.
- Provide patients with drug samples, thereby medicating them more quickly and relieving them of an expense if they cannot tolerate a new medication.
- Take the time to send appropriate letters and documents. This includes responding to patients who sent you greeting cards, forwarding medical records and test results to other physicians in a timely manner, and sending letters to family members of deceased patients.

It is important to approach these tasks with the proper mental attitude. They should not be undertaken as a way of manipulating patients. They should be done sincerely and considerately, and should demonstrate that you are a professional who is concerned about your patients' welfare. If they are done with sincerity, then they will create patient goodwill and will also set an example of appropriateness and courtesy for your staff to follow.

## Promoting to Referring Physicians

Understanding the nature of the service that referring physicians desire is critical both to design the appropriate service and to present the appropriate message. For example, what do primary care physicians desire when making referrals to specialists? Appropriate clinical care is a necessary but probably insufficient condition. Quick appointments, timely feedback, and clear and timely charting may be three additional issues. Once you understand referring sources' needs, then you can design your services to meet these needs. For example, one GI physician reserves 10 percent of his appointment slots for scheduling within 24 hours, so he can be highly responsive to referral sources. His reasoning was that the relatively few lost hours were more than compensated for by his reputation around town of being able to get patients in on short notice.

Clinical outcomes data represent one source of information that specialists can use to educate primary care physicians. Average length of hospital stay, infection rates, rework rates, mortality rates, and prescription medication costs are all examples of clinical data that specialists can use to promote their practice to primary care–referring physicians. In addition, average time to initial office visit and average time for charting and feedback are also powerful messages to give to these physicians. In these instances, the promotion message cannot be provided without appropriate information systems to supply the data.

As with the other forms of promotion, tailor your services to the customer, in this case referring physicians. Talk with current and potential referring physicians to find out what they want. The very act of doing this will set you apart from many of your colleagues, and help to develop a personal connection with potential referring physicians. Then, keep a referral database so you can determine if referral sources are changing their referral patterns, such as quantity, diagnosis, and so on. Keep in mind that just keeping the database is not enough—you must run appropriate and timely reports from it to see if changes have occurred. If

things change in negative ways, contact the referring physician to find out the reasons why. Sometimes, physicians are unaware that they have changed their referral patterns. For example, in one practice the physician gave his nurse a list of acceptable specialist practices. The nurse got into a dispute with one cardiologist's scheduling secretary, and stopped sending referrals to the practice. Both physicians were totally unaware of the change. Finally, always thank referring physicians for their referrals with a short written note.

## MARKET SEGMENTATION

Market segments, as previously discussed, are groups of people who tend to behave in a similar manner, or who have similar characteristics. Different market segments may have special needs and preferences, and this may justify developing special programs and marketing plans. For example, if people with homes in a particular ZIP code are especially likely to come to your practice, then they are behaving differently as a result of their geographical location. If a healthcare provider has more than one location, then understanding which patients go to each location may allow you to determine more precisely the services and promotion activities that are best suited to each location. Similarly, if you know that an important component of your practice consists of patients with hypertension, then you can develop programs and promotional efforts that will be particularly appealing to this market segment.

Identifying market segments is part of a marketing strategy called *target marketing*. Target marketing involves identifying one or more market segments and directing marketing efforts toward them. When physicians or healthcare organizations adopt a target marketing strategy, they do four things:

1. Identify important market segments.
2. Systematically evaluate the attractiveness of each of the segments.
3. Select one or more of the segments for special attention.
4. Position the organization by developing a specific marketing mix (the Four Ps) to establish a competitive advantage in each of the selected segments.

It also is important to note that, although you may identify one or a few market segments deserving of special attention, your practice may still be largely composed of patients drawn from outside these particular segments.

**Developing Market Segments**

The objective when looking for market segments is to identify some basis that isolates more attractive patients. Attractive may mean that they disproportionately need your services, that they disproportionately generate higher margins, that you gain particular professional satisfaction working with this segment, or that you feel an ethical responsibility to serve this segment. The issue then becomes whether you can develop specific services for or ways of communicating with a group defined by segmentation. Examining market segments defined by diseases or treatments can suggest new services to provide or new ways to communicate with potential patients. For example, an oncologist might define families of terminal patients as a segment. Developing a program to help these families deal with the eventual loss of their loved one would be a service to provide to this segment, which might differentiate this practice from its competitors. **Exhibit 7–7** contains some diagnostic market segments arranged by medical specialty. Each of these diagnostic segments can be divided into smaller segments. For example, a dermatol-

**Exhibit 7–7** Diagnostic Market Segments

Cardiology
• Post-MI
• CAGB
• Dysrhythmias
• Chronic congestive heart failure

Dermatology
• Chronic dermatitis
• Skin cancer
• Allergic dermatitis

Family Practice
• Hypertensives
• Diabetics
• Sick children
• Upper respiratory infection
• Psychosomatic illnesses
• Weight management
• Sexual dysfunction

Pediatrics
• Well babies
• Chronic ear infections
• Allergic children
• Orthopedic problems

Psychiatry
• Depression
• Anxiety/phobias
• Sexual dysfunction
• Obsessive compulsive disorder
• Rape/sexual assault
• Separation and divorce

Pulmonary
• COPD
• Asthmatics
• Industrial lung diseases
• Pulmonary fibrosis
• ICU

*Source:* Adapted from Brown, S. and A. Morley. (1986). *Marketing Strategies for Physicians.* NJ: Oradell: Medical Economic Books, pp. 181–182.

ogist may choose to focus on an *adolescent* chronic dermatitis segment, whereas an orthopedist may market to *adult* sports medicine patients.

**Exhibit 7–8** contains some generic market segments. Demographic variables are the most commonly used basis for defining market segments, because patient desires, attitudes, needs, and utilization rates often correlate with demographic variables. Demographic segmentation is commonly used to market consumer goods so marketing messages and media directly address the most promising customers. For example, it is much more likely that Mercedes-Benz ads will appear in *Architectural Digest* and *Vogue* than in *Easy Rider* because the demographic characteristics of *Architectural Digest* and *Vogue* readers are more similar to the demographic characteristics of Mercedes-Benz buyers.

Demographic variables can be important segmentation variables for a healthcare organization. Age, sex, family income, occupation, education, and race can be important because the attractiveness of medical services can vary across these segments. Women, for example, have a different distribution of diseases and procedures than men. In addition, women probably have more decision-making power regarding the treatment of children. Similarly, the medical problems associated with sports differ among age groups. Middle-age athletes experience different types of injuries

**Exhibit 7–8** Segmentation Variables

| Variable | Characteristics |
| --- | --- |
| *Geography* | City, State, Region, Zip Code, Mileage Radius, Commuting Route |
| *Demographic* | |
| Age | Under 5; 5–10; 10–13; 13–19; 19–34; 35–49; 49–64; 64+ |
| Age Category | Child; Latency; Adolescent; Young Adult; Middle Age; Elderly |
| Gender | Male; Female |
| Sexuality | Gay; Lesbian; Transgender; Bisexual |
| Family Size | 1; 2; 3–4; 5+ |
| Income | Under $20k; $20k–$35k; $35k–$50k; $50k–$80k; $80k–$120k; $120k–$200k; $200k+ |
| Occupation | Student; Labor; Technical; Professional; Farmer; Retired |
| Education | Grade School; High School Degree; Some College; College Graduate; Professional Degree |
| Religion | Athiest; Catholic; Protestant; Muslim; Jewish; Buddist; Hindu; Other |
| Ethnicity | Anglo; Hispanic; Black; Vietnamese; Philippino; Mexican |
| *Psychographic* | |
| Personality | Extroverted; Neurotic; Conscientious; Agreeable; Open to New Experiences |
| Values | Benevolence; Universalism; Self-Direction; Hedonism; Achievement Oriented; Power Seeking; Security Seeking; Traditional; Confirmity Seeking; Spirituality |
| Social Class | Lower Lower; Working Class; Middle Class; Upper Middle; Upper; Upper Upper |
| *Behavioral* | |
| Benefits | Quality; Low Price; Service; Status; Economy; Value |
| User Status | Ex-User; First-Time User; Frequent User |
| User Frequency | None; Light; Moderate; Heavy (could be expressed as numbers, 1, 2, 3, 4, etc.) |
| Attitude | Neutral; Hostile; Postive; Enthuiastic |

and have different medical needs than do teenagers. Promotional content and media also vary across these groups. Middle-age athletes may be accessed through athletic and golf clubs and softball leagues, whereas teen-age athletes can be accessed through schools, parents, and coaches.

Psychographic segmentation divides patients on the basis of social class, life style, or personality. Social class is strongly associated with preferences for consumer goods, habits, clothing, and so forth. There clearly are social class differences in the kinds of medical treatment desired and needed. People lower on the socioeconomic scale have more chronic health problems, generally have less sophisticated medical knowledge, and less disposable income. If you want to disproportionately attract this segment, then you need to develop a marketing mix that fits with this segment's characteristics. The marketing research literature is ambivalent about the real-world usefulness of personality segmentation. You may be able to devise some reasonable hypotheses, however, regarding personality segments. For example, if you have an oncology practice, you may well have a disproportionate number of situationally depressed patients. This would be a patient segment that could benefit from treatment for this problem, and might be very responsive to a practice that communicates recognition of this problem and offers integrated solutions.

Behavioral segmentation is based on attitudes toward, use of, or response to services; in this case medical services. One important behavioral segmentation variable is benefits. This means constructing groups based on what patients seek from treatment; that is, the benefits that they desire. Kotler and Clarke state that most healthcare consumers can be grouped into the following four benefit-seeking segments:[12]

1. Quality Buyers—want the best product and are unconcerned about cost.
2. Service Buyers—primarily concerned with acquiring the most caring and personal service.
3. Value Buyers—examine the price-quality trade-off. A value buyer would go to a physician who has a "reasonable" reputation and who has "reasonable" fees.
4. Economy Buyers—most interested in the least-expensive alternative.

You may find that your patients are homogeneous with respect to the benefits that they seek. If this is the case, then you are probably conveying a message to prospective patients about the benefits that you provide. This may or may not be desirable. For example, if you are trying to provide family practice services to a broad spectrum of the community, yet your patients are mostly quality buyers, then you may be unintentionally excluding a significant number of potential patients. Perhaps, for example, you are conveying an unintended message that dissuades value buyers.

## Evaluating and Choosing Market Segments

The second and third components of target marketing, previously discussed, involve evaluating the attractiveness of segments and choosing segments. Larger healthcare providers, such as hospitals and nursing homes, determine the usefulness of various market segments through marketing research. The research process typically involves many in-depth interviews and focus groups composed of patients, potential patients, and decision makers for patients (parents, guardians, etc.). The data then are evaluated, and a profile is developed of a potential purchaser's demographic, psychographic, geographical, and behavioral characteristics, and media consumption habits. Obviously, this can be a time-consuming and expensive process. An alternative approach is to look at current patients and search for prominent segmentation patterns. Concentrate on large, obvious groups defined geographically, demographically, or behaviorally, such as residence location, gender, occupation, age, diagnosis, or procedure. Don't try to create a myriad of narrow, multivariable segments, because each segment will be too small to market to effectively. Large homogeneous segments will allow you to make marketing decisions that will affect a substantial number of patients.

When evaluating whether a segment will be useful for target marketing, consider the current size and growth potential of the segment, its attractiveness, and your practice's objectives and resources. The size of a segment is important because you do not want to put time, effort, and resources into a segment that is too small to obtain a reward commensurate with your efforts. Growth potential is important because successfully marketing to a growing segment will result in practice growth. Remember, however, that a growing segment will tend to attract attention, which translates into competition. Consider also the degree of existing competition. If there are already a number of other medical practices competing for a segment, will the segment be large enough to support another provider? Do you have a competitive advantage, such that you will be able to do better in this segment than your peers?

Evaluation of the current attractiveness of a segment can be particularly important if you will be competing against nonmedical organizations or hospitals. Nonmedical competitors may be used to lower fees, and this may foreshadow an erosion of a market's profit potential. Nonmedical competition

may be encountered in segments such as smoking, weight loss, anxiety, pain management, eye care, and foot care. Consider, also, whether you will be competing with hospitals. Hospitals can be tough competitors because their enormous resources allow them to undertake expensive promotional campaigns that saturate a market with highly visible television, radio, and newspaper ads. They also can offer a service at a loss or a break-even price to attract patients who will then turn to them for other services at a later date.

Ultimately, the selection of segments is a qualitative, subjective decision. It may be based on objective data from marketing research or on intuition derived from personal knowledge of your patients coupled with a healthy dose of speculation. In the final analysis, however, it is a management decision, and it should take into account the benefit that you can add to your patients. Going back to the Four Ps, can you provide some benefit in terms of product (service), place (location, time, access), promotion (communications), or price that will give you a competitive advantage? If you cannot provide some *special* value to patients in a given segment, then you should probably not select it for special attention.

## Positioning Your Organization

The final phase of target marketing is to position yourself so that you will market to the previously identified target segment or segments. Segmenting is the difficult task. Once good segments have been identified, positioning is relatively easy. The positioning should be determined by your evaluation of the particular competitive advantages that you have vis-à-vis the segments. This should then be reflected in the specific marketing plan you construct. Dr. Smith, a psychiatrist, for example, might identify the "upscale, higher-income, better educated" segment as deserving of special attention. Note that this does *not* mean that she is necessarily restricting her practice to this segment. In this example, she is simply saying that this is a segment with particular opportunities for *her* practice, and that it fits into a mix of procedures, services and patient groups. She determines that her competitive advantages are as follows:

- She is a physician, not a psychologist or clinical social worker.
- She can prescribe medication, unlike many of her competitors.
- She can diagnose physiological problems, unlike many of her nonmedical competitors.
- She has more years of postgraduate training than competitors with other kinds of degrees.
- She has advanced training in cognitive behavioral therapy, unlike many of her medical colleagues.
- All major insurance carriers will cover her services, unlike nonmedical competitors, who are only covered by some carriers.
- Because she employs a psychologist, she can provide a complete range of mental health services, unlike many of her competitors who can only provide some of these services.
- She has a central location near the intersection of two major commuting interstates with excellent access to the wealthier parts of the region.
- She is located in a Class A office suite.

After talking with several of her patients who are in the upscale, higher-income, better-educated segment, Dr. Smith determines that they are largely quality buyers. Her marketing strategy, therefore, is to approach this

segment by appealing to the desire to obtain the best services from the most qualified provider. Her marketing plan for this segment is different only in regard to the promotion component. The services that she will provide are the *same* as those offered to all her other patients. She is not providing additional services (product), offering different hours or locations (place), or charging different fees (price) to attract this segment. She places print ads emphasizing her superior position in the provider "pecking order," including her ability to diagnose physiological causes of mental disorders and uses this to emphasize the superior quality of her services. She uses TV ads and places them on programs where viewership is heavily biased toward the better educated and upper-income segments. She decides not to advertise on radio because she can't find commercial programming consistent with the target demographic. Instead, she becomes a public radio and public TV sponsor and decides to become an active volunteer with the public TV station. She develops a Web site characterized by excellent visual design and usability, high-information content on psychiatric problems, and the synergistic potential of medications and cognitive behavioral therapy. Finally, she sets as a goal to make 12 presentations before business groups and employers with more highly educated workforces over the next 12 months.

## THE INTERNET

The Internet has rapidly developed as a source to replace or augment traditional sources of advertising. Arguably, however, the Internet provides its most important opportunities for physicians and health systems when considered more broadly for its *marketing* considerations. As noted earlier, marketing is the amalgamation of Product, Price,

Place, and Promotion. In this instance, the Internet has significance for how you operationalize Promotion, Place, and Product.

## Promotion

One promotion application to health care is obvious—have a Web site that describes the services that you offer. The key, and this is where the marketing concept is relevant, is that what you put on the Web site and how you use the Internet with your customers will change your Product and Place, and this needs to be reflected in Promotion. Advertising, one aspect of Promotion, has steadily moved onto the Internet. In 1996 Internet advertising revenue totaled $267 million. This grew to $6 billion by 2002 and $12.54 billion by 2005.[13] Newspaper readership, especially among the young, has been declining. Not only were newspapers hit by the increase in Internet advertising expenditures, but it also took a slice from other advertising media including television.[14] The implication is that you should consider replacing or augmenting traditional newspaper display ads, TV, and paper newsletters with Internet promotion. Since you can put a lot more information and higher quality information[15] less expensively on a Web site, other advertising media, such as newspapers and TV can be used to direct customers to the Web site. Production costs for high quality content, such as video (see Television above), will remain about the same, but the distribution costs in an absolute sense[16] will be greatly reduced, while exposure time increases from a few seconds or minutes to become effectively limited only by the needs of the audience. You also increase the range of access points from time watching TV or reading a newspaper to wherever the customer has Internet access, such as home, office, while traveling, and with an iPhone, anywhere there is WiFi access or AT&T wireless reception. The Internet provides a way to describe your services and yourself to prospective customers (patients, patients' families, access decision-makers) in ways that previously were either not possible or prohibitively expensive. You can take advantage of this by using video and audio to illustrate your clinical services, your patient interaction and any strengths identified in your SWOT analysis that are customer related.

## Place

Place, as you recall, captures all aspects of when and where you offer your services. The Internet gives you a presence whenever the customer wants it. In fact, it is generally the customer's need that generates the action to access your Web site or to contact you by e-mail. One of the great challenges of advertising is getting the *right* message before potential customers at the *right* time. You may have noticed that automobile ads on TV are generally annoying to you—until, you are looking for a car. Then, they take on additional salience. By definition, someone looking at your Web site is doing so for a reason. In effect, the Internet allows you to provide your message when the customer wants to see it. It also allows you to put several message strings on your website, each customized to a different potential customer.

A Place aspect to consider is using the Internet as a portal to communicate with your patients. Potentially, this can provide greater patient access to physicians and medical staff. The fear that many physicians have is that it will be overutilized by patients. The verdict is still out on this question, however, initial research indicates that this may not be the case. Lin et al.[17] reported a practice-based randomized trial comparing patients using an Internet portal with a control group.

Physicians experienced an average of 1 clinical message per day for each 250 portal group patients enrolled in the trial. Portal patients focused on providing psychosocial information, which they were less likely to send by telephone. Li's data indicated that the portal patients replaced phone calls with e-mail, and were more satisfied with the overall practice experience. Other studies have reported similar findings,[18] although some have indicated increased patient utilization.[19] E-mail correspondence is still an "early adopter" service. The American Medical Association (AMA) and American Medical Informatics Association (AMIA) have published e-mail guidelines for physicians.[20] Brooks[21] found that in a sample of 4,203 physicians 689 had communicated with patients using e-mails, but only 46 complied with at least half of 13 selected AMA/AMIA

guidelines (see **Exhibit 7–9**). Using e-mail to correspond with patients certainly changes Place characteristics. Given the current uncertainties, it may be best to conduct some limited experiments to determine its usefulness and intrusiveness in your own setting.

## Product

Effective use of the Internet results in you actually changing the product that you provide. First, it can build a more enduring relationship with your patients by providing a contact point for accessing patient support and educational programs. These programs and information, of course, do not exist because of your Internet portal, but they become feasible for you to easily inform patients about them and deliver the information to them as a consequence of the portal.

**Exhibit 7–9**  Self-Reported Adherence to AMA/AMIA Recommended E-mail Guidelines

| Policies | Physicians (n = 689) | % |
|---|---|---|
| Print e-mail communication and place in patients' charts | 331.00 | 48.00 |
| Inform patients about privacy issues with respect to e-mail | 250.00 | 36.30 |
| When e-mail messages become too lengthy, notify patients to come in to discuss or call them | 148.00 | 21.50 |
| Establish a turnaround time for messages | 111.00 | 16.10 |
| Request patients to put their names or identification numbers in the body of the message | 111.00 | 16.10 |
| Send a new message to inform patient of completion of request | 111.00 | 16.10 |
| Establish types of transactions | 110.00 | 16.00 |
| Explain to patients that their message should be concise | 70.00 | 10.20 |
| Remind patients when they do not adhere to guidelines | 55.00 | 8.00 |
| Develop archival and retrieval mechanisms | 57.00 | 8.30 |
| Instruct patients to put category of transaction in subject line of message | 48.00 | 7.00 |
| Configure automatic reply to acknowledge receipt of patient's messages | 42.00 | 6.10 |
| Request patients to use auto-reply features to acknowledge clinician's message | | |

*Source:* Brooks RG, Menachemi N. Physicians' Use of Email With Patients: Factors Influencing Electronic Communication and Adherence to Best Practices. *J Med Internet Res*, 2006;8(1):e2. http://www.jmir.org/2006/1/e2/

Examples would be educational seminars and videos relating to common problems that your patients or patients' families encounter. This is information that in the past you either did not have the time or resources to deliver, or you had to deliver them when it worked for you, as opposed to when your patients wanted to access the information.

You also change the nature of your product by providing links to other Internet resources. Here, your medical expertise is critical. You want to find high quality Web sites that add value for your patients. For example, posting links to some WebMD pages that you determine provide accurate disease information (bursitis, influenza, asthma), or links to private and public national centers of excellence, such as Cleveland Clinic, National Institute of Mental Health, American Lung Association, and so forth can really change the level of patient knowledge, and affect the quality of dialog that you have with your patients. Patients will seek this information anyway. By serving as a source you help to shape the information that they receive, and become a partner in providing it. In one study 91 percent of cancer patients reported that information that they found online helped them to communicate with their physicians.[22] By embracing the Internet as a source of information you build trust with your patients, which can be valuable when you find that they have acquired false or misleading information or have misunderstood some points. Erdem[23] has suggested proactively using the Internet by having patients "advance alert" their physicians by e-mail to information that they wish to discuss in their next visit. This could also include forwarding Web site sources to the physician. Taking this approach tells patients they are an active partner in their care, but the time implications for busy physicians might be significant.

Hartmann et al.[24] provides another example of how the Internet changes the nature of the medical product. They studied outcomes associated with an asthma Web site. Patients reported higher self-confidence, talking more during their physician visit, and having more confidence in the quality of care they were receiving. Patients also reported being more actively involved in their asthma care due to having a better understanding of their treatment options and of their role in managing their condition. Finally, patients saw that they could play a role in overcoming "physician inertia" by precipitating communication.

Finally, Koiso-Kanttila[25] identified the benefits that consumers associate with the Internet. They include speed, efficiency, control, privacy, convenience, and ease of use. All of these are attributes that can contribute to improving the physician-patient relationship, and as a consequence they truly affect the nature of the product that you offer.

### Designing the Web site

The Web site is the primary portal that patients and others use to obtain Internet access to a practice or healthcare system. Web site building is a skill that goes beyond the scope of this book. As a physician leader you will need some structure to approach the task of developing an effective Web site, and that is what this book will focus on.

Professionals should build Web sites. This said, I have met some physicians who enjoy Web site building and maintenance, and are very good at it. Web site development packages such as Dreamweaver, Go Live!, and FrontPage[26] have quick learning curves, effective tutorials, and make it relatively easy to develop a reliable and professional looking product with contingent access to pages and embedded graphics and video. I do not encourage this, however, because physicians generate revenue by practicing medicine, not as Web site designers. For the physician, however, who says, "This is fun—I really want to do it myself!," you can always contract it out later if it does not develop as you expect. It is critical, however, for physicians to be *involved* in the design of the Web site, so it will work as you need and as your users expect. Physicians have information about their patients and the nature of medical information that Web site users will access, which must be communicated to the Web site designer.

The first consideration in developing an effective Web site is to identify a Web site designer who is communicative and willing to listen to your ideas, and who develops a construction plan that provides frequent contact with you. One of the major issues that you will need to consider early on is identifying the market segments for the Web site, since these will constitute major Web site partitions (see Exhibit 7–7 for some examples) and affect Web site content, such as video and print material on the site. Second, it is highly desirable to involve a focus group[27] of patients at some point or various points in the design process. Early on, an open-ended discussion with patients about how they would use the site, what content they would find useful, media preferences (video, audio), and current access (broadband, dial-up[28]) will be helpful to brainstorm eventual content and Web site direction. Validating near-final Web site design with patient groups is also very desirable. Keep in mind that the nature of the Internet is change, so minor problems or desirable refinements identified near the end of a project can always be addressed in later Web site revisions.

The Web site designer will bring the design expertise to build a site that incorporates the standard "do's" and "don'ts" of Web design, such as preferring black text on white background whenever possible, making sure that text is in a printable (not white) color, avoiding horizontal scrolling. How do you know if a designer has these basic skills? Review Chapter 4 (Employment Methods) focusing on the discussion of work samples. Look at some of the sites that a designer has developed, and consider:

- Are the pages readable and appealing?
- Can you navigate easily or do you get lost?
- Is there consistency from one page to another (controls in the same place, consistent color coding, etc.)
- Is it quick? Slow sites frustrate users.
- Does it work equally well on several popular browsers. Try it with Safari, Firefox, Camino, Internet Explorer, and other Internet browsers.
- How well does the site convey the character of the sponsoring organization?
- Can you find the site if you put some key words into a search engine, such as Google or Yahoo?

Finally, review the discussion on References in Chapter 4. Then, talk to the Web site owner and ask her or him *why* they are satisfied or dissatisfied with the Web site and the designer, and get some war stories of what it was like working with the designer. For example, you might ask, "What went particularly well when working with . . . ." and "What were the difficulties that you had working with . . . .", or "Describe how . . . . reacted when you offered suggestions for changes, such as to page format."

One area where you can have a major impact on the quality of your Web site is to work with the designer to insure that the Web site's information architecture will work effectively with your intended users. The *information architecture* is how the information in the Web site is structured to provide intuitive access to content and to facilitate completion of tasks by users, such as completing a questionnaire, viewing a video, progressing through Web site pages, or forwarding a message to you from within the Web site. Intuitively you can appreciate that very useful and high quality information immersed in a Web site that makes it difficult to find or use the information would be a fail-

ure. The architecture level of design, as opposed to the nuts and bolts level of Web site design noted previously, is a level at which you can make a useful contribution. Danaher et al.[29] notes three primary Web site architecture designs. In the matrix design (**Figure 7–3**) users are free to pursue their own intuitive paths through the Web site's pages. The matrix provides users with the maximum amount of information and the maximum flexibility to access that information. The downside is that too many route options can

Home Page

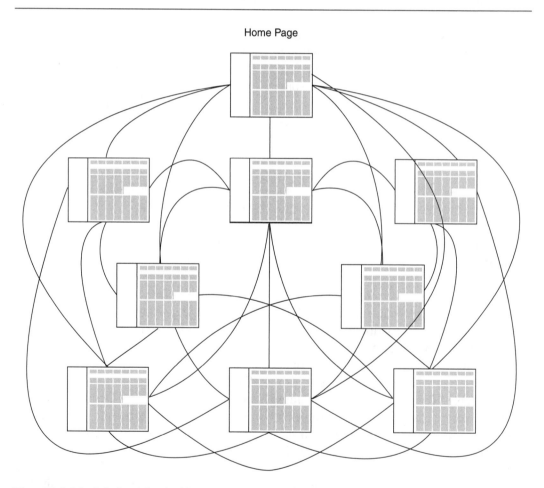

**Figure 7–3** Matrix Information Architecture.
*Source:* Danaher, B., H. McKay, & J. Seeley. "The information architecture of behavior change websites. *Journal of Medical Internet Research.* 2005;7(2):e12. http://www.jmir.org/2005/2/e12/ (Accessed July 3, 2007).

result in users literally becoming lost, and make it difficult to find the right information or then to refind it later.

In a hierarchical design (**Figure 7–4**) information is organized in a top-down manner. This avoids the confusion inherent with too many links. Computer users are generally familiar with hierarchies of folders, subfolders, and documents, so this can be an effective way to organize information into natural clusters, such as by disease, drug, treatment regimen, etc. Hierarchies become less effective if information is nested into too many levels, or if the hierarchy is not obvious or consistent with the user's mental model of the content.

A tunnel design (**Figure 7–5**) is even more structured. There is only one path through the data. Educational programs, textbooks, and movies are designed this way. You cannot get to screen 3 until you have gone through and perhaps even demonstrated mastery in screen 2. Buying an item on the

Internet is this way. The seller presents a sequence of screens (select the item, choose the color, go to checkout, choose shipping, and pay). If you truly know the best way for the user to deal with the Web site's information, then a tunnel design may be appropriate. Keep in mind, however, that a fundamental characteristic of the Internet and Web sites is *flexibility*. Users expect it, and when shoehorned into a straightjacket, they may rebel. Unless the user can see the wisdom of staying in the tunnel, you may have a valuable Web site that few will use.

A hybrid design (**Figure 7–6**) is composed of multiple architectures, so that matrix, hierarchical, and tunnel designs are matched to the information shown and the purpose to be achieved. For example, Figure 7–6 shows a tunnel that you can only access after going through a hierarchy. Notice that the user can optionally explore several Web pages from the second screen in the tunnel to acquire additional information without exiting the tunnel.

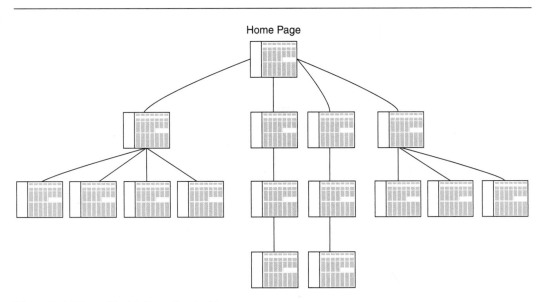

**Figure 7–4** Hierarchical Information Architecture.
*Source:* Danaher, B., H. McKay, & J. Seeley. "The information architecture of behavior change websites. *Journal of Medical Internet Research.* 2005;7(2):e12. http://www.jmir.org/2005/2/e12/ (Accessed July 3, 2007).

Home Page

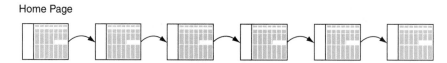

**Figure 7–5** Tunnel Information Architecture.
*Source:* Danaher, B., H. McKay, & J. Seeley. "The information architecture of behavior change websites. *Journal of Medical Internet Research.* 2005;7(2):e12. http://www.jmir.org/2005/2/e12/ (Accessed July 3, 2007).

The user works in a matrix if he or she only chooses to go down one level below the home page. Similarly, it would be possible to append a matrix off of any page in the tunnel, *if that would further the Web site's purpose at that point.*

All of this may be interesting from a design perspective, but what does it have to do with you the physician leader? You are the person with the information about how your patients and other users will most effectively access and use the parts of your Web site. The Web designer can make all of these designs work, but *you* are the one who has to tell the designer, "You know the best way for

my patients to learn how to deal with the symptoms of exercise induced asthma is to present it in this order . . . ." (tunnel design), or alternatively you may say, "Lets break it into symptoms and medications (hierarchy design) and then within each of these let's let them explore all the relevant information as they wish (matrix design), so we will provide an initial structure enhanced by choice (overall a hybrid design)."

## OTHER CONSIDERATIONS

The Web site designer will work with you on the issues of Web site size and bandwidth,

Home Page

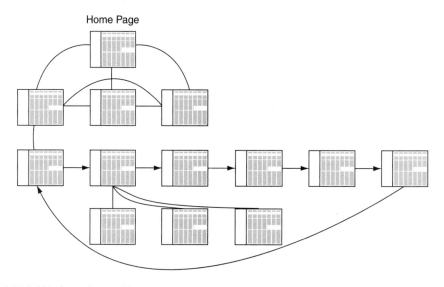

**Figure 7–6** Hybrid Information Architecture.
*Source:* Danaher, B., H. McKay, & J. Seeley. "The information architecture of behavior change websites. *Journal of Medical Internet Research.* 2005;7(2):e12. http://www.jmir.org/2005/2/e12/ (Accessed July 3, 2007).

finding a Web host and selecting a domain name. Web site size is the megabytes (MB) of data that you will need to upload to the Web host that will provide Internet access to your site. Popular Web hosts include Yahoo and Goggle, however, there are many Web hosts with less name recognition, good reliability and lower cost, so examine available options. Bandwidth is the amount of information that users will draw down through the Internet when they use your site.[30] The bandwidth that you will need will be a function of both the number of hits on your Web site and the degree to which they access data intensive information. If your Web site uses a lot of rich media, such as video and high fidelity graphics, then users will access more data which may require more bandwidth, which will increase cost.

Purchasing, also called registering, a domain name gives you exclusive use of this name. A good domain name will give users a clear indication of who you are or what you do (james.smithmd.com or giandliverdocs.com). You can register a domain name with your Internet service provider (ISP), Web host, or a Web registration company.

There are a number of ways to insure that others will find your Web site. As previously noted, one way to do this is to use other media, such as print, TV, radio, newsletters, and so forth to point to your Web site. Using traditional media is often the *best* way for healthcare providers to advertise their Web site and get potential customers to visit.

Often organizations with Web sites obsess with being findable through searches, such as on Yahoo!, Google, Ask, etc. This is less important for physicians and healthcare organizations than someone selling pants suspenders or books to the world. Think about it. Your users, for the most part, know you or know how to find you. Nevertheless, there may be some who are searching for an OBGYN in the Otay Ranch area of San Diego. Similarly, some physicians or healthcare providers may have a national reputation, and wish to use the Internet for national marketing. In these situations being findable through search engines is important. One way to do this is to register your Web site with all of the major search engines. For example, you can go to http://www.google.com/addurl/[31] to add your URL,[32] as well as comments and keywords to describe your Web site. Less important but still helpful are meta tags. Meta tags are text that is hidden from your Web site visitors that describes your Web site. They can in some instances *influence* how a Web crawler will describe your site. Web crawlers, sometimes called bots, are used by search engines to find and describe new Web sites. When a crawler finds an unlisted Web site it explores the Web site and categorizes the content. Meta tags may be helpful, since the Web crawler may use some of this language, if it also determines that the same words, phrases, and content are being used in the Web site proper. It is unlikely that you will get a high listing if you use meta tag keywords that are not also found in the body of your Web site. Once again a close working relationship with the Web site designer will insure that the words and phrases that are important for effective Web crawler description will be in your Web site, without the site reading in unfriendly or strange ways to users.

Another way to be found is to pay for an ad. The right side of any Google search results page is headed by "Sponsored Links." Often, "old media," such as the Yellow Pages, will pay for these, but sometimes individual providers sponsor them. For example, a Google search in July 2007 conducted on "CABG Surgery" produced 2,080,000 hits, however, there were only 9 sponsored links, with 7 appearing on the first page and 2 on the second page of which 3 were actual CABG surgery providers.[33] Generally, these sponsored links are paid for on a "click-through" basis. Advertisers bid in an auction for ad placement and also submit a budget. For example, if you bid $0.75 for each click-through with a budget of $750 for the month, then your ad will appear higher in the sponsored link listing than someone who has bid $0.74 and lower than someone who has bid $0.76. Given your budget, you could be shown up to 1,000 times during this time period. Once you exceed your budget, your ad will stop appearing. Successful click-through advertising balances bidding enough to appear high enough so you will appear in the first page or two, but low enough so you will get a large number of exposures.

## THE INTERNET—YOUR ROLE

Leadership, as you will recall from the discussion in Chapter 6 involves vision, inspiration, and appropriately working with others to put change in place. The physician leader's role regarding the Internet and marketing encompasses all 3 of the characteristics. The physician leader needs the vision to see beyond old ways of marketing to utilize the Internet's ability to change the very nature of the medical product, as well as place and promotional considerations. This will require inspiring others in your organization to try new things. Finally, utilizing the Internet will be most effective if you can appropriately involve yourself with the Web site designer, as well as involving other critical stakeholders, such as patients, nurses, physicians, and administrators.

## CONCLUSIONS

Success may provide the luxury of not having to overtly market. If you are in a specialty that is in high demand, or if there are relatively few competitors in your area, then you may be able to limit your marketing activities to announcing your presence, affiliating with a hospital or health system, and associating on occasion with colleagues. If you are the only hospital in town, you may be able to get away with little more than putting your name on the front of your building. Apart from these circumstances, however, marketing is a key success factor. The question then becomes whether you will do it well or poorly.

Physicians, practices, and healthcare organizations that must market their services to prosper or even survive should undertake the complete process, including performing a thorough situational analysis and SWOT analysis, developing a marketing strategy, and writing a marketing plan. These then evolve into operational marketing decisions, such as seeking to serve selected market segments, pricing, location decisions, and the like. The content of this chapter is designed to generate some insightful thinking about how your practice, hospital or health system can make use of these marketing concepts. In addition, this chapter should be helpful in allowing you to work more effectively with marketing consultants whom you may hire for specific marketing research tasks, or to work with you to develop a marketing plan.

## NOTES

1. eICU is a registered trademark of VISICU Inc.
2. Scott, J., J. Warshaw, & J. Taylor. (1985). *Introduction to Marketing Management*. Homewood, IL: Irwin Publ., 11–12.
3. For an example in which low cost was an inherent part of a practice strategy, see Norman, J. (1990). Can a practice serving the poor avoid financial quicksand? *Medical Economics* (5):79–87.
4. Hall, W. K. (1980). Survival strategies in a hostile environment. *Harvard Business Review* 58(5): 75–85.
5. Hofer, C. W. (1980). Turnaround strategies. *Journal of Business Strategy* 1:19–31.
6. Remember also that the readership of general circulation newspapers is declining and getting older.
7. Personal communication.
8. Personal communication.
9. Ogilvy, D. (1985). *Ogilvy on Advertising*. New York: Vintage Books. Ogilvy devised the slogan for Rolls Royce: "At 60 miles an hour, the loudest noise in the new Rolls-Royce comes from the electric clock." He also developed campaigns for Volkswagen, Dove soap, Hathaway shirts, and Marlboro cigarettes.
10. Generally, cable stations will charge you a fee to host your own program. In effect, they consider it an infomercial. Commercial stations may be more inclined to pay a salary or let you host the show at no charge. They contribute the production costs you contribute time, and they fill a time slot.
11. Ernhardt, J. (1989). Marketing? My patients do it for me. *Medical Economics* 2:58–64.
12. Kotler, P., R. Clarke. (1987). *Marketing for Health Care Organizations*. Englewood Cliffs, NJ: Prentice Hall, p. 244.
13. PriceWaterhouseCoopers. April 2006. *IAB Internet Advertising Revenue Report*. Available at: http://www.iab.net/resources/adrevenue/pdf/IAB_PwC_2005.pdf
14. Bradley, S., N. Bartlett. (2007). How media choices are changing online advertising. *Harvard Business School. # 9-707-458*: pg. 7.
15. Using Internet terminology this is called rich media. This includes video, audio, and large graphics.
16. In a relative sense, the cost "per viewer" may be higher since fewer people will view your Web site than an ad on the 6:00 PM local news. However, most of the local newscast viewers may not be potential customers, while most Web site visitors will be there because they sought out the Web site, so the cost per potential customer for the Web site may be *very* favorable.
17. Lin C.T., L. Wittevrongell, L. Moore, B. L. Beaty & S. E. Ross. (2005). An Internet-based patient-provider communication system: randomized controlled trial. *Journal of Internet Medical Research*, (4):47.
18. Liederman, E. M., & C. S. Morefield. (2003). Web messaging: a new tool for patient-physician communication. *J Am Med Inform Assoc*, 10(3): 260–270. Liederman, E. M., J. C. Lee, V. H. Baquero, & P. G. Seites. (2005). Patient-physician Web messaging. The impact on message volume and satisfaction. *Journal of General Internal Medicine.* 20(1):52–57. Hassol A, Walker J.M., Kidder, D., Rokita, K., Young, D., Pierdon, S., et al. (2004). Patient experiences and attitudes about access to a patient electronic health care record and linked Web messaging. *Journal of the American Medical Information Association* 11(6): 505–513.
19. Katz, S. J., N. Nissan, & C. A. Moyer. (2004). Crossing the digital divide: evaluating online communication between patients and their providers. *American Journal of Managed Care* 10(9), 593–598.
20. Kane B., & D. Sands. (1998). Guidelines for the clinical use of electronic mail with patients. The AMIA Internet working group, task force on guidelines for the use of clinic-patient electronic mail. *Journal of the American Medical Informatics Association* 5(1):104–111. See also: www.ama-assn.org/ama/pub/category/2386.html Accessed July 12, 2007.
21. Brooks, R., & N. Menachemi. (2006). Physicians' use of email with patients: factors influencing electronic communication and adherence to best practices. *Journal of Medical Internet Research* 8(1).
22. Eysenbach, G. (2003). The impact of the Internet on cancer outcomes. *Cancer Journal for Clinicians* 53(6):359–371.
23. Erdem, S., & L. Harrison-Walker. (2006). The role of the Internet in physician-patient relationships: the issue of trust. *Business Horizons* 49:387–393.
24. Hartmann, C., C. Sciamanna, D. Blanch, S. Mui, H. Lawless, M. Manocchia, et al. (2007). A Web site to improve asthma care by suggesting patient questions for physicians: Qualitative analysis of user experiences. *Journal of Medical Internet Research.* 9(1).

25. Koiso-Kanttila, N. (2005). Time, attention, authenticity and consumer benefits of the Web. *Business Horizons* 48:63–70.

26. Dreamweaver and Go Live! are published by Adobe and FrontPage by Microsoft.

27. A focus group is a group that is representative of the segment or segments in your practice that will use the Internet. They are not a random sample, but a consciously chosen sample that should be capable of providing you with useful information related to practice Web site users. Focus groups are usually composed of 5 to 10 persons who meet for 1 to 2 hours in a process guided by a moderator, but open ended enough so that participants can easily express they opinions.

28. As of March 2007, 45 percent of U.S. households had broadband access. Available at http://ncta.com/IssueBrief.aspx?contentId=3024&view=4 Accessed July 3, 2007.

29. Danaher B. G., H. G. McKay, & J. R. Seeley. (2005). The information architecture of behavior change Web sites. *Journal of Medical Internet Research* 7(2):e12. Available at http://www.jmir.org/2005/2/e12/ Accessed July 2, 2007.

30. In some instances the Web host either with or without prior notice has closed Web sites that exceed their specified bandwidth.

31. Accessed July 7, 2007. For any update to this address search on Google for "register with Google."

32. Uniform Resource Locator. The first part of the URL specifies the protocol that should be used to access the file, and the second part is the file name. Therefore, a Web address of http://robertsmithmd.com/html.index will use the http communications protocol to access the index or first Web page of the Web site, which is written in html or hypertext markup language.

33. New York-Presbyterian Hospital, Cedars-Sinai Heart Program, Rush University Medical Center. The remainder were a mixture of gastric bypass providers and medical equipment manufacturers.

## CHAPTER 8

# Negotiation

## Chapter Objectives

This chapter identifies methods to negotiate more effectively with peers, subordinates, superiors, and those outside your organization. It will give you ways to consider your own self-interest, as well as those of your adversary. Understanding these interests is central to effective negotiation. It also will provide tactics to guide you in responding to an adversary's negotiation offer.

Negotiation is the art of settling disputes between two or more parties. Physician leaders are negotiating continually with those both inside and outside their own organizations. Inside of medical practices, physicians negotiate with partners, affiliated physicians, nurses and medical assistants/extenders, and with senior-level practice managers such as business managers. Common external negotiation adversaries include insurance and managed care organizations, hospitals, landlords, suppliers, physician job applicants, and other practices. Physician leaders working in hospitals often negotiate with employees, affiliated and employed physicians, other corporate executives, and a host of external agents, such as physician groups, suppliers, consultants and insurance companies. Finally, physicians continually find themselves negotiating with patients over compliance with treatment plans, referrals, and so forth. The methods discussed in the chapter for negotiating in business situations can also be used when negotiating with patients.[1]

Arguably, what encompasses the skill of management must eventually be expressed or made operational through some form of negotiation. For example, introducing activity-based costing of medical services, information technology, use of clinical outcome measures, implementation of best practices, and critical pathways are all dependent on obtaining the cooperation of those who will have to execute these changes. Obtaining this compliance is generally a negotiated process and usually cannot be successfully unilaterally imposed.

Negotiation, as it is applied in medical organizations, is an art, not a science.[2] Many of the concepts that have become central to the art of negotiation appear at first to be self-evident. In hindsight, they are. The problem for the unskilled negotiator is utilizing the appropriate piece of "common sense" at the right time. Having a strategy, therefore, to approach the negotiation process can be helpful to ensure that you consider and incorporate your knowledge in a systematic manner.

## THE ART OF NEGOTIATION: KEY CONCEPTS

### Know Yourself

Understanding your own interests and goals is fundamental to any successful negotiation. You cannot protect your self-interest or achieve your objective if you don't have a clear idea of what you are trying to achieve from the negotiation. Understanding what you are trying to achieve requires, at a minimum, some honest introspection. Often, however, it requires collecting information or data, anticipating the business implications of various outcomes, and considering the personal and interpersonal implications of various negotiation outcomes. Generally, negotiation with another person, group, or organization is not a one-time event. Anticipating the relationship that you would like to have after the negotiation, and the atmosphere that it will create for future interactions, is a critical part of understanding what you wish to obtain from the negotiation process.

Many of the chapters in this book will give you the basis to determine what you are trying to achieve from the negotiation. For example, your performance-appraisal skills will help you set employee goals. Your financial management skills will help you identify contracting, compensation, and vendor agreement goals. Knowledge of organization change will help you identify sources of potential resistance and develop strategies to overcome this resistance. In each instance, the knowledge provides the context for negotiations with those whose cooperation will be essential for implementing change.

One of the most important considerations to identify before beginning to negotiate is your *reservation price*. This is the point beyond which you are willing to walk away from the negotiation. Sometimes, an estimate of your reservation price can be obtained directly by surveying the market. For example,

if you are negotiating to lease office space, knowing that other suitable office space is leasing for $15.00 per square foot may help you determine that under no circumstance will you go beyond $17.50. Sometimes the reservation price can be determined by examining your internal data. For example, given your space needs, perhaps you determine that you can't afford to pay more than $16.00 per square foot. Similarly, you may look at a new fee schedule from an insurer and conclude that their new fee for a standard office visit is 15 percent below any other insurers, which you conclude is beyond your reservation price. You may look at last year's revenue from a particular insurer who is converting to a capitated network. After considering the percentage of your patient base that will be involved, you conclude that you would rather not get the contract at a price, for example, of less than $0.70 per member per month. Sometimes, reservation price can be a qualitative statement. For example, a PPO medical director notes that Dr. Johnson's specialist utilization rate and cost data are outliers. She determines that her reservation price for retaining Dr. Johnson in the network is that he must be willing to participate in additional utilization training.

Another concept that is critical to understanding yourself is determining your *best alternative to a negotiated agreement* (BATNA) before you begin to negotiate.[3] Your BATNA is what you will do if the negotiation fails. Knowing your BATNA before you begin to negotiate with an adversary is important, because it places the negotiation in a larger perspective. Sometimes, negotiators may concede too much, because they aren't aware of other relatively desirable alternatives. On other occasions, negotiators fail to reach agreement, not understanding that their next best alternative is far less desirable than being somewhat more flexible in the current negotiation.

For example, your first choice for an office lease is in the Sachem Medical Arts building, which is adjacent to your primary admitting hospital. The offer is for $16.00 per square foot for a 3-year corporate lease. Your BATNA is only $14.75 per square foot, but it is located 8 miles farther away from the hospital, and the landlord is asking for a 5-year, personally guaranteed lease. This BATNA provides a context for the ensuing negotiations. Knowing your BATNA might allow you to make some concessions on price to obtain the more desirable location and lease terms, which overall would be preferable.

Returning to Dr. Johnson, perhaps the medical director's BATNA, if she can't reach an agreement with him that ensures that he will get his consulting referrals and costs under control, is to terminate his network participation. Perhaps you have plenty of other primary care physicians to cover his patients. Knowing your BATNA in this case will allow you to negotiate with Dr. Johnson with no second thoughts about compromising your goals.

## Know Your Adversary

*Adversary* is a charged word, but some term is needed to describe the person or organization with whom you are negotiating. You and your adversaries often share common interests or goals. For example, in a given negotiation your partner, spouse, or child may be your adversary, but this certainly doesn't mean they are your enemy. In fact, it is the common goals that negotiators have that often are the basis for reaching an agreement. Knowing your adversary's objectives is important to negotiating an agreement, because it will help you determine where to begin the negotiating process. Think about the considerations that might be important to your adversary. Put yourself in his or her shoes. What would you want if your places were reversed? What issues would be most important to you? Which ones might be of lesser importance? Think about the probable limits of how far your adversary may be willing to go to reach an agreement.

Begin the process of knowing your adversary by estimating his or her reservation price. What is the point beyond which he or she is likely to walk away from the negotiation? After all, you have a limit beyond which you won't go. Your adversary, similarly, has limits. How far would be too far for him or her to go on each identifiable issue? When thinking about this, consider what issues may influence the adversary's reservation price. Revisiting the lease example, your realtor estimates that the owner's financing costs for the Sachem Medical Arts building are $10.00 per square foot and that insurance, taxes, and other overhead costs for the property are about $1.00 per foot. Next, you assume that the owner will probably want to make a 10 percent margin over expenses, which adds another $1.10 per square foot. After preliminary plans are assembled, you determine that reconstruction and build-out costs for the suite will be about $1.30 per foot, which the owner will front and build into the cost. An estimate of the owner's reservation price, therefore, would be about $13.40 per foot ($10.00 + $1.00 + $1.10 + $1.30).

Similarly, you may estimate Dr. Johnson's reservation price as public censure within the PPO network if he has to consult with a mentor to review referral standards. Based on your past dealings with Dr. Johnson, you feel that he is a proud person and has a strong need for control. You guess that holding him up to scrutiny by other network physicians, even if it is for the purpose of training, would go beyond his "price."

Next, estimate your adversary's BATNA. If a negotiated agreement can't be reached, what is the adversary's probable next best choice? Evaluating the adversary's BATNA will provide information about how likely he or she is to be flexible. For example, perhaps the office leasing market is soft. If the owner does not reach an agreement with you, the BATNA may be vacant space and a loss of $11.00 per square foot per month of fixed costs for an indeterminate time. Obviously, this could have a profound effect on the owner's reservation price, your estimate of the reservation price, and both your subsequent actions.

**Be Prepared to Dance**

The term *negotiation dance* has been used by many to describe the give and take, maneuvering, and strategizing that take place between negotiating parties. The objective of negotiation is *not* to reach an agreement. Instead, negotiation is a creative discovery process. The goal is to determine whether a desirable agreement is achievable. A failed negotiation, therefore, is one in which an agreement is possible that would benefit you, and which is also acceptable to your adversary, but neither party discovered the terms or nature of this agreement so none was reached. Similarly, one form of successful negotiation is when you correctly determine that there is no mutually acceptable agreement.

Now, let's change the circumstances a bit in the lease example. Assume that the office suite that you are trying to lease is currently occupied by Ms. Jones, the owner, who is planning to use your rental income to purchase an additional office suite, where she will move her business. You estimate her BATNA to be forgoing the purchase of the other office until she can find a suitable tenant for her current space. You perceive her to be a conservative businesswoman, not one to take undue risks, and therefore unlikely to impulse buy the other suite, acquire it under unfavorable financial circumstances, or purchase the other suite while risking a loss of $11.00 per square foot for an undetermined time or renting her current suite for less than her target net income.

Conceptually, the negotiation dance takes place between the reservation prices of the adversaries, which is referred to as the zone of agreement. **Figure 8–1** illustrates the zone of agreement for the lease example in which the owner will not purchase a suite to

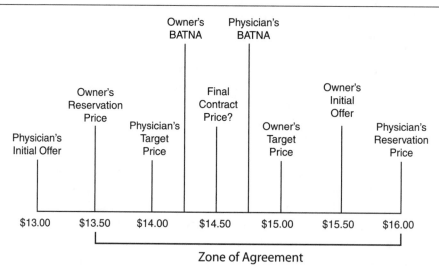

Figure 8–1  Reservation Prices, BATNAs, and Offers.

move her business unless she first obtains a renter. In this example, the zone of agreement ranges between $13.50 and $16.00 per square foot. Naturally, the owner wants to move the final contract price above $13.50, and the physician wants to move it below $16.00. This area then becomes the turf for the negotiation dance. Normally, of course, neither side knows for certain the other's reservation price, so the dance involves both identifying those boundaries and trying to conceal one's own boundary. You can see here that their BATNAs are $14.25 and $14.75, and if they are to reach an agreement it will be somewhere in this range.

## Interests Versus Positions

Conceptually, it is useful to separate a party's interests from positions. Positions are the items placed on the bargaining table. They are specific outcomes that you desire from the negotiation. "Rent of $15.50 per square foot," "$125 fee for an office visit," and "You agree not to practice within 25 miles of our location if for any reason you do not become a practice partner" are all examples of positions.

*Interests* reflect a side's needs, wants, fears, objectives, and so forth. They reflect the underlying objective that a *position* is designed to attain. You identify an interest by asking yourself, "Why am I proposing this position? What need does it satisfy for me?" In effect, interests motivate the formation of positions. On occasion, parties will have clashing positions, but their underlying interests may not conflict or be less in conflict than you would guess based on their respective positions. When this occurs, and one or both parties realize this, there is an opportunity to move the negotiation toward agreement. Similarly, it is possible that there is an agreement (positions) that will satisfy the

most important interests of both sides, even if each must be less than fully satisfied regarding secondary interests.

Always begin a negotiation by considering your interests and trying to get your adversary to do the same. Starting with positions gets you "dug in" to them. You become less open to alternative solutions. You confound the *underlying* need with *one way* to obtain it. A position gives a *single* solution of how your needs might be met, but it disregards the possibility of other solutions that might still meet your interests, but that may also do better at meeting the adversary's interests. Fundamentally, your position is *your* solution to the problem. Positional negotiating is inefficient, because it often leaves value on the table because you may not discover other options. You can look for new positions with confidence, if you have done your homework as noted previously by identifying your own self-interests, reservation price, and BATNA, as well as considering these issues for the adversary.

Keep in mind, also, that future relationships often are a hidden interest in a negotiation. Generally, negotiating with other organizations, partners, employees, patients, and the like, are not one-time events. One of the issues that you should anticipate is the relationship you will have after the negotiation. What will the atmosphere be like in future interactions coming out of this negotiation? It is very possible to win the immediate negotiation, because you can, but to create a very adversarial, hostile work environment for the future. Now, take a look at the Application Exercise in **Figure 8–2** to consider the personal relevance of these concepts. Think about some alternative positions that either of you could take that may come closer to being mutually acceptable

Returning to Dr. Johnson's situation with the medical director, **Figure 8–3** shows their

Think of an issue on which your position and another physician's position might differ.

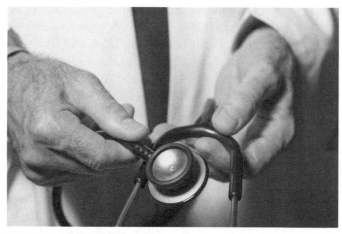

What are *your* interests, which are driving this position? What might be some of the *other* physician's interests, which might be driving his or her position?

**Figure 8–2** Application Exercise: Positions and Interests that Matter to You.

respective positions and interests. Although their respective positions are in conflict, the same degree of disharmony is not found in their respective underlying interests. Dr. Johnson wants to remain on the PPO panel, and the medical director wants to keep him. Dr. Johnson is concerned about appropriate medical care, and so is the medical director. It is apparent that the way each party is expressing its interests in terms of specific positions is really the major source of conflict. Perhaps Dr. Johnson views the PPO's referral guidelines as endangering him and his patients. As a result, additional training is irrelevant. His opposition to Dr. Antonio as a mentor could be founded in his interests of need for control and embarrassment avoidance. They may also be founded in some past experiences with Dr. Antonio.

The medical director, on the other hand, has operationalized her interests in terms of three particular positions: provide Dr. Johnson with additional education, mentor him over an extended time period to be certain that the training "sticks," and change or leave. As an effective negotiator, she should be willing to modify her positions, as long as she does not sacrifice her interests. Similarly, if Dr. Johnson's interests can be protected while satisfying the PPO administrator's interests, he may be willing to modify his positions. Thinking about the negotiation from the perspective of interests as opposed to positions may give each side the opportunity to modify its position without compromising what is dear or losing face. As a negotiator, then, one of your most fundamental tactics should be to recast the discussion away from positions and toward interests. You cannot, however, be naive about this. There will be times when interests are so divergent that it makes the chance of identifying mutually

# Interests

# Positions

## *Dr. Johnson*

**Retain a Sense of Personal Control**

**Continue with the group**

**Provide Appropriate Medical Treatment**

**Malpractice "Defensibility"**

**Avoid "Public" (peer) Criticism**

**Referrals were medically appropriate.**

**Bad luck with comorbid conditions.**

**Additional supervision is not necessary.**

**Additional training is irrelevant.**

**Risk adjustment data are not accurate/complete/descriptive.**

## *Medical Director*

**Reduce Unneeded Referrals & Associated Costs**

**Retain Johnson if Possible**

**Maintain "Control" over Outcomes**

**Provide Appropriate Medical Treatment**

**Retrain Dr. Johnson on referral standards**

**Have Dr. Antonio mentor Dr. Johnson**

**Change or Leave**

**Figure 8–3** Interests and Positions of Two Adversaries.

---

acceptable positions unlikely. If that is the case, using interests as a lens to focus your thinking about the negotiation should allow you to determine this sooner as opposed to later. Ending a negotiation that has little or no possibility of being successfully concluded also is of value.

## INTEGRATIVE AND DISTRIBUTIVE NEGOTIATING

In its simplest form, negotiating is the process of distributing a fixed resource between two competing adversaries. For one side to win something, the other side must

lose something. This circumstance is frequently referred to as a *zero-sum-game* because for me to gain $50, you must lose $50, and the sum of the two is $0. This *distributive* or *competitive approach* to negotiation assumes that the size of the pie is fixed and that each side can only gain at the expense of the other side. The goals, therefore, of the competing parties are in direct conflict. A distributive negotiating situation can arise when:

- There truly is a single issue to be negotiated.
- Resources *are* limited, each side truly *does* need more, and each side can only get it at the expense of the other.

- One or both sides envision negotiation as a confrontational, "macho" exercise (to many, the essence of negotiation is "I win, you lose").
- One or both sides won't take the time or are unwilling to expend the effort to see whether there is an alternative to this approach.

Recognize that sometimes the world really is this way, and two adversaries truly are in a zero-sum contest. When you are in this situation, it is important to behave accordingly. However, many of the situations in which you will be negotiating as a physician don't exclusively fit this model. For example, think of your negotiations with a partner, colleague, patient, or hospital administrator. As noted, you must live with these adversaries after the negotiation is completed, and approaching it distributively may not be in your best long-term or overall interest. Imagine, for example, that you extract an exploitive partnership agreement out of a young associate, because you can given his life circumstance and your relative power in the situation. What will be the consequences long term? Most likely, the atmosphere in the practice will be characterized by retribution, confrontation, and conflict. Is that really in your self-interest? Is that really in your economic, lifestyle, or satisfaction self-interest? When there are several issues on the table, some are more important to you than others, and the ordering of the interests of the parties varies (you and your adversary may both have the same priority for issues 1 and 2, but your 3rd issue is the adversary's 5th, his 3rd is your 4th, etc.), then you are in an *integrative* negotiation situation.

It's important to understand how to negotiate under both distributive and integrative conditions.

## Negotiation Under Distributive Conditions

An important goal in distributive negotiating is to get a good estimate of the adversary's reservation price and BATNA, and then perhaps to influence them. Data to help you evaluate this include:

- Indications of time pressure that the adversary is under
- Cost to the adversary if the negotiation fails
- Adversary's perception of how much you need to reach an agreement or value a particular negotiating point

Naturally, adversaries are hesitant to reveal critical information, so often the data available will be problematic. An action you can take to affect your adversary's perceptions is selectively presenting information. For example, you could mention that your current lease rate is $12.00 per square foot without disclosing that the current renewal offer is $15.00 per foot. Consciously choosing emotions, verbal language, and body language also can create an impression. Although it may be appropriate to provide less-than-full information and to consider carefully how you present information, it is not appropriate to lie. Beyond the ethical considerations, reputations travel. In addition, substantial lies can invalidate a legal agreement.

As the negotiation proceeds, generally each side will make concessions. Concessions recognize the legitimacy of the other side's interests as represented in its positions, as well as value gained through concessions that the adversary has made on other issues. Generally, concessions that successively decline in size indicate that the side is nearing its target or reservation price. Effective negotiators will gauge the size of concessions relative to the initial offer. High initial offers create more negotiating room and hence are generally associated with larger concessions.

Sometimes, "hardball tactics" occur during distributive negotiations. These tactics attempt to force the adversary to do something that he or she doesn't want to do. They change the focus of the negotiation away from content and interests toward context and pressure. Many people find these tactics to be offensive and perhaps unethical. At a minimum, they are dangerous to use, because they can hurt your reputation, cause the adversary to break off negotiations, or create an incentive to get even. The following are some examples of hardball tactics:

- *Good Cop/Bad Cop*—Two or more negotiators work in collaboration. One takes a threatening, belligerent, and perhaps extreme bargaining position. He or she temporarily leaves the negotiation (e.g., for a previously arranged meeting). The good "cop" takes over, expresses sympathy for the opponent having to deal with the bad cop, and then proposes that they try to reach an agreement before the bad cop returns. This tactic often is transparent and can easily alienate the opponent.
- *Lowball/Highball*—This involves making a very low (or high, whichever would be more favorable to the adversary) initial offer that will not be honored. If the opponent accepts the offer, he or she is told that there are additional elements to the negotiation that had been "overlooked." Auto dealers use this tactic so buyers will return before accepting another dealer's offer. This gives the first dealer another shot at the sale. Sometimes this tactic becomes "bait and switch" when the buyer learns that the product really isn't available, but a similar one with a few more bells and whistles (and a higher price) is ready for sale.

- *Nibbling, Salami Slicing, Nickel and Diming*—This involves asking for a small concession after one side thought an agreement had been reached. The classic example is a customer who asks for a free tie after the tailor has taken measurements and written up the ticket on a suit. The cost of the tie is small relative to the suit, so there is great pressure to comply. This tactic creates ill will for a small gain, and may result in future retribution.[4]
- *Chicken*—This is bluffing with a very threatening position. An important cardiac surgeon threatens to move his or her surgeries to another hospital unless some changes are made to the physicians' lounge. You may feel strongly that the surgeon is bluffing, but can you take the chance? The problem with this tactic is that the stakes are high and a bluff may be called. If the bluffer doesn't follow through, he or she will lose all credibility. Once again, future retribution is another possible outcome.
- *Intimidation*—This involves using threats, false anger, guilt, and the like. These tactics can be used to distract the opponent from the basis of negotiation by focusing on context.
- *False "Facts"*—This should not be confused with less-than-full disclosure. This tactic is dangerous, because there is no fallback position if your opponent challenges you to support your facts.

Your response to a given hardball tactic will depend on the specific circumstances, including your BATNA. All responses, however, are dependent on you being able to recognize the tactic for what it is: an attempt to shift the focus from the content of the negotiation to contextual issues, and thereby gain an advantage. Here are some specific ways to counter hardball strategies:

- Ignore them. Change the subject, or pretend it didn't happen. For example, responding in a calm manner can be disconcerting to an opponent who is ranting and raving (intimidation).
- If an opponent confronts you with data that you suspect may not be correct, it is always appropriate to ask for substantiation or time to collect your own data. Separate this from the "people" issue of trust by asserting that, "I always verify factual assertions that materially affect negotiations."
- Diffuse a hardball tactic by confronting your opponent with it. Fisher and Ury give an example of responding to a Good Cop/Bad Cop situation, "Say, Joe, I may be totally mistaken, but I'm getting the feeling that you and Ted here are playing a good guy/bad guy routine. If you two want a recess for any time to straighten out differences between you, just ask."[5]
- Respond in kind. Once your adversary understands that you can be equally extreme or irrelevant, he or she may move on. For example, a janitorial service offered to clean a hospital's new outpatient clinic for $2.00 per square foot per year. The physician manager immediately responded, "I was thinking more on the order of $0.10!"

"Where did you get that number from?" the service negotiator replied.

The physician manager then responded "Look, instead of us just throwing numbers around, why don't we talk about this in terms of what it costs *you* to provide this service, and what we *pay* for it at our other locations?" Combining an equally extreme counteroffer with a quick proposal to change the *basis* of negotiation often results in moving the discussion away from unsubstantiated, arbitrary positions to one based on objective criteria.

In summary, distributive negotiating is a win–lose approach in which negotiators try to reach agreement by influencing beliefs about what is possible, while at the same time trying to obscure their own real interests as they attempt to ascertain their opponent's interests.

## Negotiating Under Integrative Conditions

Integrative negotiation is characterized by a recognition that the parties will have to live together after the negotiation. The issues in integrative negotiations may first appear to be win–lose, but what separates this from a distributive process is how the opponents respond. The negotiation atmosphere is characterized by a sincere interest in trying to understand the adversary's real interests and objectives. This is not to say that the two sides are not advocates. They are, but both sides also recognize that they may be more personally successful through a mutual understanding of interests. Because each side has an interest in the other understanding its interests, there is a freer flow of information between the two parties than in a distributive negotiation. Lewicki and colleagues have identified four steps in the integrative negotiation process.[6]

### 1. Identify and define the dimensions of the problem.

Several points characterize an integrative strategy for defining the dimensions of a problem. First, there is an attempt to define the problem in terms that are mutually acceptable to both parties. For example, in negotiating a pharmaceutical supply contract, the dimensions may be cost, timeliness, quality, and service, not my price or your price, my timeliness performance or your timeliness standards, which are positions. Once both parties agree on the *dimensions* to be negotiated, then they can formulate positions on each dimension.

Second, the problem should be stated as a goal to be attained, as opposed to a statement of a specific solution. For example, "Our objective is to reduce our inventory costs" is a goal. It doesn't specify or foreclose options for reaching it. Whereas, "We will give you an exclusive contract in exchange for lower unit prices. Now, let's negotiate those prices" is a *solution*. Exchanging exclusivity for price may be the ultimate solution that you mutually reach, but by stating this as an objective, it cuts off discussion on other perhaps superior ways of achieving your interest, which is to reduce inventory costs.

Third, problem identification needs to be depersonalized as much as possible. When one side or the other has ownership, this can generate defensiveness. A personalized statement would be "Your pharmaceutical sales people are always pushing too much stock on us and overestimating order lead time." A depersonalized statement would be "There is a difference of opinion on necessary inventory and when orders need to be placed to attain appropriate inventory levels while controlling costs."

Fourth, separate problem identification from finding a solution. If the two occur at the same time, then negotiators may jump into problem solving before fully evaluating the scope of the negotiation. Integrative negotiating is characterized by exchanges that go back and forth over the range of issues to be resolved. For example, "I'll give you this on Issue A, if you give me that on Issue B." Discussing solutions before the full range of issues to be resolved has been identified can result in having to revisit prematurely reached solutions.

### 2. Bring interests to the surface.

Next, the integrative process focuses on interests. By examining the problem at this deeper level, you move behind positions, which are really particular attempts to satisfy underlying interests. Because there generally are several positions that can satisfy

an interest, this increases the chance of reaching a solution. Fisher and Ury provide an excellent example of how moving beyond positions to interests can result in a solution that is better for both parties:[7]

> Consider the story of two men quarreling in a library. One wants the window open and the other wants it closed. They bicker back and forth about how much to leave it open: a crack, halfway, three quarters of the way. No solution satisfies them both.
>
> Enter the librarian. She asks one why he wants the window open. "To get some fresh air." She asks the other why he wants it closed. "To avoid the draft." After thinking a minute, she opens wide a window in the next room, bringing in fresh air without a draft.

This example points out several advantages of redefining the problem in terms of interests. While the problem remained defined as positions, it was likely that neither side would be happy because any opening dissatisfied one party and even half-open dissatisfied the other party. The librarian's intervention was successful because she focused on the question of why. Why was each party unhappy? This refocused the dispute in terms of the underlying interests.

### 3. Generate alternative solutions.

The third aspect of integrative bargaining is generating alternative solutions. Four methods of generating alternatives are expanding the pie, log rolling, cost cutting, and brainstorming. Conflicts often arise because there simply are not enough resources available. By making the pie bigger (i.e., allocating more resources), conflict can be reduced. A hospital wishes to reduce the number of artificial hips that are used from 11 to 3. It estimates that this will save $1 million over 3 years. Surgeons, however, are resisting the change. Some initially will have longer operating times, because they are beginning at the start of the learning curve. In addition, they will have to receive training on unfamiliar hips. Finally, they are concerned about who will make the choices, whether quality will be sacrificed to price, and having flexibility to change as new devices come on the market. Expanding the pie in this instance may mean that the hospital returns some of the cost savings to the surgeons in a legal way.[8] In this instance, the hospital addressed the physicians underlying concerns. They committed to reinvest 60 percent of the savings to improved facilities, orthopedic program development, funding orthopedic research, and marketing the orthopedic program. They created a hip selection committee with physician majority staffing to address the control issue.

Log rolling involves trading off issues so that both parties achieve some success in the issues that are most important to them. To log roll, however, it is necessary for each party to have different priorities on several issues, *and* for communication to be open enough so that each side can see this, and believe it. Sometimes, log rolling requires that complex issues must be decomposed into component parts. For example, "value" to these surgeons might be achieved through favorable committee assignments, and preferred surgery times that could go along with the agreement.

Underlying all of these approaches is brainstorming. All too often, original ideas are prematurely rejected or never given full consideration. Brainstorming overcomes these problems by separating the generation of ideas from their evaluation. Brainstorming is generally a group idea generation process, but it can be done individually. The basic rules of brainstorming include the following:[9]

- No idea is too ridiculous to be stated. Everyone is encouraged to state any idea irrespective of how extreme, ridiculous, or outlandish.

- Each idea that is presented belongs to the group, not the person stating it. This allows members to build on the ideas of others without getting into issues of personal credit.
- No idea can be criticized. The purpose of the session is to generate ideas, not evaluate them. (See also the discussion of brainstorming in Chapter 6.)

Once the ideas have been generated, they are evaluated. Many of the ideas will be of no value. Some, however, may have an element that had not previously been considered. Others, when taken in combination, may provide the basis for a new way of looking at the negotiation.

### 4. Choose Specific Solutions that Address Both Sides' Interests.

The final integrative negotiation stage is to evaluate the options that have been generated and to choose the best alternatives. Try to focus the negotiation process away from a confrontation of personal wills and arbitrarily held positions, and toward using objective external criteria. Fisher and Ury refer to this approach as principled negotiation. Examples of external objective standards include market price, precedent, scientific judgment, professional standards, efficiency, cost, law, moral standards, equal treatment, tradition, and reciprocity. Using external standards to guide a negotiation reframes it into a more objective problem-solving process. This moves the focus of the negotiation toward a discussion of determining what would be an objective, fair basis to formulate an agreement and away from personal, arbitrary positions. Reaching an agreement that *both* sides see as fair has a lot to offer to everyone, if each side has to "live" with the adversary after the negotiation. It also provides a basis for each party to change its position without losing face or feeling foolish.

Returning to our real estate example, Ms. Jones, the owner, initially offers the physician a rate of $15.50 per foot. Several days later, the physician responds as follows:

My agent has surveyed several other "Class A" office suites in this part of town that are either on the market now or that have rented in the past 6 months. The price has ranged between $13.00 and $14.00 per square foot. Please correct me if I'm wrong on this, but this seems to be the market range. Is there some reason, perhaps some characteristic of your suite that would warrant going outside this range?[10]

You have reframed the discussion into what is externally fair and away from a direct contest of wills. Ms. Jones is now in the position of having to do one of the following:

- Produce alternative data that supports her offering price of $15.50. Perhaps, for example, she believes that you and your agent are not being truthful, or that your data are not valid for some other reason.
- Identify an alternative objective standard, such as her internal costs, irrespective of market price.
- Offer a justification for why her office suite may merit a higher rent, such as it's on a lakefront, or has particularly good interstate access.
- State that she will not be governed by any standards; this simply is her price.

If Ms. Jones chooses the last strategy, then the negotiation can be quickly concluded. You would then know that from the owner's perspective, there is no basis to modify her position. You must choose between accepting the offer at $15.50, which is lower than your reservation price, but higher than your BATNA, or walking away from this negotiation. On the other hand, any of the first three alternatives can provide a basis for you and

Ms. Jones to modify your positions and reach a negotiated agreement.

Let's assume that Ms. Jones does produce some valid conflicting data. For example, perhaps her justification is that the office suite is on a lakefront, and generally waterfront properties do have higher rents. Now you must decide whether looking at ducks between breaks in your busy schedule is worth the additional cost. If it is, then you probably should try to obtain some waterfront rental price data to justify accepting her offer, or to justify a counterproposal. If it is not, then the negotiation will quickly conclude. Negotiating on the basis of principle (in this case fair market price) creates this efficiency. If, on the other hand both sides' negotiation standard is, "This is what I want because I want it," it could take considerable time and mutual wasted effort to discover that you can't reach an agreement.

Returning now to Dr. Johnson, the administrator made the following comments to him after he disputed the validity of the case mix data:

There were 14 cases that you referred on to consultants that easily fit within our guidelines for nonreferral. These guidelines were initially developed by a national panel and then reviewed and modified by local board-certified PCPs. In addition, we have been modifying these standards over the last 3 years based on our local network experience. Our incidence of malpractice claims is well below national standards, and lower than that of local PCPs outside our network. Finally, our clinical outcomes data show that our PCPs are providing excellent quality of care.

I agree with you that the standard for these decisions should be outcomes, and I'm willing to impartially look at the particulars of your case-mix. We have a case-mix committee and we can refer this on to them, or if you want, you and I can discuss your case-mix concerns prior to me referring your observations to them. If there are additional case-mix issues to consider, then I want to know this, because we are constantly striving to improve our processes.

The administrator, therefore, is negotiating on principle, which in this case is having the best possible case-mix adjustment process. If Dr. Johnson's reaction is that case-mix data are irrelevant, then the administrator can quickly conclude the negotiation. On the other hand, if Dr. Johnson identifies some truly distorting aspects of the case-mix adjustment, then the medical director has stated her willingness to consider and incorporate this information. Finally, if Dr. Johnson accepts the validity of the case-mix data, then this can change the focus of the negotiation to how he can become skilled in using the referral guidelines. His long-term interest probably is best served by learning to live in this new world. If the administrator successfully depersonalizes the process by negotiating on principle, then this may give Dr. Johnson the room to identify his true self-interest, and to act on it. If, however, he is *really* saying, "This is what I want, because I want it!," and he leaves this PPO over this issue to work with another, the "new world" will eventually catch up with him again. Hopefully, given time and a depersonalized negotiation process, he also will see this last consequence.

Let's apply some of these ideas to a negotiation between a hospital that wants to introduce an activity-based cost management system (see Chapter 1) into its breast cancer program. Some of the physicians oppose this, because they believe that it would be intrusive, create more paperwork for them, and jeopardize their ability to make clinical decisions. Addressing the physicians' underlying interests, the hospital proposes providing more administrative and clinical support to develop and maintain the ABC system. They also extend an offer to the physicians to be-come part of the ABC system development team,[11] and to provide compensation for this time. The hospital proposes an oncologist-dominated ABC oversight committee to address their concern that administrators will dictate clinical decisions through policy. Finally, a brainstorming session containing representatives from all interested parties (administration, oncologists, oncological surgeons, nursing, quality control, etc.) generates some breakthrough ideas, such as moving the breast cancer program in the hospital organization structure up to departmental status, so it prepares its own budgets. This allows the program to protect its own self-interest, while creating incentives to better manage costs, which is the hospital's primary interest.

**Possible Reactions to All of This**

Invariably, there are some whose reaction to these ideas can be summarized as, "But how do I win! I don't give a damn about the other side; I want the most that I can get!" Sometimes in life you are stuck in situations where you can't win, unless the other guy gets something that he wants. If he doesn't get something, then *you* won't get *anything*. Keep in mind that you are in this situation of negotiating with someone else, because there is something that you want, which the *other* side controls. After all, if you could get what you are seeking in the negotiation by simply taking it yourself, then you probably already would have. Remember, it is possible for you to lose or gain, the other guy to lose or gain, and for both of you to lose or gain! Lose–lose outcomes do occur! Sometimes, walking away by rejecting a less-than-ideal agreement will make you feel good, but are you really better off?

"But when I try to act cooperatively, the adversary doesn't act accordingly!" This is not unusual. Sometimes your initial negotiation discussions have to be educational. If this truly is an integrative situation, then sometimes you have to bring the adversary around to the ideas of discussing interests, not getting locked into positions, or creatively thinking of mutually beneficial outcomes. William Ury expressed this better then most,

> The problem is that while you would like to discuss each side's interests and how to satisfy them, the other side is likely to insist on their position. While you may be flexible, they may stonewall. While you may be attacking the problem, they may be attacking you.[12]

An approach that some suggest for dealing with this situation is called the broken record technique. Many physicians are old enough to remember vinyl records, and can remember what happens when a record becomes badly scratched: it repeats, and repeats, and repeats. Here is the mantra:

- Focus on finding their interests—repeatedly, insistently and in many ways. Ask, "Why do you want that," or "Why not do this? It seems to satisfy what you are looking for," or "What do you need or want out of this negotiation?"
- Set an example—express your interests and stay away from positions. Repeatedly do this so they can see what you are talking about, and how this is different from being positional.
- Openly talk about the distinction between positions and interests—don't consider this to be secret knowledge that will provide a tactical advantage. It's not. It only is to your advantage when the adversary similarly sees it to his or her advantage to think and act this way.

- Restate their position out loud—over and over again. Sometimes, people don't really hear what they are saying, until it is verbally stated back to them. "What you are saying to me is . . .," or "Correct me if I'm wrong, but you are saying that . . . ."
- Take a timeout—sometimes, an adversary needs time to think about what they have said, and what you are saying to them. They may feel uncomfortable dealing with new ideas and feel under pressure to reply. Give them some time. "Maybe we should both think about this more. How about taking a break until tomorrow or for a few days?"
- Recycle back through these ideas—in effect you are saying the same things in many different ways. Be persistent. If necessary, recess for an extended period of time, such as several days or weeks.
- Avoid the temptation to strike back—striking back will only increase the adversarial atmosphere of the negotiation, and provide a rationalization for the adversary to continue being positional.
- Don't give in—persistence is an important negotiation skill. Keep your eye on your objectives. If you give in, then you lose, and that is not an acceptable outcome. It is important to remember that integrative negotiating situations also have some distributional aspects. In other words, if you don't look out for your own self-interest, then no one else will. An integrative process is a way to achieve the most that *you* can, because it will produce solutions that might not have been considered, and help you and the other side to find agreements and avoid deadlocks. Still, within the context of log rolling, creating new ideas, and trading this for that, you need to focus on obtaining the best outcome you can for yourself, while recognizing that the adversary is doing the same, and that both of you are in this negotiation because each has something to gain from the other.

- If all else fails, and you see no hope of reaching an integrative solution, then move to your BATNA. In this instance BATNA stands for "*b*etter *a*lternative *t*han any *ne*gotiated *a*greement with this adversary!"

## THE PRISONERS' DILEMMA: A METAPHOR FOR MANY NEGOTIATION ISSUES

At this point you may be saying to yourself something like, "I understand what you are saying, but there is *something* about all of this that makes me feel uneasy." If you are like many physicians and negotiators, that vague uneasy feeling that you have involves the issue of trust: "How will my adversary react to integrative (cooperative) overtures?" After all, this could be taken as a sign of weakness, and you may fear that you might be taken advantage of. The other side of this is temptation; your temptation to try taking advantage of an adversary who is acting cooperatively. After all, you might be able to take advantage of this cooperative adversary and win really big? That is your goal, isn't it? To win big?

Fears about how the other side will react in the face of cooperative overtures are a common negotiation phenomenon. For example, take trash recycling. If everyone in the community recycles and you don't separate your plastic from your aluminum, then you win big. You get the benefit of a clean community without the effort of recycling. If, however, others start following your example, then you soon have a dirty community and everyone loses. Oil cartels are faced with the same dilemma. As long as the cartel holds the price and production restrictions, then all of the cartel members win. If one starts selling crude under the table, as Nigeria did in the 1980s, they make out very well. Inevitably, the increased supply pushes the price down, others defect to compensate for declining

prices, and all lose. An interesting example of this happened with the cotton crop in the United States. A serious disease was decimating the crop. Some seed companies reengineered the seed, but all the farmers in a contiguous geographic area had to plant the new seed for it to control the disease, and the new seed had a 20 percent lower yield. Imagine the temptation for a farmer, all of whose neighbors have planted the new seed. If he plants the old seed, he's pretty well protected from the disease, but he gets a 20 percent greater yield than his neighbors. If everyone starts thinking this way, then the disease comes back and everyone loses. Immunizations for communicable diseases present a similar dilemma.

All of these situations are examples of a common negotiation situation called the prisoners' dilemma.[13] It addresses the question of whether trust and cooperation will be reciprocated or taken advantage by the competitors in a negotiation. A prisoners' dilemma occurs under the following conditions:

- Each side can choose to cooperate or defect.
- The reward for defecting is greater than the reward for cooperating, if others cooperate.
- If all defect, then all lose.

Richard Axelrod[14] was a University of Michigan researcher who designed an interesting experiment that examined responses to a prisoners' dilemma. He designed a competition for computer programs to see if there were better strategies when working under prisoners' dilemma rules. Competitors were expert strategists from political science, sociology, economics, psychology, and mathematics who wrote computer programs that faced off against each other in a round robin tournament. Pairs of programs battled each other for 200 rounds in which each round was a simple decision: cooperate or defect. The payoff matrix for each round is found in **Figure 8–4**. The goal of the game was to win as much as possible across the 200 rounds of the game.

The experts wrote programs that utilized a range of different strategies. Some programs chose each move (cooperate or defect) randomly. Others used complex exploitative strategies that calculated an opponent's defection rate based on previous rounds, and then defected just a little more frequently. Axelrod noted several characteristics of the better programs. All of the eight top-ranked programs were nice; that is, they started off cooperating. The best of the "mean" entries scored 401 points, and the lowest of the "nice" entries received 472 points. When nice entries played against other nice entries, they averaged almost 600 points, which suggests the premium that may be possible for finding integrative solutions. Another common characteristic of the best programs was that they were provocable. They punished defection by defecting themselves. In other words, they were not martyrs. The best programs were also forgiving. They didn't hold grudges. Defection was not an irredeemable

sin. They gave the opponent the opportunity to resume cooperation. Finally, the best programs clearly communicated whether they were cooperating or defecting. Complex strategies can be difficult for the opponent to decipher and could result in unintended defections. The best programs signaled clearly when they cooperated, and when they defected.[15]

The program that achieved the most success was called *Tit for Tat*. This program cooperates in the first round and thereafter does whatever the opponent did on the preceding round. If the opponent defected on the previous round, then *Tit for Tat* defects on the next round. If the opponent cooperated on the previous round, then *Tit for Tat* cooperates on the next round. This strategy was nice, provocable, forgiving, and clear. Axelrod had a number of interesting comments about the programs, which sound all too much like the actions of real people in the heat of negotiation:[16]

> . . . the entries were too competitive for their own good. In the first place, many of them defected early in the game without provocation, a characteristic which was very costly in the long run. . . . Even expert strategists from political science, sociology, economics, psychology, and mathematics made the systematic errors of being too competitive for their own good, not being forgiving enough, and being too pessimistic about the responsiveness of the other side.

Axelrod, encouraged by the success of the first tournament, held a second one. Entrants were given a report describing *Tit for Tat* as well as the conclusions regarding niceness, provocability, forgivingness, and clarity. Sixty-two entries were received from six countries. Once again, *Tit for Tat* proved to be the most successful program. Next, Axelrod tried to determine whether *Tit for*

|  | Other | |
|  | **Cooperate** | **Defect** |
|---|---|---|
| **Cooperate** | 3 to Other<br><br>3 to You | 5 to Other<br><br>−5 to You |
| **Defect** | −5 to Other<br><br>5 to You | −2 to Other<br><br>−2 to You |

**Figure 8–4** Prisoners' Dilemma Payoff Matrix.

*Tat's* success was due to similar competitors' "knocking each other off." In other words was *Tit for Tat* robust? Could it do well in different, narrower environments? Axelrod constructed six hypothetical tournaments. *Tit for Tat* won five and finished second in the sixth. He commented:[17]

> What accounts for *Tit for Tat's* robust success is its combination of being nice, retaliatory, forgiving, and clear. Its niceness prevents it from getting into unnecessary trouble. Its retaliation discourages the other side from persisting whenever defection is tried. Its forgiveness helps restore mutual cooperation. And its clarity makes it intelligible to the other player, thereby eliciting long-term cooperation.

Axelrod's final conclusion gives much to ponder if you place it in the context of humans instead of computer programs. Arguably, this is a legitimate context, because the programs were written by humans and certainly represented many of the habit, values, and preferences of their authors:[17]

> *Tit for Tat* foregoes the possibility of exploiting other rules (programs). While such exploitation is occasionally fruitful, over a wide range of environments the problems with trying to exploit others are manifold. In the first place, if a rule defects to see what it can get away with, it risks retaliation from rules that are provocable. In the second place, once mutual recriminations set in, it can be difficult to extract oneself. And, finally, the attempt to identify and give up on unresponsive rules (such as *random*) or excessively uncooperative rules often mistakenly led to giving up on rules which were in fact salvageable by a more patient rule like *Tit for Tat*. *Being able to exploit the exploitable without paying too high a cost with the others is a task which was not successfully accomplished by any*

> *of the entries in round two of the tournament.* [emphasis added]

In a nutshell his last sentence summarizes the problem that many have with integrative negotiating. We want to "exploit the exploitable." We are attracted to maximizing and we proceed accordingly. The problem arises when we learn through hard experience that the adversary is a moving target. They are not easily exploitable, and in the process of learning this we throw away the opportunity to attain real, valuable, although not ideal gains. In effect, we claim the southeast cell in Figure 8–4.[18]

Clearly the prisoner's dilemma has some characteristics that are problematic in real negotiations. To mention a few, each player knows with certainty whether the other has defected or cooperated in the previous round. In real life, you often don't know with certainty whether cooperation really is cooperation or artfully disguised defection. Reward contingencies in real negotiations will vary greatly from the ratios used in the game, and this obviously could have a major impact on behavior. Finally, negotiators in real life can talk to each other before they make or respond to an offer. They can express intentions, propose commitments, and threaten. All these considerations should give pause about the generalizability of Axelrod's *specific* findings.

Nevertheless, there do seem to be some lessons that could be cautiously drawn and applied from this research:

- Trust is critical to succeeding in integrative situations. It's easy to lose and hard to regain. Unless you are given reason to believe otherwise, it may be beneficial to begin negotiations assuming that the adversary will be willing to be cooperative.
- Retaliation for a violation of expectations is a reasonable response. Don't, however,

overreact. Be certain of your facts, and carefully choose your reaction so it is appropriately proportional to the violation. Remember, the objective of retaliation is not to obliterate your adversary. You don't want to start the escalation to a nuclear war over a border dispute. The objective is to simply convey the message that you know when a defection has occurred, and you won't be taken advantage of.

- Don't hold a grudge. If it appears that your opponent is willing to move from confrontational to cooperative negotiations, be willing to respond accordingly. This is difficult to do. Memories of past violations of trust are hard to forget or forgive. Nevertheless, effective negotiators learn from past experiences, and move forward with cooperative negotiations when the adversary *demonstrates* that this trust is merited.
- Clear communication is critical. Although the content of the negotiation may be complex, strive to communicate in direct, unambiguous language and signals. Don't give confounding messages, such as nonverbal cues that contradict written and verbal messages. Every dimension of a negotiation communicates information including:
- meeting personally or negotiating over the phone
- using an attorney and when you use an attorney
- if face to face, the clothing that you wear (business attire or casual)
- language, eye contact, tone, and gestures

Finally, don't be greedy. Even if the immediate negotiation is limited and there is little chance that you will have future dealings with your adversary, think long and hard about being exploitive. Even if you don't believe in fate, karma, balance in the universe, or "what goes around comes around," your reputation will precede you.

## CASE ANALYSIS: THE BLACK BOOK

Paul Grant, MD, and Larry Jones, MD, partners in Down East Internal Medicine, Ltd., were simultaneously facing a professional and business crisis. Two years ago, they made their first foray into managed care by contracting with Portland Shipbuilding and Down East Dreadnoughts, both major local employers, to provide capitated services. As a result of obtaining these contracts, they greatly expanded their practice. They hired three additional nurses, two secretaries, and two nurse practitioners and doubled their office space by acquiring an adjacent, vacant suite. Finally, they hired two physicians to work as employees. Fran Sorella, MD, was fresh out of residency. Her career plan was to work for a while before making any permanent commitments. Erik Klaameyer, MD, was retiring from the Navy at age 51. He was looking to begin a new career, but he wasn't sure that he wanted to stay in Portland for his next career or, for that matter, to be in a small private practice.

Both physicians were only interested in an employment relationship, and both were happy to sign 2-year employment contracts. Drs. Grant and Jones saw this as an opportunity to profit substantially while still paying Sorella and Klaameyer equitable salaries. Grant commented "I figured that if one or both became successful, and we got along, we could work out a partnership arrangement later. If it didn't go well, I could hire someone else."

Eighteen months later, the effects of international peace struck. Portland Shipbuilding, a subsidiary of a major conglomerate, closed its doors as a result of the Navy canceling all its new construction contracts. Down East Dreadnoughts also lost all its new construction contracts and was barely staying alive doing ship repairs. As a result, Down East layed off 70 percent of its hourly employees. With the decline in employment, Drs. Grant and Jones saw an immediate and precipitous decline in cash flow from their managed care contracts as their per-member–per-month covered lives declined. In addition, they noted that copayments were becoming more difficult to collect, indemnity insurance patients were increasingly reluctant to schedule annual physicals and preventive care, and receivables were increasing. At about this time, Dr. Sorella decided that she didn't like the climate and would be moving to the southwest. She gave 6 months' notice.

Dr. Grant saw the handwriting on the wall. The first thing that he did was to ask his business manager to run a breakeven analysis (see Chapter 1 for a discussion of breakeven analysis) to see how the projected loss in revenue would affect the practice. After he reviewed the analysis, he said:

> The results were sobering. If things continued the way we were projecting, we would be losing over $20,000 a month within 6 months. We had to make some immediate changes, so Larry and I sat down with the breakeven analysis spreadsheet to see what changes we could make to our expenses, with the goal of survival. We also saw the specter of bankruptcy in the background.

The first to go would be Dr. Klaameyer, whose contract would not be renewed. Both physicians figured that they could absorb his declining case load. Next to go were the physician extenders and unneeded clerical support. Still, however, they had a projected annual loss of almost $165,000. This left two major areas to cut: their own salaries and rent. Currently, they were renting 6,000 square feet at $20 per square foot for a total annual payment of $120,000. They no longer needed this amount of space. In addition, with the decline of the local economy, the

bottom had fallen out of commercial real estate rents. Office space that had rented for $20 per square foot and more could now be leased for $13 to $14 per square foot. Dr. Grant commented:

> We decided that we would try to renegotiate our lease. We would get the best deal that we could. Any remaining shortfall would have to be taken out of our salaries. We were both willing to take substantial salary hits to keep the practice going, but we also both agreed that at some point it wouldn't make sense, and that we might have to choose other alternatives, such as Chapter 11 bankruptcy, or even Chapter 7, and move elsewhere.[19]
>
> We felt that the building owner would be willing to work with us. We had been in the building for 7 years, and they had always been cooperative in the past. Plus they were local, and all of us had this siege mentality that if we could stick together, we might all be able to weather the storm.
>
> Then the other shoe fell! We receive a certified letter telling us that the building was in foreclosure. In hindsight, that shouldn't have been a surprise. This was a high-rise, Class A office building, but occupancy was only about 50 percent, and I knew that several occupants were really hurting financially. The new owners were Conglomerated Insurance Company of America (CICA) out of Los Angeles! How do you negotiate with an insurance company? What are their interests, and what do they want? We had this image of an administrative bureaucracy that would be difficult if not impossible to negotiate with. This was a real blow. We felt that we needed advice; some help in understanding how CICA would look at what we would propose, so we turned to our attorney.

Their attorney, Duncan Foster, suggested that CICA's goal was to position the property for sale. A property generating more revenue would support a higher selling price.

This meant that CICA would try to increase occupancy, which of course would have to be accomplished at current market rates. Another element of value in commercial real estate was lease lengths. All other things being equal, a building with longer occupant leases was worth more than one with shorter leases. Foster commented, "I think that your strategy of renegotiating the lease is viable. If we can come up with a plan that makes sense given *today's* real estate reality, CICA will probably listen. Yesterday's real estate circumstances are history."

"How do we do this?" asked Grant.

"Well, I would begin by constructing a black book," responded Foster.

"What's that?"

Foster continued:

A black book is something that we use in bankruptcy negotiations, and that is where you fellows are. If your numbers are correct, you will go under unless CICA will work with you. A black book contains the alternatives that are available and spells out the financial implications for the other side given each alternative. For example, what will CICA receive if they accept your proposal, and what will they receive if you go into Chapter 7? Then they can make an informed choice.

We need to provide a breakeven analysis showing that at the right rental rate you will be a viable long-term tenant that will be financially stable. That's important because long-term leases are probably important to CICA. Next, we can show them how much revenue they will receive from you if they accept your proposal, and what they are likely to get if you file for Chapter 7 bankruptcy. That's important because those are the choices that they will have.

Two days later, Jack Duggan, a senior vice president at Maple Leaf Realty Group, a regional commercial real estate firm, contacted Dr. Grant to inform him that his firm would be managing the property for CICA. Dr. Grant scheduled a meeting with him to tell him about the practice's financial problem. Dr. Grant stated:

My objective for the meeting was to tell Duggan about our financial problem and then to *listen*. I wanted to learn as much as possible about Duggan's and CICA's goals for the building, and what might be their underlying interests. Duggan either played his cards close to his vest or simply didn't know much about CICA's plans for the building. I suspect more the latter than the former. I threw out some of Foster's hypotheses—that they would be interested in retaining tenants at current market rates and trying to fill the building as much as possible for a resale. Duggan said that filling the building and dealing with the reality of current market conditions made sense under any circumstances. The meeting concluded with my promise to have a proposal to him in 1 week.

Grant, Jones, and Foster then met to identify their interests and what they guessed would be CICA's interests (**Exhibit 8–1**). This would form the basis of the proposal that they would make. Appendix 8A contains a copy of the black book that Foster and Dr. Grant assembled for Jack Duggan. In addition, Dr. Grant wrote a cover letter to Mr. Duggan describing the history of the practice, the impact of the local financial crisis on the practice, his desire to consider any alternative that made financial sense, and the need to conclude the negotiation in 30 days.

Upon receipt of the proposal, Mr. Duggan called Dr. Grant and told him that he would pass the proposal on to his contact at CICA and that he hoped to be back to Dr. Grant in 1 week to 10 days. Two weeks elapsed with no word from Mr. Duggan. Dr. Grant called him, and after several unreturned phone calls over

**Exhibit 8–1**  Interests of Down East Internal Medicine, Ltd., and Assumed Interests of CICA

---

*Interests of Down East Internal Medicine, Ltd., partners*
- Preserve the personal assets of Drs. Grant and Jones
- Reduce operating costs
- Achieve financial stability under projected financial conditions
- Preserve the practice for Drs. Grant and Jones if possible
- Conclude negotiations expeditiously, so that in the event they fail, Drs. Grant and Jones can expeditiously pursue other alternatives

*Assumed interests of CICA that could affect negotiations*
Probable
- Generate maximum rental income for property
- Raise current building occupancy rate
- Minimize concessions to Down East Internal Medicine, Ltd.
Possible
- Sell property in an expeditious manner; avoid a "fire sale"

---

3 days, Duggan's secretary called and said that the proposal was still under consideration. In the meantime, Dr. Grant, being aware of the importance of a BATNA, contacted a real estate agent to begin a preliminary search for more affordable space. During these discussions, Dr. Grant learned that CICA also owned several other properties around town and that it had developed a reputation as an exceedingly slow decision maker. He also met with Mr. Foster again to position the practice for either Chapter 11 or Chapter 7 bankruptcy.

Twenty-eight days after Mr. Duggan received the black book proposal, he called Dr. Grant and told him that CICA was making a counterproposal. The next day the counterproposal arrived by express mail. The letter in **Exhibit 8–2** contains CICA's counterproposal. Grant, Jones, and Foster then met to analyze it. Its content indicated that they had anticipated CICA's interests. All the terms related to the themes of living with current market rates, trying to fill the building, and cooperating with Down East in a financial workout that would be mutually advantageous. The annual rent of $45,000, or $15 per square foot, was perhaps a little above market,

but this only translated into $3,000 more per year than Down East's proposal. Dr. Grant commented, "I'm sure there is $3,000 worth of slop somewhere in our numbers. I just hope that it's slop in our favor! We can always take it out of our salaries. . . . We won't let this go over that small an amount."

CICA's counterproposal to be able to move the practice around in the building or perhaps even out of the building was obviously related to its desire to seek large tenants, who might take a whole floor. Dr. Grant continued:

This could be a problem. You just can't move a medical practice on that short a notice, especially if we had to find another building. On the other hand, flexibility would be very important to them, if one of their fundamental goals is to fill the building. Maybe they would provide more than 60 days notice; probably any move would be to another suite in the building. It would be in their self-interest to do that. Probably they will never ask us to move. Larry and I didn't like it, but we could live with it.

The year extension was no problem. Our breakeven showed that we could reach financial stability, so what's an additional year

**Exhibit 8–2**  CICA Counterproposal

---

Paul Grant, MD
Down East Internal Medicine, Ltd.
1100 Corporate Drive, Suite 705B
Portland, Maine

Dear Dr. Grant:

CICA management has evaluated your proposal and authorized me to make the following offer:

1. The annual rental shall be $45,000.
2. Down East Internal Medicine, Ltd., shall vacate suite 705B and relocate in suite 705A.
3. Down East Internal Medicine, Ltd., shall cover any building costs necessary to separate suites 705A and 705B.
4. Down East Internal Medicine, Ltd., agrees to be relocated elsewhere within the building at CICA's expense with 60 days notice during the remainder of the lease, should CICA find it desirable to do so. If no suitable space is available, CICA shall cover reasonable moving expenses. Build-out costs and other expenses associated with moving to another building would not be borne by CICA.
5. Down East Internal Medicine, Ltd., agrees to extend the length of its lease for an additional year with a 4% rent increase in this third year.

Please contact me if there are any other issues to resolve.

Very truly yours,

*Jack Duggan*

Jack Duggan
Sr. Vice President
Maple Leaf Realty Group

---

to us given what we gain? The net effect on the cost of the deal, however, makes their numbers look a lot better. Our proposal had a total value to them of $84,000 in rental payments over 2 years. We were on the hook for $240,000 over 2 years. Adding the third year along with the 4 percent escalation and the $15 per foot price brought the value of their counterproposal to $136,800. Finally, they weren't proposing any personal guarantees. They were willing to leave this as a corporate debt. That could have been a big stumbling block.

Dr. Grant called Mr. Duggan the next day and indicated that he would accept the proposal. He asked whether the move notifica-

tion could be increased to 90 days. Duggan stated that he did not have personal authority to make that change and implied that it would be tortuous to reenter the CICA bureaucracy. He then stated:

I doubt that we could get CICA's approval on a new tenant in less than 60 days. In all practicality you will probably get plenty of notice. If you don't have any other issues, then I will proceed to have this agreement drafted into an amendment to your current lease.

Dr. Grant agreed. It took CICA 6 weeks to get him the amendment and an additional 3 months before a fully endorsed copy sporting the signatures of three CICA vice presidents was returned to him. Although it was frustrating to wait this long for the paperwork, it also provided an unintended assurance that they would not have to relocate on very short notice.

## CONCLUSION

Physician leaders constantly encounter situations that require negotiation skills. On occasion, negotiations can be distributive, and when that is the case, distributive skills are appropriate. On many occasions, an integrative strategy will result in both sides achieving more than if they had adopted a win–lose approach. Identifying interests, as opposed to becoming fixated on positions is a good place to begin any negotiation process. Being "nice," "provocable," "forgiving," and "clear" are reasonable guidelines to pursue unless given reasons to proceed otherwise.

Negotiation is an art, not a science. A physician who wishes to succeed in this art must use common sense and an insightful understanding of the adversary to shape his or her negotiation positions. The physician also must use good judgment and humility to know when all that can be achieved has been achieved. Summarizing a few more points:

- Know yourself—your BATNA, reservation price, what you hope to achieve (goals).
- Know your adversary. What are their (likely) aspirations, BATNA, reservation price, and goals?
- Will there be an ongoing relationship, or is this a one-time deal? Some negotiations have ongoing but not obvious effects on other relationships or events.
- Resolve to think in terms of interests first and not get locked into positions.

Finally, preparation should be proportional to the importance of the negotiation. If the negotiation involves trivial issues, then the actions described in this chapter may be excessive and not justified based on the likely benefit. If, on the other hand, the subject of the negotiation is important, then the ideas proposed in this chapter will help you to achieve better negotiation outcomes, and justify the work involved in using them.

## NOTES

1. See, for example, Sachs, G. "STEP-BD Program Update." Proceedings of the 12th Annual Santa Fe Psychiatric Symposium. Santa Fe, New Mexico, June 28–30, 2006. In this instance, negotiation concepts were used to gain greater compliance with a bipolar disorder treatment plan.
2. That said, there are scientific studies of negotiation concepts discussed in this chapter. It seems, however, that negotiation concepts and paradigms have been identified by practitioners, and that research has been conducted to validate or invalidate these observations. See for example: Kim, P, & A., Fragale. (2005). Choosing the path to bargaining power: An empirical comparison of BATNAs and contributions in negotiation. *Journal of Applied Psychology* 90(2):373–381. O'Connor, K., J. Arnold, & E. Burris. (2005). Negotiators' bargaining histories and their effects on future negotiation performance. *Journal of Applied Psychology* 90(2): 350–362. Velden, F., B. Beersma, & C. DeDreu. (2007). Majority and minority influence in group negotiation: The moderating effects of social motivation and decision rules. *Journal of Applied Psychology* 92(1):259–268.
3. Fisher, R., & W. Ury. (1991). *Getting to Yes. Negotiating Agreement Without Giving In.* (2nd ed.). New York: Penguin Books, p. 83.
4. Perhaps, for example, the tailor will leave a few stitches out or use a somewhat inferior fabric, neither of which will become apparent during the "warranty period." From the tailor's perspective, this may create equity.
5. Fisher & Ury p. 130.
6. Lewicki, R. (1994). *Negotiation.* Burr Ridge, IL: Irwin, pp. 83–110.
7. Fisher & Ury p. 40.
8. Simply paying them could be construed as a kickback.
9. Gibson, J., J. Ivancevich, J. Donnelly, & R. Konopaske. (2006). *Organizations—Behavior, Structure, Processes,* (12th ed.). New York: McGraw-Hill Irwin, p. 472.
10. Remember, it's always appropriate for adversaries to obtain their own data. "Giving them permission" makes this impersonal, and demonstrates that you are truly negotiating from principle.
11. Physician participation in the ABC process would be absolutely essential since they have critical information about core activities.
12. Ury, W. (1993). *Getting Past No: Negotiating Your Way From Confrontation to Cooperation.* New York: Bantam Books, p. 76.
13. The term comes from a situation that police can use with two alleged criminals. Put them in separate rooms and offer each a better deal if they implicate the other first.
14. Axelrod, R. (1984). *The Evolution of Cooperation.* NY: Basic Books.
15. For example, if a program is calculating the adversary's defection rate and then defecting itself at a slightly higher rate, a defect or cooperate on the preceding round is not a clear message of the intent to cooperate or defect.
16. Ibid, 40.
17. Ibid, 54.
18. I have conducted prisoners' dilemma games with over 2,000 physicians. Invariably, fewer than 10 percent win more than they would have won from consistent cooperation (northwest cell Figure 8–4).
19. Chapter 11 provides a court-defined "breathing space" for the organization to restructure its finances. Chapter 7 results in liquidation of the organization's assets.

# The Black Book Proposal

## PROPOSAL FOR LEASE MODIFICATION

Down East Internal Medicine, Ltd., proposes to reduce the annual rent for the remaining 2 years on its lease with Conglomerated Insurance Company of America (CICA) to $42,000 per year, payable in 24 monthly installments of $3,500. This adjustment is being requested because of the effects of the local economic downturn on our practice's financial condition. To facilitate this proposed rent reduction, Down East Internal Medicine, Ltd., also proposes to vacate suite 705B and move all its operations into its original location in suite 705A. If this proposal is acceptable, then the proposed annual rent of $42,000 would represent a rate of $14 per square foot, which is representative of current market conditions. This would also provide CICA with the opportunity to lease suite 705B.

Under this proposal, we project that the landlord will receive at least $42,860 more than it would recover under Chapter 7 bankruptcy, as illustrated in **Exhibit 8A–1**.

Before making this proposal, Down East Internal Medicine, Ltd. has developed a plan to make severe reductions to its expenses, which will amount to approximately $621,000 over a 12-month period. This is illustrated in **Exhibit 8A–2**. Of this amount, 12.6 percent would be due to the proposed lease modification. The largest reductions will come from eliminating salaried physician and medical professional positions as well as administrative salary reductions on the part of the two partners, Drs. Grant and Jones. The proposed rent reduction will be the final reduction to fixed costs, which will allow the practice to break even.

The alternative, which we have discussed with legal counsel, is Chapter 7 bankruptcy.

**Exhibit 8A–1** Financial Comparison of Proposal and Chapter 7 Bankruptcy

| | | |
|---|---:|---:|
| Landlord Recovery Under Proposed Lease Arrangement: | | |
| Rent: 2 years at $42,000 | | $84,000 |
| Landlord Recovery Under Chapter 7 Bankruptcy: | | |
| Value of fixed assets per tax return | $23,147 | |
| adjustment for market value | $(13,888) | |
| Accounts receivable | $52,687 | |
| Adjustment for bad debt and write-offs | $(15,806) | |
| Projected legal and administrative costs | $(5,000) | |
| Total | | $41,140 |
| Net CICA gain for lease modification proposal | | $42,860 |

**Exhibit 8A–2** Projected Expense Reductions

| Operating Expenses | Projected Next 12 Months | Prior 12 Months | Reduction |
|---|---|---|---|
| Advertising—Marketing | $2,065 | $2,065 | $— |
| Advertising—Yellow Pages | $1,049 | $1,049 | $— |
| Credit card discounts | $1,475 | $1,475 | $— |
| Bank service charges | $396 | $396 | $— |
| Interest expense | $472 | $472 | $— |
| Travel—Business related | $1,000 | $6,894 | $(5,894) |
| Licenses—Professional | $600 | $600 | $— |
| Licenses—Business | $3,385 | $5,924 | $(2,539) |
| Other taxes and licenses | $2,000 | $2,555 | $(555) |
| Business meals | $2,876 | $4,578 | $(1,702) |
| Food/entertainment—Marketing | $1,000 | $5,498 | $(4,498) |
| Legal expenses | $2,578 | $2,578 | $— |
| Accounting expenses | $500 | $500 | $— |
| Other professional expenses | $2,487 | $6,500 | $(4,013) |
| Rent—Office space | $42,000 | $120,000 | $(78,000) |
| Rent—Equipment | $4,000 | $7,500 | $(3,500) |
| Office supplies | $6,895 | $10,598 | $(3,703) |
| Medical supplies | $26,597 | $35,895 | $(9,298) |
| General overhead | $3,548 | $3,548 | $— |
| Computer repair/maintenance | $1,124 | $1,124 | $— |
| General repair and maintenance | $1,206 | $1,206 | $— |
| Payroll taxes—Employer total | $10,370 | $20,740 | $(10,370) |
| Postage | $2,276 | $2,731 | $(455) |
| Health insurance | $6,000 | $12,000 | $(6,000) |
| Professional liability insurance | $16,000 | $26,000 | $(10,000) |
| Insurance—Other | $972 | $972 | $— |
| Salaries—Medical | $300,000 | $700,000 | $(400,000) |
| Salaries—Physician management | $— | $50,000 | $(50,000) |
| Salaries—Front office staff | $93,000 | $123,000 | $(30,000) |
| Telephone | $4,259 | $4,685 | $(426) |
| Total | $540,129 | $1,161,082 | $(620,953) |
| Percentage expense reduction due to lease proposal | 12.6% | | |

If the fixed assets (Exhibit 8A–1) are liquidated, an optimistic recovery would be $9,258.80. If Down East Internal Medicine, Ltd., must proceed with bankruptcy, it is likely that the accounts receivable will suffer significantly as a result of the loss of a continuing practice to pursue collection. In addition, the legal and administrative costs of even a straightforward Chapter 7 corporate liquidation would be at least $5,000.

The practice under the proposed arrangement will be a viable, competitive entity, and it will be in a position to rebuild its patient base. It retains several strengths that will ensure that it will be able to meet the revised lease terms:

- an excellent clinical reputation
- two well-respected physicians with full case loads
- a managed care contract with a local shipyard, which may produce additional revenue as the shipyard recovers
- established referral sources
- an experienced business manager
- extremely efficient collection of receivables
- extensive marketing and promotion expertise and practice visibility
- an excellent location for attracting patients throughout the greater metropolitan area
- no debt other than to the partners

In conclusion, the proposed annual rent of $42,000 will result in the landlord receiving substantially more financial benefit than would be received under the bankruptcy alternative. The partners are committed to staying in practice if this is financially feasible. We have developed a plan that, with your cooperation, will make this feasible.

To proceed with the necessary restructuring, it is essential that we know as soon as possible whether you will accept this proposal. I propose that we determine whether we can reach an agreement within 30 days. If the negotiations extend much beyond this time, we will begin to incur losses that will be unacceptable, and we will have to consider other alternatives.

## CHAPTER 9

# Organizational Integration

## Chapter Objectives

The goal of this chapter is to help you get the parts of your practice, hospital, or healthcare system to work together as an integrated whole. Often, this is the physician leader's biggest challenge. Self-interests and inertia work against implementing the larger vision of coordinating around organizational goals instead of local, personal, and parochial objectives. This chapter provides an organizational structure context, so you can identify likely parts of the organization that need attention, discusses issues that inhibit integration, such as differing values in parts of the organization, and presents specific methods for achieving integration. Finally, many practices and healthcare systems are acquiring other practices and hospitals. Integrating a new organization, therefore, is a specific integration challenge in itself. This chapter discusses strategies for integrating acquisitions and provides a case example.

## INTRODUCTION

*Integration* is the process of coordinating the parts of your practice, hospital, or healthcare system so it works together in a coordinated manner. More specifically, it is the process of motivating the *people* in the organization's parts to work toward this end. Integration is important to healthcare organizations, because it is a strategy for reducing costs and improving the quality of outcomes. If, for example, a hospital's nurses, medical staff, laboratories, pharmacy, housekeeping, and billing work more effectively with each other, so patients on average are discharged 4 hours sooner than a competitor across town can achieve, this provides a competitive advantage. If, in addition, this integrated performance across jobs, departments, and professions results in patients not waiting 2 hours in the radiology department or 3 hours

for their physician to discharge them, then patient satisfaction also improves.

The examples just cited make it sound as though employees and departments want inefficiencies to occur. Far from it. Generally, these inefficiencies occur as a result of employees, groups, or departments trying to do what they do exceedingly well. They do it so well, in fact, that it is done to the exclusion of any other person or group's needs, including perhaps the patient's! For integration to occur, the achievement of employee, departmental, and professional goals must be subordinated to the larger organizational need. When this doesn't happen, and organizational units such as pharmacy, radiology, surgeons, and respiratory therapy try to excel in achieving their own narrow objectives and overall organization productivity suffers, this is called *suboptimization*.

As the size and diversity of an organization's product and service offerings increase, integration becomes more difficult to achieve. Diversified healthcare organizations have the most to gain from achieving integration. Consider a diversified healthcare system that provides tertiary-level hospital services, outpatient surgery, outpatient physician services including primary and specialty care, nursing home services, and insurance, including indemnity, preferred provider organization (PPO), and health maintenance organization (HMO) products. Each of the products and services is contained in a separate part of this healthcare system, such as shown in **Figure 9–1**. Now, consider all the ways in which each part can perform its mission so it looks good, but at the same time hurts the performance of another part of the health system or the overall system. Primary care physicians may shift costs to specialists by referring to them for procedures that they themselves could conduct. Similarly, specialists may choose to use the hospital's surgical facilities as opposed to their own, if as a result they can shift costs to the hospital. The insurance company may be going after market share through low rates, and as a result is flooding the system with more patients than the primary care physicians can handle. Tertiary hospital ser-

vices might discharge early, thereby increasing costs to specialists and the insurance division.

Because integration is concerned with how to get the parts to work together, you will have to understand the choices in how to assemble the parts if you are to achieve this objective. In the smallest organizations, each part is a separate job description. For example, in a solo private practice, the front office staff may comprise one person who performs all front office functions, such as answering the telephones, scheduling, insurance billing, and so forth. In this instance, it is relatively easy to achieve front office integration, because it occurs within the brain of the office manager. In this type of organization structure, the challenge will be to integrate the roles of the office manager and the physician.

As organizations get larger, the size and degree of organizational unit specialization increase. The front office of a large multispecialty practice might be divided into several functions, such as, scheduling, collection, billing, or insurance, each of which is one part of the job description of the business manager in the solo practice. Each of these functions might well have a supervisor, and several persons may be employed within

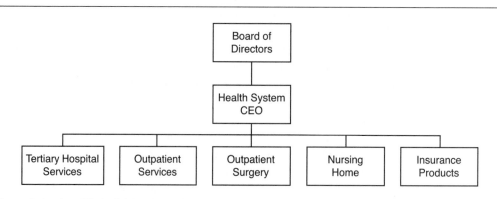

**Figure 9–1** Diversified Divisional Health Care Organization.

each function. In addition, the large, multi-specialty practice probably has front office functions that the solo practice does not have, such as managed care contracting and information systems management.

## STRUCTURE

The manner in which the parts of the organization are pieced together is called the organization's *structure*. An organization's structure should help it solve problems. If the organization's internal or external environments change, the structure often must change in response. Perhaps one of the most dramatic examples of this has been the decline in the number of solo practitioners and the growth of ever-larger single specialty and multispecialty practices. Fundamental changes in the economics of medicine that place a premium on better utilization of fixed costs and competition for managed patient contracts have resulted in practices changing their structure.

Understanding the way in which the parts of a healthcare organization are assembled, or its structure, helps answer the following questions:

- *Where do you draw the boundaries that define the specialized parts of the organization?* These lines are the boxes that appear on an organization chart. The boxes represent the grouping of human resources. In effect, these boxes or boundaries determine who works closely with whom, and what boundaries or barriers must employees span in order to exchange information to work together.
- *What type of measurement and reward systems will be needed?* As noted in Chapters 5 (compensation) and 6 (management), employees ultimately do what is in their self-interest. Similarly, they will work in the aggregate toward those goals that they believe are in their group's, practice's, service line's, or hospital's self-interest, if they don't conflict with their personal self-interest. By creating boundaries, you also create the need to think about the rewards that are created for these organizational units. For example, if you reward a finance department for keeping costs under control, you should not be surprised when it limits resources to a pathology laboratory that is exceeding its expense budget. Unfortunately, this may occur even though the laboratory also is exceeding its net income goal by an even larger amount! If departments, and consequently their employees, are given goals and rewarded for keeping costs down and not for encouraging growth in net income, then you shouldn't be surprised by the wayward consequences.
- *How do you integrate the parts of the organization so that their individual contributions combine to achieve the organization's overall goals?* This objective can be achieved if you think carefully about how you draw the subunit boundaries, how you measure performance, and how you structure the rewards that define the relationship among employees, groups, and the organization.

There are three fundamental strategies for organizing all organizations, including those in healthcare: *functional structure*, *divisional structure*, and *matrix structure*. Each structure has strengths that address some integration challenges and weaknesses with others. A functional structure arranges the human resources by their function, or what they do. **Figure 9–2** illustrates a hospital that is functionally organized. Employees are grouped into organizational units by what they do. All the medical services such as ICU, and surgery, are grouped together and report to the

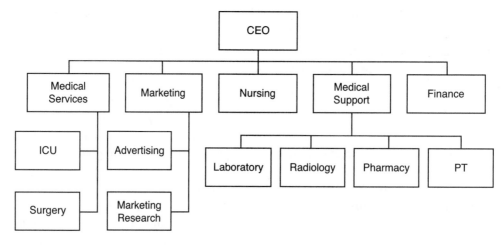

**Figure 9–2** Functional Hospital Organizational Structure.

medical services vice president. Similarly, marketing, nursing, and medical support services each have their own "boxes," so that people who work in these functional areas are grouped, work, and led together. As you descend into the organization structure, you can see that functions may be broken into smaller subareas. Medical support, for example, has four major groupings within it: laboratory, radiology, pharmacy, and physical therapy. Marketing is broken into advertising and marketing research.

**Figure 9–3** illustrates the functional structure of a multispecialty practice, which also utilizes committees. Once again, the basis for grouping people together is what they do. Notice that on occasion different aspects of the same operational process may be organizationally divided, and this is where lack of integration can get you into trouble. Both marketing and information systems, for example, appear in the business administration and internal medical planning committee functions, because there are marketing and information systems issues that both must address. Contracting appears under both business administration and external med-

ical planning. Finally, there probably needs to be communication and coordination between research and grants (internal medical planning committee) and medical school relations (external medical planning committee). The issue that determines whether this structure is working for the practice is whether these committees and functional units operate as though they are in isolated smokestacks, or whether they transfer information across the vertical functional lines and work together as a team.

The organization chart also indicates the specific jobs that should have primary integration responsibility. The medical administration director is responsible for integrating across the medical specialties (functions) of primary care, orthopedics, cardiology, oncology, gastroenterology, and nursing. The leaders of the internal planning committee and the external planning committee are responsible for integrating across the committees that they supervise. The chief executive officer (CEO) is responsible for integrating across business administration, medical administration, internal medical planning committee, and the external medical planning

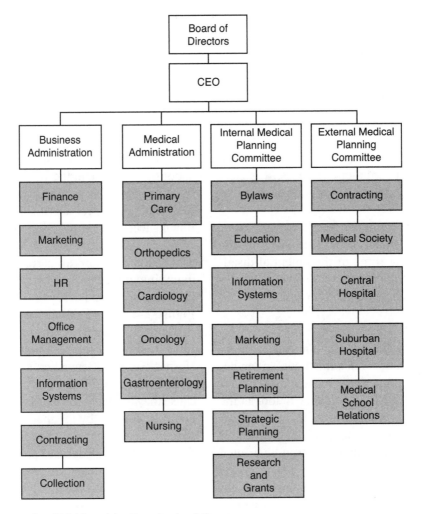

**Figure 9–3** Functional Multispecialty Organizational Structure.

committee. Often, integration at this level will be addressed through meetings chaired by the CEO and attended by all of these functional directors and leaders.

Functional designs have the following potential advantages:

- *Economies of scale and high efficiency are possible.* Because all those performing a function are grouped together, they can work closely with each other, and the fewest number of employees will be needed.

- *Similar employees will develop collegiality and bootstrap each other's skills.* Similar backgrounds, education, and training, coupled with common department goals, develop group cohesiveness. Employees who work together all the time know each other's strengths and weaknesses and can compensate for, adjust, and develop each other accordingly.

- *Performance standards are easy to set.* Everyone in a department is working toward the same goal, and the goals of the department are defined by the homogeneous function. Marketing is evaluated on marketing performance. All of the cardiologists work together and can set their own internal quality and cost standards, and so on.

- *Decision making and lines of authority are simple and clear.* If, for example, the director of information systems has a question about cardiology services, it is clear where he or she can go for an answer.

When a functional design is being used, the goal is to achieve these advantages while not incurring some of the potential disadvantages of this structure. The potential disadvantages include the following:

- *Members within a function can become insulated from the rest of the organization.* The horizon within a functional group becomes the function. Cardiologists, for example, will have a tendency to look at the practice, hospital, or health system from the cardiology perspective, and human resource professionals will have their own functional perspective. This within-group perspective can lead to narrow thinking, poor communication, and focus on achieving functional performance instead of focusing on overall organizational (practice, hospital, health system) goals. For example, the information systems group develops information systems that meet its own needs regarding capital acquisition cost, maintenance budget, software budget, staffing, and functionality, but doesn't fully meet user (physicians, nurses, administrators, patients, etc.) needs.
- *There may be a tendency for "buck-passing."* Because no single function is responsible for a complete product, failure often results in everyone pointing a finger at another function. Pulmonology's failure to meet performance criteria may result in

this department blaming information systems for producing misleading or incomplete outcome data reports and contracting with local coal mines. No one is willing to take responsibility, because no one really *has* responsibility for the *overall* product.

In a functional structure, the ability of the CEO to integrate across functions to prevent suboptimization, and the willingness of the functional unit heads to think and act beyond their functions become critical to organizational success.

When the product mix or geographical dispersion of an organization creates too many integration problems in a functional design, a divisional design is an alternative. **Figure 9–4** shows a simplified[1] organization chart for the General Hospital system. You can refer to some of the components, such as Hospital Services, Senior Services, HealthNet, and Insurance Products as companies, because they have a functional structure within them, as denoted by the marketing (M), finance (F), and contracting functions (C). Since hospital services, insurance products, senior services, and primary care services are so different from each other, they require a degree of specialization in order for each to function effectively. There also may be regulatory and professional reasons to keep some of the companies, such as Insurance Products and HealthNet Outpatient Care as separate distinct organizations, with their own functional structures.

To illustrate this point further, consider the archetype of divisional organizations: General Motors Corporation. Why have a Chevrolet Division, Cadillac Division, Saturn Division, and so on? Consider the marketing problem for a moment. It certainly would be possible to have marketing people working back and forth across Cadillac, Chevrolet, and Saturn marketing projects. If, however, you want to get really good at

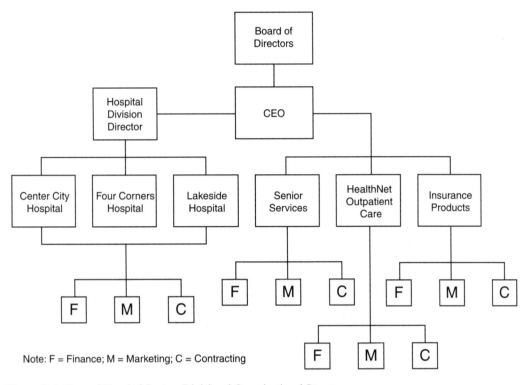

Note: F = Finance; M = Marketing; C = Contracting

**Figure 9–4** General Hospital System Divisional Organizational Structure.

marketing Cadillacs, you probably need to spend a lot of time understanding the Cadillac product and the Cadillac customer. The Cadillac customer is seeking different product attributes than the Chevrolet customer, and as noted, the key to successful marketing (product, place, price, and promotion) is knowing your customer and then developing a product or service to meet their specific needs. If you really want to get good at marketing Cadillacs, given the complexity and expense of marketing cars, you probably have to specialize in this product line. Repeating the functions across different product or geographical companies creates specialization and allows an organization with complex customer mixes[2] to match this complexity in its product mix. In a divisional structure, a whole product line or region is now an organizational unit, so the lines of responsibility also

are clearly established. If corporate is dissatisfied with Cadillac's productivity, it is clear where to look. Cadillac can't blame Chevrolet or Saturn. This structure, therefore, makes "buck passing" more difficult, because a unit has clear responsibility across all functions for a product or geographical area. Returning to Figure 9–4, note the separate divisions for hospital services, nursing home, insurance products, and primary care. Just as with General Motors, the products and services that each unit provides are so different that specialized marketing, finance, and contracting are necessary.

The potential disadvantage of this structure is that, once again, suboptimization may occur. In this case, however, the suboptimization may arise from the divisions themselves. Divisions may achieve their objectives at the expense of the organization. In the early 1980s, Cadillac tried to increase its sales by developing a "low-end" product. The Cimarron was a restyled Chevrolet Cavalier that sold for substantially less than other Cadillacs but about $4,000 more than the Cavalier. Not only was the Cimarron a poor product in terms of quality and design, but it also achieved some of its sales at the expense of Oldsmobile and Buick products. Thus, Cadillac's success was achieved to some degree at the expense of Olds and Buick. When the outpatient services division opens an outpatient surgical center that competes with the hospital division's inpatient surgical services, that also is suboptimization, if the net impact on the healthcare system is detrimental.

Finally, a divisional structure has a lot of potential for unneeded personnel and resources. If all the marketing personnel and their support equipment and systems across the several General Motors divisions were consolidated into one huge marketing function, it is likely that fewer positions, computers, secretaries, and water coolers would

be needed. It is likely, however, that marketing quality would suffer as a result of the lack of specialization, and the unwieldy size of the homogeneous marketing unit. The goal, of course, is to achieve the specialization that divisionalization can achieve without too much redundancy. The role of top management in a divisional structure is to coordinate the roles of the different divisions. Top management sets overall divisional goals, helps define product and service parameters, provides financial resources, and allocates them to the divisions. All this is done with the objective of minimizing both suboptimization and unnecessary duplication.

Some organizations have developed a structure that combines aspects of both functional and divisional structures into a matrix. **Figure 9–5** illustrates a matrix structure for an aircraft manufacturer. The columns contain the traditional functions of manufacturing, marketing, engineering, research and development, information technology, and human resources, and a functional director

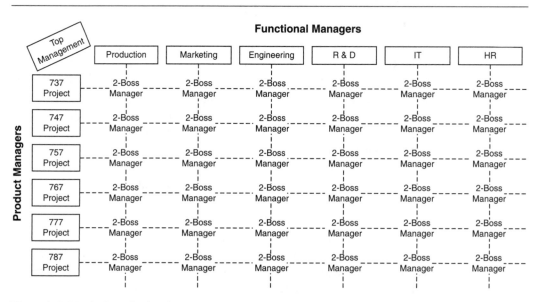

**Figure 9–5** Matrix Organizational Structure.

heads each. The rows represent the different aircraft projects that are underway, such as the 737, 747, and 757 projects, and a project director leads each project. Inside the matrix is the 2-Boss Manager, who reports to a functional director on a career basis, and a project director on an operational basis.

Each project director is responsible for a complete project across all functions. The project director, therefore, is market focused or *externally* focused meaning that he or she is focusing on producing the best possible product for the customer. Each functional director is responsible for a function across all projects. The functional director, therefore, is internally focused, and is concerned with the most efficient allocation and utilization of resources. Functional directors and the project directors are on the same organizational level, so consequently neither side of the matrix is superior or subordinate to the other. This means that for the organization to be successful both sides must cooperate.

For example, suppose a sales agent returns from southeast Asia with an opportunity to make a new sale of 737s. He or she needs some additional sales and marketing assistance to put together a proposal. The 737 project director, who is responsible for all aspects of the 737 project including sales, does not have the line authority to move marketing and sales personnel across projects. The functional marketing director is aware of all of the marketing resources and their scheduling across all of the projects. He is aware that the needed marketing resources could be drawn from the 747 and 777 projects. In order to do this, however, an agreement must be reached between the 737, 747, and 777 project directors. The skills required for success in this type of structure include being flexible, adaptable, and willing to look at a problem from a *corporate* perspective. Correspondingly, a project director who has the

attitude, "What's mine is mine," won't do well in this structure. The strength of a well-run matrix is that it simultaneously focuses on external market sensitivity and internal operational efficiency.

Notice that top management is totally *outside* the matrix. Top management should not resolve issues between the two sides of the matrix. To do so would remove the need for discussion, negotiation, and ultimately integration across the two sides of the matrix. If top management provides the solutions, then the name of the game becomes "get to top management first." Instead, top management's role is to provide organization strategic direction and financial resources, and to stay out of day-to-day operational decisions.

The downside of a matrix is that it adds complexity and requires additional skills. As noted, matrices require leaders and employees to be flexible, adaptable, and be able to effectively negotiate, all of which may necessitate training and development. In addition, they require dual reward, financial, and appraisal systems to create incentives for leaders to run their parts of the organization well, but also to focus on overall organizational success. All of this creates potential for confusion and questions of "who's in charge?" Poorly run matrixes can result in too much talk, too many meetings, and not enough action.

Matrix organizations require a high level of integration. Why create a structure that is so highly dependent on successful integration? The answer lies in the types of industries where matrixes have emerged. Generally, these industries utilize sophisticated, expensive technology that is in a constant state of change. To succeed, they must be constantly changing and redeploying their expensive resources and personnel to where they are most urgently needed. Aircraft manufacturing (Boeing), shipbuilding (Northrop Grumman

Newport News), and space exploration (National Aeronautics and Space Administration) are three industries that have successfully applied matrix structure concepts—health care is a fourth.

Many integrated healthcare systems need to pay close attention to operational efficiency, which can best be managed functionally. Clinical and business information systems, for example, need to be effectively managed across the entire organization. Human resources costs need to be controlled, and personnel need to be assigned to where they are most needed. Financial controls need to be applied across all programs and departments to create a level financial playing field. At the same time, rapid changes in medical technology, contracting, and the desires of patients create value in closely managing critical product and service lines so they are customer focused. For example,

coronary surgery, emergency department, oncology, maternity, insurance products, primary care, and hospital delivered services are product lines that are critical to a healthcare system's success in the marketplace. Someone needs to be paying undivided attention to each of these "profit centers." After all, patients and employers (i.e., customers) have no intrinsic interest in the underlying functional support systems. Their concern is with the medical service.

**Figure 9–6** illustrates a hospital matrix in which information systems, support services, cardiac services, and quality assurance (QA) cut across the major "product lines" of the health system's hospitals and outpatient physician services. Patients come to this organization for the services offered by the product lines, and the product line directors are therefore patient focused. They are interested in providing the most efficient highest

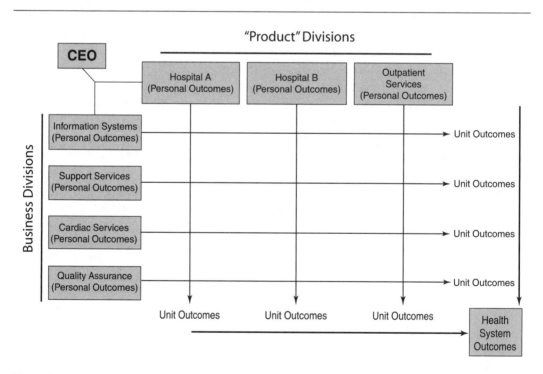

**Figure 9–6** Matrix Organizational Structure and Compensation Incentives.

quality services possible. If they are left to their own devices, however, they might create organization-wide inefficiencies (suboptimizations), such as redundant cardiac service facilities and standalone information systems that only meet local needs. The "row" directors are concerned with producing the most effective and efficient systems from a total organization perspective. QA, therefore, should provide system-wide procedures, evaluations, and guidance, but do it while being sensitive to the market focus and physician focus of Hospital A, Hospital B, and Outpatient Services. The reward, measurement, and support systems will be critical to the success of this matrix, because they are the systems that create the operational balance. See Figure 5–2 and the related discussion in Chapter 5 (Compensation) for a discussion of the motivational aspects of matrix designs. This matrix will have to be staffed with people who understand this integrated mission, and who are committed to it and responsive to the reward system. Consequently, employee selection and development become critical, so the right people with the right mindset staff the matrix.

**Figure 9–7** contains a matrix for the department of nursing at Abbott Northwestern Hospital. Notice, once again, that each side of the matrix is attending to a different need. The columns are patient focused and the rows are system focused. Notice also, that this chart tells nothing about the rest of Abbott Northwestern's structure. Different parts of a larger organization can have a local structure that meets local needs. Matrix units, for example, can exist in an organization that is otherwise departmental, functional, or matrix.

If the healthcare organization is structured functionally, there may be little coordinated emphasis on realizing the potential of each

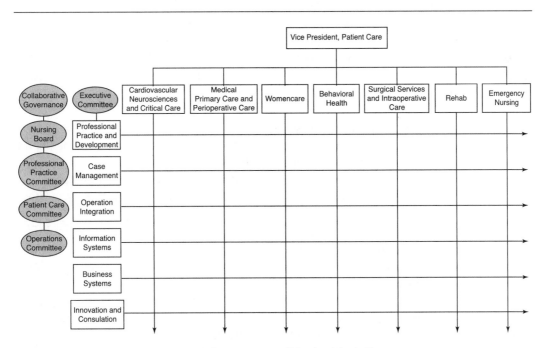

**Figure 9–7** Abbott Northwestern Hospital Department of Nursing Matrix Structure.
*Source:* Abbot Northwestern Hospital and VHA, Inc.

service line. Information systems may tend to be designed with the needs of the information systems staff (function) foremost. Alternatively, organizing only around products and services could easily result in overspending on resources and suboptimization across product and service lines, as each one tries to maximize its position in the organization through highly customized and duplicative functional spending. For example, why should oncology use the hospital's information system or electronic medical record if oncology can develop its own that will best serve oncology's needs? Without the control of a functional constituency, no one will say, "Hold it! We need to talk about this. Perhaps we can make it work better for you!" Under these circumstances, a matrix structure could offer some obvious strengths by simultaneously attending to both the functional and the product/service axes. This situation points out, however, that a matrix structure must be more than a drawing on a piece of paper. Critical to a matrix's success is that those on the matrix's sides and in the matrix must truly behave in an appropriate manner. Communication, negotiation, cooperation, a desire to achieve organizational goals (i.e., to act in an integrated manner) become essential. The key to achieving these behaviors are measurement and reward systems that create personal incentives to act in appropriate ways.

In summarizing all three structures, note that integration becomes a central concern for each one. What needs to be integrated varies with each structure. In a functional organization, integrating across functions is the challenge; in a divisional organization, the challenge is to integrate across divisions (products and locations). The challenge in a matrix organization is to integrate within and across functions and products/services. Understanding the type of structure that you have will help you identify where you need

to develop organizational integration. Finally, given the integration issues that you identify, you may want to consider changing the organizational structure to one that more directly complements the nature of your medical products and services.

## FACTORS INHIBITING INTEGRATION

You have seen that the nature of the organization's boundaries can either help or hinder integration. There also are other sources of inadequate integration. At a generic level, four additional factors that inhibit integration are:

1. *Complexity.* This occurs when there is a large volume of information that must be exchanged for integration to occur, but the support systems are not adequate. Because of the inadequate information exchange, two or more parts of the organization cannot optimally coordinate their actions. An example would be the coordination required to reduce waits for testing and special services in a hospital. Each unit, such as radiology, has its own schedule, as does the attending physician and the patients, based on where they are in their respective treatment protocols. Coordinating all this activity to reduce average patient waiting time is a complex data exchange and scheduling problem. As a result, it often doesn't occur effectively.

2. *Differentiation.* This occurs when different subunits in the organization have different values, attitudes, and behaviors. Differentiation can arise from a number of differences, including education, professional orientation, and goals. Historically, differentiated groups include physicians, administration, and nursing.

3. *Poor informal relations.* When differentiation goes on for an extended period of

time, a history of distrust and animosity can build, so that it takes on a life of its own. In some hospitals, for example, this has occurred between physicians and administration. Administrators assume that physicians simply don't understand their perspective on decision making, never will understand, and have no interest in understanding. As a result, physicians are viewed as adversaries, and often are not brought into the decision-making process. Similarly physicians can develop pessimistic attitudes toward administrators. This becomes part of the organization culture when new physicians, nurses, administrators, etc. are taught by "old-timers" about the evils of the other constituencies.

4. *Physical size and distance.* Obvious examples include a multiple hospital system with facilities and personnel spread across a region. Similarly, within a facility, the physical distances between patient beds, physician offices, laboratory, physical therapy, administration, and so on can inhibit integration. Information systems have great potential to reduce size and distance barriers. Electronic medical records, integrated clinical and financial databases, e-mail, local area networks of personal computers, personal digital assistants, and image digitizing and transmission all reduce this integration problem.

## INTEGRATION MECHANISMS

There are a number of standard approaches to overcoming integration barriers that are applicable to healthcare organizations. These are summarized in **Exhibit 9–1**. Probably the most basic approach to integration is to establish a management hierarchy. In effect, you create a job whose responsibility is to create integration. For example, the position of medical support director in Figure 9–2 has responsibility for coordinating across laboratory,

pharmacy, radiology, and physical therapy. When the amount of work that managers must do to integrate becomes too great, they can be "extended" by adding staff positions. The staff's role is to work with the organization units, gather information, report back to the integrating manager, and to help the integrating manager and each unit coordinate with the others.

Rules and procedures are an effective integration strategy when integration is required around routine matters. Establish a rule, for example, that says "Whenever antivenin inventory reaches 35 percent of nominal, contact purchasing to order more" or "Whenever an account goes into 90 days past current, audit it and take some action within two business days." **Figure 9–8** illustrates a patient flow process for diagnosis-related group (DRG) 209 that integrates the functions that need to be coordinated if the DRG is to be treated in an efficient and effective manner. Similarly, critical pathways can be considered as sophisticated integration methods.

Goals and plans are another integration tool. A hospital system's management services organization (MSO) sets a goal of improving its competitiveness for acquiring contracts with large regional employers in 8 months. The MSO determines that it will do the following to achieve this goal:

- Train physicians to understand how they affect financial outcomes.
- Train reception staff to send triage patient calls to appropriate levels.
- Acquire contracting and cost projection software.
- Train employees and physicians in the use of the software and the assumptions that it makes.
- Develop a patient education process, so that patients will understand when to call, thereby eliminating many unneeded office visits.

**Exhibit 9–1** Integration Methods

| Tactic | Advantages | Disadvantages |
|---|---|---|
| Management Hierarchy | Links together all of the organization's functional parts. | Can become overloaded and can break down. Not very flexible or easily changeable. Narrow span of control can create bureaucratic complexity and slow down decision making. |
| Staff | Can supplement hierarchy and help it to perform more integration. Easily changeable. | Cost. Also can create its own integration challenges. |
| Rules & Procedures | Economical way to achieve integration around routine issues. | Limited to routine issues. Can't handle complexity. Heavy use can create dysfunctional outcomes. |
| Plans & Goals | Can handle nonroutine issues that rules and procedures cannot. | Cost in time and effort. Can be too static for a dynamic environment. |
| Meetings, Committees, Task Forces | Can deal with a large number of unpredictable problems and decisions. | Cost in personnel time. People involved need skills in group decision making. |
| Integrating Roles | Can deal with a large number of unpredictable problems and decisions. | Can be difficult to find people with the right characteristics to fill this role. Requires effective personal influence skills. |
| Measurement & Reward Systems | Can self-motivate behavior directed at integration. | Unmeasured activities or outcomes will be ignored or undermined. Can produce dysfunctional or suboptimized outcomes. |
| Selection & Development Systems | Acquires or develops integration skills in personnel who are already valuable for their functional or product line skills. | Can be expensive and time consuming. |
| Information Systems | Insensitive to physical distances. Dynamic and changeable. Can address all sorts of integration challenges. | Financially costly. Can become an integration challenge itself if not designed with all users in mind. Security issues. |
| Changing Departmentalization | | |
| *Functional* | Facilitates integration within functions. | Does not facilitate integration across functions. |
| *Divisional (Market, Product, Geography)* | Promotes integration within and among functions inside each market, product, geography area. | Does not promote integration between each market/product/geography area. |
| *Matrix* | Promotes integration between each side of the matrix thereby integrating functional and market, product, geography units. | Expensive. Can generate conflict and tension. Requires highly developed interpersonal, communication, and negotiation skills. |

*Source:* Adapted with permission from P.F. Schlesinger, et al. (1992). *Organization: Text, Cases, and Readings on the Management of Organizational Design and Change.* Burr Ridge, IL: Richard F. Irwin, pg. 119.

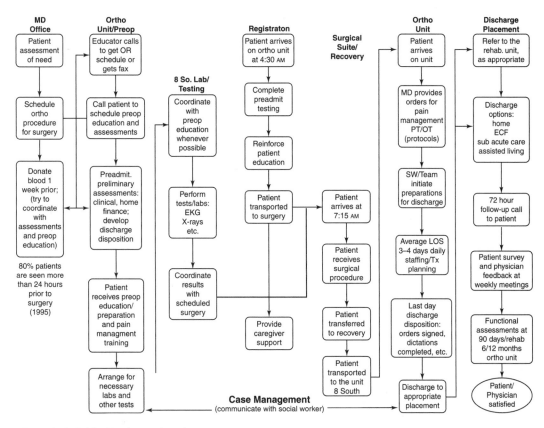

**Figure 9–8** Critical Pathway Flowchart.
*Source:* Courtesy of Memorial Health Systems, South Bend, IN.

Setting the goal has increased integration. For instance, physicians who understand the business aspects of their medical decisions are more likely to practice in a manner consistent with the assumptions being made in the projection software. Similarly, those working with the software will be more likely to make reasonable assumptions if they work with business-knowledgeable physicians during the model building phase. By establishing these integrated goals, the physician services office begins training physicians in the business aspects of medicine. Simultaneously, the information systems unit begins evaluating managed care decision support software.

Committees and task forces can be effective ways of using current staff to make integrated decisions. By drawing physicians and administrators from various medical specialties and management functions across the healthcare organization to staff a committee, you can bring a wide range of perspectives to the table. Figure 9–3 illustrates a multispecialty practice that uses committees as part of its standard structure. Committees and task forces also provide flexibility because, by their nature, they are temporary structures. A task force is a temporary grouping of personnel who are given a specific goal to achieve. After the goal has been reached, the task force is dissolved. Sometimes task forces are referred to as project teams. Once again, this is a temporary unit that will be dissolved after the mission has been accomplished. They can expand and contract in size, add members to bring in additional relevant constituencies and skills, and even go away if the need for them no longer exists. Often, physicians feel that committee work is frustrating and inefficient. When contrasted with the alternative of creating a full-time position or positions to do the work of the committee, it can be an efficient, low-cost option.

Integrating roles are usually used when integration is difficult to achieve but is nevertheless very important. Generally, integrating roles have no direct authority over the areas to be integrated. This prevents "railroading." Instead, integration is achieved through personal influence and leadership skills. Often, the physician staff office in a hospital system performs this function. Another approach to using integrating roles is to create a project manager position to integrate services across a product line. An oncology project manager could, for example, integrate all inpatient and outpatient oncology services across a healthcare system. This position's perspective would cut across professions, specialties, and organizational units with the goal of improving the cost and quality of oncology services. If this position becomes permanent, then the structure has evolved into a matrix.

Measurement and reward systems are two of the most powerful integration tools. The goal is to assess personnel and subunits based on their cooperation and achievement of joint goals. Giving employed physicians incentives that are congruent with healthcare system goals, such as lower costs and improved clinical outcomes is one example of how a reward system can integrate two parts of the organization. It is important to carefully consider the nature of the incentives to

individuals. Assume that whatever is not measured won't occur. Providing rewards without thinking about the *system* effects can foster suboptimization. Independently rewarding physicians based on outcomes, laboratories on reduced turnaround time, and administrators on lowered costs, without considering how these measurement and reward systems may interact can create a suboptimized outcome.

Selection and development systems are long-term approaches to improving integration. Managers and physicians can be selected based in part on whether they have the interpersonal skills and attitude necessary to work cooperatively. Similarly, providing team development and employee development training can improve current employees' integration skills. Promotion across functional lines and systematic job rotation across functional or divisional lines are two commonly used ways to develop employees' abilities to think in integrated terms. Physicians, nurses, pharmacists, and others with clinical experience who acquire business skills (marketing, financial management, etc.) can make excellent managers, because they can see both the business and medical aspects of a problem.

Information systems, such as electronic medical records, and integrated medical and financial databases can easily overcome distance problems. In addition, they provide a substantial increase in the ability to integrate across the medical/business boundary.

Finally, you can modify organizational boundaries to include interdependencies. Patient-centered units in which diagnostic and treatment facilities are located under unit control can increase the integrated delivery of services. Moving from a functional structure to a divisional structure based on medical services increases the integration around the service. Often, the move from a functional to a divisional structure is a result of increased size and the need to specialize in the delivery of services. As healthcare systems grow in size and diversity of products and services, the evolution into a divisional structure is an appropriate response. For healthcare systems that have particularly important integration issues across both function and product/ service lines, adopting a matrix structure may be an appropriate response.

## SMALL PRACTICE STRUCTURES

The challenge of integration also applies to small practices. The structural choices available to small healthcare providers, however, are different. Solo physicians or very small private practices sometimes adopt a simple structure. This structure is often *so* simple that none of the participants perceive that there is any structure at all! Quite simply, everyone reports to the physician manager. As a result, the physician manager becomes the focus of all the upward and downward practice communication. If Joanne, a secretary, has a problem that she can't resolve herself, Dr. Smith, the physician manager, is the one she will contact. Dr. Smith then will have to do something about it, even if it is nothing more than telling Joanne to work it out with one of the other secretaries. This type of structure can provide the physician manager with a lot of information about daily practice operations, especially if the physician manager is willing to listen to employees and they feel that the physician manager is responsive to reasonable requests.

One of the primary responsibilities of the physician manager in the simple structure is integration. The physician manager becomes personally responsible for making certain that employees' contributions fit together, so that the totality of their efforts results in a smooth-running, coordinated, and produc-

tive office. The problem with this scenario is that it takes too much physician time. An alternative is the office manager structure (**Figure 9–9**). In this structure, the office manager takes over some of the management responsibilities that were previously assumed by the physician manager, and performs the front-line management tasks. In effect, this is the simplest of functional organizations. The office manager directs the daily activities of office staff, sets priorities, implements standard office policies, and coordinates the efforts of the front office to produce integrated, effective group performance. The physician manager's management role is to supervise the office manager, focus on long-term planning, and assist the office manager in problem solving and procedure revision on more significant front office issues.

Effective communication between the physician manager and the office manager is essential to the success of this structure. Weekly meetings often form the basis for vertical integration between the physician manager and the office manager. For example, if the accounting reports indicate that expenditures for supplies seem to be rising, the physician manager would ask the office manager to determine the reasons why and discuss and propose solutions. The office

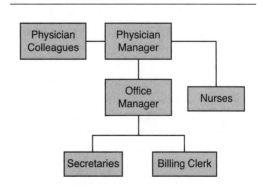

**Figure 9–9** Office Manager Structure.

manager would be responsible for implementing changes and keeping the physician manager informed of progress made in controlling these expenditures. The structure in Figure 9–9 depicts the physician manager as representing his or her physician colleagues, and serving as a buffer between the other physicians and business operations.

If the office manager is not capable of making decisions that are generally consistent with the physician manager's management philosophy, you will find yourself micromanaging and constantly reviewing your office manager's daily decisions. You effectively will be operating as though there were no office manager, yet you will be paying a salary for one! In addition, the office manager will come to resent the micromanagement, and the office manager's subordinates will realize that he or she is a figurehead. All this will tend to create dissension and dissatisfaction. This scenario points out the need for employees to have the right skills to operate with the level of independence required by the structure. If you find yourself in the position of reviewing all of an office manager's decisions, you should ask yourself some hard questions, such as these:

- Are you perhaps too perfectionistic?
- Are you able to recognize that there may be more than one effective solution to a problem?
- Is it possible that the office manager's solutions to problems could be as effective as your solutions?

If, after sincerely considering these questions, you conclude that the problem lies with the office manager, then you need a new office manager. Unfortunately, with this type of practice structure, you may not notice that the details are going unattended until a major problem develops. The delegation of power and authority through an office manager

structure can provide you with great power, because it effectively multiplies your presence. Unfortunately, delegation is a double-edged sword that can wound you seriously if your office manager is inadequate.

The office manager structure suffices for many private practices. Larger practices, however, will find it necessary to evolve additional structural elements to deal with the complexity and quantity of information in such functional areas as marketing, information systems, collection, billing, and human resources. In effect, they evolve into fully developed functional structures.

As functional structures in practices grow, partners often take responsibility for supervising one or more functions. One physician might take on quality management, another assumes responsibility for leadership in human resources, another oversees financial issues, and so forth. By dividing the management responsibilities in this manner, the partners achieve two objectives: they reduce the amount of time that each partner devotes to practice management, so that no one is unduly burdened, and each partner develops a relative degree of expertise in one or two functional areas, with the result that the practice as a whole acquires more total management expertise.

When physicians functionally specialize, it is important for them to integrate across functions. On occasion, the partners should meet with the objective of achieving integration. Each partner should familiarize the others with what is happening in his or her functional area of responsibility. These meetings also should focus on integrated goal setting for the functional areas. Often, one physician will act as a managing partner, making daily business decisions and chairing the cross-functional partner meetings. If the physicians rotate their supervision, such as every 18 months or 2 years, over time physician leadership will develop a great deal of skill, depth, and flexibility on business issues. Through job rotation, they will come to see business problems from different functional perspectives, which will allow them to make more balanced business decisions.

## Integrating Acquisitions

A healthcare system acquires a hospital in a neighboring city. Several gastroenterology practices merge to form one larger and hopefully stronger practice. These are both examples of a trend in healthcare, which began in the 1980s and continues to this day. Providers coalesce into larger organizations. One reason for this, which was discussed in Chapter 1, relates to the issue of cost. *Theoretically*, larger organizations can make better use of their fixed costs due to potential economies of scale and their ability to fully utilize them. In addition, their purchasing power should allow them to reduce variable costs by buying in larger volumes and eliciting lower prices through more competition from vendors. By reducing costs, larger organizations should be able to offer lower prices, which should generate higher volume, and still create a profit. As many, however, have experienced (see United Family Practices Ltd.: Appendix 6–A), the potential efficiencies of larger organizations often fail to materialize, because they fail to integrate the parts of the organization, so they don't become more effective than the sum of their separate parts.

Integration of acquisitions creates special challenges in addition to those that normally occur within an existing organization. Often, the acquired hospital or practice has a past history of competition with the acquiring organization. Similarly, organizational cultures often clash. Organizational culture is a somewhat imprecise term, which nevertheless captures some vital issues. It is the pattern of values, assumptions, expectations, and beliefs that characterize an organization. Edgar Schein has defined it as:

> . . . a pattern of basic assumptions— invented, discovered, or developed by a given group as it learns to cope with problems of external adaptation and internal integration—that has worked well enough to be considered valid and, therefore, to be taught to new members as the correct way to perceive, think, and feel in relation to those problems.[3]

One company in particular stands out as a successful integrator. GE Capital, a subsidiary of GE, has integrated over 100 acquisitions into its organizational structure. As a consequence, they have developed integration best practices, so that integration can be a replicable process. These best practices can be summarized into six integration principles.[4]

1. *Begin the integration process as soon as possible.* GE Capital actually starts during the due diligence phase.[5] Their experience was that considering integration issues during due diligence was helpful in deciding whether to proceed with the deal. Operationally, what this means is that planning for integration should take place *prior* to actually signing the papers. This will result in putting the integration plan into effect sooner than if no planning is completed until after the acquisition occurs.

2. *Integration management is a full-time job.* Because integration is an ongoing process and not a stage in the acquisition, someone must manage it. Although there may be a team of executives focusing on aspects of the acquisition—HR, clinical integration, and IT—one person must be

responsible to be certain that all parts of the integration are successful across *all* functions and *all* business lines. This is best achieved by giving this job to one person and then holding him or her accountable for integration results.

3. *Make key decisions soon.* Being acquired often means that employees' jobs will change, some will no longer have jobs, and for the survivors of the acquisition, life as they know it will be different. The uncertainty and anxiety created by an acquisition can be debilitating. Employees may spend their time worrying about the future instead of doing their jobs well now and working hard to integrate into the new organization. It is best to decisively make the necessary changes sooner versus later. Because most acquisitions involve restructuring, it is important to do this soon and let people know if they will still have a job. There will never be a "right time" for this message, so don't try to find it. By making the decisions sooner, you change the focus from a debilitating fear about what might happen, to actively working on the future.

4. *Make decisions with respect.* Be straightforward with employees. When decisions have been made, let them know. If you don't know the answers to questions, then say, "We don't know" or "We will have an answer by . . .." Use outplacement, severance pay, and other ways to make the transition easier. It is the ethical thing to do, and it also conveys a very powerful and important message to those employees you will retain. It says that you treat people fairly and with respect.

5. *Integrate technical systems and organizational cultures.* It's clear that technical systems such as medical information systems, accounting systems, and purchasing procedures need to be integrated.

Organizational cultures also need to be integrated. GE Capital does this through frequent meetings in which employees from both organizations are encouraged to discuss the positive aspects of their company and to brainstorm how these could be used to improve the new organization. There is an emphasis on openly discussing organizational values and standards. For example, a hospital with a reputation for very physician-centric values and culture acquired one with a reputation for very patient-centric values and culture[6]. Integration efforts focused on each group verbalizing exactly what these values meant on a day-to-day operational basis. In reality, there were many commonalities with a few substantial differences. This helped the acquired employees to understand where their world would remain the same, where it would differ, and identified some areas for the acquiring hospital to consider changing its procedures.

6. *Integrate around short-term projects.* This is consistent with the discussion of change management methods (Chapter 6) in which Rapid Cycle Improvement is used to introduce change. Focus groups and team meetings that discuss organizational values and integration objectives are necessary places to begin integration, but ultimately people start acting in integrated ways and really learn what this means when they have to do something. Get people working together on projects with important business purposes (not make work) and with defined near-term completion schedules.

## CONCLUSION

The "take away" from this chapter for both physicians in private practice and those working in healthcare systems is to ask three questions:

1. What information must be communicated across the organization in order to achieve clinical, business, or other important outcomes?
2. Who (persons, groups, teams, organizational units) needs to work together effectively in order to achieve clinical, business, or other important outcomes?
3. Are there organizational barriers that are impeding the communication of this information or the cooperation of these persons, groups, teams, or organizational units?

The answers to these questions will identify the integration challenges that you face. The methods discussed in the chapter provide tools to address these integration challenges. Integration issues, however, generally can't be segregated to just this context. Additional relevant considerations include how you address the situation as a leader, and how you address resistance to change through change management methods. Both leadership and change management are discussed in Chapter 6. The Northeast HealthCare case in Appendix 9–A illustrates the interrelationship between leadership, change management, and integration considerations. Please read this case before proceeding.

## NORTHEAST HEALTHCARE CASE ANALYSIS

Nutmeg, Northeast HealthCare, and clinic managements have two barriers to overcome. First, what is the best way to make the case for the merger, so the physicians will vote to do this? Second, once the merger is agreed upon, how is the integration actually achieved? Recall the United Family Practices case. They merged, but they didn't successfully integrate,

and this was the challenge facing Dr. Anderson. The immediate challenge at Northeast HealthCare relates to some of the barriers to integration discussed in the case. The business case can be made in a logical rational way focusing on marketing and financial issues, but pushback should be anticipated around the issue of differentiation. The Lyme Clinic has a strong osteopathic tradition. The Norwich Clinic is multispecialty, while the other two are primary care. Some of these differences may be substantial enough to be classified as "poor informal relations." In addition they currently have no meaningful electronic links through databases or other automated information exchange. This could be addressed in the future, but for now this is a barrier. Many of the physicians don't fully trust clinical information systems, and some may oppose the merger if they see this as an inevitable consequence.

The managerial skills to address these questions were discussed in Chapter 6. The leader participation model suggests that clinic leadership approach these issues using a facilitative approach, meaning that they actively participate in discussions, educational seminars, and all other forms of communication with the physicians prior to the vote. Appropriate change management methods include creating urgency, utilizing a broad-based change implementation team, developing and concretely expressing a vision of what the future practice would be capable of, acting assertively by aggressively communicating the reasons for change to the physicians, and decisively addressing resistors' positions. Some short-term wins might be achieved on easily achievable clinical integration projects prior to the vote.

If the merger resolution passes, then the integration methods in Exhibit 9–1 are a good checklist of ways to achieve this goal. First, consider management hierarchy and the basis for departmentalization. What are the best ways to structure the new practice so that working relationships are contained within organizational boundaries versus across them? Creative use of goals and plans, as well as linking successful completion to reward systems (measurement and reward systems) are powerful ways of using self-interest to integrate. Information systems will be necessary to take advantage of the new structure, but they also should be designed so that they further clinical and business outcomes. Finally, long-term, selecting physicians and staff (selection and development systems) who are more inclined to work effectively as part of an integrated team, and developing physicians' leadership and business skills, as well as their ability to develop integrated clinical system (TQM, best practices, and critical pathways) will "make the change stick," which was the final change objective described in Chapter 6 and Exhibit 6–3.

## NOTES

1. The real organization chart would show many more functional units, some of which would be unique to each division, such as laboratory, radiology, and pharmacy within the hospital division.
2. Meaning that the customers are looking for very different kinds of products or services.
3. Schein, E. (1985). *Organizational Culture and Leadership*. San Francisco: Jossey-Bass, p. 9.
4. Ashkenas, R., L. DeMonaco, & S. Francis. (1998). Making the deal real: How GE Capital integrates acquisitions. *Harvard Business Review*, January–February: 165–178.
5. This is a phase in an acquisition during which an acquiring organization can examine the financial records and internal operations of the prospective acquired organization to determine whether assertions and financial records are truthful. If the acquired organization's financial information, for example, is not correct or is misleading, then the acquiring organization can back out of the deal. Depending on the terms of the due diligence, the acquiring organization may have to pay a financial penalty to terminate the acquisition.
6. Personal communication.
7. This is not the real name of this healthcare system. Similarly, the names of the institute, clinics, and medical corporations have been changed to provide anonymity.

# Northeast HealthCare

Northeast HealthCare[7] is composed of several large hospitals and affiliations with regional groups of outpatient and multispecialty practices. Outpatient services are provided through institutes, which are really umbrella organizations for physician groups, which actually provide the patient service (**Figure 9A–1**). For example, the Nutmeg Medical Institute provides primary and multispecialty care through the Lyme, Suffolk, and Norwich Medical Clinics. These three medical clinics are owned by their member physicians, and nominally report to the medical director in the Nutmeg Medical Institute. The Nutmeg medical director has no "line control" over the clinics, which means that the only way he or she can affect the clinics actions is through personal influence. The Nutmeg Medical Institute employs the staff and owns the hard assets used by each of the clinics, and these are organized into the Lyme, Suffolk, and Norwich Medical Corporations.

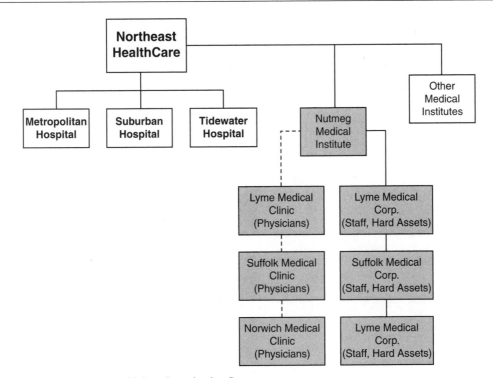

**Figure 9A–1** Northeast HealthCare Organization Structure.

The Nutmeg Medical Institute is a not-for-profit business, and the medical clinics are for profit. This working arrangement has endured since the 1960s.

The healthcare environment is changing. Pressures to assess and improve clinical outcomes, reduce duplication, leverage capital assets and fixed costs, improve clinical and business efficiency and effectiveness, and retain more referrals within the Northeast HealthCare system are all creating pressure to increase clinical and business integration. In addition, MassCare, a very large regional healthcare system with an international reputation, a successful record of offering a wide range of insurance products (HMO, PPO, POS), world-class quaternary hospitals, and leading regional tertiary hospitals is beginning to purchase and develop contractual relationships with primary and multispecialty practices in Northeast's market area. MassCare views Northeast HealthCare's geographic region as a new source of patients to feed to its high-reputation hospitals.

The Nutmeg Medical Institute is proposing to the Lyme, Suffolk, and Norwich Medical Clinics that they merge. If they can do this, then they would potentially achieve several benefits:

- Improve clinical outcomes—their size would make it more feasible to establish true programs of excellence and compete for greater market share. As one practice they would be able to identify and adopt best practices, develop local standards of care, and have the resources to adopt quality improvement methods.
- Improve financial outcomes—reduce administrative duplication, develop and implement business system best practices, increase revenues through programs of excellence, and develop a focused brand.
- Increase control—as a larger organization, the physicians would be more influential in the Northeast decision-making process.

Because its member physicians own each of the medical clinics, a merger would require a majority vote of each of the clinics. Nutmeg Institute's leaders and Northeast HealthCare's leaders strongly believe that a merger is in everyone's best interest. They have begun discussions with the leadership of each of the medical clinics about merging.

# CHAPTER 10

# Business Law

## Chapter Objectives

This chapter will provide you with an understanding of fundamental business law concepts. As a result, you will be able to prevent disputes, avoid lawsuits, and anticipate the legal consequences of your actions. Physicians may be concerned about legal exposure that is unique to their status as physicians, such as medical malpractice, kickbacks, and the Stark Law. In addition to these, physicians and their organizations also have legal exposure to litigation, as would any other person or business.

This chapter is organized around the following potential sources of liability or conflict:

1. Torts
2. Contracts
3. Employment issues, including equal employment opportunity, employee contracts, contractor agreements, and the Fair Labor Standards Act
4. Malpractice, which is a particular type of tort
5. Kickbacks

After reading this chapter, you will understand how the legal system approaches these potential sources of litigation. As a result, you will be able to conduct your daily affairs with due consideration to their possible legal implications.

Americans are living in an increasingly litigious society. Many explanations have been offered for this, including a declining respect for authority, an ever-increasing number of lawyers, a rise in consumerism, and an evolving interpretation of what constitutes negligence. As a physician, your relationships with your patients expose you to the risk of malpractice litigation. As a physician manager, your organization's arrangements and dealings with insurance companies, landlords, suppliers, employees, contractors, partners, and so on all have potential legal ramifications.

Legal considerations are best handled in anticipation of events. If you are aware of the potential legal consequences of an action, then you often can avoid a legal confrontation or, at a minimum, place yourself in a more favorable legal position. This strategy is called *preventive law*, and it is analogous to preventive medicine. By eliminating or minimizing problems before they occur, you may avoid the courtroom and all the expense and personal disruption that are associated with this ultimate form of decision making. This chapter will help you recognize when you are entering territory with legal implications. In addition, by understanding the legal aspects of your actions, you will be able to communicate more effectively with your attorney. You should, of course, consult your attorney regarding situations with obvious legal implications, such as a contract, lease, or employment dispute. There will be many daily situations, however, in which understanding the principles of law will allow you to make good operational decisions to avoid litigation exposure, as well as help you determine when you should involve your attorney.

Legal problems can arise from a number of different sources. When a wrong has been committed that harms a person, this person can seek to recover monetary damages from the wrongdoer. If the harm was committed through the breach of a contract, then contract law governs the process. For example, if you have a contract with a cleaning service and you feel that its performance is inadequate, then your recourse will be governed by the content of the contract, and how contracts are interpreted under contract law. When there is no contract, then the wronged party may seek recovery under tort law. For example, if a patient or member of the general public happens to fall in your parking lot, he or she may seek to recover damages under tort law, because there is no contract between the two of you. Employment and malpractice cases are, respectively, specific types of contract and tort cases. For example, contract law will govern firing an employee who has a contract with the practice. Tort law generally governs malpractice cases, although some cases are filed as a breach of contract between the patient and the physician.

**Figure 10–1** outlines the general structure of U.S. law. Statutory law is the result of statutes enacted by state legislatures, ordinances enacted by municipalities, and laws passed by Congress. Common law, derives from the decisions of judges:

> Common law . . . makes itself up as it goes along; it sets precedents but they are never unalterable, because they are derived ultimately, not from a book of rules, but from a judge's intuitive feeling for equity

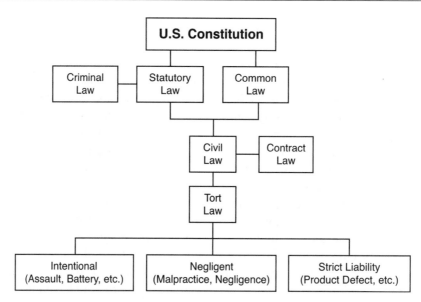

**Figure 10–1**  The U.S. System of Laws.

and fair play. . . . Common law assumes a freely developing pattern that is nevertheless consistent with itself, like the development of a living language.[1]

Criminal law protects society's interest in order, safety, and the integrity of its institutions by defining and prohibiting unacceptable behavior. By definition, criminal law is statutory because it derives from the actions of legislatures and Congress. Civil law also protects society's interests, but it does so by defining the rights and obligations of one person or business vis-à-vis another. Civil law can be constitutional, statutory, or common (case or case based). Kickbacks can be a violation of either criminal law (Medicaid Anti-Kickback Statute 42 U.S.C. §1320a-7b), civil law (Stark Law 42 U.S.C. Section 1395nn), or both.

## GENERAL TORTS

### Definition

A *tort* is a civil wrong that has been committed against another party or another party's property, but is not due to a breach of contract. A tort is distinct from a crime, which is an intentionally harmful act that is committed against society. As a result, individuals bring tort actions, whereas crimes are prosecuted by the state. Those responsible for a tort are referred to as *tortfeasors*; those responsible for a crime are referred to as *criminals*. An act can result in both a tort and a crime, as exemplified by the O.J. Simpson cases. Simpson was prosecuted by the state under criminal law, and by the injured parties under tort law. It also is possible for there to be a crime with no tort, such as the case of a physician who misrepresents his or her personal property assets to the local tax collector in an attempt to reduce tax liability. Because no individual has been harmed,

there is no tort. Finally, there can be a tort with no crime. For example, if a patient inadvertently takes the wrong coat from a waiting room, this is the tort of conversion. This is not a crime, however, because the motivation necessary for theft is absent.

### Liability

The simple fact that a person is harmed or injured does not in itself mean that a tort has occurred. For a tort to occur, there has to be a basis for liability. The following considerations can be used to establish a basis for liability.

### Voluntary Action

The tortfeasor's voluntary actions or voluntary failure to act must have contributed to the harm. Actions resulting from immediate peril or fear generally are considered involuntary acts. For example, if you jump back at the sight of a snake and inadvertently strike another person, the action would probably be considered involuntary.

### Intent

Some torts require the demonstration of intent, whereas other torts do not. In tort law, the issue of intent relates to whether the tortfeasor intended to commit the act, not whether harm was intended to the other party. To prove intent, it is necessary to demonstrate that the actor either knew or believed that certain results were likely to follow his or her actions. This knowledge is determined on an objective basis, meaning what a reasonable person would be expected to know or would expect to occur under the circumstances. The following example illustrates the role of intent:

> As a practical joke, Jack pulls a chair out from under Jill as she begins to sit, causing

her to fall and sustain a hip fracture. Although Jack actually meant Jill no harm, a court could reasonably find that he knew with substantial certainty that Jill would attempt to sit down where the chair had been and could fall and be injured. Hence, Jack had the knowledge required to support a finding of intent for tort liability. His intent was to do an act that he could have reasonably foreseen would cause injury to another.[2]

## Causation

For a tort to be sustained, it must be demonstrated that there was a causal relationship between the wrongful act and the harm. State laws vary regarding how directly the act must be related to the harm for causation to be demonstrated. The following example illustrates how the causal chain can become extended:

> George Nesselrode was a passenger in an airplane made by Beechcraft Aircraft Corporation. A few minutes after taking off, the plane crashed and all occupants were killed. Action was brought by George's widow against Beechcraft on the theory that it was at fault in failing to prevent the improper installation of certain parts in its airplanes, in consequence of which the parts could be installed in reverse or backwards, and this improper installation had caused the fatal crash. . . .
>
> Judgment [was] against Beechcraft Aircraft Corp. Although no harm would have occurred if third persons had not made an improper installation, the fact remained that the prior failure of Beechcraft to give proper warning was a substantial factor in bringing about the harm. It therefore could not claim that the installation was an act that broke the causal chain. As a substantial contributing factor, the manufacturer was liable even though the wrong installation was the proximate cause and was the act of a third person.[3]

Notice that motivation is largely irrelevant, other than perhaps as a way of demonstrating intent.

## CLASSIFICATION

Torts can be classified into three basic groups:

1. Intentional torts result from intended acts, such as assault, battery, malicious prosecution, and defamation.
2. Negligence torts result from unintended acts, such as negligence and malpractice.
3. Strict liability torts result from a liability regardless of fault or culpability. Examples include product liability cases in which the manufacturer is held strictly responsible for defective goods. For example, if a piece of glass is found in a can of soda, the manufacturer would be held strictly liable for any personal injuries suffered regardless of how the glass got in the bottle.

The following discussion elaborates on some of the torts that a physician might reasonably encounter, as either the victim or the tortfeasor.

## INTENTIONAL TORTS

### Assault

*Assault* is an act (more than words) that creates the apprehension of an immediate harmful contact. The important elements for demonstrating assault are the tortfeasor's action, his or her intent, the perception of fear or apprehension on the part of the assaulted person, and the causal relationship between the assaulted person's fear and the tortfeasor's actions. For example, Mr. Smith is dissatisfied with Dr. Jones's services. He confronts Dr. Jones and points an unloaded pistol at her while threatening to shoot. Assault has occurred because Smith committed an act that a reasonable person would assume would create fear or apprehension whether or not the gun was actually loaded. Dr. Jones had those fears, and they were the proximate result of Smith's actions.

## Battery

*Battery* is intentional, unjustified touching of another person's body. The contact does not have to cause actual physical harm. Battery has occurred even if the action is only offensive or insulting. For example, Dr. Brown intentionally and without consent unjustifiably kisses and fondles Ms. Arnold. Even though no physical harm is done to Ms. Arnold, a battery has taken place. Defenses against assault and battery suits include consent and privilege. Consent exists if the allegedly wronged party implied or expressly stated that the actions were permissible. Privilege might exist if the alleged tortfeasor acted in self-defense or in the defense of others or of property. The level of force must be reasonable given the circumstances and cannot be retaliatory.

## Intentional Infliction of Emotional Distress

This involves disturbing someone's peace of mind through outrageous behavior. The words or actions must be exceedingly severe, otherwise, torts could be claimed based on fictitious psychological damage. Physicians could be exposed to a suit through overly aggressive bill collection procedures that might include abusive or insulting language and threats of violence. Sexual harassment also can result in this tort.

## Invasion of Privacy

This is an infringement of the right to be left alone. Invasions of privacy fall into four categories. The first is intrusion into another person's private affairs or solitude. The second is disclosure of private, embarrassing facts. The third is publication of information about someone that places the person in a false light. The fourth is the unauthorized use of someone's name or likeness for commercial purposes. For example, a physician can become exposed to an invasion of privacy suit by revealing confidential information about a patient to a third party (e.g., a social acquaintance at a party or even a professional colleague if a proper release has not been obtained from the patient).

## Abusive Discharge

This tort occurs when an employee who does not have a written contract is discharged for a reason that violates public policy. For example, Dr. Wilson discharges Ms. Blakely because she has become pregnant and he fears that her attendance and job performance will deteriorate. This violation of public policy regarding sexual discrimination could be prosecuted under the equal employment laws and as a tort by Ms. Blakely.

## Disparagement or Trade Libel

This occurs when there are false, injurious statements made about a competitor's reputation. This tort injures the business reputation of the victim and often disparages the conduct of a competing commercial enterprise over time. For example, Dr. Li makes condescending and untruthful remarks about Benevolent Daughters Hospital or about another physician's clinical skills.

## Interference with Contract

This tort requires that a contract exists between two parties, a third party knows about the contract, and the third party induces one of the other two parties to breach the contract, or prevents one of the other parties from fulfilling the contract. For example, Fred Kane is a physical therapist with 6 months remaining on his employment contract with Dr. Jones. Dr. Blanco is aware of this contract, but mentions to Fred that he would give him a higher salary if he joins his practice now. Fred leaves and goes to work for Dr. Blanco. Dr. Jones sues Dr. Blanco for interference with contract, and Fred for breach of contract. It is important to note that it is not necessary for Dr. Jones to prove that Dr. Blanco maliciously intended to harm her. What is important is that Dr. Blanco knew that there was a contract, and that his actions interfered with the completion of that contract.

### Malicious Institution of Civil Proceedings

This occurs when an individual initiates legal proceedings that are both unwarranted and unsuccessful. The plaintiff must show that the tortfeasor lacked probable cause to institute the legal proceedings. In essence, someone cannot instigate a frivolous legal action in an attempt to "even things out."

### Defamation

This occurs when a reputation is injured as a result of false statements. If the statement is in writing, then this is called *libel*. If the defamation occurs verbally or by acts or gestures, then it is called *slander*. In most cases, the truth is a successful defense, even if the motivation was less than benevolent and even if the accused believed the statements to be false at the time they were made. Defamation can be a particular concern when one is providing a reference for a former employee.[4] Stick to the facts regarding an employee's job performance. In this regard, your performance appraisal records could be critical to

a successful defense (see Chapter 3). It generally is permissible to provide information about a former employee that might on its face appear to be defamatory, if the information will help you protect an important interest. Important interests have been defined to include a legal or moral duty to speak, defend your own reputation, warn others of a prospective employee's misconduct or mismanagement, and protect the interests of a third party such as the prospective employer.

Conveying negative information is a privileged right that may be lost under some circumstances, including the following:

- You did not believe the reference you gave to be true.
- You had no reasonable grounds for your beliefs about the employee, even though you held your beliefs in good faith.
- The information you gave was not an appropriate response to the third party's inquiry.
- You gave information to a person who had no need for it.
- You gave information out of *malice*, which in a legal sense means recklessly, with an improper motive, with an absence of good faith, and with an intention to do harm.

Here are some guidelines to follow when providing references:

- If the employee is being dismissed, explain why, and let the employee review his or her personnel file.
- Tell the employee that, if he or she chooses to use the practice as a reference, you will respond truthfully.
- Have the employee sign a form prepared by your attorney consenting to the release of information (have your attorney prepare a standard release form and keep copies in your office so that they can be

used as needed). Do not release information if the employee refuses to sign the form. If the employee refuses to sign the form and subsequently uses you as a reference, tell the inquirer that you cannot supply information until the former employee signs a release.

- Do not use a release supplied by the other employer. It might not provide you with the appropriate legal safeguards, as would a form drafted by your attorney.
- State that your evaluation of the former employee is your opinion, and provide a full and accurate discussion of the facts supporting your opinion.
- If you forward a written recommendation, be certain to mark the outside envelope *confidential* or *personal.*
- Do not volunteer information that has not been requested.
- Some employers will give employees who are discharged for inadequate job performance a generic written reference stating that the employee had been a "good employee." Never do this because it could be used against you by the former employee as evidence of wrongful discharge.

## NEGLIGENCE TORTS

Negligence is the most common kind of tort. *Negligence* occurs when a person or company fails to act with reasonable care under the circumstances. For an injured person to be able to recover for negligence, the following five elements must be demonstrated:

1. *The defendant had a duty to exercise reasonable care.* What constitutes reasonable care is often a subject of contention in the litigation. Generally, the standard that is applied is what an imaginary reasonable person might do under the circumstances. Obviously, this type of standard is going to vary from one occasion to another, and ultimately the issue of reasonableness is only determined by the resolution of the lawsuit.

2. *The defendant breached the duty to behave reasonably.* The standard of performance is not perfection. Rather, the standard is reasonable performance by the defendant under the circumstances. Generally, the more serious the hazard, the more care the defendant must exercise.

3. *Cause in fact.* The plaintiff must demonstrate that the injury would not have happened but for the defendant's acts or omissions.

4. *Proximate cause.* This concept deals with the foreseeability of the consequences of the defendant's act. (The term *proximate* is a lamentable choice of words because the issue has nothing at all to do with closeness in time or place. The issue relates to how far courts will extend culpability in a chain of events.) Proximate cause exists when there is no intervening cause or chain of causes between the defendant's actions, and the harm that occurred to the plaintiff. For example, Andrews is injured in an accident while a passenger in Hill's car. Hill removes Andrews from the car and lays him by the side of the road. Roberts, a passerby, moves Andrews into the roadway, where he is struck by Thompson's car. Hill's alleged negligence is not the proximate cause of the injuries suffered by Andrews as a result of being struck by Thompson's car, although his actions are the proximate cause for the injuries suffered in the original accident.

5. *Injury, damage, or loss.* The plaintiff must demonstrate that personal injury, property damage, or economic loss actually occurred as a result of the act.

The following example illustrates how the elements listed previously can combine to form a tort. As a result of a snowstorm, the entrance to Dr. Framingham's office has become slippery. Dr. Framingham has a contract with a cleaning service to provide snow removal. Dr. Framingham learns that the entrance was slippery when he arrives at his office. Before the cleaning service comes to clean the entrance, Mr. Sparacio slips on the icy entrance and breaks his leg.

Under these circumstances, it is likely that Dr. Framingham was negligent. Courts have generally held that it is a business's duty to provide a safe entrance. The fact that the cleaning service may or may not have responded does not relieve Dr. Framingham of this duty to the public to provide a safe entrance. Therefore, Dr. Framingham breached this duty. The snow at the entrance was the cause in fact of the accident, and the consequences of leaving the entrance covered with snow were foreseeable and known by Dr. Framingham. Finally, Mr. Sparacio did suffer an injury. As a separate issue, Dr. Framingham may be able to bring an action against the cleaning service based on the wording of the cleaning contract. For example, if the contract stated that snow would be removed before the office opened in the morning, then the cleaning service may have breached the contract with Dr. Framingham, and be liable to him for monetary damages.

Aside from negligent malpractice, which is discussed separately, a physician's greatest exposure to negligence torts lies in the physical state of his or her office. People are very creative in their ability to misuse items and act without forethought. It is essential to examine how patients physically flow through your office and your physical facilities, and then to rectify any potential hazards. The goal is to prevent injuries, not simply provide a reasonable care defense. The following suggestions might be helpful:

- Have all trash removed from your premises (not just your office) as quickly as possible.

- Hallways and entrances should be routinely cleaned and maintained.
- All office furniture should be routinely inspected for loose legs, loose backs, exposed wires, and so on.
- Consider eliminating toys from your waiting room. Playing correlates with activity, and activity correlates with injury. If you must have toys, examine them for sharp edges, points, ingestibility, breakability, or any other potential danger. Instead of toys, stock your waiting room with children's books, and encourage parents to read to their children or let them read.
- Be certain that the receptionist understands that he or she has a responsibility to keep order in the waiting room.
- Be certain that all appropriate safety equipment is properly located and maintained. For example, have an adequate supply of properly placed fire extinguishers, be certain that exit signs are visible, and routinely check safety equipment such as ground fault interrupters, pressure relief valves, and locks.

## MALPRACTICE

*Malpractice* is the tort of negligence as it applies to a professional. For a patient to demonstrate malpractice, he or she must prove by a preponderance of the evidence that the five elements necessary for any tort are present:

1. *Duty.* There was a bona fide physician–patient relationship, and the physician owed the patient a duty to provide a certain standard of care.
2. *Breach of Duty or Standard of Care.* The patient must demonstrate that the physician did not provide a reasonable standard of care.
3. *Causation in Fact.* The injury would not have happened but for the physician's actions.

4. *Proximate Cause.* The consequences of the physician's actions would be foreseeable by a reasonable, prudent person.
5. *Injury, Damage, or Loss.* The injuries caused by the physician resulted in a physical, financial, or emotional loss.

These points are elaborated here.

## Duty and Breach of Duty

Unless there is a physician-patient relationship, there can be no malpractice liability. Once a physician-patient relationship has been formed, however, the physician has an obligation to care for the patient until treatment is completed or the relationship is terminated in a professionally appropriate manner. Failure to properly terminate a physician–patient relationship can result in a charge of abandonment. Proper termination includes providing the patient with reasonable notice, assisting the patient in finding another physician (when requested or when appropriate), and providing medical records when the new physician has presented a signed patient record release.

Obviously, the physician must be particularly concerned about the abandonment issue if the patient is in an emergency or crisis situation. Special caution is called for if the patient has been diagnosed with a mental illness, because an abrupt termination of the case may exacerbate feelings of loss and abandonment and may precipitate suicidal or other irrational behaviors. Once it has been established that there is a physician–patient relationship, the standard of care then becomes an issue. The physician owes the patient a certain quality of care, but at the same time the physician is not required to guarantee a favorable outcome. A physician generally is not negligent for errors in judgment except where the treatment falls below accepted standards of care.[5] Historically, the standard of care applied in a given malpractice case usually has been related to the standards of the local community, and to the specialty and school of medicine practiced by the physician. This standard, however, usually is established through the use of expert testimony. Historically, local experts testified to the standard of care provided in the community. Over the years, the locality rule has eroded, so that experts from outside the defendant's practice area can be used as expert witnesses. As a result, the standard of care is now often regional or even national.

The demise of the locality rule has been due to a number of circumstances, including the hesitancy of local physicians to testify against one another, the adoption of national uniform standards for certification, residency, continuing education requirements, development of national best practices, standards of care, and critical pathways.[6] As a consequence, there has been a tendency to homogenize and thereby raise the legal standard of care. Within a specialty, a physician is held to the standard of care of other specialists in the specialty. A primary care physician, for example, is not required to provide the quality of care that would be provided by a specialist. The standard of care for a primary care physician, however, might well require a referral to or consultation with a specialist in a given set of circumstances. The standard of care also is related to the physician's school of medical thought. An osteopathic gynecologist is not held to the same standard as an allopathic gynecologist, and vice versa. There is a presumption that patients understand that different schools of medicine may practice differently, and that they will take this into consideration when selecting providers.

Finally, the physician has a duty to provide the patient with the opportunity to consent. If the patient did not consent to a treatment, the physician could be liable for an intentional tort, such as assault or battery. Obviously, it is always best to obtain written consent from the patient, the spouse, or a legal guardian. Consent, however, may be implied in several circumstances, such as these:

- There are extensive discussions between the physician and the patient, as demonstrated by the subsequent actions of both parties.
- An emergency arises, and the physician cannot obtain consent.
- Adjunct treatment is required because of a procedure to which the patient has consented.

If the physician obtains the consent of the patient, but the patient has not been properly informed of the potential consequences of the treatment, then the physician has not obtained *informed* consent. Informed consent becomes an issue when the patient alleges that he or she was not provided with sufficient information to make a knowledgeable decision. Some courts have found that the degree of disclosure is determined by the standard of care generally applied by other physicians in similar circumstances. Some states, however, have adopted legislation requiring discussion of risks if a reasonable person in the patient's position would attach significance to the information. Finally, consent only becomes an issue if a reasonable person would have made a different decision as a result of the withheld information. Discuss the content of your state's consent laws with your attorney.

Consent also can be a question when the patient is a minor. Generally, it is best to obtain written consent from the parent of any patient who is younger than 18. Minors can provide consent under certain circumstances, including emergency treatment (when the life of the patient is at risk) and when the minor is emancipated, which can occur as a result of marriage, a court decree, or a failure of the parents to be legally responsible for the child.

### Causation in Fact

The burden of causation requires that the plaintiff demonstrate by a preponderance of the evidence that the physician's care was the cause in fact and the proximate cause of the damage done to the patient. The courts have tended to take two approaches to determining the question of cause in fact.[7] Using the "but-for" standard, the question is whether the harm would not have occurred but for the actions of the physician. If the harm would not otherwise have occurred, cause in fact is taken to be demonstrated. A second standard that courts have applied concerns whether the physician's actions were a substantial factor contributing to the patient's damage. If, for example, there were two causes of the patient's harm, then the substantial factor test would associate liability with the source of each cause. Generally, the plaintiff has the burden of proof to demonstrate cause. It can shift to a defendant, however, if one physician is seeking to limit his or her liability with respect to a codefendant.

### Proximate Cause

The issue of proximate cause is related to the foreseeability of the consequences of the physician's actions. Negligence can only be found if the consequences were foreseeable by a reasonable, prudent person. If the consequences were not foreseeable, then the physician did not have a duty to protect the patient from them, even though the physician may have caused them to occur in fact. The old parable "For want of a nail, a shoe was lost; for want of a shoe, a soldier was lost; for want of a soldier, a battle was lost; for loss of a battle, a war was lost" demonstrates the need for the concept of proximate cause. Still, a physician can be negligent because he or she sets a chain of events into motion. The proximate cause standard, however, requires that the physician be an instrumental cause of the injury in the chain of events, as opposed to simply creating conditions in which the harm was possible.

Another way in which cause can be demonstrated is through the doctrine of *res ipsa loquitur*, which is a Latin phrase meaning "the thing speaks for itself." *Res ipsa loquitur* allows a jury to reach a conclusion based on circumstantial evidence without the plaintiff having to demonstrate that the defendant actually caused the harm. This doctrine is often applied, for example, when a foreign object has been left inside a patient. The fact that the object is there is sufficient to demonstrate causation. *Res ipsa loquitur* has also been used to demonstrate cause for injuries outside the area of treatment. For example, a patient receives burns during a procedure on a part of the body even though it is distant from the operated site, or a patient develops paralysis after receiving anesthesia. "It speaks for itself" that the harm was done while under the physician's care.

Courts also have applied this doctrine when many people have had control over a patient's unconscious body, such as during the preparation for, conduct of, and recovery from surgery. In this type of situation, it would be difficult if not impossible for the patient to identify the *specific* person responsible for the harm. *Res ipsa loquitur* shifts the burden of proof to the defendant, who must then demonstrate by a preponderance of the evidence that he or she did *not* cause the harm.

For *res ipsa loquitur* to be applied by a court, the plaintiff must demonstrate that:

- the injury is of a type that ordinarily doesn't occur unless there is negligence.
- the injury was caused by something that was within the control of the defendant.
- the plaintiff did not contribute to the cause of the injury.

## Damages

For malpractice to be proven, the plaintiff must demonstrate that harm has occurred. The harm can be in the form of financial, emotional, or physical injuries. Compensation can be required for past and future medical costs, loss of income, funeral expenses, pain, mental suffering, and so on. The legal objective is to provide an award of money damages in recompense for the harm done to the plaintiff. In addition, courts occasionally assign punitive and exemplary awards over and above the plaintiff's actual losses, although these awards are usually limited to outrageous, malicious, or intentional acts.

## Defenses Against Malpractice

There are several defenses to a charge of malpractice. One strategy is to challenge the basis of the tort by claiming that the plaintiff failed to demonstrate that a duty existed, that the standard of care was not breached, that the physician's actions were not causally related to the harm, or that the patient suffered no harm. In addition, the physician can raise substantive defenses, which relate to the facts of the case, and procedural defenses, which relate to the legal basis of the complaint.

Substantive defenses include the contributory negligence and the comparative negligence defenses. Contributory negligence occurs when a patient contributes to the harm that occurred. For example, a patient who fails to follow the physician's directions or provides false or incomplete information may be found to be contributorily negligent. Contributory negligence is a complete defense, which means that if it prevails it will preclude any recovery by the plaintiff. Attorneys may hesitate to use this defense even if it is available, because a jury may resent an attempt to equate a minor indiscretion on the part of the patient with a major dereliction on the part of the physician.

Comparative negligence defenses try to apportion the negligence between the plaintiff and the physician. It is not a complete monetary defense, and the award of damages would be in proportion to the harm found to be attributable to the physician. For example, if it was determined that the physician was responsible for 80 percent of the damage, which was assessed at $100,000, then the physician would be liable for $80,000.

Historically, case law has recognized the doctrine of contributory negligence, but state legislatures have been replacing this doctrine with comparative negligence statutes. The two doctrines are mutually exclusive, and only one will be in force in any given jurisdiction.

A third substantive defense is called *assumption of risk*. This occurs when the plaintiff knows and appreciates the risk and voluntarily assumes the risk. Obviously, demonstrating that the patient gave informed consent is essential to this defense. Except where informed consent is present, this defense is usually not successful. Generally it is recognized that the physician has superior knowledge of the risks involved and is better able to weigh information in making medical decisions.

A procedural defense relies on a failure to comply with legal procedures. One procedural defense is to claim that the statute of limitations has expired and that the physician thus has been released from liability. A person who alleges injury must initiate legal action before the expiration of the time period stated in that state's statute of limitations. Some

states start the clock on the date when the alleged malpractice occurred. Because some injuries may not be observable for years, it is possible for patients to lose the right to sue before becoming aware of the problem. As a result, many states have adopted statutes that start the clock when the patient discovers or should have discovered the injury.

Some physicians have attempted to limit their liability by having patients sign forms releasing them from liability. These forms generally are worthless because, as a matter of public policy, a person cannot contract away liability for negligence. A release can be valid, however, in the case of experimental or inherently dangerous treatment. Under these circumstances, the release must be signed before the beginning of treatment, and it must pertain to the consequences of properly performed treatment. It will not constitute a defense for improperly or negligently *performed* experimental or inherently dangerous treatment.

In addition to legal malpractice defenses, you can implement financial defenses. One such defense is called *insolvency planning*.[8] The goal is to make your assets as judgment proof as possible. Because some aspects of insolvency planning may be inconsistent with prudent estate and financial planning, it is essential to consult your attorney and appropriate tax and financial planning consultants so you can balance these competing interests.

Another financial defense is to maintain sufficient malpractice insurance and periodically reevaluate your level of coverage. Joint ownership of assets can also hamper creditors, especially in states that recognize the concept of tenancy by entirety. This requires that the asset be transferred to both a wife and a husband, so that one party's interest cannot be transferred to a third party. Creditors of both the husband and the wife, however, can execute a judgment against this type of ownership. Some states have homestead laws that protect a portion of an owner's equity from a judgment. Retirement plans are also protected from creditors, although distributions from a plan can be subject to a judgment.

## CONTRACTS

The objective of this section is to provide a basic understanding of how contracts are formed and interpreted by the courts. Whenever you are in doubt regarding the meaning of a contract, or whenever a contract includes a substantial commitment of time, money, personnel, or other resources, you should have it reviewed by your attorney. A *contract* is a legally binding agreement between two or more parties. Examples of contracts include agreements with your employees, your partners, your suppliers, the telephone company, and your bank. Contracts can be in written or verbal form. As a general rule, you should not enter into any significant contract without first having it reviewed by your attorney. You will probably have to enter into many contracts, however, and it would be time consuming, expensive, and cumbersome to have your attorney review all of them. For example, you engage a security service to install an alarm, a water company to supply bottled water to your office, an employment agency to provide a temporary secretary for this afternoon, a store to supply a wingback chair, and a painter to repaint a chipped file cabinet. All these transactions are contractual, yet probably none of them is of sufficient magnitude to warrant the inconvenience and cost of forwarding it to your attorney for review. It is important, therefore, to appreciate how contracts are formed, interpreted, and enforced so you can identify dubious or potentially disadvantageous situations, and selectively use your attorney.

For a contract to exist, the following must occur:

- The parties must be competent.
- They must reach a mutual agreement.
- Consideration must be provided.
- What has been contracted for must be legal.

*Competence* means that all parties are legally capable of entering into the agreement. Minors, the insane, and individuals who are intoxicated may be considered incompetent to enter into contracts. Entering into a contract with a minor is particularly dangerous, because the adult party may be held to the terms of the contract, whereas the minor may withdraw at any time. For example, if you treat a minor without the consent of a legal guardian, you may not be able to hold the minor financially accountable, although the minor will be able to hold you to an acceptable standard of care. Although state law may hold the parent financially responsible, you then would have the problem of locating and collecting from the parent.

*Mutual agreement* means that there was both an offer and an acceptance. An offer means that you intend to be legally bound if the offer is accepted. Because offers may be preceded by preliminary negotiations, it is important to indicate clearly whether you are making an offer or merely expressing an intention to make an offer at some future time. For example, Dr. Cook may state to Dr. Jackson "I'm interested in selling my practice for $100,000. Would you be interested in buying it?" This is merely an inquiry, not an offer to sell. Dr. Jackson cannot force the sale by producing a check for $100,000. If, however, Dr. Jackson responds by stating "I will buy your practice for $100,000," that would constitute an offer. If Dr. Cook accepts the offer, a contract would then exist. Phrases such as "Would you be interested in," "I understand that you are looking for," and "How would you feel about" do not constitute offers. Because communications can become complex and the price of misunderstanding can be so great, it is always best to label an inquiry as such.

An offer can be terminated in several ways. The offerer can revoke it at any time before the other party accepts it. For example, if Dr. Jackson offers Dr. Cook $100,000 for the practice, Dr. Jackson can revoke the offer at any point before Dr. Cook accepts it. The revocation must be received before the offer is accepted for it to be valid. An offer can be terminated by a lapse of time. For example, an offer can state when it will expire. If the offer contains no stated expiration time, a court will consider the offer valid for a reasonable length of time. What constitutes a reasonable length of time will depend on the facts and circumstances of the case. An offer will terminate upon rejection or counteroffer. Once an offer is rejected, the person who rejected it cannot change his or her mind and then accept it. If an acceptance is conditional (e.g., "I will accept the offer if . . .") or if the person to whom the offer is made changes some of the terms, the result is considered a counteroffer, not an acceptance. The original offerer, now the offeree, is free to accept the counteroffer, thereby binding the other party to a valid contract or to reject it.

Once the person to whom the offer is made accepts the terms of the offer and conveys this acceptance to the offerer, the contract is binding. Communication of acceptance can take place in several ways. If the offer dictates the method of communication, such as by certified mail, then the acceptance must be communicated in that form. If the offer states that the acceptance must be made within a certain time, then once again the acceptance must occur within that time. Generally, an acceptance is considered valid when it is placed in the mail prior to or on the date specified in the offer. To avoid problems with any offers that you make, you should always specify the manner of acceptance and when the offer expires.

*Consideration* is the exchange that takes place as a result of the agreement. *Something must be given and something received in order for a contract to be valid.* For example, consideration exists if you agree to purchase bottled water for your office at $7.50 per jug. Generally, courts are not concerned with the adequacy of consideration; if you strike a bad deal, you will be stuck with it. Consideration does not exist if one party is not truly committed to provide something. For example, an agreement that states "If Dr. Cook determines that he needs bottled water, he will purchase it for $7.50 per jug from the Gulch Water Company" would be considered an illusory promise. It would not demonstrate consideration because Dr. Cook is not promising to purchase water.

Finally, for a contract to exist the subject matter must be legal. If a contract is in violation of any statutes or public policy, it is not enforceable. For example, Dr. Hazek contracts with Johnson Construction Company to enlarge his office. As part of the contract, he requires that Johnson Construction Company remove the fire doors after the project is completed, and a certificate of occupancy issued, so the building will no longer be in compliance with the building code. This is a violation of local ordinance, and cannot be enforced under contract law.[9]

Similarly, contractual terms requiring the violation of public policy will also be unenforceable. The term *public policy* is a loose one, but it generally means "protecting from that which tends to be injurious to the public or contrary to the public good, . . . or any established interest of society."[10] Contracts that obstruct justice, corrupt public officials, are immoral, are offensive to public decency, restrain trade, or discriminate on the basis of race, religion, sex, age, disability, or national origin may violate public policy. For example, if the only two urologists in town contract to fix the price of urological services, this may be construed as a restraint of trade. If one of the urologists then violates the agreement, the other could not enforce it, because the content of the agreement violated public policy. In addition, both urologists might be prosecuted under federal or state antitrust laws.

As you can see, the four requirements of a valid contract do not include the necessity of a written document. With certain notable exceptions, verbal contracts generally are enforceable if they are agreed to by competent parties and reflect mutual agreement, consideration, and legal content. Obviously, verbal contracts can be troublesome, because memory can be faulty and selective. To protect your own interests, you should insist on a written contract whenever the worst possible outcome from a business arrangement is more burdensome than arranging for your attorney to prepare a contract.

Certain types of contracts must be in writing to be enforceable:

- Contracts for the sale of land or an interest in land (in some states, a verbal lease of less than 1 year is enforceable)
- Contracts for the sale of goods in excess of $500
- Contracts that by their terms cannot be fulfilled within 1 year
- Suretyship contracts (promises to pay for the debts of others)

When a written contract is drafted, it is critical that you or your attorney anticipate all possible consequences of the arrangement and ensure that the contract provides for adequate resolution. If a dispute should arise, a court will apply the *four corners rule* to resolve it. This means that the court will look first to exactly what is contained within the four "corners" of the contract. Irrespective of what you intended, the contract will be literally interpreted. (There can be exceptions to the four corners rule. For example, if the contract is ambiguous or contradictory, the court may look to "parole" evidence, which is evidence outside the contract, to determine the intent of the parties.)

Consider the following example. Dr. Rodriquez was working for Dr. Smith. Dr. Rodriquez left Dr. Smith's practice, opened her own practice, and incorporated as Darla Rodriquez, MD, PC. Dr. Rodriquez's contract with Dr. Smith had stated that she, Rodriquez, would pay Smith 15 percent of all fees *received by her* for any patients transferred from Smith's practice for a period of 6 months. This was in consideration for Smith having provided referrals to Rodriquez, and otherwise assisting in building Rodriquez's practice. Rodriquez's practice, Darla Rodriquez, MD, PC, paid Rodriquez a salary of 60 percent of collected fees. Rodriquez then paid Smith 15 percent of her salary from transferred patients, or 15 percent of 60 percent of transferred patient collections for 6 months. Smith objected on the basis that this was simply a subterfuge. Smith maintained that, because Rodriquez "was the corporation," the arrangement was simply a sham to avoid paying 15 percent on all fees collected from transferred patients. Rodriquez refused to comply, and Smith sued Rodriquez.

Judgment was for Rodriquez. The contract clearly stated that the 15 percent payments were payable by Rodriquez on fees *collected by Rodriquez.* The fact that she interposed a corporation between herself and Smith did not change the clear language of the contract. The court reminded Smith that if his intention was to have Rodriquez pay a fee on all collections for transferred patients, whether by her or by a corporation employing her, then this should have been so stated in the contract.

Attorneys are skilled at anticipating what can go wrong, drafting language to clarify what the resolution will be if something should go wrong, and positioning their client so that, if a dispute does occur, the client will be in a strong position. Nevertheless, it is important, in any business arrangement, that your attorney fully understand your objectives, your exposure if the other party fails to fulfill the terms of the contract, and protections that you feel you need if the arrangement does not prove to be satisfactory.

You are the ultimate consumer of your legal services, just as you are the consumer of an accountant's services or any other professional consultant. If an attorney does not fully appreciate your needs or drafts a document that does not fully meet your needs, you are the one who will ultimately have to live with the consequences. It is critical, therefore, that you have an effective *dialog* with your attorney.

## EMPLOYMENT ISSUES

Many aspects of the employer-employee relationship have legal implications. The most basic legal consideration in the employer–employee relationship is the employment contract. Other legal considerations include employment discrimination, worker's compensation laws, and the Fair Labor Standards Act. Once again, it is important for you or your business manager to appreciate the legal issues involved so you will know when to involve an attorney, and be able to make daily decisions that are not legally risky.

### Employment Contracts

As is the case for other contracts, an employment contract can be written or verbal. Both written and verbal employment contracts can be for a set term or at will. A *set*

*term* means that the contract is in force for a stated length of time. *At will* means that the contract can be terminated by either party at its will, which in the extreme can be for good reason, bad reason, or no reason at all.

There are four major reasons why you might want to have a written employment contract with an employee. First, a written contract will decrease the chance that either party will misunderstand the mutual commitments. The process of negotiating the employment contract will require both parties to think about most aspects of the employment relationship, including compensation, vacation time, sick leave policy, work schedules, and termination. If disagreements are discovered in the contracting process, then they can be resolved before they lead to a dispute.

Second, if you want a long-term commitment from an employee, it generally should be put in writing. To be enforceable, the contract must be put in writing if it is for 1 year or longer. For example, if you have a skilled radiology technician and you want to be certain that the employee doesn't leave on the spur of the moment, you could negotiate an employment contract stating that the employment would last for an agreed period of time, such as 1 year.

Third, you can include in the contract a noncompetition clause that will restrict the employee's ability to work with competitors after leaving your employment. Obviously, the issue of competition only is relevant for physicians or other skilled professionals. Generally, courts have found these clauses to be valid as long as they are limited to a reasonable time period and a reasonable geographical area. The standards of reasonableness vary with state law and local tradition. In the previous example, the 15 percent fee on transferred patients that Dr.

Rodriquez was to pay Dr. Smith for 6 months might well be considered reasonable in many jurisdictions. A contract precluding practice in the same city for 5 years generally would be considered unreasonable. It is important to remember that the employee has a right to earn a living and that noncompetition clauses contradict the spirit of antitrust laws, which are based on the notion that open, robust competition is beneficial for society. As a result, courts will not enforce a noncompetition clause that unduly restricts this right. Some courts have struck down overbroad noncompetition clauses, whereas others have determined and then applied appropriate geographical and time restrictions. A local attorney's advice is essential to determine what might be a reasonable noncompetition restriction.

Fourth, an employment contract can increase a practice's financial security by committing revenue-generating employees to long-term employment. Practices that employ several physicians can coordinate the lengths of their contracts so that the expiration dates are staggered. This makes it more difficult for the employed physicians to conspire and decimate a group practice by leaving en masse. Other revenue-generating employees, such as nutritionists, physical therapists, physician assistants, and nurse practitioners should also be considered for employment contracts.

The wording of the termination clause in an employment contract is important. An improperly worded termination clause will restrict your ability to fire an employee. For example, the following termination clause was contained in a nurse's employment contract:

This Agreement will be in effect for one year from the date upon which it was made and entered into. This Agreement can be terminated before the end of one year:

1. at any time by the Employee with 30 days written notice;
2. at any time by the Company for inadequate job performance.

During the term of the contract, Nurse Roberts developed strong antiabortion attitudes. He did not allow them to interfere with his job performance, but his participation in public demonstrations and the extremeness of his attitudes caused Dr. Smith, his employer, to feel uncomfortable with Nurse Roberts. Dr. Smith no longer wished to employ him, but because his job performance had been adequate Dr. Smith was committed to retaining him for the remainder of the contract.

From your perspective as an employer, the most favorable termination clause is one that states that the employee serves at your will, and that you may terminate the employee for any reason or for no reason and at any time. Although this provision sounds harsh, it can be both legal and highly desirable from your perspective. There are few things as frustrating as not being able to fire an employee immediately when you feel that it is necessary and justified. There are also few things that are as destructive to the morale and effectiveness of an office as a dissatisfied and malevolent employee. Clever employees can be malevolent in passive-aggressive ways that are difficult to document, which can make it hard to show cause for terminating them on the basis of job performance. It is desirable to retain the prerogative to terminate an employee at your will whenever you want.

Because employees, generally, are interested in job security, they naturally will hesitate to sign contracts with strong at-will provisions. They often will seek to limit your ability to terminate them, or at a minimum they will seek severance benefits. Kahn and colleagues propose some provisions that attempt to balance the legitimate needs of physicians to terminate employees with the desires of employees for security:[11]

- There should be a fixed length for the term of the agreement, such as 1 year, 2 years, and so on.
- The employer should retain the right to terminate the employee in case of an employee's disability that prevents the employee from carrying out his or her duties, or a failure of the employee to obey orders.
- The employer should retain the right to terminate the employee immediately for misconduct, with no severance benefits. Misconduct is to be defined at the sole and unrestricted discretion of the employer.
- The employer should retain the right to terminate the employee for any reason, with notice (e.g., 2 weeks).
- The employee should retain the right to resign at any time for any reason, with notice to the employer (e.g., 2 weeks).
- In the case of physician employees, they should agree not to work for a competing practice for a fixed period of time in a stated geographical area.

These termination provisions still give the physician wide latitude to terminate the employee for inadequate job performance or any other reason, yet they provide some measure of job security and financial security for the employee. They also limit the ability of the employee to work for a competitor or to be stolen by a competitor for a higher salary during the term of the agreement.

**Exhibit 10–1** contains a checklist of items that should be considered for inclusion in any employment contract. You can use this checklist to help ensure that you explore all relevant issues with the employee or applicant and with your attorney. In general, you only should enter into written employment contracts with valued employees and only

after carefully considering the consequences and having the contracts drafted by an attorney. A written contract will be more restrictive than an unwritten agreement simply because the employee will ask for restrictions that would not occur to him or her with an unwritten agreement. The difficulties and frustrations associated with any restrictions on your ability to terminate hourly employees, for example, should not be underestimated.

Often, the security offered by a long-term contract is illusory. Even if you are able to enforce a contract so an employee stays contrary to his or her own true wishes, your victory is almost always pyrrhic. Employees serving against their wishes will take their dissatisfaction out on you, your practice, and your patients, and a written contract will provide you with no effective defense against this form of retribution. It is better to replace employees who simply provide services, such as secretaries, business managers, and nurses, than try to keep them against their will.

Decisions regarding revenue-generating employees are more difficult. The following are three strategies for dealing with revenue-generating employees who are serving against their will:

1. Release them, and consider the lost revenue the price for your own well-being and that of your employees and patients.
2. Negotiate a price for the employee to buy him- or herself out of the contract.
3. Enforce the contract, grit your teeth, and bear it. If you pursue this alternative and the employee leaves, you may seek an injunction barring the employee from working for or becoming a competitor. Courts, however, generally recognize that slavery has been illegal for quite some time, so they are unlikely to force the employee to go back to work for you. Under these circumstances, you may seek monetary damages.

**Exhibit 10–1** Employment Contract Checklist

- *Offer and acceptance of employment.
- *Contract expiration date.
- *Compensation, including formulas for determination, payment schedules, bonuses, insurance, retirement plan, employer contributions to retirement plan, and any other compensation related issues.
- Termination. For cause: state specifics such as theft, drug use, inadequate job performance, etc. If employment is at will this should be clearly stated. State entitlements to any compensation or access to benefits at termination and, if so, under what circumstances.
- Statement that the employee is in fact an employee *for all purposes* including taxation, unemployment compensation, etc.
- (Only if relevant) Statement that the practice may purchase at its cost insurance (life, disability, etc.) on the employee with the practice as a beneficiary, and that the employee will cooperate in this process.
- Provide a list of the major duties and responsibilities of the position and a disclaimer that they may be changed at management's discretion.
- Statement requiring full-time, exclusive employment and that any other employment will require your written approval.
- Discipline procedures, or if desirable to you, reference to the employee handbook.
- Noncompetition—State reasonable time period and geographic area.
- Nondisclosure of confidential information, such as business plans, patient information, etc.
- "Zipper clause" ("This is the whole of the agreement").
- (Only if relevant) Statements regarding actions that the employee must take, such as professional license, etc.
- Procedure for amending the contract.
- Successors in interest—Statement that the contract will remain in force if the practice is sold.
- Statement regarding breach of the contract and remedies for a breach.
- Severability statement—If any part of the contract is found to be illegal, the remaining legal parts will remain in force.
- Procedure for providing notice to the other party (by certified mail, where, etc.).
- Governing law ("This contract shall be governed according to the laws of the state of . . .").

*These items must be included in some form.
*Source:* Adapted from Kahn, S., B. Brown, & B. Zepke. (1988). *Personnel Director's Legal Guide, 1988 Cumulative Supplement.* New York: Warren, Gorham, and Lamont, pp. S2-53–S2-54.

You would have an obligation, however, to mitigate the damages by attempting to replace the employee. The damages that you may be able to recover would be the lost income less the damages that were mitigated, plus your costs for replacing the employee.

For example, Dr. Temple leaves Dr. Nova's practice in violation of her employment agreement. Dr. Temple generated $200,000 in gross receipts and continues at this rate after leaving. Dr. Nova hires a replacement, at a cost of $20,000 in search fees, who generates $100,000 during the time remaining on Dr. Temple's contract. Dr. Nova would likely recover damages of $120,000. If Dr. Nova does not attempt to mitigate the damages, the court may decide that there would have been none and may choose to assign no damages. On the other hand, if Dr. Nova made a good-faith effort to find a replacement but none was available, Dr. Nova may be awarded $220,000. Your choice of strategy for dealing with contract-breaking employees should depend on a number of issues, including the precedent that you want to set for other employees, the value of the employee's revenue to the financial health of the practice, and your own peace of mind.

### Employment at Will

Employees with no written or stated verbal contract that specifies a term of employment are employed at will. An at-will arrangement, however, implies a contract. When a legally competent employee agrees to provide labor in exchange for compensation, there is consideration, mutual consent, and legal content, so a contract exists. Traditionally, at-will arrangements allowed employers to terminate employees for good cause, bad cause, or no cause at all. Over the years, however, courts and legislatures have placed limits on the employer's ability to dismiss employees.

Most states currently have laws that restrict the employer's ability to terminate at-will employees unless there is good cause. One type of restriction relates to abusive or retaliatory discharge. This occurs when the discharge is in retaliation for an employee's refusal to violate public policy. For example, many states do not allow dismissal for whistle blowing, or for failure to perform an illegal activity, such as refusing to commit perjury to protect the employer, refusing to commit bribery, failure to submit false insurance claims, and refusing to falsify records. Many states have made it illegal to dismiss an employee for filing a worker's compensation claim, for refusing to take a polygraph test, or for fulfilling military or jury duty obligations. In addition, federal and state antidiscrimination laws also limit the employer's ability to dismiss at-will employees on a racial or sexual basis.

An ex-employee's allegation that dismissal was in violation of public policy certainly doesn't mean that a court will uphold this allegation and assign damages. It does mean, however, that the employer may have to provide some evidence for dismissal that refutes the claimed violation of public policy. Documentation of inadequate job performance or insubordination, for example, would be a cornerstone for a successful defense under these circumstances. The need to provide a defense in the first place exemplifies the erosion of the employer's traditional at-will prerogative to terminate an employee for any reason or no reason.

Another challenge to the employer's at-will termination prerogative arises from the concept of implied terms in the employment agreement. Courts have found that oral statements made to the employee, as well as written documents other than the employment contract, can become part of the employment agreement. This, then, makes dismissal conditional upon good cause. For example, some courts have held that an employee handbook can become part of the employment contract. In *Toussaint v. Blue Cross and Blue Shield of Michigan,* the court found that statements in the company's personnel manual indicating that employees would only be terminated for cause had become part of the employment contract, because the personnel manual was reviewed with the employee during the selection interview.[12] Other implied terms have been found in oral statements made at the time of hiring, such as "You'll always have a job here as long as you do as I say," and "I won't fire an employee until I give him or her three chances to improve."

Another attack on at-will employment is application of the doctrine that good faith and fair dealing is implied in any contract. Some courts have interpreted good faith and fair dealing to mean that the employer has an obligation to provide employees with due process, and to base terminations on just cause. If the employer has to justify the dismissal or provide an appeal process or a forum for the employee to contest the dismissal, then the at-will option is obviously compromised. This doctrine has been used, for example, to invalidate terminations whose purpose was to avoid paying wages by coercing an employee to write a resignation letter.

It should be noted that there is wide variation in how far courts will go to find implied contract provisions. For example, a California court held that "merely exchanging pleasantries about the company during an interview did not imply a promise by the employer of job security."[13] Similarly, many courts have held that company handbooks and other written documents are simply unilateral statements. Because there is no "meeting of the minds," there is no contract.

There are several things that you, as an employer, can do to preserve your at-will option to terminate employees insofar as your jurisdiction permits:

- Make no statements in the employment process that could be construed as making an exception to at-will employment. For example, don't say "You'll have a job here as long as you perform well," or "If your work isn't satisfactory, I'll give you a chance to improve."
- Never give an applicant a policy manual or handbook during the employment process. If you do, it may be argued later that its contents *as of that date* were part of the reason that the applicant accepted the job, which will make it part of the employment contract. As a consequence, the employee may not be subject to revisions of the employee handbook.
- Tell the job applicant that the terms of employment are at will, and explain what that means. Some companies have new employees sign a document at the time of employment in which they acknowledge and accept their at-will status.
- Always document reasons for discharge. Inadequate job performance, absenteeism,

and insubordination are among the legitimate reasons for termination, and they can be used to refute allegations of abusive discharge or of an implied contract.
- Have your attorney check state laws and court interpretations and inform you of illegal grounds for termination in your state.
- Always review the facts of a termination with your attorney before you terminate an employee. Do this even if you feel that the facts are clear and your behavior is fully justified. Your attorney may have suggestions regarding how to document the facts and orchestrate the termination to provide you with maximum defensibility.
- Review personnel manuals, employment applications, training materials, and so on for any language that could be construed as limiting your at-will termination authority. These documents should contain a clear statement that employment is at will. In addition, each manual or handbook should contain a disclaimer stating that nothing in it is intended to create or modify a contract with an employee.
- If you create any documents specifying a code of conduct, always include a disclaimer in which you state that the document is *illustrative*. This will give you latitude, because it is impossible to anticipate all the creative ways in which employees can violate the spirit of a policy without clearly breaching its specific content.
- Review the performance-appraisal suggestions in Chapter 3. Using these ideas will strengthen your legal defensibility.
- Apply your discipline and termination procedures with consistency.
- Be honest with yourself regarding the real reasons why you are terminating an employee. Sometimes, feelings of anger or betrayal may result in you doing something that isn't legally defensible. If you are honest with yourself, you will avoid a questionable termination.

## Equal Employment Opportunity

Federal and state legislation precludes employers from discriminating against employees on the basis of race, religion, sex, national origin, age, or disability. This legislation encompasses all aspects of employment, including hiring, promotion, compensation, access to training, discipline, and termination. Employers covered by this legislation cannot use a person's race, religion, sex, national origin, age (if over 40 years), or disability status to influence an employment decision.

The primary federal equal employment opportunity (EEO) laws are the 1964 Civil Rights Act (in particular, Title VII), the Age Discrimination in Employment Act of 1967 (ADEA), the Age Discrimination Act of 1975, and the Americans with Disabilities Act (ADA). Other relevant pieces of federal legislation include the First, Fifth, Thirteenth, and Fourteenth Amendments to the U.S. Constitution, various executive orders issued by the President, and the Equal Pay Act of 1963.

The Equal Employment Opportunity Commission (EEOC) was created as a result of the Civil Rights Act of 1964. Its mission is to administer Title VII of that act as well as federal age discrimination legislation. The EEOC interprets the meaning of civil rights legislation, provides guidance to employers, and enforces the legislation through prosecution in federal court. As a result of its central position in drafting, interpreting, and enforcing EEO legislation, the EEOC's interpretations, published in its guidelines to employers, are important.

Many medical practices will not be subject to federal EEO regulation because of their size. The Civil Rights Act of 1964 and the ADA only cover employers that have 15 or more employees working each day for 20 calendar weeks or more in the current or preceding year. The ADEA and Age Discrimination Act of 1975 only apply to companies employing 20 or more employees for 20 calendar weeks or more in the current or preceding year. In addition, these two acts only provide protection to employees who are 40 years old or older. Because most federal discrimination enforcement emanates from these acts, many medical practices are effectively exempt from federal EEO regulation. Many of these same practices, however, will be subject to state EEO laws. Because these laws vary considerably from state to state, it is essential that you contact your attorney to understand the compliance requirements in your particular state. In addition, some cities, such as New York City and San Francisco, have developed their own civil rights legislation, and once again you should seek guidance from your attorney.

Although the following discussion of federal civil rights legislation only applies directly to those healthcare organizations that are covered by the various civil rights laws just noted, smaller medical practices nevertheless may want to be familiar with federal guidelines. First, many state laws are based on the EEOC's interpretations of federal legislation. Understanding the EEOC's perspective may help physician managers comply with state legislation. Second, the EEOC's perspective strikes a good balance between society's need for fair and equal treatment of applicants and employees, and the employer's need for competent, qualified personnel. Finally, the EEOC's thinking, as embodied in its recommendations to employers, generally is consistent with good personnel management and employment methods. Thus understanding the EEOC's position may help physician leaders institute more effective personnel management and employment methods.

The primary source of federal EEO enforcement is Title VII of the Civil Rights Act of 1964. Various EEOC publications provide the employer with specific guidance regarding how to hire, compensate, terminate, and otherwise deal with employees without discriminating. The following sections are designed to provide you with an overview of how to comply with the EEOC's recommendations as stated in its guidelines.

### Employment Methods

It is important to understand the technical definition of the word discrimination as it relates to employment. One form of discrimination is called *disparate treatment*, which occurs when the employer bases an employment decision on race, color, religion, sex, age, or national origin. In effect, disparate treatment occurs when the employer willfully discriminates by choosing to treat people differently based on an illegal standard. For example, using different selection procedures for applicants of different races would constitute disparate treatment. Requiring one race or sex group to have higher scores than another in order to be employed would constitute disparate treatment. Using different interview questions for different applicants can also be construed as disparate treatment. Disparate treatment is volitional and intentional discrimination, because the employer intends to treat applicants differently. Disparate treatment per se is illegal, and there are no affirmative defenses to a demonstration of disparate treatment.

Another condition that *may* constitute discrimination is called *disparate impact*. Disparate impact occurs when selection rates are different for protected classes, even though everyone has been treated the same. Disparate impact focuses on outcomes. Specific-

ally, if the selection rate of a protected class is less than 4/5ths of the selection rate for the group with the highest selection rate, this constitutes disparate impact. For example, assume that all men and women applying for a position receive the exact same tests and interview questions. If the selection rate for women for this job is 60 percent and the selection rate for men is 40 percent, this would constitute disparate impact, because the selection rate for men is less than 4/5ths of the rate for women. The critical value in this case would be 48 percent ($60\% \times 4/5 = 48\%$).[14] Disparate impact in and of itself is *not* illegal. Its significance is that it shifts the burden of proof to the employer to prove that the employer is using job relevant employment methods that assess important aspects of the job. In other words, *demonstrating validity is an affirmative legal defense should disparate impact occur*. This reasoning makes provision for the fact that abilities are not uniformly distributed across all protected classes and across all geographical regions. In effect, the disparate impact is justified based on the skills exhibited by applicants on a job-relevant selection process.

The distinction between disparate treatment and disparate impact is important when assessing litigation risks. The rewards and opportunities for those claiming disparate treatment are much greater than for those claiming disparate impact. Allegations of disparate impact are tried before judges, and generally the awarding of punitive damages are not allowed. Since passage of the Civil Rights Act of 1991, allegations of disparate treatment can be tried before juries and punitive damages are allowed. Plaintiffs and their attorneys, therefore, are much more interested in disparate treatment cases, because juries are more sympathetic to plaintiffs, and the large dollar awards occur when punitive awards can be granted.

Another opportunity for plaintiff litigation is to sue under common tort law. As seen, a tort is a civil wrong and not a violation of statutory law, such as the Civil Rights Acts of 1964 and 1991. Employment torts can occur when someone incurs "pain and suffering" as a result of not being hired, or being terminated. Because there are often no caps on tort damages, there has been a shift in litigation away from statutory claims to common law torts. Tort claims are wrongs against a *person*, and they are naturally more relevant to allegations of disparate treatment: "You treated me wrong and therefore I suffered," as opposed to a facially neutral process, which simply resulted in the "wrong" numbers.

Hospitals and practices that adopt the employment methods proposed in Chapter 4 will largely eliminate allegations of disparate treatment, because the methods discussed there are standardized and structured across all applicants. Compare this to the hospital or practice that is using unstructured or semi-structured interviews with no stated scoring standards. It is very likely that under these latter conditions applicants were treated differently, even though there may have been no malevolent intent. Being unable to recall what questions were asked, or being unable to state definitively why Applicant A was hired over Applicant B is almost certainly a losing argument. Similarly, the structured job based performance appraisal methods and documentation standards presented in Chapter 3 provide a strong defense against allegations of termination based on disparate treatment.

The employment methods discussed in Chapter 4 also provide hospitals and practices with a strong defense for allegations of disparate impact. First, by definition, these cases will be tried before a judge who is more likely to understand technical selection issues and be less swayed by emotional and sentimental arguments than a jury. Second,

published tests of GMA and Conscientiousness are widely validated and these data can be used as a legal defense applying the concept of validity generalizability.[15] Third, validation of any other locally developed methods, such as structured interviews, or work samples, can be used as a legal defense. Remember, in an allegation of disparate impact demonstrating the validity of the employment methods used against job relevant criteria is a legal defense.

Finally, using valid employment methods can lower the risk of litigation, because you will be more likely to make successful hiring decisions! Sharf and Jones report that one survey of EEOC claims filed showed that only 7.7 percent of the charges were related to hiring and 47.2 percent were related to discharge. Stated another way, *the risk of litigation is almost seven times greater for discharge decisions than for hiring decisions.* The implication is that employers can significantly reduce their exposure to litigation by making better hiring decisions, thereby avoiding the need to discharge employees. They also note that only 0.3 percent of all charges filed with EEOC in 1997 had any relation to testing. They conclude:[16]

The use of demonstrably job-related employment tests is a winning strategy for minimizing the risk of employment litigation. Forty-plus percent of employee decisions in the private sector (*Fortune* 100 companies) are based on the results of employment tests. Litigation challenging employment test use, however, occurs in less than one-half of 1 percent of all discrimination claims. So the tides have turned from the post-*Griggs* (*Griggs v. Duke Power Company*) days, when employers abandoned the casual use of employee tests. Legally defensible employment testing is now one of the safest harbors offering shelter from the howling gales of class-action EEO litigation. (pg. 314)

Finally, the best and least expensive legal defense is always prevention. Even if an employment method is job related, you always want to consider how it will *appear* to the applicant. An employment method that doesn't look job related will raise questions in the applicant's mind. A litigious leaning applicant may suspect that the test or interview is merely a subterfuge to reject on an illegal basis. It is a good idea, therefore, to think twice before using a selection method that appears to be irrelevant. If you decide to use it anyway, then precede its use with a brief statement concerning why you are asking the applicant to perform this task. You might say, for example, "This questionnaire measures some job-related tendencies, such as your ability to get along with others and your desire to work."

## Promotion

The same general issues that arise in the selection of employees also arise in making promotion decisions. For example, it is illegal to make a promotion decision based on an employee's race, religion, sex, national origin, or age (disparate treatment). Documentation of disparate impact can arise from a number of sources, including a pattern of promotions for a particular race or sex, age category, and so forth, and use of inconsistent promotion standards. Once the disparate impact has been demonstrated, the employer's task is to document the validity of the promotion decision. Evidence that promotions were made using valid and consistently applied performance appraisal procedures is a legal defense.

## Sexual Discrimination

Several additional points need to be discussed regarding sexual discrimination. Obviously, there are some jobs in which a person's gender *is* relevant to job performance, such as the preference for an actress for a female role in a play. In this instance, being female is a bona fide occupational qualification (BFOQ). Because of the potential for abuse, the EEOC has interpreted BFOQs very narrowly. For example, a BFOQ would *not* exist in the following circumstances:

1. An employer refuses to hire an applicant based on the preferences of coworkers, clients, or patients. It is not permissible to reject a man for a nurse or receptionist position, for example, simply because staff or patients might object or perhaps feel uncomfortable.
2. An employer refuses to hire an applicant based on assumptions about a certain gender, such as "Women are more likely to be sick, or to have higher turnover rates, or be better with patients."

Discrimination on the basis of pregnancy also is prohibited under Title VII. You cannot terminate or refuse to hire or promote a woman solely because she is pregnant. In addition, it is illegal to set a mandatory pregnancy leave requirement. Pregnancy must be treated as any other short-term disability. Women who take a pregnancy leave have a right to reinstatement once they are able to perform the work, just as other employees do with other short-term disabilities. Health-care organizations not covered by Title VII still may have to comply with state regulations regarding pregnancy, so it is important to consult with your attorney on this matter. See also the discussion later in this chapter of the Family and Medical Leave Act of 1993 for additional legal requirements regarding pregnancy.

## Sexual Harassment

The EEOC has defined *sexual harassment* as unwelcome sexual advances, requests for sexual favors, and other verbal or physical conduct of a sexual nature when:

- Submission to such conduct is made either explicitly or implicitly a term or condition of an individual's employment
- Submission to or rejection of such conduct by an individual is used as the basis for employment decisions
- Such conduct has the purpose or effect of unreasonably interfering with an individual's work performance or creating an intimidating, hostile, or offensive working environment[17]

In addition to back pay and injunctive relief, plaintiffs often file tort claims in state court for assault, battery, wrongful discharge, invasion of privacy, false imprisonment, and emotional distress. These tort claims create the possibility for both compensatory and punitive damages, and extremely offensive cases have resulted in jury awards exceeding $1 million.

Sexual harassment can occur in two different ways. *Quid pro quo* sexual harassment occurs when the employer provides, withholds, or offers job-related benefits based on compliance with sexual requests. "If you don't sleep with me, you won't get a pay raise," or "If you won't go out with me tonight, then I'll give you extra work to do" are two blatant examples. Sexual harassment also occurs if an employer acts in this way, even if it is not overtly stated.

More common, and more difficult to define and address, is sexual harassment arising from a *hostile working environment*. This occurs when unwelcome sexual conduct interferes with the employee's job performance or creates an intimidating, hostile, or abusive work setting, even though there is no threatened loss of benefits. Examples can include fondling, abusive language, requests for sexual favors, and sexual jokes *if*, according to

the U.S. Supreme Court, these are "sufficiently severe to alter the conditions of . . . employment and create an abusive working environment."[18] Generally, an isolated comment, obscenity, request for a date, or invitation to dine does not constitute a hostile environment. *There are instances, however, where a single incident, because of its nature, has constituted sexual harassment.*

A danger is that two sincere individuals can see the same situation differently, especially if they differ greatly in power, such as a physician and an employee, or an administrator and a subordinate. What Dr. McClain views as voluntary and uncoerced, Ms. Wellington may perceive as unwelcome. In the eyes of the law, an event can be both voluntary and unwelcome at the same time. People also vary in their sensibilities. Repeated sexual jokes and gestures can create an atmosphere of discrimination that may be offensive to an employee, although the harasser may not perceive this. Finally, although men have historically been the harassers, sexual harassment is just as illegal and offensive when a woman conducts it.

To reduce the chance that sexual harassment will occur and to provide the strongest possible defense should it be alleged, implement the following policies. First, distribute a written policy to all employees that clearly defines and prohibits quid pro quo and hostile work environment harassment. Defining both forms is very important. Some individuals may be harassing and not know it or may rationalize it by giving it another definition, such as flirtatious or humorous. Specifically prohibited are sexual advances, requests for sexual favors, intimate relationships between supervisory and subordinate employees unless they are married to each other, and verbal or physical behavior that may be offensive. Emphasize that this is extremely important and set a personal example by your own behavior. Provide a clear procedure for an employee to complain directly to the "top," such as the managing physician or, in a healthcare system, a senior executive. State that all incidents will be taken seriously, quickly resolved, and documented. Put this policy in any employee manual, conduct training with all employees when it is first implemented, and be certain that it is reviewed with all new employees.

If an event occurs, it is essential to investigate and act on it immediately. Take *every* complaint seriously, irrespective of who is involved. Harassment can be subtle and encompass a wide range of activities. It is not just young attractive women who are harassed. Some cases may turn into a "he said–she said" confrontation, and it becomes difficult to identify what really happened. Sometimes, communication and mutual conciliation between the parties will resolve the matter, but in many cases this will fail. *Generally, courts hold that you as the employer are not responsible for sexual harassment if, once notified of an occurrence, you follow your procedures and take appropriate action.* This can include firing the offender, but a strong written reprimand with a threat of future dismissal can be sufficient.

Be certain that you thoroughly and accurately document each employee's job performance on a regular basis and determine pay raises, promotions, discipline, and termination on well-documented performance appraisals (Chapter 3) or published seniority or time-in-position standards. This can provide the basis for a legal defense. Finally, have your attorney review your harassment grievance procedure, and seek legal guidance whenever an employee alleges harassment.

## Age Discrimination

The general standards that have been discussed also apply to age discrimination. Employers who are covered by the ADEA cannot discriminate against an employee who is 40 years old or older on the basis of age. The standard defense to a charge of age discrimination is to document that the job action was based on job performance. If the charge relates to giving preference to a younger applicant, then the defense is to document the superior performance of the younger employee in the employment-selection process or on the job.

The ADEA also recognizes the concept of bona fide occupational qualifications. As with sexual discrimination, relatively few BFOQs are accepted as legitimate. Generally, these are related to public safety and to instances in which youth is essential to authenticity, such as a youthful part in an advertisement intended to promote the sale of a product to youthful consumers. Age-related BFOQs largely are irrelevant to medical practices.

A medical practice typically encounters the issue of age discrimination when an older person applies for a clerical or technical position. In these instances, utilization of the employment methods and strategies discussed in Chapter 4 will provide the basis for a sound defense based on business necessity, if an age discrimination suit is brought. More importantly, using these methods will ensure that you will hire the best available applicant.

## The ADA

The ADA makes it illegal for employers to discriminate against a disabled person *who is otherwise qualified for a job*. It applies to hiring, firing, promotion, compensation, training, or any other conditions or terms of employment. The ADA covers individuals who:

- Have physical or mental impairments that substantially limit a major life activity, such as standing, talking, walking, seeing, or speaking.

- Have a record of such impairment, including those who have recovered from problems such as cancer and drug addiction, or who are asymptomatic but test positive for a condition, such as HIV.
- Are regarded as having an impairment, such as obesity or disfigurement, when the employer cannot state a job-related reason for an action. (The inference is that the employer would then be acting on the basis of a stereotype or fear. This provision also precludes, for example, rejecting an applicant with a chronically ill child on the assumption that this would affect the applicant's attendance record.)

Generally, people with contagious diseases, including AIDS, are covered by the ADA, if their condition does not impose a significant health or safety risk to employees or patients. Former drug addicts and alcoholics also are considered disabled. The employer, however, may set attendance, performance, and behavior standards for all employees. An alcoholic who violates these policies cannot use his or her alcoholism to avoid or mitigate discipline or termination. Stated another way, the condition of alcoholism is not a basis for termination, but alcoholic behavior certainly is.

Perhaps the ADA's most controversial provision is the requirement for employers to make reasonable accommodation to employ otherwise qualified disabled applicants. Reasonable accommodation can include making facilities accessible; restructuring jobs; modifying access to employment methods; adjusting work schedules; acquiring or modifying equipment, procedures, or training materials; and providing qualified readers or interpreters. The employer, however, is not required to make accommodations that would create an undue hardship to itself.

Undue hardship occurs when the accommodation would require significant expense or difficulty, taking into account the organization's size and financial resources and the nature of the job. If this sounds vague, it is. It is safe to say, however, that a large hospital system will be held to a standard different from that of a smaller private practice.

For example, Alistair, who is otherwise qualified to be a practice's business manager, uses a wheelchair. He cannot reach all the vertical files, the chair can't enter some of the business areas because of the positioning of furniture and equipment, and the computer desk is too low for him to use with the chair. Reasonable accommodation may mean purchasing lateral files, moving furniture, and putting blocks under the computer desk. These accommodations would probably not constitute an undue hardship, nor would it be permissible to let these accommodations influence the evaluation of Alistair's qualifications for the job.

Marie is also otherwise qualified for the position. She lost her sight in an auto accident, however, and she would need a full-time reader, which would cost about $50,000 per year. This almost certainly would constitute an undue hardship for many practices, but what about a healthcare system generating several hundred million dollars annually?

The real-world cost of most accommodations is small. In one study, Sears found that 69% of their reasonable accommodations cost nothing, 29% cost less than $1,000, and only 3% cost more than $1,000.[19]

The ADA specifically excludes coverage for homosexuality, bisexuality, transvestitism, transsexuality, pedophilia, exhibitionism, voyeurism, gender identity disorders, compulsive gambling, kleptomania, pyromania, sexual behavior disorders, and disorders resulting from using illegal drugs. State and city laws, however, may cover some of these classifications. For example, New York, California, Massachusetts, New York City, and San Francisco have employment discrimination legislation that precludes discriminating against homosexuals.

To ensure that your organization does not violate the ADA, be certain that all employees with personnel management responsibilities are trained in ADA requirements. In a practice setting, have one managing physician responsible for reviewing all personnel decisions that affect the disabled. This physician's responsibility is to understand enough about the ADA to recognize when the practice is entering dangerous territory and to contact your attorney to avoid or minimize the exposure.

Conduct a thorough job analysis before filling any position, and be certain that the job description clearly defines the tasks that are essential. Review all selection procedures for their job relatedness. Don't use employment tests or other selection criteria that adversely affect the disabled, unless the methods are job related and there are no other choices.

As a physician, you may be called on to provide physical examinations for other employers. Always ask the employer for a job description. Don't make blanket statements about an individual's general suitability for a job. Don't make any final employment decisions for an employer. Instead, specify the tasks that an individual can't perform or perform safely. The employer then can make a balanced employment decision.

## The Fair Labor Standards Act

This act, also known as the *wage-and-hour law*, was enacted by Congress in 1938. Provisions of this act have been copied in so many state laws that the application of its provisions is nearly universal. Among other things, the act sets a national minimum wage, and it also requires the payment of time and a half for overtime in excess of 40 hours per week. Not all employees are covered by the overtime provision of the act. Employees who are not covered by the overtime provision are referred to as *exempt employees*. Exempt employees are those who are employed in a bona fide executive, administrative, or professional capacity. Definitions of executive, administrative, and professional employees are found in **Exhibit 10–2**. Classification of some positions as exempt can be difficult, and, given that there may be significant financial implications, you should consult your attorney for the latest interpretations of exempt status for problematic positions. There are many positions in a healthcare organization that could be classified as exempt, including business manager, office manager, and various nursing and technical positions as well as all physician employees.

It is important to document all time worked by nonexempt employees. Nonexempt employees can claim to have worked overtime, and if you do not have adequate documentation of their actual work hours, you may have to pay time and a half. The employer has a duty under the Fair Labor Standards Act to keep accurate work records. **Exhibit 10–3** lists the data that should be kept for 3 years for each nonexempt employee. Although the Department of Labor only requires that these records be kept for 2 years, an employee can bring an action for willful violation of the Fair Labor Standards Act for 3 years. It is safest, therefore, to retain these records for 3 years after employment ends. To maintain accurate records on the hours each employee works, nonexempt employees should complete time sheets for

**Exhibit 10–2** Fair Labor Standards Act: Definitions of Executive, Administrative, and Professional Employees

---

*Executive Employees*
- Normally supervises two or more employees.
- Has authority to hire and fire, or whose recommendations in that regard are given serious consideration.
- Primary duty involves managing the practice.
- Regularly exercises discretionary powers.
- Receives salary compensation of at least $455 per week.

Also, any employee who receives $455 per week and who manages a department or who supervises two or more employees is considered an executive.

*Administrative Employees*
- Primary duties consist of office or nonmanual work directly related to management policies or the general operation of the business.
- Exercises discretion and independent judgment on a regular basis.
- Regularly and directly assists executives, performs specialized work, or possesses specialized knowledge and exercises these skills under general supervision only.
- Receives salary compensation of at least $455 per week.

*Professional Employees*
- Requires advanced knowledge acquired through a course of specialized intellectual instruction.
- Performs work that is original and is dependent on the employee's imagination and talent.
- Teaches for an educational institution.
- Performs work that requires the exercise of consistent discretion.
- Performs work that is predominantly intellectual and varied in character.
- Receives salary compensation of at least $455 per week.

*Source:* Adapted from U. S. Department of Labor.
www.dol.gov/esa/regs/compliance/whd/fairpay/fs17b_executive.htm. Accessed July 10, 2007.

---

each payroll period. Because nonexempt employees who work unauthorized overtime must be compensated for this time, do the following to prevent unauthorized overtime:

- Establish and distribute a policy stating that a supervisor must authorize in writing all work beyond normal work hours.
- Don't suggest, pressure, or condone coming in early, working late, or taking work home unless you intend to pay for it.
- Notice when employees arrive and leave. If they are coming in early or staying late, find out why.
- Audit time sheets, and be certain that they are being accurately kept.

- Remember, it is ultimately management's responsibility to make certain that time sheets are accurate, and that employees only work the hours that you intend.

These are primarily business manager responsibilities, nevertheless, if you are a practice's physician leader it is your responsibility to pay attention and supervise the business manager closely enough so you will be aware of these issues.

**Family and Medical Leave Act of 1993**

Under the Family and Medical Leave Act of 1993 (FMLA) covered employers must

**Exhibit 10–3** Fair Labor Standards Act Record-Keeping Requirements

- Employee's full name and social security number
- Address, including zip code
- Birth date, if younger than 19
- Sex and occupation
- Time and day of week when employee's workweek begins
- Hours worked each day
- Total hours worked each workweek
- Basis on which employee's wages are paid (e.g., "$6 an hour," "$220 a week," piecework)
- Regular hourly pay rate
- Total daily or weekly straight-time earnings
- Total overtime earnings for the workweek
- All additions to or deductions from the employee's wages
- Total wages paid each pay period
- Date of payment and the pay period covered by the payment

*Source:* U. S. Department of Labor.
www.dol.gov/esa/regs/compliance/whd/whdfs21.htm. Accessed July 10, 2007.

provide eligible employees with up to 12 workweeks of unpaid leave for covered life events during any 12-month period. These events include:

- Birth and care of an employee's newborn child
- Placement with the employee of a child for adoption or foster care
- Caring for an immediate family member (spouse, child, or parent) with a serious health condition
- Taking medical leave when the employee is unable to work because of a serious health condition.

Generally, the FMLA covers any employer with 50 or more employees who have worked each working day for the past 20 or more calendar weeks in the current or preceding calendar year. All work sites within 75 miles will be used to determine eligibility, so if you have several offices within 75 miles, then eligibility will be determined based on the total number of employees.

Employee eligibility is determined by the following tests: (1) has been employed by the employer for at least 12 months; and (2) has been employed for at least 1,250 hours of service during the 12-month period immediately preceding the commencement of the leave. Either the employer may require or the employee may choose to substitute accrued paid vacation leave, personal leave, or family leave for any part of the 12-week FMLA mandated time. In addition, the employee is required to provide at least 30 days notice for predictable events, such as the birth or adoption of a child.

## ANTIKICKBACKS AND ANTIREFERRALS LEGISLATION

Antikickback and antireferral legislation exist in both the criminal and civil varieties. The Medicaid Anti-Kickback Statute (42 U.S.C. §1320a-7b) makes it a felony (crime) to receive direct, indirect, overt, or covert compensation in exchange for referrals or for recommending any kind of treatment or service for Medicare, Medicaid, or any other federally funded healthcare program. This legislation outlaws a number of relationships and actions including kickbacks, bribes, rebates, discount arrangements, and manufacturers providing gifts and business courtesies. Penalties can be assessed of up to a $25,000 for each violation and up to 5 years in prison or both. In addition, civil monetary penalties may also be levied.[20] This statute is interpreted with a "one-purpose" test, meaning that even if the financial arrangements have several legitimate purposes, if one goal is to influence referrals, then the arrangement is illegal. Interpretation of whether a particular arrangement is in violation of this statute is not simple. Whenever you enter into any arrangement with another physician, practice, or healthcare organization to which you make or receive referrals, it is essential to consult an attorney knowledgeable in this body of law. For example, a radiology group and a family practice group that forms a limited liability company in which family practice physicians would share in the revenue derived on scans from patients that they refer would certainly need to consult with an attorney. Similarly, some relationships in which hospitals fund physicians' practices or business opportunities with the potential oucome of increasing physicians' referrals to the hospital are likewise questionable.

A safe harbor is a provision of a statute or regulation, which excuses liability for otherwise prohibited acts. Some forms of leases, ambulatory surgery centers, and ventures in rural areas, may be safe harbors, if the facts fit clearly into the safe harbor definitions in the Medicaid Antikickback Statute. Situations that don't fit into the safe harbors may still be legal, but clearly, an expert's opinion is needed to avoid prosecution.

In contrast to the Medicaid Anti-Kickback Statute, the Stark Law (42 U.S.C. Section 1395nn) is civil legislation. Penalties are monetary (up to $15,000 per infraction). The issue of motivation or intent to influence referrals is *irrelevant*. The issue is simply whether the financial arrangements between two healthcare organizations violate Stark. Stark focuses on the issue of physician self-referral, which occurs when a patient is referred to a facility in which the referring physician has a financial interest. Under Stark, however, this self-referral may mean the physician's own practice. It applies only to physicians who make referrals of Medicare and Medicaid patients for specific medical services to entities with which they have a financial relationship. Specifically, you need to answer three questions when you make a referral:[21]

1. Does this arrangement involve a referral of a Medicare or Medicaid patient by a physician or an immediate family member of a physician?
2. Is the referral for a "designated health service"?
3. Is there a financial relationship of any kind between the referring physician or a family member and the entity to which the referral is being made?

If your answer is "no" to any of the questions, then Stark does not apply. If it is "yes" to all three, then you need to determine whether your relationship falls into one of the stated exceptions. However, understanding Stark's definitions of referral, designated health service, and how value is determined are critical to correctly answering the questions and determining whether you fit into an exception. For example, Stark defines the word referral so broadly that

. . . if a physician creates a plan of care, the physician is deemed to have referred the patient to whoever provides services pursuant to the plan, even if the physician does not explicitly mention the particular provider. For example, if a physician indicates that a patient requires crutches, but does not name a particular vendor, the physician is deemed to have "referred" the patient to the ultimate provider of the crutch.[22]

Stark only applies to particular designated health services (DHS), which are noted in **Exhibit 10–4**. Physicians who offer any of these services must determine whether they have any financial relationships with referring physicians. Unlike the antikickback statute, Stark also applies to payments *within* a professional corporation. To qualify for several exceptions, such as for intraoffice referrals and referrals to other physicians in the same group, a group practice must meet the Stark definition of a group practice. The following are the considerations:

- Two or more physicians must be *legally* organized, such as in a partnership, professional corporation, etc.

- Each physician working in the group must offer a similar range of DHSs. If one does not, such as for example a part-time consulting physician who offers few or none of the DHSs, then the group would fail the test and all DHS referrals would violate Stark.

- The group must function as an integrated business. Markers include centralized financial controls, such as a single compensation and salary structure, centralized integrated billing and financial reporting, and integrated quality control and utilization review. The practice can be organized into cost centers, but physicians can't be compensated based on the volume or value of their DHS referrals. Physicians can, however, share in the overall profits of the group, some of which would be as a result of fees collected for the DHS services.

- The group must use a single taxpayer ID number and at least 75 percent of all services provided by each W-2 physician employee and owner must be billed under this ID. A concern, therefore, is whether some group members are moonlighting or offering services through another tax ID. In

---

**Exhibit 10–4**   Stark Law Coverage

*Designated Health Services*
Clinical laboratory
Physical therapy
Occupational therapy
Radiology and other diagnostic servcies (MRI, CAT, etc.)
Radiation therapy services and supplies
Durable medical equipment and supplies
Parenteral and enteral nutrition
Prosthetics and orthotics
Home health services
Outpatient prescription drugs
Inpatient and outpatient hospital services

*Source:* Adapted from Glaser, D. (2004). Stark laws, safe harbor regulations, and anti-kickback statutes. *Sports Medicine and Arthroscopic Review.* 12(4):248–249.

addition, group members must provide at least 75 percent of the group's patient encounters. If independent contractors provide more than 25 percent of the group's patient encounters, then this fails the Stark definition of a group practice. This provision eliminates "virtual" groups.

- A preset formula must be established regarding the distribution of the group's expenses and income prior to receiving payment for services that generated them. Notice the "accrual thinking" embedded in this rule (see Chapter 1). The implication is that you can't retrospectively change internal practice compensation formulas. You can, however, do this prospectively. The driver is the financial formula at the time the service is offered.

In order to refer patients to your own practice for DHSs, such as X-rays and clinical laboratory services, you must qualify as a group under Stark, *and* satisfy the additional following requirements:

- In-office ancillary services must be personally furnished by a group physician or someone who under the Medicare/Medicaid definition is directly supervised by one of the group's physicians.
- The office in which the in-office ancillary services are being provided also must offer unrelated non-DHS services. Centralized facilities, such as an MRI or CT office must, therefore, also offer a normal range of non-DHS services.
- Billing for ancillary services must be under the performing or supervising physician, under the group tax ID, or by another group whose ownership is exactly the same as the ancillary service provider.

Finally, the financial transactions must take place at "fair market value." This means that prices must be based on other external transactions by uninterested parties in the same community. Other provisions of the Stark Law provide exceptions for preventive services, make allowances for small non-monetary compensation such as holiday gifts, and govern compensation that hospitals might offer to practices to support recruiting new physicians. In addition, lease arrangements between physicians and the renter of the facility providing DHSs, physician incentive plans, personal service arrangements, and bona fide employment relationships also are governed, and when properly structured do not preclude referrals. The complexity of the legislation and published guidelines makes legal advice essential.

### Independent Contractor Agreements

An *independent contractor* is one who contracts to render personal services as well as provides the means to perform those services. Consulting physicians, psychologists, social workers, physical therapists, nurses, and a number of other types of workers sometimes are engaged as independent contractors by healthcare organizations. The distinction between an independent contractor and an employee has important financial and tax considerations for the employer. For example, independent contractors are not covered under the Fair Labor Standards Act or worker's compensation laws. Employers also do not have to withhold federal and state taxes on wages, pay the employer's share of FICA, or pay federal and state unemployment taxes for independent contractors. Because of these financial considerations, federal agencies including the Internal Revenue Service (IRS) may closely examine independent contractor agreements.

Often, the distinction between an employee and an independent contractor is hard to ascertain. Federal agencies, such as the Department of Labor and the IRS, have an interest in classifying workers as employees, because that generates more taxes and creates more federal control. The costs to a practice or health system can be substantial if it treats workers as independent contractors, and the IRS or the Department of Labor subsequently determines them to be employees. The IRS, for example, often seeks to collect FICA taxes not withheld plus interest and penalties. As a result, whenever you are considering treating someone as an independent contractor, it is important to discuss this with your attorney. Your attorney should prepare all contracts that you execute with independent contractors.

The overriding issue when determining whether a worker is a contractor or an employee is the degree of control exercised by the employer. There are a number of tests that have been established to determine contractor or employee status. **Exhibit 10–5** contains some tests used by the IRS. Imagine that passing each test results in one check mark on the employee or the contractor side of a ledger. The preponderance of the checks may determine the worker's status. The word *may* needs to be stressed, because of the predisposition of federal agencies to decide in favor of employee status. Ultimately, both the courts and federal agencies look to the reality of the relationship, as opposed to simply counting the number of characteristics

---

**Exhibit 10–5** IRS Tests To Determine Contractor or Employee Status

*Factors Contributing to Employee Status*

A good example would be a practice business manager.

- The employer has the right to direct and control the individual's performance, including the means, methods, and details of achieving the results. This control does not have to be actually exercised; it simply has to be available to the employer. (The business manager largely determines his or her own daily actions, sets priorities, and governs the front office, but nevertheless is under the potential control of the physician.)
- The employer can discharge the individual.
- The employer furnishes tools and other equipment for performing the work.
- The employer furnishes a place to work, and the individual regularly works there.

*Factors Contributing to Contractor Status*

An example would be contracting with an accountant to provide financial services, such as bookkeeping, financial statement, etc.

- The employer only determines the end to be accomplished, not the means to reach the end. (The practice does not influence how the financial statements are prepared.)
- The individual furnishes his or her own tools and normal workplace. (The accountant does the work largely in his or her own office, although he or she may on occasion visit the practice.)
- The individual represents him- or herself to the public as available to perform similar duties for others, including being a contractor for others in the same type of business. (The accountant has other clients.)
- The individual does not in fact spend most of his or her time working for one employer.

*Source:* Adapted from Kahn, S., B. Brown, & B. Zepke. (1988). *Personnel Director's Legal Guide*, 1988 *Cumulative Supplement.* New York: Warren, Gorham, and Lamont, pp. S3-16–S3-17.

associated with contractor or employee status. The IRS will issue a declaratory ruling for tax purposes, which is an *opinion* about whether a particular worker is an employee or contractor. IRS, however, will not be bound by this decision in the future. Asking IRS for a declaratory ruling may put you on an investigation list. If you are subsequently investigated and it is determined that the worker is an employee and you have been treating the worker as a contractor, you still may be assessed penalties and interest in addition to the back taxes owed.

The use of independent contractor arrangements also can create some insulation from liability. Because an independent contractor operates outside the control of the employer, this can provide a defense for the employer in tort cases, such as malpractice. To assert this defense, however, the employer cannot lead a third party, such as a patient, to believe that the contractor is an employee. To ensure that the provider is perceived as an independent contractor, all letterheads, pamphlets, and publications should clearly indicate the provider's contractor status. In addition, request for treatment or financial forms signed by patients should clearly state that the provider is an independent contractor and not under the supervision or control of your practice or hospital. Since in fact you may want to exercise control and may be ethically bound to provide control, you may be best off recognizing this as an employment situation and employing the individual as a part-time employee.

## SELECTING AN ATTORNEY

Because the law permeates all aspects of business, it is essential to have an attorney who is readily available. The time to develop a relationship with an attorney is *before* you find yourself in a crisis. Consult your attorney whenever you are considering any action with legal implications or receive any document with legal implications. The following documents and actions, among others, require a legal consultation:

- Written employment contracts or verbal employment agreements
- Contracts with vendors, suppliers, or independent contractors with large financial considerations, or where the "worst-case scenario" is quite bad
- Participating agreements with insurance companies
- Notification that a lawsuit has been or will be filed against you or your practice
- Termination of an employee
- Apparent violation of any employment contract or vendor, supplier, or contractor agreement
- Injury to any patient, employee, contractor, or member of the general public on your premises
- All leases and other contracts relating to real property
- Any allegations of illegal discrimination (race, sex, age, etc.)

Recommendations from other physicians or healthcare professionals can be helpful in identifying potential business attorneys. Interview attorneys before making a decision. Many attorneys will not charge a fee for this type of consultation. Finally, once you select an attorney, you should continue to evaluate the quality and timeliness of his or her work. If you become dissatisfied, discuss this with the attorney; if there is no change, select another attorney.

It is not essential to retain a lawyer or legal firm that specializes in medical practices for your general legal needs. Larger firms have the advantage of being able to offer attorneys who specialize in various parts of the law, such as tax law, malpractice, and employment law. This also can work to your disadvantage.

For example, if you call with a question regarding a contract, but that also may have tax implications, the firm's contract lawyer may consult with the firm's tax lawyer, and you will be billed for both attorneys. Is this kind of intrafirm consultation really required? In some instances it may be, but at other times it may be a strategy for "running the billing clock." In addition, you may find it more difficult to establish a personal relationship with an attorney in a larger firm. If you like developing personal relationships with your attorney or accountant, such as golfing or socializing, then you may be more satisfied with a smaller firm that gives you personalized attention. Keep in mind that you may be a medium or large account to a small firm, whereas you may be a small account to a large firm. A small firm or an attorney with a general business practice will generally possess adequate knowledge to handle most business law questions, and the firm or attorney can always refer you to a legal specialist when necessary, such as for a complex arrangement with potential anti-kickback or Stark implications as previously discussed.

Fees should be discussed in your initial meeting with the attorney. Generally, the attorney will be your legal representative, file annual corporate papers, and do specified other tasks for a flat fee, which will vary with your geographical location. Additional tasks, such as providing an opinion on a contract, representing you in litigation, or giving advice on how to terminate an employee are generally handled on an hourly basis. Hourly fees will vary with geography and with the experience of the attorney.

## CONCLUSION

By reading this chapter, you should have gained an understanding of the legal responsibilities and implications associated with the business side of a healthcare organization. You should have a basic understanding of contracts and torts that you can use to identify potentially threatening or litigious situations. You should understand the theory of malpractice. You should be able to deal with employment and personnel matters so you don't inadvertently forego your employer prerogatives, while at the same time comply with federal legislation, such as the Fair Labor Standards Act and the Civil Rights Act of 1964. You should be vigilant to issues involving kickbacks and referrals. Finally, you should have developed an awareness of how to avoid legal conflicts in the daily operation of your health care organization, understand the role of a business attorney, and be able to recognize situations in which you should seek legal counsel.

## NOTES

1. Maurer, V. (1987). *Business Law: Text and Cases*. San Diego: Harcourt Brace Jovanovich, pg. 5.
2. Ibid, pg. 74.
3. Ibid, pg. 163.
4. Kahn, S., et al. (1988). *Personnel Director's Legal Guide, Cumulative Supplement*. New York: Warren, Gorham & Lamont, pp. S2-27–S2-28.
5. Szalados, J. (2007). Legal issues in the practice of critical care medicine: A practical approach. *Critical Care Medicine* 35(2):S45.
6. Fineberg, K. et al. (1984). *Obstetrics/gynecology and the law*. Washington: Health Administration Press, pp. 21–22.
7. Ibid, 43–47.
8. Solomon, R. (1997) Malpractice: Can you really protect your assets? *Medical Economics* 66(21): 129–131.
9. Often, contracts contain a "severability" clause. Any part of the contract that is subsequently found to be illegal can be severed from the con-

tract leaving the remainder of the contract in force.

10. Anderson, R., et al. (1987). *Business Law*. Belmont, CA: South-Western Publishing, p. 271.

11. Kahn, S., et al. (1988). *Personnel Director's Legal Guide, Cumulative Supplement*. New York: Warren, Gorham & Lamont, pp. S2-42–S2-43.

12. *Toussaint v. Blue Cross and Blue Shield of Michigan*, 408 Mich. 579, 292 N.W. 2d 880 (1980). See also *Hetes v. Schefman & Miller Law Office*, 393 N.W. 2d 577 (1986).

13. Kahn et al., *Personnel Director's Legal Guide* (1988). New York: Warren, Gorham & Lamont, pp. S5–S25.

14. Federal authorities give "strong deference" to this 4/5ths rule, but there are exceptions where they will determine that a selection rate higher than 4/5ths does constitute disparate impact and a rate below 4/5ths does not. Nevertheless, this is a good rule of thumb. This rule is stated in the EEOC's Uniform Guidelines on Employee Selection.

15. This is an accepted validation strategy stated in the EEOC's Uniform Guidelines on Employee Selection (1978).

16. Sharf, J.C., & D.P. Jones. (2000). Employment risk management. In Jerard F. Kehoe (Ed.), *Managing Selection in Changing Organizations*. Jossey-Bass, San Francisco: pp. 271–318.

17. Equal Employment Opportunity Commission, Guidelines on Sexual Harassment in the Workplace (1978). 29 C.F.R., Sec. 1604.11, *Federal Register*. 43:74676–74677.

18. *Meritor Savings Bank v. Vinson*, 477 U.S.57 (1986).

19. Reno, J. & Thornburgh, D. (1995). "ADA—not a disabling mandate." *The Wall Street Journal*. July 26, 1995, A12.

20. Hubbell, T., A. Mauro, & D. Moar. (2006). Health care fraud. *American Criminal Law Review, American Law Review*. 43 AM.Crim. L. Rev. 603.

21. Gosfield, A. (2003). The stark truth about the Stark law: Part I. *Family Practice Management*. 10(10): 28.

22. Glaser, D. (2004). Stark laws, safe harbor regulations, and anti-kickback statutes. *Sports Medicine and Arthroscopic Review*. 12(4):248.

## CHAPTER 11

# Quality Improvement

## Chapter Objectives

Quality is a concern that has become a preoccupation of U.S. business. It is difficult to pick up a copy of the *Wall Street Journal, Business Week,* or *Fortune,* or for that matter the *Journal of the American Medical Association, New England Journal of Medicine,* or *American Medical News* without seeing an article on or reference to the importance of quality. Historically, quality has been of paramount concern to physicians. The life and death nature of healthcare services, coupled with their complexity, results in quality being an obvious element in the success of any healthcare organization. The question, however, is how to achieve it. In the past, healthcare organizations placed heavy reliance on the ethics and goodwill of healthcare providers and the internal health system control of collegiality. This hasn't worked well enough.[1]

Formal quality improvement methods have significantly improved quality in many diverse industries including automobiles, aircraft manufacturing, and health care. Quality improvement methods have evolved over the years. Currently, the popular methods used in healthcare organizations include LEAN[2] and Six Sigma. These were preceded by continuous quality improvement (CQI), quality improvement (QI), and initially total quality management (TQM). Each of these quality approaches requires extensive training and mentoring, as well as conducting a project in the given quality discipline in order to become a certified and competent practitioner. For example, Six Sigma has several competency levels. The lowest, Green Belt, typically requires 2 weeks of full-time training plus conducting a quality improvement project. A chapter, such as this one, must have a more modest objective than formally developing your skills in any specific area of quality improvement. Instead, the goal is to acquaint you with how practitioners of quality improvement methods *think* about quality. It turns out that how quality improvement proponents think about quality can itself be a powerful source of change. As a physician leader, you can go quite far creating useful change, if you can capture this quality improvement mindset. This leads to two limited but nevertheless useful chapter objectives:

1. Developing a willingness on your part to look around you, see problems through the lens of quality, and use quality *concepts* to make meaningful improvement, even if not through a formal quality improvement program using formal quality improvement methods.
2. Considering obtaining formal quality training, or bringing formal quality improvement methods such as LEAN and Six Sigma to your practice or healthcare system.

## TOTAL QUALITY MANAGEMENT (TQM) CONCEPTS

The term "TQM" per se is somewhat controversial in the healthcare community. To some people, it congers up painful memories of large cumbersome quality improvement projects. TQM, however, was the first modern formal approach to quality improvement, and as such its philosophy and methods are fundamental to more recent evolutions, such as LEAN and Six Sigma, so we will begin here. Two employees working for the Hawthorne Works of Western Electric in the 1930s, the manufacturing division of AT&T, defined the fundamental nature of TQM. AT&T, and the Hawthorne Works in particular, had a long history of industrial engineering and management research. Walter A. Shewart, an engineer on a team investigating quality and control problems, discovered the significance of understanding, measuring, and displaying variability. **Figure 11–1**, for example, con-tains a control chart that reports the percentage of samples of a hospital's charts containing one or more errors. An error, for example, might include a missing signature, incomplete insurance verification information, illegibility, and so forth. The UCL line is the upper control limit, which is statistically defined in this case as two standard deviations above the mean. Variability above or below a UCL is considered out of tolerance.

The importance of variability is that it can be used to identify the *sources* of quality problems. For example, what happened in months 9, 12, and 18? Were these months in which new employees were working? Was there a volume increase, or were new management procedures implemented? Once variance is identified, then causes can be sought, problems identified, and variance reduced. If, for example, the variance in Figure 11–1 is associated with new employees, then the cause might be inadequate training. Changing the training should result in increased quality.

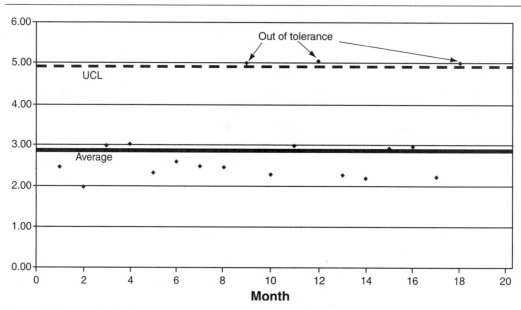

**Figure 11–1** Control Chart.

This example illustrates that work is performed through *processes*. In this case, the process defines when and by whom charts are completed. Often, quality problems occur because the work process has been poorly designed or not designed at all. By studying variation and changing the process through which work is performed, quality can be dramatically improved. Focusing on the *process* as opposed to the *individual* is central to TQM. Notice that this is a different emphasis than taken in Chapter 3, where the focus was on performance appraisal and controlling quality through the contribution of the individual. More on this later.

The control chart in Figure 11–1 illustrates one of the tools that TQM practitioners use to display variability and describe quality. This is one of the TQM tools that Sashkin and Kiser[3] have referred to as the seven old tools; the other six are charts, fishbone diagrams, run charts, histograms, scatter diagrams, and flowcharts. Several of these tools

are discussed and illustrated later. In each case, an example is provided in the context of receivables collection.

**Figure 11–2** illustrates a *Pareto chart*, named for Vilfredo Pareto, an economist who first noted that a few individuals control most of the wealth. A Pareto chart displays the number of quality problems by their source. Figure 11–2 displays a practice's out-of-tolerance receivables (90+ days) by various causes. One widely noted observation is that most problems are attributable to a limited number of causes or sources. Pareto charts, therefore, can be helpful to determine where your effort can have the greatest payoff. In this case, understanding why practice policies are not being enforced and fixing this problem appears to be the first place to direct effort.

**Figure 11–3** contains a *fishbone diagram*, also called a *cause-and-effect diagram*. The diagram represents hypotheses regarding the major sources of the effect noted at the end

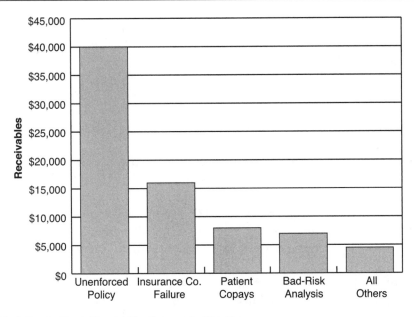

**Figure 11–2** Pareto Chart: Receivables Sources in 90+ Days.

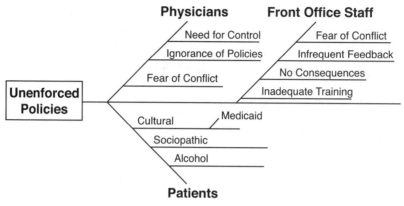

**Figure 11–3** Fishbone Diagram.

of the diagram. Constructing a fishbone diagram helps stimulate thinking about a problem. Because it is difficult to represent the interaction among various causes (bones), fishbone charts should not be taken too literally. Displaying information this way can be useful to summarize the results of brainstorming and to express logical thinking about a problem.[4]

A run chart shows quality trends over time. **Figure 11–4** contains a *run chart* for the receivables in 90+ days. A run chart can be particularly helpful in collection management, because it will allow you to detect when a change has occurred. The physician leader then can inquire and direct corrective action. For example, the chart shows that something happened in July. The control level at approximately $10,000 was exceeded in that month, and a steady climb in receivables ensued. If the practice regularly utilized a run chart, this would probably have been noticeable in July and certainly by August.

Shewart's work centered on developing statistical methods for identifying and displaying variability in the manufacturing process. W. Edwards Deming, also at Western

Electric at that time, extended Shewart's work into a general theory of management. Deming was instrumental in developing statistical tools and display methods, and he trained a generation of engineers and managers in their use. He observed, however, that the ability to use these tools did not ensure that quality would necessarily improve. Deming, who became the personification of the TQM philosophy, recognized that control charts, statistical analyses, and exhortations to improve quality don't solve quality problems by themselves. Improvements in quality only occur when managers and employees are willing, as well as able, to *use* the information to change the production process.

As he examined his successes and failures, Deming concluded that the management and organizational contexts within which the TQM tools were used were critical to successful quality improvement. He summarized the management characteristics that he felt were necessary for quality to flourish as his 14 Points.[5] They define the parameters of the TQM management philosophy, and provide insight into the physician leader's role in quality improvement.

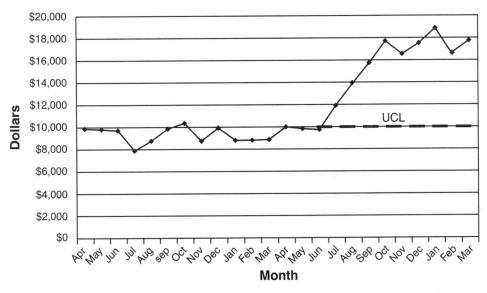

**Figure 11–4** Run Chart of Receivables in 90+ Days.

1. *Create constancy of purpose for improvement of product and service.* Deming stresses that quality should be the primary goal, not profit. Profit is a by-product that will flow from quality. Although this may sound naive, it can be expressed in another way: Quality is a less direct but more certain route to obtain profits. Replace short-term reaction to problems with a long-term commitment to solve the underlying causes of problems.

2. *The whole organization must adopt the new philosophy.* All employees including top management, not just selected pockets, levels, or work teams must accept the central importance of quality. It must permeate the organization from the highest level down to the bottom. If this doesn't occur, TQM can result in limited successes on the more easily defined quality problems. There will not be the opportunity, however, to improve in unexpected areas, where quality problems

are not obvious, or to improve beyond what is now considered acceptable.

3. *End dependence on inspection; understand the purpose of inspection.* Mass inspection assumes that quality can be added on at the end by correcting errors. Errors are wasteful, because it is much more expensive to fix a mistake than to build the product right or provide the service correctly to begin with. The most important purpose of inspection, therefore, is to identify the reasons for poor quality. Generally, this can be achieved much more easily and effectively by sampling rather than by inspecting all output.

4. *Identify best source suppliers, and don't awarding business on price alone.* The primary criteria to use when selecting suppliers should be their willingness to meet customers' needs and their willingness to work toward improving quality. Price should be considered, but only as a secondary issue. Many healthcare

organizations are wrestling with this issue. In a sense, short-term, immediate cost savings may be incompatible with long-term quality improvements, which ultimately may be more frugal *and* effective. In addition, multiple suppliers increase variance.

5. *Constantly improve, and continue to improve production and service systems forever.* Quality improvement must be an ongoing process. It never ends, and there is no improvement level beyond which quality is considered excessive.

6. *Institute training.* Deming recognized the need to train workers in statistical control methods and the use of quality control tools. He also stated that all workers must be fully trained in the technical skills needed to perform their jobs. Finally, he noted that it is necessary for managers to have training in management and organizational skills, because these are essential to create a climate in which TQM can flourish.

7. *Teach and institute leadership.* This means developing managers' skills to create a vision of what could be, gather the necessary resources, obtain the cooperation of others, and design management systems, including TQM. It means creating a culture in the organization that truly values quality. See Chapter 6 for discussions of leadership and change management.

8. *Drive out fear.* For quality to flourish, employees at all levels must feel secure. They must know that making or finding errors will not lead to retribution. Telling the truth, pointing out a problem, and thinking of new ways to do the job will not occur if employees believe that they will be punished overtly or covertly as a result of their acts. Deming viewed regular performance appraisals as fear in-

ducing and detrimental to quality, because they focus on and tie compensation to short-term job performance. Deming's position on performance appraisal is not at odds with ideas expressed in Chapter 3 of this book. If the physician leader uses the performance appraisal process to identify areas of improvement and then provides effective training and skill development opportunities along with goal setting and related rewards, then performance appraisal becomes a positive helping process.

9. *Break down organizational barriers.* Sometimes, work groups, teams, departments, divisions, and so forth will compete with each other. This can be over budgets, personnel, reputation, or power. Often, even if they don't compete with each other, they don't work effectively as an integrated team with an undivided interest to satisfy the customer's (patient's, patient's family, etc.) needs. Organizational barriers will prevent the integrated delivery of healthcare services. They must be removed. Strategies for improving integration were discussed in Chapter 9.

10. *Eliminate exhortations and slogans.* Quality cannot arise from short-term motivational and inspirational "highs." If workers want to do better, but don't have the tools to do it or are working in an organizational culture that punishes it, then exhortations to improve are viewed as hypocritical. If, on the other hand, employees are truly motivated to improve quality and work in a climate in which this is rewarded and not punished, exhortations and slogans will be viewed as superfluous if not demeaning.

11. *Eliminate numerical production quotas.* When production goals become the primary goal, quality will suffer even if

quality standards are met. Production quotas will replace the emphasis on stretching quality beyond the current standard. Instead, the emphasis will be stretching production statistics beyond the current standard while producing standard quality.

12. *Remove barriers to developing pride of skill.* Providing adequate training, high-quality materials and tools, and an organizational culture that encourages developing skills and producing a high-quality product will enable employees to develop pride in their product or service. Employees who take pride in their work will have a built-in incentive to improve quality, because it will increase their personal satisfaction.

13. *Encourage education and self-improvement.* Beyond using the tools and methods of quality control, Deming believed that employees need to learn how to work together as a team. They need to learn new behaviors and ways of interacting. Skills, such as team building, leadership, and change management, can help employees develop these skills.

14. *Take action to accomplish the transformation.* Top management must put these ideas into action. Managers cannot leave it up to lower-level employees, because the key to improving quality is to involve the whole organization in a culture of quality improvement. Only top management has the stature and resources to animate the whole organization toward a common quality objective.

In Deming's view, TQM does not exist until these 14 points are endemic to the organization. This goes beyond platitudes and grand statements by top-level management. These policies must be truly incorporated into every employee's way of thinking about his or her job. Deming's approach to quality goes far beyond the use of statistical tools and control procedures, which are necessary but insufficient in themselves for quality to flourish. Implementing variance charting and other quality tools is the easiest part of instituting TQM principles. The most difficult part is to develop an organizational culture in which quality is central, whether this is operationally accomplished through TQM methods, Six Sigma, or any other tactical approach. Organizations that don't successfully institute the culture of quality generally have limited success, because employees at a fundamental level do not truly have a reason to excel toward quality.

The discussion of quality to this point describes a process to achieve it. There is another element to add, however, that focuses on the purpose of quality. Deming proposed that the purpose of quality is to produce a product or service that "meets the demands of the market." [6] In other words, *the purpose of quality* is *to obtain customer satisfaction.* Defining quality by focusing on the customer's needs should sound familiar. This is consistent with the definition of marketing in Chapter 7. A marketing approach starts with customers' needs. Products and services then are developed around these needs, and they are then priced, placed (distributed), and promoted, and the organization is staffed so they meet customers' needs. This contrasts with a selling approach, in which a product or service is developed because it meets *your* needs, with the subsequent goal being to convince the customer why he or she needs to buy it. If you approach quality improvement purely to satisfy your own internal needs, then this results in quality improvement, but not necessarily the customer-focused quality improvement that Deming proposed.

Joseph Juran further developed Deming's idea of satisfying customers' needs as the focus for quality through what he calls the Juran Trilogy. The Juran Trilogy comprises quality planning, quality control, and quality improvement. The idea behind quality planning is to build quality into the product or service at the outset, as opposed to plating it on by catching mistakes before they reach the customer. A quality-control process focuses on "fire fighting," such as identifying and fixing the sporadic spike, sometimes referred to as *special variance*. Special variance is due to intermittent causes. For example, why does the success rate at a fertility clinic suddenly "spike down" by 50 percent over a 3-month period? Once the spike has been detected, the search for personnel, material, and procedural causes can proceed. Notice, however, that this says nothing about, nor does it address, the adequacy of a clinic's "normal" in vitro fertilization success rate. Quality improvement then focuses on the *normal* success rate.

Juran discusses marketing research as intrinsic to successful quality planning. Specifically, marketing research is a process for identifying the quality needs of customers. It is a method of finding out what features are important, and how your product or service compares with those of your competitors. It allows you to build in the quality from the *customer's* perspective, as opposed to finding out after the fact that your service does not fit the customer's needs or wants. Notice, also, that this differs somewhat from Deming's focus on reducing errors, by defining the errors in the external context of the customer.

Juran describes a road map for quality planning that focuses squarely on meeting customer needs:[7]

- *Identify the customers.* Customers are those who will be affected by your efforts. For a healthcare organization, the definition of the medical customer is complex and may include patients, patient families, insurers,

employers, government, and primary care physicians. A primary care physician is the cardiologist's customer. Similarly, the cardiologist may be a customer to the hospital's billing staff, ICU nurses, and laboratory. Not all constituencies are equally important, but all are relevant. This intertwined customer list lends additional importance to Deming's observation that quality must be endemic to the entire organization. Customers are *everywhere. You never know where the most value will be added through quality improvement.* Patient customers will be affected by several processes, such as admitting, scheduling, billing, and discharge, which in turn may be reciprocal customers to each other. If quality is defined as meeting customer needs, then you also must consider the needs of these internal customers.

- *Determine customers' needs.* Do this in *their* language, so that they can communicate effectively with you. As a physician leader conversant in business thinking and language, you should be able to solicit this information from business customers, such as insurers; finance, marketing, and management administrators; and others. Your medical background also will allow you to solicit the needs of medical customers, such as referring physicians, staff physicians, pharmacy, nurses, patients, and so forth. This ability to communicate across both sides of what previously was a fence is a unique strength of the physician leader.

- *Translate those needs into your language.* Here, the role of the physician leader becomes particularly important. As a physician who understands the language of business and the perspective of management, you can be a particularly skilled translator because you also understand the issues from a medical perspective.

- *Develop a product (service) that can respond to those needs.* Physician leaders need to be able to work with other healthcare professionals to develop services that meet internal and external customer needs. As the professional with the optimal management and medical perspectives, the physician leader has a critical role.
- *Optimize product or service features so that they meet your needs as well as external customers' needs.* Here, Juran is talking about balancing the needs of the various constituencies. Physician leaders, once again, are uniquely qualified to balance the medical and business considerations of a problem.
- *Develop a process that is able to produce the product or service.* A practice, hospital, or healthcare system can develop treatment protocols and a process for revising them based on clinical outcomes, cost outcomes, and research. Similarly, it can conduct patient attitude surveys, focus groups, and brainstorming to systematically assess patient and physician perceptions, and it can use these findings to further develop the treatment protocol *beyond clinical outcomes*.
- *Optimize the process, don't suboptimize it.* Just because customer needs can be identified does not mean that all employees will work toward their achievement. Suboptimization (see Chapter 9) occurs when various constituencies deviate from the organization's goals to meet their own needs. The surgeon, for example, who insists on stocking a lens or valve that is not demonstrably superior, and the MIS department that insists that all computer consultants be under its direct supervision may both be suboptimizing. Joint planning, avoiding subunit goals, evaluating managers on overall *organization* success and customer satisfaction instead of department goals, and obtaining participation

from all constituencies are ways to avoid suboptimization.
- *Prove that the product works under operating conditions.* For example, put the treatment protocol into effect for a sample of patients. See the discussion on obtaining short-term wins and rapid cycle improvement in the Leading the Change Process section of Chapter 6. Observe clinical, cost, and patient satisfaction outcomes. Are they as expected? If they are not, study the problem again. If they are, then:
- *Transfer the process to the operating forces.* Put the changed process into operation, and use it according to the operating plan. The plan also should have feedback mechanisms so that, as conditions change and as the definition of quality evolves, quality can be continuously improved.

Envisioning quality as encompassing internal and external customers and variability assessment tools leads to the possibility of intervening in the quality process at several points. These checkpoints are places where quality can be assessed and inserted into the process. Because the customer first defines quality, quality checkpoint 1 (QC1) is the opportunity to assess customer satisfaction. Examples of QC1 assessments include patient surveys, interviews, and focus groups. Because parts of the organization are the customers of other organizational parts, these same methods are appropriate for internal use. In a hospital, for example, a QC1 assessment occurs when ICU physicians, nurses, and respiratory therapists participate in a focus group to comment on ICU procedures. Similarly, patient data that incorporate quality-of-life measures would constitute a QC1 assessment. Organizational climate surveys are another form of QC1 data. QC1 data are a particularly important quality issue for medical procedures with aversive side effects, such as with bone marrow transplantation or chemotherapy.[8]

QC2 is located at the point of service delivery. Control tools such as Pareto charts, run charts, and other ways of describing clinical and cost outcomes and their variability focus on this checkpoint. Many organizations concentrate all their quality efforts at QC2, without appreciating that performance at this point is an input to QC3 and an outcome of QC1. Reinfection, mortality, morbidity, time, number of procedures, and an almost limitless number of financial variables are all ways of assessing QC2 quality.

QC3 is located at the point where materials come into the organization. These materials can be physical, such as antibiotics, syringes, and MRI machines, but they also can be human. For example, using effective employment methods (see Chapter 4) to hire the best staff is a QC3 issue that can pay substantial dividends at QC2 and QC1. Consider the costs of using work samples, simulations, role plays, and tests for hiring administrative and professional personnel. Think of all the ways that a higher caliber of employee manifests itself downstream in higher quality at QC2 and QC1.

QC4 moves the quality process back one more step to the supplier. For example, some auto manufacturers work closely with their vendors and suppliers, to the degree that they help them design parts and develop their management systems. Ford, for example, has greatly reduced the number of engineers designing engine seals and gaskets by moving the design work back to the parts supplier. The Ford engineers then assume the role of coordinators, integrators, and project leaders. Developing this close relationship with the supplier pays off in better-fitting parts that are more reliable and are delivered reliably when they are needed, not before and not late.

Working with suppliers that are willing to consider designing their product to satisfy their customer's (i.e., the healthcare organization's) needs is the basis for Deming's admonition to end the awarding of contracts on price alone. Because the cost of rework increases at each successive step, quality that can be designed before your organization acquires the product or service is the least expensive way to add value. For example, a supplier that studies a hospital's utilization patterns and packages sutures and heart valves in more useful quantities may be a better choice than the low-cost vendor. Similarly, healthcare organizations that work with internship programs and universities to develop physicians with management skills as well as medical skills may acquire higher-quality physician leaders than healthcare systems that try to train physicians in management skills in mid-career.

## TEAMWORK: THE CORE OF TQM AND ORGANIZATION INTEGRATION

In a hospital or medical practice, internal customers reside in different functional parts of the organization. The challenge is to integrate these different parts. As we noted in the discussion of organization structure (Chapter 9), different parts of an organization have different perspectives, goals, and incentives. This can result in suboptimization, or the achievement of local goals at the expense of the organization's goals. Complex processes, such as medical treatments, cut across many different organizational groups. How, then, do you integrate these diverse groups, which have different immediate goals, perspectives, and even languages? A fundamental TQM concept for addressing this integration problem is the idea of a quality team. Quality teams are assembled cutting across organizational boundaries. They include members from all groups that contribute to or affect a process. Because even processes in fairly small practices cut across organizational boundaries, teams become important because no one can see the whole process. In this way, differing perspectives can be focused on a problem or process. Often, quality teams are assembled to tackle a specific problem. In this case, their members should include all constituencies that are affected by the problem.

Traditional management thinking says that employees must be responsible for their personal behavior and that there should be consequences as a result. Traditionally, managers used the performance appraisal process to evaluate and document job performance and then, as a consequence, to make compensation and promotion decisions. Traditional-management thinking is more short-term focused; TQM is more long-term focused. Traditional-management thinking assumes that, if there are no short-term evaluation consequences, employees will lose focus and not excel. TQM, on the other hand, assumes that relieving employees of short-term performance requirements will free them to look at their jobs in a larger and longer-term perspective.

*Empowerment*, or pushing decision making and involvement down to lower levels, is essential for team-based TQM to succeed. Employees with high-growth needs (high need for achievement, recognition, responsibility, etc.) who are flexible and adaptable and have or desire to possess strong interpersonal skills are good candidates for empowered jobs. These also are the characteristics of employees who can flourish in a TQM type of environment. Employees who seek achievement for achievement's sake, and an internal sense of satisfaction do not need the regimentation of a short-term focused appraisal system to structure their performance.

In contrast, some employees obtain little or no satisfaction from the work itself. They are rigid and set in their ways, have limited in-terpersonal skills, and do not wish to develop the range and depth of their talents. These employees will be frustrated by empowered jobs, and will have great difficulty adapting to the fluidity of a quality improvement environment. In addition, they may take advantage of a system that does not pay close attention to short-term performance through regular performance evaluations.

What is necessary, then, for a TQM culture to flourish is a synergy of management systems. For teams to function effectively, employment methods must first select employees with the interpersonal skills, independence, and need for achievement required in a TQM system. Training must be supplied so that employees develop the technical skills and management skills including quality improvement skills, necessary to work effectively in groups. Finally, management systems, such as performance-appraisal and compensation systems, must complement the long-term perspective that is an inherent part of a TQM management philosophy. The eventual goal is to blur the line between improving quality, and the definition of an employee's job. Both should be viewed as one and the same.

A final element of the culture that is necessary for successful TQM teams to develop is to use the scientific method for problem solving. Problems are identified, data collected and displayed using TQM or other quality improvement tools, hypotheses are formed, processes are adjusted in response to the data and hypotheses, effects are observed, and processes are adjusted again, if necessary. Finally, conclusions are reached, and the process of hypothesis generation, testing, and system implementation and improvement *continues forever*. This is a process that healthcare professionals generally feel comfortable with, because it is the basis for the sciences of their professional disciplines.

## SIX SIGMA

Six Sigma utilizes statistical process control with the objective of pushing performance out six standard deviations (sigmas) above the mean, or 3.4 errors per million opportunities for a defect. For example, let's look at those hospital charts found in Figure 11–1. Using a Six Sigma analysis, draw a sample of charts, say 500, and note the number and type of errors. Assume that you find three charts with no signatures, two with incomplete insurance verifications, and two with illegible notes at some point in the chart. A Six Sigma analysis shows that this process is operating at 4,667 errors per million operations:

$$[(\text{Total Errors}) \div (\text{Sample Size} \times \text{Classes of Defect Opportunities})] \times 1,000,000$$

or

$$[(3 + 2 + 2) \div (500 \times 3)] \times 1,000,000$$
$$= 4,667$$

This is operating at approximately 4.1 sigmas. The goal then would be to improve the process to get it down to six sigmas or 3.4 errors per million operations.

Six Sigma programs are based on extensive quality training throughout the organization, with its practitioners being classified into various categories based on their training and their role in quality improvement. Green Belts retain their normal jobs, but also function as quality improvement team members, or as a part-time Six Sigma team leader. Their role is to bring Six Sigma concepts to daily business operation. Black Belts take on full-time quality improvement roles, usually for 18 months to 2 years. Often, they are very successful middle managers or rising stars. They take the lead in working on critical quality improvement opportunities. They lead projects, and work with and coach teams

of Green Belts. Master Black Belts serve as coaches and mentors to Black Belts. Master Black Belts have developed true expertise in statistics and Six Sigma analysis tools and methods. Champions are senior managers who sponsor a Black Belt's project, so that Six Sigma projects receive high organizational priority and respect. Six Sigma teams are cross-organizationally staffed and focus on solving quality problems with a customer focus. The strategy used is consistent with TQM described previously: and is expressed in the acronym DMAIC (Define, Measure, Analyze, Improve, Control).

- Define—consider the problem from a customer perspective. Identify root causes. Usually Black Belts will guide the team to focus on satisfying customer needs.
- Measure—collect data in terms of outcomes, such as results, defects, and the like.
- Analyze—examine the procedures and methods used to do the work. Consider how machines and tools are used, and the impact of the quality-of-input materials.
- Improve—devise solutions. Often, this requires "unfreezing" to get people to kick free of old habits, ways of doing things, and thinking about problems. Often, several competing solutions may be identified, and these need to be sorted through by focusing back on the customer-based quality criteria. Ultimately, the project champion will need to approve the solution. This phase also includes implementation, where the change management methods discussed in Chapter 6 can be applied. As with any type of change, don't count on Six Sigma change to "sell itself."
- Control—this makes the change stick. Continuing to monitor outcomes, identifying a few critical indicators of success for management to track, ensuring that the performance-appraisal and goal-setting process is consistent with the new process,

and selling the changed process through the change management methods discussed in Chapter 6 are all ways of making sure that things won't digress back to their old ways.

## CASE ANALYSIS: HIGHER QUALITY AND LOWER COSTS IN DIALYSIS[9]

Recognizing the potential to save lives, the Joint Commission on Accreditation of Healthcare Organizations now requires hospitals to set up quality improvement programs. Only a handful, however, have implemented the measurement systems, developed the protocols, and fostered the teamwork needed to make it work. More often, attempts bog down in endless meetings and fractious infighting. Even rarer is the small medical practice that can muster the vision, resources, expertise, and commitment to adopt a rigorous continuous quality improvement (CQI) program. For those that do, however, the payoff can be huge. Just ask Ernie Rutherford, MD.

Five years ago, Dr. Rutherford set out to improve performance at five dialysis centers that he owns and operates with partners Joan Blondin, MD, and Herschel Harter, MD, in and around Monroe, Louisiana. A Deming devotee with no formal business training, Dr. Rutherford was convinced that statistical process control and CQI could work the same wonders for medicine that it has for industry. Four years into the program, the results have far exceeded Dr. Rutherford's expectations. Mortality rates have dropped from about 23 percent (close to the national average) to 11 percent. Hospitalizations are down 40 percent. Patients report feeling better than they have in years. At the same time, marginal costs per dialysis treatment have fallen 35 percent, netting an additional $500,000 this year for the dialysis centers.

Dr. Rutherford believes that his approach is significant for other reasons as well. As physicians are being asked to take more and more

risk, statistical process control gives them a powerful tool for understanding and controlling risk. It will help physicians who master it retain control of medicine. "If you can get rid of variation [in a process], you can predict how it will perform. If you can predict, you can take risk."

Others are interested in Dr. Rutherford's approach. He has presented his results to meetings of the Renal Physicians Association and is working with a local hospital to develop treatment algorithms for congestive heart failure. Representatives from other dialysis centers and the Healthcare Financing Administration's (HCFA's) renal network have visited Dr. Rutherford's centers to find ways to improve quality. Even the Institute of Medicine has taken a look.

The key is to focus on quality, not cost, Dr. Rutherford says. "If you focus on cutting costs, quality will go down. If you focus on improving quality, costs will eventually go down." That's largely because improving quality through process control also means eliminating waste and duplication of effort to fix mistakes. Implementing quality improvement with strict process controls is not a simple task, however. Dr. Rutherford and his colleagues had to overcome both technical and cultural hurdles that have halted CQI programs at other facilities.

### The Scientific Method

Dr. Blondin describes CQI as "just the scientific method applied to business." CQI proposes that products (in this case the health and functioning of patients with end-stage renal disease) are the result of processes. For the product to improve, the process must change. That's where the scientific method comes in. First, the process is defined. This step is analogous to generating a hypothesis and designing an experiment. At the North Louisiana Dialysis Center, teams of physicians, nurses, nutritionists, and technicians develop algorithms, or detailed flowcharts, of standard treatment procedures for processes ranging from controlling blood chemistry to treating malnutrition. These algorithms then are tested on groups of patients.

Second, the capabilities of the process are measured. Quality indicators, including hospitalizations, complications, adverse drug events, and blood chemistries, are monitored. Once a process is standardized, over time normal variation in its outcomes can be established. These data track the results of the experiment and function as control charts. They are collected in a computerized patient record system.

Third, the process can be changed. Results quickly become evident on the control chart. They may move an indicator up or down, or they may reduce or increase the normal variation of the process. Likewise, monitoring of control charts can alert physicians and staff that a change has crept into a process.

If data points leave the normal variation range or establish a trend above or below the median, it's time to look for the cause. "What we're doing now is practicing evidence-based medicine," Dr. Rutherford says. "We don't have to guess anymore. We have the data. Dialysis lends itself well to process control because the same procedure is done over and over, allowing opportunity to measure outcomes and improve processes." He believes, however, that it can work with other types of medical practice, particularly managing chronic diseases.

### Physician Leadership

One element that is missing from many hospital CQI programs is strong physician involvement, according to Dr. Rutherford. Often, administrators are the first to be trained, and physicians are the last to be brought in. That's a mistake because physicians control 80 percent of the resources and are positioned to make the greatest impact. They often catch on to CQI quicker than others because they have scientific training, Dr. Rutherford adds.

Physician leadership proved critical at the North Louisiana clinics. To train staff in CQI basics, Dr. Rutherford brought in the training team from Hospital Corporation of America. Physicians and key staff were flown to seminars for advanced training, one of which was taught by Deming himself.

The total training cost exceeded $70,000, which represents a large investment for a small practice. Because CQI is predicated on teamwork, however, everyone must be trained, physicians especially. "At first I thought that if we had one or two people trained they could tell us what to do," Dr. Harter says. "But everyone at the top has to know it. If you don't understand the system, you can't critique the process."

Once implementation began, leadership played an even bigger role. Typically, the transition to CQI means an initial drop in productivity as the charting process and the need to come up with measurement criteria are piled on top of regular duties. For the North Louisiana clinics, this lasted about 18 months, says Jennifer Bennet, RN, who directs the program. The first set of algorithms took 6 months to complete. The process required bringing five physicians to consensus with input from all staff involved.

By all accounts, Dr. Rutherford's vision pulled the clinics through. "There was more than one occasion when I dropped into a chair in his office and said 'I quit,'" Bennet says. Dr. Rutherford was steadfast in his faith that the system would work.

After several months, it became clear that recording and properly interpreting data were problems. Dr. Rutherford brought in statistician Ray Carrey, Ph.D., for advice. One problem was that the clinics chose some complex processes to chart as they launched the program. Biological processes in homeostasis proved particularly difficult to chart and measure. "If we had it to do over, we would start with some simpler processes," Dr. Rutherford says.

Learning to use software to produce algorithms, which are flowcharts of every step in a given process, and to generate control charts was also a challenge. The clinics began with one big advantage, however: They already were using computerized patient records. Without them, retrieving data for control charts from paper patient records would have been impossible. "You couldn't hire enough monks to do it," Dr. Rutherford says.

Once the technical hurdles were cleared, the program began to show results. Results inspired confidence, and now enthusiasm for the program is palpable. Dr. Bennet commented, "Everyone is excited. They're saying, 'What are we going to do next?'"

**Drive Out Fear**

As significant as teaching the technical end of CQI was, fundamental changes had to be made to make the process work. The first was changing the working relationships among staff and physicians. In place of hierarchical arrangements, where nurses and technicians exercised little judgment and always deferred to physicians' orders (even when they knew the order was wrong), Dr. Rutherford fostered a culture of cooperation. "Free input from all parties is needed to understand and get control of every part of the process," he noted.

"Staff have to know they won't be punished for speaking up. Drive out fear—that's the most important thing in the beginning."

It's crucial for two reasons. First, for CQI to work, the collective knowledge of everyone on the team must be tapped and codified. When quality teams meet to develop algorithms, everyone has an equal say. Of course, once an algorithm is developed, it must be approved by consensus of all physicians on staff.

Second, staff must feel comfortable defending the algorithm once it is in place because success depends on keeping processes regular. The CQI method of looking at patient treatment as a process with normal statistical variation has become so ingrained that nurses will ask physicians, "Are you sure you want to make a decision based on just one data point?"

The algorithms don't take authority from physicians; rather, they represent a consensus on the best current method for dealing with a problem. Physicians can override them. The algorithms are subject to constant review and update. In practice, they free physicians from making many routine adjustments by spelling out how staff should deal with problems. "They've cut down a lot on phone calls, and the calls I get now are usually the ones I really need to get," Dr. Harter says.

Dr. Blondin concurs: "It is one of the most effective ways of extending physician practice that I have seen. It allows me to concentrate on the problems that really require a physician's attention." Ironically, removing physicians from constant interaction with patients has improved results in some ways. Before CQI, physicians saw patients every time they were dialyzed, usually three or four times a week. Generally, they'd write prescriptions based on the patient's vital signs that day.

"We thought we were practicing high-quality medicine, but what we were really doing was tampering with the system," Dr. Rutherford says. "One day blood pressure would be high, and a doctor would write a prescription for that. The next day it would be low, and a different doctor would write a prescription for that. Before you knew it, the patient was on three different blood pressure medications when he or she didn't really need any."

The HCFA now requires physicians to see patients at least once a week. "We see them, but we leave our prescription pads behind." Dr. Rutherford's goal is to leave day-to-day operations to staff as much as possible, reducing direct physician intervention to quarterly meetings with care teams. "I'd like to meet with them and say 'Great work, people, you did well.' We're not there yet, but we're getting closer."

**Break Down Barriers**

Some of the most spectacular results have been the direct result of breaking down traditional barriers between departments and completely rethinking how care is delivered. For example, malnutrition was known to be a significant factor in hospitalizations and mortality, so the North Louisiana centers shifted the focus of care toward nutrition services.

All staff are more aware of patients' nutrition needs. The centers now employ one nutritionist for every 100 patients, about twice the usual ratio. "What's different is that physicians and nurses believe in nutrition," says nutritionist Kathy Baker. Most important, an algorithm has been developed to spot malnutrition early, determine causes, and aggressively treat it with everything from diet to treatment for depression to parenteral feeding. The centers' high use of parenteral feeding drew attention from the HCFA at first, but the centers were able to demonstrate that it lowered costs by preventing hospitalizations.

Another improvement was an increase in the average length of time on dialysis by 30 to 40 minutes per session. Often, dialysis centers try to save money by shortening sessions. Dr. Rutherford and his colleagues, however, found that longer sessions improved patients' health and quality of life and saved money by reducing hospital stays.

The centers can afford longer dialyses because they have cut overhead. Here again, knocking down traditional barriers between departments played a major part. For example, reuse of artificial kidney filters jumped when the reconditioning department started working with the dialysis units to get the filters into reprocessing within 3 to 5 minutes after use instead of 30 to 45 minutes. It became easier to clean them, and reuse leaped from 8 to 45 times per filter. The centers also cut costs by settling on one supplier for non-biocompatible filters and one for biocompatible filters. That eliminated inventory costs and emergency shipping costs for overnight delivery of out-of-stock filters.

CQI not only has improved quality but also has brought the staff together around the centers' central mission: saving lives. "The most exciting thing has been the involvement and participation of staff and patients," Dr. Blondin says. Dr. Rutherford adds "It's been gratifying both professionally and personally."

**CONCLUSION**

The physician leader's most important role in improving organizational quality is to help create an organization culture in which customer-focused quality is paramount. There is no magic to doing this. Skillfully applying your knowledge about organization structure, employee motivation, leadership, performance evaluation, selection, and compensation and reward systems and having a vision of what a quality-focused organization looks like are essential. In addition, if you believe that formal quality improvement methods could be beneficial, then your role as a leader would involve acquiring method specific expertise, such as in Six Sigma, for yourself and your organization as did Drs. Rutherford, Blondin, and Harter.

---

## NOTES

1. See, for example, Millenson, M. (1999). *Demanding Medical Excellence*, Chicago: University of Chicago Press, for an early but still relevant discussion of historic quality problems in healthcare and attempts to improve quality.
2. LEAN is a quality improvement process based on Toyota's manufacturing process called the Toyota Production System. It is based on changing the organization's culture to one with a central focus on quality. In this instance, the process analysis focuses on identifying value added steps, and eliminating waste by eliminating those steps that don't add value.
3. Sashkin, M., & K. Kiser. (1993). *Putting Total Quality Management to Work*. San Francisco: Berrett-Koehler.
4. Bounds, G., et al. (1994). *Beyond Total Quality Management*. New York: McGraw-Hill, p. 382.
5. Deming, W. E. (1986). *Out of the Crisis*. Cambridge: Massachusetts Institute of Technology, Center for Advanced Engineering.
6. Deming, W. E. (1972). Report to management. *Quality Progress*, p. 41.
7. Juran, J. (1988). *Juran on Planning for Quality*. New York: The Free Press, p. 14.
8. See, for example: Skeel, R. (1989). Quality of life assessment in cancer clinical trials—It's time to catch up. *Journal of the National Cancer Institute* 81:472–473; or Moinpour, O., et al. (1989). Quality of life end points in cancer clinical trials: Review and recommendations. *Journal of the National Cancer Institute*, 81:485–495.
9. *American Medical News*, May 13, 1996. Reprinted with permission.

## CHAPTER 12

# Final Thoughts

## INTEGRATING THE PHYSICIAN MANAGER'S MANAGEMENT SKILLS

The issue of integration was discussed as the challenge of getting the parts of a healthcare organization or system to work in a synergistic, coordinated manner. Similarly, physician leaders need to use their management skills in an integrated fashion. One of the difficulties of presenting a survey of business issues is that to organize the process so the content would be most understandable, the book had to be divided into homogeneous chapters. As a result, the chapters are organized around specific content, such as finance, performance appraisal, marketing, and so forth. The physician leader's job, however, is more than the sum of each of the chapters in this book.

In reality, the lines between the knowledge areas discussed in this book either do not exist or are at best indistinct. Leadership blends into motivation. Motivation blends into performance appraisal and negotiation. Financial information blends into marketing and integration. Quality management becomes marketing, integration, motivation, and leadership. Part of the skill of being an effective physician leader is developing the intuition to look beyond the immediate situation to envision additional implications of your actions.

## THE PHYSICIAN MANAGER'S PERSONAL CHALLENGE

In life, what usually creates the most pain, disappointment, and difficulty are your own expectations or, perhaps better stated, unrealistic expectations of one's self and others. What happens when expectations are unrealistic? They play havoc with emotions, thereby interfering with interpersonal relationships, feelings about one's self, and with an ability to act in a rational, problem-centered manner. Fear, anger, anxiety, and a need for retribution begin to control your life, and you act in ways that are ineffective and self-defeating.

Many physicians initially have unrealistic expectations concerning the demands of running a business, or working in a large healthcare organization. For some, reality causes them to adjust their expectations to more realistic levels. Other physicians, however, begin with unrealistic expectations and never give them up. They continue to assume that their expectations are realistic, and that the world simply isn't cooperating! Understanding and mastering the personal and emotional aspects of managing and working with others are essential for the physician leader to succeed. What, then, are typical expectations that physician leaders have that may affect their ability to act effectively? They basically fit into two categories. The first category is expectations of others, including employees and associates as well as yourself. The second category is expectations regarding how the business world operates.

## EXPECTATIONS OF OTHERS AND SELF

For practice-based physicians, owning and running a practice is an exciting, motivating process. Similarly, physician leaders in management positions in larger healthcare organizations generally have challenging, responsible positions with considerable organizational visibility. In both types of settings, physicians frequently are involved in important decisions at the highest levels of their organization. It is easy for physicians in these positions to become caught up in the excitement of their jobs. It also is easy for them to fall into the trap of expecting others, especially employees, to have similar feelings and degrees of commitment.

Others may initially be equally enthusiastic, but their enthusiasm often fades. No one will care as much about "your baby" or your project as you do, and no one will be as willing as you to sacrifice and struggle when times are difficult. For practice-based physicians, this also can be a problem with other partners, who perhaps don't have as large a financial stake, or who simply don't have the same degree of psychological investment as you do.

Others' lack of caring may manifest itself in a number of ways. For example, your receptionist might walk through the waiting room and fail to pick up a candy wrapper that is lying on the floor. On a more serious plane, one of your partners might promise to review the practice's aging analysis on Saturday, but instead spends the entire weekend on a camping trip. Perhaps you have a report for the hospital CEO on the integration status of the hospital that your system acquired 2 months ago. Your assistant leaves at 5:00 PM and never informs you that it won't be finished in time for your 8:00 AM meeting tomorrow with the CEO.

These incidents have two levels of significance. First, you should be concerned, because someone did not perform a task that should have been performed. In this regard, providing immediate feedback along with a clear statement of your future expectations can address the performance issue. At another level, however, you may be exasperated, perhaps even exhausted, if these are the latest in a series of events that are symbolic of an uncaring, irresponsible attitude. When this happens, you may have an emotional reaction, such as disappointment, anger, or perhaps even hopelessness.

Routinely expecting others to have the same degree of investment or insight into how their actions affect others is simply setting yourself up for disappointment. Although you probably accept that it is unrealistic to expect that employees who have no ownership or who don't share in the rewards of top management should have the same degree of commitment that you have, it is always disappointing when they don't.

Employees work for the goals that are important to them. Expectancy theory, discussed in Chapter 6, suggests that you should not expect employees to work as though they were owners or top-level executives, when they will not in fact enjoy the rewards or benefits of these positions. Many nonexempt employees, especially, will perceive demands beyond the ordinary perhaps minimal duties of their jobs as inequitable. Generally, employees who perceive inequity will regain equity indirectly, for example by being cold or uncaring toward a patient or leaving for the day with a project incomplete. Unrealistic expectations of others will result in disappointment, doubts about your own management ability ("If I was a good manager, he never would have . . ."), and employee turnover.

When a partner or other executive behaves in ways that you perceive as unfair or irresponsible, then feelings of disappointment, anger, and even betrayal are common. What should you do about the situation? You don't have many choices. Either you can look the other way, knowing that this may perpetuate if not reinforce the behavior, or you can immediately discuss the matter with the other individual. If you choose to discuss the problem, consider undertaking this discussion at both the factual and the emotional level. Tell the partner or peer about your expectations, and how his or her actions made you feel. If you were disappointed or angry, let him or her know this. This will be helpful to you because you will reduce your frustration by "getting it off your chest." It also tells the partner or peer that the behavior has affected you, and the discussion process may help clarify any misperceptions regarding mutual expectations. The ideas in the negotiation chapter will be helpful for handling these discussions, but they won't decrease your disappointment or frustration.

Usually, directly addressing the circumstances will result in both parties adjusting their behaviors and expectations. Suppose, however, that the other individual is a partner who continues to behave in ways that you perceive as inequitable. Assuming that you have tried to clarify your expectations, you then may conclude that the transgressions were the result of conscious decisions. Your partner simply doesn't care about your feelings or what you need. In effect, your partner is not functioning as a partner. When circumstances reach this point, you may need to consider getting a "divorce," such as the situation that we saw at Oregon Sports Medicine with Drs. Able, Baker, and Cane in Chapter 1.

This is the time to focus very sharply on your own interests and to weigh the financial and personal value of continuing the relationship against the frustration, inconvenience, and financial costs, as well as benefits, associated with dissolving the business relationship. Once again, the underlying theme is that people work for themselves. If a group practice is such that one party will tolerate a disproportionate share of the burden, then another party will invariably take advantage of this situation. Conducting civil war to regain equity almost certainly will lead to a dysfunctional organization. If you and your partners cannot work together without feelings of unfairness, then it may be best to recognize this reality and end the relationship.

You should, however, place your dissatisfaction into perspective. As practices have become larger and physicians find themselves working in larger healthcare organizations, work life has become much more complex. Simply having more people around, all of whom carry their own perspectives, agendas, and personal and organizational self-interests, ensures that the level of potential discord in organizations in which physicians now are finding themselves will be greater than in the past. Physicians are beginning to experience more of the frustrations of organizational life that much of the rest of society has been living with for most of the 20th century. Holding out for a standard of perfection and perfect agreement, and allowing relatively minor levels of disagreement, transgression, or inequity to destroy a *generally* beneficial situation is self-defeating. Before you enter into civil war, organizational, or professional suicide think long and hard about the cost-benefit relationship.

The belief that you will be truly in control, and that you can force events to occur the way that you wish is a fantasy. You can influence events to varying degrees, but you cannot control your practice, employees, or healthcare organization as if it were an extension of yourself. The larger the organization of which you are a part, the more it takes on a life of its own that to some extent meets the competing needs of employees, partners, departments, shareholders, patients, the community, and to some degree, yourself. You cannot be everywhere all the time, and when and where you are absent, these other constituencies may make decisions based on their needs; decisions that are not always to your liking.

Someone once said that running a business is like being in a war. You are going to have casualties, and the casualties may be your needs and desires. The goal is to take acceptable casualties in relation to the objectives you achieve. No secretary will be perfect. Some fees will not be collected, and some telephone messages will be lost. Occasionally, charts will be misfiled. Others whom you counted on for political support will defect. Employees, partners, and patients will not live up to their promises. The list of daily failures can appear endless, if you choose to count them. If you are of a mind to, you can create an inexhaustible list of events over which to become upset. What you must keep in mind, however, is whether, in spite of these failures, you are achieving the objectives that are really important to you and to your organization. This is not to say that you should be unconcerned about setting high performance standards because, if you don't set them, no one will. Instead, this is a call for balance and realism. Effective managers know when to push. They push when it makes a real difference, and they back off when it doesn't. Effective managers also know when it's important to care, and when to shrug their shoulders, and recognize that tomorrow is another day.

It also is vitally important for you to examine your own need for perfection. A perfectionistic attitude can result in pushing for perfection at the wrong times or in the wrong places. Virtually every element of a physician's development and training encourages perfectionism. Perfectionism is adaptive in the practice of clinical medicine, because inattention to detail can significantly affect the well-being of patients. Medicine attracts people who are intellectually oriented toward facts and details, and enjoy pursuing cause-and-effect relationships. The demands of medical education tend to eliminate those who are not concerned with nuances. Finally, the physician-patient relationship is an unequal one. The patient is in a dependent position, which tends to reinforce the physician's expectation that his or her requests will be followed unquestioningly.

Unbridled perfectionism can result in striving for that last 10 percent, when it really doesn't matter. If you don't choose when to be demanding, you will waste a lot of energy fighting battles of no great consequence, and you will create a tense, confrontational work environment for no good reason.

## BUSINESS EXPECTATIONS

It is important to have a realistic understanding of the relationship between your practice, hospital, or healthcare system and others. In many ways, business relationships are like the criminal-justice system. In the criminal-justice system, each side advocates its strongest possible position. The competition of ideas and facts, as filtered by the law, reveals the truth, which is determined by a judge or jury. In the business world, each business seeks to maximize its own gain by offering its most competitive products or services. Business law, business ethics, standards of practice, and community standards serve as the law in this competition, and the marketplace, which is both jury and judge, will determine the value of the competing services. Integrative cooperation between adversaries, such as noted when suppliers work with hospitals to achieve mutual gain, only occurs when it is to both parties' advantage.

In the current healthcare environment, your gain is generally a competitor's loss, and vice versa. In addition, everyone in your business environment is trying to survive, and someone else's survival might be at your expense. Every time you turn around, someone will be trying to take money out of your pocket. Employees expect pay raises, cities increase taxes on revenues and personal property, suppliers raise their prices, insurance companies increase their premiums while simultaneously tightening their claims payment criteria, some patients will not pay for services, equipment will break, new forms of providing and organizing healthcare services will evolve, competitors will move into the market, others will consolidate . . . the list is endless.

This sounds like the law of the jungle, and it is. For many physicians, however, these business realities have been masked by a forgiving jungle in which there has been a plentiful supply of patients at fees that were tolerant of business inefficiency. Tigers can become fat and complacent when the food supply is abundant. Many healthcare organizations expect that revenues will always flow irrespective of the competition and changing market conditions. "It will never happen here" is still a common refrain in many regions, and in many healthcare organizations.

For some physicians in some specialties, or in well-positioned healthcare systems, this may continue to be the case, for a time. Others, however, are finding a market in which increasing competition or declining patient demand requires them to run a leaner, more effective medical business now.

This book provides some insight into the skills and methods that physicians can use to lead leaner, more effective medical businesses, whether it is in a practice, hospital, or other healthcare delivery organization.

# Index

Note: Tables, figures, and exhibits are denoted by *t*, *f*, and *e*.

## A

Abandonment, charges of, 363
Abbott Northwestern Hospital, Department of Nursing Matrix Structure, 341, 341*f*
ABC. *See* Activity-based costing
Absenteeism, 161
  pay dissatisfaction and, 183
  termination and, 375
Abusive discharge, 359
Abusive working environment, 380
Acceptance
  leadership and, 230
  leading meetings and, 243
Accommodations, reasonable, Americans with Disabilities Act and, 382
Accountability, employee, 120–121
Accounting functions, keeping physical handling of cash separate from phases of, 70–71
Accounting statements, financial statements, reports and, 22–36
Accounts
  placement of, in collection, 96–98
  problem, managing, 104–106
Accounts payable, 22
Accounts receivable manager, effective collection and, 76
Accrual basis accounting, 24, 25, 27
Accrued expenses, 28
Accrued revenue, 27
Acid test ratio, 33
Acquisitions, integration of, 349–350
Actions, expectancy theory and, 247
Activity-based costing, 46–47
  negotiation analysis and data from, 50*e*
Actual volume, 42
ADA. *See* Americans with Disabilities Act
ADEA. *See* Age Discrimination in Employment Act of 1967
Adjunct treatments, 364

Administrative employees, Fair Labor Standards Act and definition of, 384*e*
Administrative positions, filling, 148
"Advance alerts," via e-mail, 294
Adversaries
  integrative cooperation between, 414
  knowing, 305–306, 326
Advertising/advertisements, 40, 257
  billboard, 274, 275*e*
  click-through, 300
  direct mail, 262, 274, 275*e*
  image, 267
  Internet, 291–300
  job, 141
  magazine, 274, 275*e*
  newspaper, 274, 275, 275*e*, 276–278, 292
  paid, 274–278, 279*f*, 280
  patient characteristics and, 277
  radio, 274, 275*e*, 276–277, 283
  television, 262, 274, 275*e*, 276–278, 283, 291, 292
  unpaid, 280–284
  Web page, 274, 275*e*, 299
  Yellow Pages, 276
Age discrimination, 376, 381
Age Discrimination Act of 1975, 376
Age Discrimination in Employment Act of 1967, 376, 381
Aggressive patient collections, sequence and timing of, 102*e*
Aging, unacceptable, 77
Aging analysis, 77
Aging history database, 80, 81*e*, 106
Aging reports
  physician manager and examination of, 73
  reviewing, 106
Agreeableness, 149
AIDS, Americans with Disabilities Act and, 382
AIDS services, promoting, 275
Alcohol abuse, 161
Alcoholics, former, Americans with Disabilities Act and, 382
Alliances, point plan development and, 203

Alternative solutions, generating, 313–314
AMA. *See* American Medical Association
American Lung Association, 294
American Medical Association, e-mail guidelines recommended by, 293, 293*e*
American Medical Informatics Association, e-mail guidelines recommended by, 293, 293*e*
*American Medical News,* 393
Americans with Disabilities Act, 376, 381–383
    exclusions under, 382–383
AMIA. *See* American Medical Informatics Association
Amphetamines, 162
Anger, 412, 413
Annual appraisals, conducting, 121–123, 126–128. *See also* Performance appraisals
Annuities, 13
    present value, 14*t*
Anorexia, 260
Antikickback legislation, 385–388, 391
Antireferral legislation, 385–388
Applicant pool, 138, 166
Application forms, 147, 157–158, 180*e*
    with at-will statement, 159*e*
Appraisal system, physician performance and, 133
*Architectural Digest,* 288
*Area Wage and Salary Survey* (BLS), 202
Assault, 358–359
Assertiveness
    change process and, 240
    collecting from patients and, 83
Asset decisions
    importance of, 11
Assets
    on balance sheet, 22, 23*e*
    joint ownership of, 366
    selling, turnaround strategy and, 271
Assumption of risk, 366
Asthma care, Web sites and, 294
Attacking marketing strategy, 267
Attorneys
    collection methods used by, 97–98
    effective dialogues with, 370
    selecting, 390–391
AT&T wireless reception, 292
At-will employment, 158, 370, 374–375
At-will statement, application form with, 159*e*
Authorization procedures, insurance collection and, 99
Autocratic decisionmaking, 228
Average collection period, 34
Axelrod, Richard, 318, 319, 320

**B**

Baker, Kathy, 408
Balance sheets, 22
    balancing, 22–23
    for private practice, 29, 29*e*, 31
Bandwidth, Web site and, 298, 299
Bankruptcy, 74
    black book and, 322, 323–326
    patients and, refusing to be intimidated by threats of, 84
    problem accounts and, 104
Barbiturates, 162
Base pay, determining, with point system, 198*t*
BATNA. *See* Best alternative to a negotiated agreement
Battery, 359, 380
Bay of Pigs decision, 231
Behavioral cost information, capturing, 46–47
Behavioral goals, 126
Behavioral segmentation, market segments and, 288*e*, 289
Benchmark jobs, 190, 196
    identifying, 192, 198
    inflation and, 202
    point system and, 197
    two, point evaluation of, 198*t*
Benefits, 183, 206–208
    physician compensation and, 210
Benefit-seeking segments, 289
Bennet, Jennifer, 405, 406
Benzodiazepines, 162
Berra, Yogi, 126
Best alternative to a negotiated agreement, 304–305, 306*f*, 315, 318
    hardball tactics and, 311
    interests *vs.* positions and, 307
    leasing, reservation price and, 305–306
Best practices, 352
    national uniform standards of, 363
Betrayal, 412
BFOQs. *See* Bona fide occupational qualifications
Bias, positive leniency, 127
Big 5 personality factors, 149, 151*e*, 161
    psychological, 169, 170
Billboard advertising, 274, 275*e*
Billings
    average daily, 34
    insurance, 98–99
Billing strategies, 90–92
    defined, 90
    full-payment strategy, 91–92
    insurance pay-patient statement strategy, 90

modified strategies, 91
patient payment-file insurance strategy, 90
patient prepayment strategy, 92
preventing patient payment problems, 92
Black Belts, Six Sigma and, 404
Black Book case analysis, 321–326
bankruptcy negotiations and, 323–326
Black book proposal
financial comparison of, and Chapter 7
bankruptcy, 328, 328*e*
for lease modification, 328–330
projected expense reductions, 328, 329*e*
Blondin, Joan, 405, 407, 409
Blood testing, 162
Bluffing, 311
Board of directors, *332*
Body language, negotiating and, 310
Boeing, 339
Bona fide occupational qualifications, 379
age discrimination and, 381
Boston Consulting Group strategies, 268–270, 268*e*
Bots, 299
Boundaries, organizational structure and, 333
Brainstorming, 313, 314, 316, 401
leading meetings and, 243
Breach of contract, between patient and physician,
356
Breach of duty, malpractice and, 362, 363–364
Break-even analysis, 7, 10, 322, 323
Bribes, 386
Broken record technique, 317
Brooks, R., 293
Browsers, 295
Buck passing, 336, 337
Budgets and budgeting. *See also* Control and
budgeting
click-through advertising and, 300
financial control and use of, 39–46
flexible, 42
pro forma, 264
static, 42
Bulimia, 260
Bureau of Labor Statistics, 195
*Area Wage and Salary Survey,* 202
wage and salary survey, 192
for office and administrative occupations,
193–194*t*
Business courtesies, 386
Business expectations, 414–415
Business law, 355–391, 414
antikickbacks and antireferrals legislation,
385–390

classification of torts, 358
contracts, 367–370
employment issues, 370–385
general torts, 357–358
intentional torts, 358–361
malpractice, 362–367
negligence torts, 361–362
selecting an attorney, 390–391
Business manager
case application: hiring of, 172–179
goal-setting discussion between physician and,
118–119
job analysis by, 140, 141
job description factors, selection factors, selection
procedures, 172*t*
narrative self-evaluation by, 121, 122*e*
performance appraisals and, 110
point evaluation of, 198*t*
practice job description, 112*e*
résumé of applicant (disguised), 173*e*
structured interview questions and responses,
176–178*e*
structured telephone interview format and
evaluation, 174*e*
Business realities, perspective on, 414
Business skills, internal marketing and, 263–264
*Business Week,* 393
"But-for" standard, 364

**C**

CABG. *See* Coronary artery bypass graft
Cafeteria-benefits plan, 207, 249
Calendars, computer-based, 103
California Psychological Inventory, 175
Camino, 295
Cancellation fees, 85
Cancer patients, online information sources and, 294
Cannabinoids, 162
Capital asset planning, 2, 11–21
net present value and internal rate of return,
12–16, 18, 21
payback analysis, 11–12
Capital equipment, depreciation of, 24
Capital purchasing, examples of, 11
Cardiology practice compensation issues, 212*t*
Careerbuilder.com, 142
Caring, others' lack of, 412
Carrey, Ray, 407
Cascading goals, 117–118, 118*e*
Case analyses/case studies
Black Book, 321–326
building and using CVP model, 9–11

Case analyses/case studies (*continued*)
  business manager's equity, 208–209
  collection, rewards and behaviors, 82–83
  collection report data usage, 100–102
  financial statements for private practice, 28–33
  general hospital MRI system, 8
  higher quality, lower costs in dialysis, 405–409
  hiring business manager, 172–179
  Oregon Sports Medicine, 50–57
  personality disordered patients and triangling,
      85–86
  selection failure—a personal perspective, 179
Case-mix adjustment, 128
Cash, diversion schemes and, 66
Cash accounting, 25
Cash basis accounting, 24
Cash control
  methods, theft reduction and, 161
  physical manager's role in, for small practice,
      72–74
  short-term, 2
  successful, 61
Cash Cow phase, within Boston Consulting Group
      strategies, 268e, 269
Cash disbursements journal (abridged), 69e
Cash flow statement, 22, 26e, 70
Cash management, 62–65, 106
  daily activity by provider, 62
  daily activity by provider sheet, 64e
  daily receipts/adjustments, 62
  daily receipts and adjustments sheet, 63e
  gross receipts report, 63, 65
  in private practice, 61–106
Cash management procedures, applied, 70–72
  check signing authority in hands of practice
      owner, 71–72
  depositing to checking account on daily basis, 71
  disbursements for practice expenses made with
      prenumbered checks, 71
  petty cash account maintenance, 71
  separating physical handling of cash from
      accounting function, 70–71
  separating posting of procedures/payments from
      checkbook management, 71
  staff vacations and deterring cash diversion
      schemes, 72
Cash problem, hypotheses about, 100–102
Cash receipt and disbursement reports, physician
      manager and examination of, 73
Cash receipts and disbursements journals, 66, 68–70
Cash receipts journal, 68e
Causation, torts and, 358

Causation in fact, malpractice and, 362, 364
Cause-and-effect diagram, 395
Certification, national uniform standards of, 363
Certified ophthalmic technicians, 196
*Challenger* space shuttle, 231
Chamber of commerce, wage-and-salary data
      through, 192
Change implementation plan, 238e
Change implementation teams, 239
Change management, 399
Change process, leading, 237–240, 242–245, 398
Changes, making them stick, 242–243
Chapter 7 bankruptcy, 323
  financial comparison of black book proposal and,
      328, 328e
Chart of accounts, 67e
Charts, 395
Chavez, Cesar, 226
Checkbook accounting, 24
Checkbook management, separating posting of
      procedures/payments to patient accounts
      from, 71
Checking account deposits, daily, 71
Checks, prenumbered, cash disbursements for
      practice expenses paid with, 71
Check signing authority, in hands of practice owner,
      71–72
Chicken tactic, 311
Chief executive officer, 253, 334, 334f, 335
  cascading goals and, 118e
  functional structure and, 336
Churchill, Winston, 226
Church newsletters, press releases distributed to, 282
CICA
  black book case analysis, 321–326
  counterproposal, 325e
  interests of, 324e
Civil law, 357
Civil proceedings, malicious institution of, 360
Civil Rights Act of 1964, 378, 391
  Title VII of, 376, 377, 379
Civil Rights Act of 1991, 377, 378
Claims, denied, 98, 100
Clarke, R., 289
Clerical positions, filling, 148
Clerical salaries, 40
Cleveland Clinic, 266, 294
Click-through advertising, 300
Clinical outcomes
  data, 286
  Northeast HealthCare and improvement in, 354
  treatment protocols and, 401

Cocaine, 162
COLA. *See* Cost of living
Colleagues
  leading, 225–251
  motivating, 245–250
Collection administrators
  collection and role of, 82
  collection plan developed by, 104
  collection roles, problem areas and, 75*e*
  denied claims and, 100
  meaning of term, 76
  recurrent treatment patients and, 89
  small claims court and, 97
Collection agents, cost and recovery rate and, 97
Collection database, 61, 103–104
  screen, 103*e*
Collection fees, 87
Collection letters
  guidelines for, 93
  sample first, 94*e*
  sample second, 95*e*
  time standards and, 103
Collection management, 74
  run charts and, 396
Collection period, average, 34
Collection plan
  areas within, 104
  effective, 74
Collection plan (partial) sample, 107–108
  collection steps and sequencing, 108
  copayment collection procedures, 108
  insurance billing procedures, 108
  patient education process, 107
  patient intake process, 107
  problem account detection, 108
  verifications and preauthorizations, 107
Collection report data, using: case example, 100–102
Collection reports, 61, 103
Collection(s)
  accounts placed in, 96–98
  business manager applicant and knowledge of, 175
  cash basis, physician compensation based on, 213
  defined, 74
  from insurance companies, 98–102
  of overdue patient balances, 92–96
  patient intake process and, 86–87
  from patients, 83–86
  in private practice, 61–106
  rewards and behaviors: case analysis, 82–83
  roles and problem areas, 75*e*
  roles and responsibilities, 74, 76–77, 80, 82

steps and sequencing, collection plan (partial) sample, 107–108
  work sampling and, 164–165
Colleges, recruiting at, 143
Collegiality, physician appraisal process and, 134, 135
Collusion, reducing possibilities of, 73
Colonoscopies, 258
Commercial real estate, 322, 323
Commissions, 6
Common law, 356–357
Communication skills
  negotiation and, 321
  structured interviews and, 153
Community bulletin announcements, 280
Community newsletters, press releases distributed to, 282
Community standards, 414
Comparative negligence, 366
Compensation
  control and, 50
  costs, 6
  of employees, 183–215
  employee's conclusions about fairness of, 188–189
  equity as theory and strategy for determining, 184–186
  incentives, matrix organizational structure and, 340, 340*f*
Compensation plans
  cafeteria, 207
  constructing, who should be part of, 184
  coverage, 202
  effective, 183
  equity used for construction of, 186–190
  job evaluation methods and, 190–191
  motivation and, 245
  physician, 210
  physician, development of, 212–214
  point system of job evaluation and, 197–199
Compensation process, practical considerations in, 202–203
Compensation system, fair and equitable, job descriptions and, 113–114
Competence, contracts and, 367
Competition, 260
  market segments and, 290
Competitive advantages, determining, 291
Competitive approach, to negotiation, 309
Complexity
  integration and, 342
  of work life, 413
Computer-based calendars, 103

Computer operator/secretary
    job description for, 140*e*
    point evaluation of, 198, 198*t*
    selection factors, 140*e*
"Concierge" practices
    growth in, 92
    personalized attention with, 258
Conformity, groupthink and, 244
Congress, 357
    laws passed by, 356
Conscientiousness, 149
    personality factor of, 148
    published tests of, 378
Consent, 364
Conservation, 5–6
Consideration, defined, 368
Constitution (U.S.), 376
    U.S. system of laws and, *356*
Consultants
    compensation plans designed by, 184, 215
    job analyses done by, 114, 141
    media, 278
    selection method development and, 155–156
    wage-and-salary surveys conducted by, 192
Consult Group leadership style, 230*e*, 231
Consult Group situation, leading meetings and, 244
Consult Individually leadership style, 230*e*, 231
Consulting, leaders and, 226
Continuing education requirements, national uniform
    standards of, 363
Continuous quality improvement, 393, 405
    saving lives and, 408
Contractor agreements, 355
Contractor status, IRS tests for determination of,
    389, 389*e*
Contracts, 355, 367–370
    competence and, 367
    defined, 367
    employment, 370–374
    enforceability of, 368
    four corners rule and, 369
    interference with, 359–360
    written, 369
Contribution margin, 6
Contributory negligence, 365–366
Control and budgeting, 2, 36–46
Control charts, 394, 394*f*, 395, 406
Control(s)
    budgets and projections used as, 44
    collection process and, 77
    defined, 36
    postacquisition analysis and, 36, 38–39
Cook, James, 237

Cooperation, fostering culture of, 407
Cooptation, overcoming resistance and, 241*e*, 250
Copayments
    collecting, 82
    collection plan (partial) sample, 108
Coronary artery bypass graft, 46, 258
Cortina, J., 148, 149
Cost cutting, 313
Cost driver, 5
Cost of living, 202
Cost-of-living adjustments, 201
    inflation and, 202
Costs
    of accommodation, 382
    fixed, 3–5, 6, 11
    mixed, 6
    reducing, turnaround strategy and, 270
    variable, 3, 5–6, 11
Cost-volume-profit, 242
Cost-volume-profit analysis. *See* CVP analysis
Cost-volume-profit relationship, cost reductions and,
    271
COT. *See* Certified ophthalmic technicians
Court costs, 87
CPI. *See* California Psychological Inventory
CQI. *See* Continuous quality improvement
Credit card balances, 33
Credit card payments, 83
Credit card statements, 71
Creditors, joint ownership of assets and, 366
Credit side, in cash receipts journal, 69
Criminal-justice system, business relationships *vs.*, 414
Criminal law, 357
Criminals, 357
Critical incidents file, 116–117, 126
    excerpts from, 116*e*
Critical pathway flowchart, *345*
Critical pathways, 352
    national uniform standards of, 363
Cronshaw, S. F., 153
Cross-reactions, with drug testing, 163
Cryogen expenses, general hospital MRI system case, 8
Current assets, 33
Current liabilities, 33
Current ratio, 33
Customer needs
    determining, 400
    identifying, 257
    quality planning and, 400–401
CVP analysis, 2–11
    case: building and using CVP model, 9–11
    case: general hospital MRI system, 8
    fixed costs and, 3–5, 6

mixed costs and, 6
utility of, 2–3
variable costs and, 5–6
CVP model, building and using, 9–11

**D**

Daily activity by provider, 62, 64*e*
Daily activity reports, forwarding of, to physician manager, 73
Daily receipts/adjustments report, contents of, 62
Damages
  malpractice and, 363, 365
  negligence and, 361
Danaher, B. G., 296
Deadlines, for employee goals, 126
Debit side, in cash receipts journal, 69
Debts
  collecting via telephone, 95–96
  collection mechanics around, 92–93
  tests of liquidity and, 33
Debt-to-equity ratio, 34
Decide leadership style, 230*e*, 231
Decision making
  financial information used in, 31, 33
  functional designs and, 336
  involving others in, 227
Decisions, understanding medical and financial components of, 1
Decision Significance factor, 233*t*, 234*t*, 235
Declaratory rulings, 390
Deductibles, collecting, 82
Defamation, 360–361
Deferred expenses, 27–28
Deferred revenue, 27
Defined benefits plan, 208
Defined contribution plan, 208
de Gama, Vasco, 237
Delegate leadership style, 230*e*
Delegation
  leadership and, 226, 228
  leading meetings and, 243
Delinquency
  patient reasons for, 83–86
  time standards for collection activities and, 102–103
Delinquent accounts, placing in collection, 96–98.
    *See also* Collection(s)
Demand, 262–263
Deming, W. Edwards, 396, 397, 398, 399, 400, 402, 405
Demographic variables, market segments and, 288, 288*e*
Denied claims, 98
  examining, 100
Dental insurance, 207

Department of Labor, 389
Dependent variables, 5
Depreciation, 23–24
DER ratio. *See* Debt-to-equity ratio
Design
  of Web sites, 294–298
  of Yellow Pages advertisements, 276
Designated health services, 387, 388
Development, leading meetings and, 243
Development driven model, 235
  leader participation model and, 233*t*
DHS. *See* Designated health services
Diagnosis-related group, 5, 343
Diagnostic market segments, 287*e*
Dialysis, case analysis: higher quality and lower costs in, 405–408
Dialysis center example, 7–8
Differentiation, integration and, 342
Differentiation marketing strategy, 266–267
Dimensions of problem, integrative negotiating and identification of, 312–313
Direct mail advertising, 262, 274, 275*e*
Disability
  equal employment opportunity and, 170
  prohibiting discrimination on basis of, 376
Disability insurance, 207
Disappointment, 412, 413
Disbursements
  cash flow statement, 26*e*
  journal, 69*e*
  typical, 66, 68–70
Discharge, abusive, 359
Discipline
  job performance improvement and, 132
  problem accounts and, 105
Discount arrangements, 386
Disease information, via Internet, 294
Dismissals, legal guidelines related to, 360–361
Disparagement, 359
Disparate impact, 377
Disparate treatment, 377, 378
Distribution, 263
Distribution plan, for a psychiatrist, 271*e*
Distributive conditions, negotiation under, 309, 310–312, 317
Diversified health care organizations, 332
  divisional, 332*f*
Diversions of funds, case illustrations, 72
Divisional organization, integration and, 342
Divisional structures, 333
  moving from functional structures to, 346–347
DMAIC (Define, Measure, Analyze, Improve, Control), 404–405

Documentation, defending legal challenges to
personnel decisions and, 123
Dog phase, in Boston Consulting Group strategies,
268e, 269
Domain name, selecting and registering, 299
Down East Internal Medicine, Ltd.
black book case analysis, 321–326
interests of, 324e
proposal for lease modification, 328–330
Dreamweaver, 294
DRG. *See* Diagnosis-related group
Drug abuse, 161
Drug addicts, former, Americans with Disabilities
Act and, 382
Drug testing, 162–163
Duty, malpractice and, 362, 363–364
Dysfunctional reward contingencies, incentive plans
and, 203–204

**E**

Earnings, retained, 22
Eating disorders, 260
e-claims software, 99
Economies of scale, with functional designs, 335
Economy buyers, 289
Education
encouraging, 399
expenses, 40
in point system of job evaluation, 217, 218t
EEO. *See* Equal employment opportunity
EEOC. *See* Equal Employment Opportunity
Commission
Effectiveness, efficiency *vs.*, 42
Efficiency, 314
effectiveness *vs.*, 42
flexible budgets *vs.* static budgets and, 42
EIA tests. *See* Enzyme immunoassay tests
eICU, 262
Electronic claims submission, 98, 99
Electronic medical records, 204, 205, 343
e-mail, 343
AMA/AMIA guidelines, self-reported adherence
to, 293, 293e
consultations via, 258
Embezzlement, 161
reducing possibilities of, 73
Emotional distress, 380
intentional infliction of, 359
Emotional stability, 149
Employee behavior
employee accountability for, 120–121
Employee compensation, 6

Employee contracts, 355
Employee Polygraph Protection Act of 1988, 161,
162
Employee relations climate, equity and, 186–187
Employees
at-will, termination of, 374
critical incident file and, 116–117
development of, 229, 230
equity in compensation and, 184–186
exempt, 383
feedback about performance appraisal for, 115–116
goal setting for, 126–127
leading, 225–251
motivating, 245–250
nonexempt, 383, 384, 412
performance appraisal for, 109–111
with similar backgrounds, group cohesiveness
and, 335
at top of pay range, strategies for, 200–201
written employment contracts with, 370
Employee selection
basic principles, 143–144
example of, 144–147
factors in, 139–141
Employee status, IRS tests for determination of, 389,
389e
Employers, physician performance and, 133
Employment, at-will, 158, 374–375
Employment agencies, 142
Employment contract, checklist for, 372, 373e
Employment gaps, investigating, 157
Employment issues, 370–385
age discrimination, 381
Americans with Disability Act, 381–383
employment at-will, 374–375
employment contracts, 370–374
employment methods, 377–379
equal employment opportunity, 376–377
Fair Labor Standards Act, 383–384, 384e, 385e
Family and Medical Leave Act of 1993, 384–385
promotion, 379
sexual discrimination, 379
sexual harassment, 379–381
Employment methods, 137–180, 377–379
additional testing, 158–163
drug testing, 162–163
honesty/integrity tests, 161–162
performance and skills tests, 158–160
application form, 157–158
case applications
hiring a business manager, 172–175, 178–179
selection failure—personal perspective, 179

concluding remarks, 179–180
equal employment opportunity, 170
job description: identifying selection factors, 139–141
overview, 137–139
recruiting, 141–143
references and recommendations, 165
résumé, 156–157
selecting physicians and other professional employees, 168–170
selection procedures, 147–155
   basic principles, 143–144
   developing, 143–147
   example of, 144–147
   significance of findings on, 148–149, 151, 153–155
selection strategy, 165–168
testing, design and conduct related to, 155–156
uses for, 180*e*
validity of, 378
work samples, 163–165
Employment sequencing, steps in, 166, 167*e*
Employment torts, 378
Empowerment, 403
EMRs. *See* Electronic medical records
Entrances, cleaning and maintaining, 362
Environmental issues, external marketing and, 260–261
Enzyme immunoassay tests, 162, 163
Equal employment opportunity, 170, 355, 376–377
Equal Employment Opportunity Commission, 376, 377, 378
Equal Pay Act of 1963, 376
Equal treatment, 314
Equipment, lease *vs.* purchase decisions, 21–22
Equipment acquisition
   NPV and IRR analyses of, 15*e*
   value of money concept, 14–16
Equipment costs, general hospital MRI system case, 8
Equity
   achieving, importance of, 215
   case application, 208–209
   motivation and, 246
   physician compensation plans and, 210
   as theory and strategy for determining compensation, 184–186
Equity level of jobs, pay ranges and, 199–200
Equity perceptions, unrealistic, 209
Erdem, S., 294
Errors
   control chart and, 394, 394*f*
   evaluation, 127–128

Ethics, 414
Evaluations. *See also* Performance appraisal
   errors in, 127–128
   of physician performance, 132–135
   reading, 136
   revenue collection and, 76
Excel. *See* Microsoft Excel
Executive employees, Fair Labor Standards Act and definition of, 384*e*
Executive orders (presidential), 376
Executive recruiters, guidelines related to, 142
Exempt employees, 383
Exhortations, eliminating, 398
Expanding the pie, 313
Expectancy, 247
Expectancy theory, 412
   cafeteria compensation and, 207
   components of, 246–247
   equations related to, 248
   motivation and, 246–250
   understanding, 250
Expectations
   business, 414–415
   of others and self, 411–414
   partners and, 412–413
   unrealistic, 411
Expenses
   accrued, 28
   deferred, 27–28
   net income and, 24
   prepaid, 28
Experience, in point system of job evaluation, 217
External equity
   comparisons, 187*e*, 188, 189, 190
   data, obtaining, 192, 195–196
   job evaluation methods for achievement of, 190–191
Externally focused physician compensation plans, 213
External marketing factors, 259*e*, 260–263
   competition, 260
   demand, 262–263
   distribution, 263
   environmental issues, 260–261
   life cycle, 261–262
External market opportunities and threats, 257, 259
External objective standards, examples of, 314
Extroverts, meetings and, 245
Eye contact, negotiation and, 321

**F**

Facilitate leadership style, 230*e*, 231
Facilitate situation, leading meetings and, 244

Facility fees, negotiating, 47
Failure in selection, case application, 179
Fair Labor Standards Act, 355, 370, 383–384, 388, 391
  definitions of executive, administrative, and professional employees, 384e
  record-keeping requirements, 385e
Fair market price, negotiating on, 315
Fairness of compensation, 184–186
Fake Good Scale, 179
False "facts" tactic, 311
False imprisonment, 380
False-positive errors, expense of, vs. expense of false-negative errors, 146
Family and Medical Leave Act of 1993, 379, 384–385
  events covered under, 385
Fear
  driving out, 398, 407
  tortfeasor's actions and, 358
Fee collection, motivating employees about, 76
Feedback, 412
  immediate, performance appraisal and, 115–116
  operating plans and, 401
Fees
  attorney, 391
  executive recruiters, 142
  large, patient education and, 89
  prepayment of, 27
Fee schedule, reservation price and, 304
Fifth Amendment, 376
Finance charges, 87
Financial advisors, effective use of, 47, 50
Financial control
  budgets used for, 39–46
  short-term, 2
Financial hardship cases, collections and, 84
Financial losses, theft/embezzlement and, 161
Financially literate physician leaders, pivotal role of, 1, 39
Financial management, 1–57
  activity-based costing, 46–57
  capital asset planning, 11–21
  control and budgeting, 36–46
  CVP analysis, 2–11
  financial statements, reports, and accounting systems, 22–36
  lease vs. purchase decisions, 21–22
  uses for ratios, 36
Financial mission, medical mission and, 57
Financial outcomes, Northeast HealthCare and improvement in, 354

Financial statements
  for private practice, 32e
  reports, accounting statements and, 22–36
Firefox, 295
First Amendment, 376
First-level outcomes, expectancy theory and, 247, 249, 250
Fishbone diagrams, 395, 396, 396f
Fisher, R., 313, 314
Five Ws, of newspaper reporting, 280
Fixed costs, 3–5, 6, 11
  controlling, 3–4
  examples of, 3
  integration of acquisitions and, 349
  volume and, 4–5
Flexibility, in leadership, 228
Flexible budget, 42
  group practice, 43e, 44
  for MRI facility analysis, 45e
Flowcharts, 395, 407
FMLA. See Family and Medical Leave Act of 1993
Focus groups, 401
  Web site design and, 295
Force, expectancy theory and, 247
Ford Company, 402
Foreclosures, 322
Fortifying and protecting marketing strategy, 267
Fortune 100 companies, psychological test profiling and, 170
Fortune magazine, 393
Four corners rule, 369
401k plan, 208
Four Ps
  differentiation strategy and, 266
  evaluating and choosing market segments and, 290
  of marketing, 257, 258
  marketing plan and, 259, 271
  target marketing and, 287
Fourteenth Amendment, 376
4/5ths rule, federal authorities and "strong deference" to, 392n
Fraud, 73
Friendships, equity and, 185
Front office jobs, filling, 148
Front office staff, 332
  collection and role of, 80, 82
  collection problem areas and, 75e
  preventing patient payment problems and, 92
FrontPage, 294
FTE. See Full-time equivalent
Full-payment strategy, 91–92
Full-time equivalent, 7

Functional designs
  advantages with, 335–336
  disadvantages with, 336
Functional directors, 339
Functional hospital organizational structure, 334*f*
Functional organizations, integration and, 342
Functional responsibilities, 221, 223
Functional structures, 333
  moving from, to divisional structures, 346–347
  of multispecialty practice, 334, 335*f*
Fund diversions, case illustrations, 72
Furniture in office, inspecting, 362
Future value, calculating, 14

### G

Gaming, of quantitative performance measures, 129
Gaps in employment, investigating, 157
Gastroenterology practice, outpatient ABC analysis
  of procedures, 47, 48–49*e*
Gay newspapers, advertising in, 274, 275
GE, 228
GE Capital, 349, 350
Gender
  equal employment opportunity and, 170
  prohibiting discrimination on basis of, 376
General hospital MRI proposal
  NPV and IRR analyses, 17*e*
  NPV and IRR analysis at 85th percentile of
    projected volume, 19*e*
  at 115% of projected volume, 20*e*
General hospital system divisional organizational
    structure, 336, 337*f*
General mental ability, 153, 158, 161, 163, 165, 168
  measures incrementally added to, 148
  measuring, 147
  tests for, 148, 378
General Motors Corporation, 336–338
Geography
  advertising and, 274
  market segments and, 288*e*
Gerstner, Louis, 228
Gestures, negotiation and, 321
Gifts, 386
GMA. *See* General mental ability
Goal Alignment factor, 233*t,* 234*t,* 235, 236
Goal Alignment situation, leading meetings and, 244
Goals, cascading, 117–118, 118*e*
Goal setting, 249
  characteristics of, 126–127
  integration and, 343–344
  performance appraisals and, 117–119
  physician compensation and, 211, 213

Going rate, for jobs, 188
Go Live!, 294
Good cop/bad cop tactic, 311, 312
Good faith and fair dealing, at-will employment and,
    374–375
Google, 295, 299
Graphics, high fidelity, Web site, 299
Green Belts, Six Sigma and, 393, 404
*Griggs v. Duke Power Company,* 376, 377, 378
Gross receipts report, 63, 65, 65*e*
  physician manager and examination of, 73
Group Expertise factor, 233*t,* 234*t,* 235
Group practices
  budget analysis for, 40–46
  flexible budget, 43*e,* 44
  integrative opportunities for members and, 210
  static budget, 41*e*
Group Think, 231
  leading meetings and occurrence of, 244
Growth potential, of market segment, 290
Grudges, negotiation and, 321
Guerrilla warfare, 267

### H

Hall, W. K., 270
Hallways, cleaning and maintaining, 362
Halo effect, 185
Halo error, 128, 129
"Hardball tactics"
  countering, 312
  examples of, during distributive negotiations, 311
Harter, Herschel, 405, 406, 409
Hartmann, C., 294
Harvesting marketing strategy, 267–268
Hawthorne Works of Western Electric, total quality
    management and, 394, 396
Hay Aptitude Test Battery: Number Perception, 158
Hay Associates, 184
Healthcare Financing Administration (HCFA), 405
Health insurance, 207
  equity and, 185
Health maintenance organizations, 258, 332
Health system CEO, 332*f*
Heroin, 163
Hierarchical information architecture, 297, 297*f*
Highway systems, marketing plan and, 261
Hiring. *See also* Employees, 146
  business manager, 172–179
  organizing process of, 166
  physicians and other professional employees,
    168–170
  selection procedures for, 147–149, 151, 153–155

Hiring decisions, discharge decisions and, 378

Histograms, 395

History reports, physician manager and examination of, 73

HIV, Americans with Disabilities Act and, 382

HMOs. *See* Health maintenance organizations

Hogan Assessment Systems, 155

Hogan Personality Inventory, 149
  partial, section from, 152*e*

Holidays, 206

Homestead laws, 366–367

Homosexuals, prohibiting discrimination against, 383

Honesty/integrity tests, 161–162

Hopelessness, 412

Hospital Corporation of America, 406, 408

Hospital organizational structure, functional, 334*f*

Hospitals
  point plan development and, 203
  wage-and-salary surveys and, 196

Hostile working environment, 380

HPI. *See* Hogan Personality Inventory

Human resources (HR) staff, interviewing job applicants and, 156

Hunter, John, 147, 148, 149, 161, 163, 165

Hybrid information architecture, 297, 298*f*

**I**

IBM, 228

Illness burden, 128

Image advertising, 267

Image digitizing and transmission, 343

Immaturity, 161

Importance of Commitment factor, 233*t,* 234*t*

In basket, 180*e*

Incentive plans, 203–206

Incentives
  job performance improvement and, 132
  reward systems and, 346

Income statement, 22, 24, 25*e*
  Oregon Sports Medicine, 52–53*e*

Income taxes payable, 33

Incremental validity, 147, 161, 165

Independent contractor agreements, 388–390

Independent variables, 5

Indirect expenses, general hospital MRI system case, 8

Individual equity comparisons, 187*e*, 188, 189, 190

Inflation, 202
  general hospital MRI system case, 8

Infomercials, 258

Informal relations, poor, integration and, 342–343

Information architecture
  hierarchical, 297, 297*f*
  hybrid, 297, 298*f*
  matrix, 296, 296*f*
  tunnel, 297, 298*f*
  Web site, 295–298

Information systems, 346
  matrix structures and, 342

Informed consent, 364

Infrequent treatment patients, patient education and, 89

Ingenuity, in point system of job evaluation, 217, 221*t*

"Initiating structure," 227–228

Injuries, negligence and, 361

Insolvency planning, 366

Inspection, understanding purpose of, 397

Inspiration, leadership and, 226

Institute of Medicine, 405

Instrumentality, expectancy theory and, 247

Insubordination, 161
  termination and, 375

Insurance billing procedures, collection plan (partial) sample, 108

Insurance commission, 99

Insurance companies, collecting from, 98–102

Insurance coverage, patient education and, 87

Insurance expenses, 40

Insurance pay-patient statement strategy, 90

Insurance products, 332, 332*f*

Insurers, physician performance and, 133

Intake procedures, financial hardship cases and, 84

Intake process, 86–87

Integrating roles, 346

Integration
  of acquisitions, 349–350
  around short-term projects, 350
  best practices and principles of, 349–350
  defined, 331
  factors inhibiting, 342–343
  management, 349–350
  mechanisms for, 343, 345–347
  Northeast HealthCare case analysis, 351–352
  of physician manager's skills, 411
  small practice structures and, 347–350
  teamwork and, 402–403

Integration methods, advantages and disadvantages with, 344*e*

Integrative conditions
  negotiation under, 310, 312–316, 317
    bringing interests to the surface, 313
    choosing specific solutions that address both sides' interests, 314–316

generating alternative solutions, 313–314
identifying and defining dimensions of
  problem, 312–313
Integrative negotiating, 47
Integrity tests, 148, 149, 153, 161–162
  legal issues related to, 162
  strengths and weaknesses of, 161–162
Intent, torts and demonstration of, 357–358
Intentional torts, 358–361
  abusive discharge, 359
  assault, 358–359
  battery, 359
  defamation, 360–361
  disparagement or trade libel, 359
  intentional infliction of emotional distress, 359
  interference with contract, 359–360
  invasion of privacy, 359
  malicious institution of civil proceedings, 360
Interdependencies, organizational boundaries and,
  346
Interest rates, 13
Interests
  application exercise, 308*f*
  of both sides, specific solutions for, 314–316
  bringing to the surface, 313
  physician compensation plans and positions *vs.*,
    210–211
  positions *vs.*, 307–309
  of two adversaries, 309*f*
Interference with contract, 359–360
Internal equity
  comparisons, 187, 187*e*, 188, 189, 190
  job evaluation methods for achievement of,
    190–191
Internal job postings, 143
Internally focused physician compensation plans,
  213
Internal marketing factors, 259*e*, 263–265
  financial resources, 264
  personal goals, 264–265
  professional and business skills, 263–264
Internal organizational strengths and weaknesses,
  259
Internal rate of return, 2, 11, 12–21
  control and, 36
  equipment acquisition and, 15*e*, 16
  general hospital MRI proposal, 17*e*
  general hospital MRI proposal analysis at 85th
    percentile of projected volume, 19*e*
  general hospital MRI proposal at 115% of
    projected volume, 20*e*
  Microsoft Excel formula for calculation of, 18

Internal Revenue Service, 208, 388, 389
  declaratory rulings, 390
Internet, 291–300
  browsers, 295
  designing Web site, 294–298
    related considerations, 298–300
  flexibility and, 297
  leadership role and, 300
  place, 292–293
  portals, 292–293
  product, 293–294
  promotion, 292
  Web page advertising, 274, 275*e*
Internet Exlorer, 295
Internet service provider, 299
Interpersonal issues, physician selection and, 169
Interpersonal skills, structured interviews and, 153
Interpolation, base compensation rates determined
    for nonbenchmark jobs through, 196
Interviews, 138, 147, 180*e*
  structured, 148, 149, 151, 153, 154*e*, 169
Intimidation tactic, 311
Introverts, meetings and, 245
iPhone, 292
IQ (or intelligence), job success and, 147
IRR. *See* Internal rate of return
Irresponsible patients, collection process and, 84–86
IRS. *See* Internal Revenue Service
ISP. *See* Internet service provider

**J**

Janis, Irving, 244
Job analysis, 138
  obtaining information about, 112–113
Job applicants, time consumed in selection of, 179*t*
Job descriptions, 138
  accurate, performance appraisal and, 111–115
  annual appraisal and, 121
  identifying selection factors, 139
  physician performance and, 133
  for position of computer operator/secretary, 140*e*
  practice business manager, 112*e*
  ranking job evaluation method and, 191
  using, identifying selection factors, 139–141
  writing, 113–114
Job evaluation methods
  for achieving internal and external equity,
    190–191
  ranking, 191–192, 195–196
Job evaluations, point system of, 197–199, 217–223
Job history, examining, 157
Job offers, 179

Job performance
    collection and, 80
    evaluating, 110
    false and true positives and negatives, 145, 145*f*
    improving, 132
    providing clear explanations/expectations for, 119–120
    variability in, 144
Job-relevant information, on application forms, 158
Jobs
    benchmark, 190, 192, 196, 198
    compensating, 186–187
    external equity comparisons among, 187*e*, 188
    individual equity comparisons among, 187*e*, 188
    internal equity comparisons among, 187, 187*e*
    ranking, 191–192, 195–196
    red circling of, 196
    restructuring, 132
Joint Commission on Accreditation of Healthcare Organizations, 405
Joint ownership of assets, 366
Jones, D. P., 378
Jones Reproductive Clinic, 266
*Journal of the American Medical Association,* 393
Juran, Joseph, 399, 400, 401
Juran Trilogy, 400
Jury duty obligations, 374

**K**

Kahn, S., 371
Kennedy, John F., 231
Keywords, 299
Kickbacks, 355, 357, 391
King, Martin Luther, Jr., 226
Kiser, K., 395
Knowledge, in point system of job evaluation, 217, 218*t*
Knowledge, skills, and abilities, 114, 139
Koiso-Kanttila, N., 294
Kotler, P., 289
KSAs. *See* Knowledge, skills, and abilities

**L**

Lancaster, James, 237
Language
    negotiation and, 321
    in performance evaluations, 123
    translating customer needs and, 400
Laparoscopic gastric bypass surgery, 262
Large healthcare organizations, compensation plans in, 184
Late payment charges, 85

Law, 314. *See also* Business law, 414
    civil, 357
    common, 356–357
    criminal, 357
    preventive, 355
    statutory, 356
Layoffs, 322
Leader participation model, 229, 235, 236, 237
    development driven model, 233*t*
    time-driven model, 234*t*
Leaders
    motivation of employees and colleagues and implications for, 248–250
    situational issues for, when considering selecting leader style, 232*e*
    successful, characteristics of, 227
    successful, decision making by, 229
Leadership, 226–232, 235–237, 399
    aspects of, 226
    Internet and, 300
    management *vs.,* 226–227
    motivation and, 411
    situational approach to, 228
    teaching and instituting, 398
Leadership styles, 230*e*
    matching of, to situations, 228
Leading
    change processes, 237–240, 242–245
    meetings, 243–245
LEAN, 393, 394, 409*n*
Leaner medical businesses, 415
Lease modification, black book proposal for, 328–330
Leases of office space, renegotiating, 322
Lease *vs.* purchase decisions, 21–22
    analysis of, 21*e*
Legal challenges, to personnel decisions, documentation and, 123
Legal consultations, situations requiring, 390
Legal fees, 83, 87
Leniency errors, 127
Letterman, David, 277
Letters to the editor, 280, 283–284, 284*e*
Lewicki, R., 312
Liabilities, on balance sheet, 22, 23*e*
Liability torts, strict, 358
Libel, 360
    trade, 359
Lie detector tests, 161
Life cycle, external marketing and, 261–262
Life goals, 250, 264
    second-level outcomes and, 247

Life insurance, 207
Likelihood of Commitment factor, 233*t,* 234*t,* 235, 236
Lin, C. T., 292, 293
Lind, James, 237
Line responsibilities, 221
Links, sponsored, Web site, 299–300
Liquidity, 33
Liquidity ratios, 33–34
Loans payable, 22
Local area networks, 343
Local environmental issues, marketing plan and, 260–261
Locality rule, demise of, 363
Location, 258
    market segments and, 286
Locum tenens arrangement, physician selection and, 170
Log rolling, 313, 314, 317
Long-term treatment, patient education and, 89
Loss, negligence and, 361
Lowball/highball tactic, 311
Low-cost provider marketing strategy, 266
Low-cost providers, 258
Loyalty, equity and, 185
Lying, 161

**M**

Magazine advertising, 274, 275*e*
Mailing lists, of local newspaper, television, and radio reporters, 281
Malice, 360
Malpractice, 355, 362–367, 390
    causation in fact, 362, 364
    damages, 363, 365
    defenses against, 365–367
    duty and breach of duty, 362, 363–364
    proximate cause, 363, 364–365
Managed care contracts, 321, 322
Management
    leadership *vs.,* 226–227
    top
        in matrix organizations, 339
        total quality management and, 399
Management reports, 61
Management services organization, 343
Market growth rate, 268, 268*e*
Marketing, 257–300, 411
    concluding remarks about, 300
    Four Ps of, 257, 258
    overview of, 257–259
    quality and, 399

selling *vs.,* 257
    target, 286–287
Marketing mix, 258, 259, 263, 289
Marketing plans, 259*e,* 271–272, 300
    developing, 259–266
        situational analysis, 260
    external factors, 260–263
        competition, 260
        demand, 262–263
        distribution, 263
        environment, 260–261
        life cycle, 261–262
    internal factors, 263–265
        financial resources, 264
        personal goals, 264–265
        professional and business skills, 263–264
    physician compensation and, 211
    for a psychiatrist, 271*e*
    revising, 272
    SWOT analysis, 265–266
Marketing strategies (generic), 266–271
    attacking, 267
    Boston Consulting Group strategies, 268–270
    differentiation, 266–267
    fortifying and protecting, 267
    guerrilla warfare, 267
    harvesting, 267–268
    low-cost provider, 266
    turnaround, 270–271
Market price, 314
Market rate, for jobs, 188, 190
Market segmentation, 286–291
    developing market segments, 287–289
    evaluating and choosing market segments, 289–290
    positioning your organization, 290–291
    variables, 288*e*
Market segments, 263, 300
    developing, 287–289
    diagnostic, 287*e*
    identifying, 286–287
    for Web site, 295
Matrix information architecture, 296, 296*f*
Matrix organizational structure, 338*f,* 338–342
    compensation incentives and, 340, 340*f*
    comprehension incentives and, 204–205, 205*t*
Matrix organizations
    integration and, 339–340, 342
    limits of, 339
Matrix structure, 333
    Abbott Northwestern Hospital Department of Nursing, 341, 341*f*

Measurement and reward systems, 346
Media. *See also* Advertising/advertisements
    rich, 299, 301*n*
    strengths and weaknesses in use of, 274, 275*e*
    Web site advertising and, 299
Media consultants, 278
Media outlets, press releases sent to, 281–282
Medicaid Anti-Kickback Statute, 385–386
Medical associations, wage-and-salary data through, 192
Medical Group Management Association, 68, 77, 213
Medical histories, equal employment opportunity and, 170
Medical mission, financial mission and, 57
Medical office management software, 61, 62, 65, 70, 80
    aging analysis and, 77
    collection database and, 104
Medical technology, marketing plan and changes in, 261
Medicare, physician performance and, 133
Meetings
    closing, 245
    leading, 243–245
    planning and managing, 245
Megabytes (MB), Web site size in, 299
Memorial Hospital (Houston), 6
Mental illness, abrupt terminations and, 363
Mental impairments, Americans with Disabilities Act and, 381, 382
Merit, 202
    salary based on, 200
Merit system, 201
Meta tags, 299
Methaqualone, 162
Method of payment forms, 87
    sample, 88–89*e*
MGMA. *See* Medical Group Management Association
Minimum wage, 383
Minors, contracts and, 367
Mixed costs, 6
"Moab Management," being on the lookout for, 119–120
Modified billing strategies, 91
MOMS. *See* Medical office management software
Money, time value of, 12–15
Monster.com, 142
Morale, building, problem accounts and, 105
Moral standards, 314
Mortality rates, 128
Motivation, 245–250
    incentive payments and, 203–206

    leadership and, 226, 245–250, 411
    performance appraisals and, 110
MRI facility
    CVP analysis, 9*e*
    flexible budget analysis, 45*e*
    payback analysis, 12*e*
    postacquisition analysis after year 1, 37–38*e*
    projections, 10*e*
MSO. *See* Management services organization
Multispecialty practices
    functional structure of, 334, 335*f*
    growth of, 333
Mutual agreement, 367
    verbal contracts and, 369

**N**

National Aeronautics and Space Administration, 340
National Institute of Mental Health, 294
National origin, prohibiting discrimination on basis of, 376
Negative information, conveying, 360
Negative net income, 10
Negative owner's equity, 23
Negligence
    comparative, 366
    contributory, 365–366
    defined, 361
Negligence torts, 358, 361–362
Negligent malpractice, 362
Negotiation, 303–326
    art of: key concepts, 304–309, 326
    black book case analysis, 321–326
    defined, 303
    under distributive conditions, 309, 310–312, 317
    of employment contract, 370
    integrative, 47
    under integrative conditions, 310, 312–316, 317
    interests *vs.* positions, 307–309
    know your adversary, 305–306, 326
    know yourself, 304–305, 326
    overcoming resistance and, 241*e*, 250
    principled, 314
    prisoners' dilemma and, 318–321
Negotiation analysis, with use of ABC data, 50*e*
Negotiation dance, 306–307
Nepotism, 141
Net billings, 34
Net income, 4, 24
    cash flow statement, 26*e*
    negative, 10
    salary and, 35
Net present value, 2, 11, 12–21
    control and, 36

of equipment acquisition, 15–16, 15*e*
general hospital MRI proposal, 17*e*
   at 115% of projected volume, 20*e*
   at 85th percentile of projected volume, 19*e*
Net revenue, 15
   accrual basis, physician compensation based on,
      213
*New England Journal of Medicine,* 393
Newsletters, 274, 276
   Web site advertising and, 299
Newspaper advertising, 258, 274, 275, 275*e*,
      276–278, 292
   for business manager applicant, 172
   for job applicants, 141
Newspaper readership, declining, 292
Newspaper reporting, five Ws of, 280
News release, sample, 281*e*
News story, with local physicians, 283*f*
Niblling tactic, 311
Nickel and diming tactic, 311
"90-day clock" on claims, 91
90806 procedure, revenue growth and, 66
NMT. *See* Nuclear medicine technologist
Nominal group technique, leading meetings and,
      244
Noncompetition clauses, 370–371
Nonexempt employees, 383, 384, 412
Nonmedical competition, market segments and, 290
Nonsupervisory responsibility, in point system of job
      evaluation, 217, 219–220*t*
Normal success rate, 400
Northeast HealthCare
   case analysis, 351–352
   organization structure, 353*f*, 353–354
North Louisiana Dialysis Center, 405
Northrop Grumman Newport News, 339
"No-show" rates, 87
NPV. *See* Net present value
Nuclear medicine technologist, 192
Number comparison task, 160*e*
Numerical production quotas, eliminating, 398–399
Nursing home, 332, 332*f*
Nursing/technology line of positions, rank ordering
      of, 191*t*

### O

Offeree, 368
Offers, 306*f*
   terminating, 368
Office and administrative occupations, Bureau of
      Labor Statistics wage and salary survey for,
      193–194*t*
Office hours, 258

Office manager
   effective collection and, 76
   effective communication between physician
      manager and, 347*f*, 347–348
   integrating roles of physician and, 332
Office manager structure, 347, 347*f*
Office space, leasing, reservation price and, 304,
      305
Ogilvy, David, 278
Ohio State University, 227
"One-purpose" test, 386
Online recruiting, for job applicants, 142
Operating costs, general hospital MRI system case, 8
Operating plans, 401
Operational inefficiency, integrated healthcare
      systems and, 340
Opiates, 162
Opportunities, examples of, 265
Opposition, groupthink and dismissal of, 244
Optimizing process, customer needs and, 401
Oregon Sports Medicine, 413
   analyzing departure of one physician from,
      54–55*e*, 57
   case analysis, 50–57
   income statement, revenue analysis, and salary
      calculation, 52–53*e*
   projection calculation worksheet, 56–57*e*
Organizational barriers, breaking down, 398
Organizational goals
   leadership and, 226
   working toward, 227
Organizational integration, 331–354
   structure and, 333–342
Organizational structures, technical systems
      integrated with, 350
Organization charts, 333, 334, 334*f*
Organization integration, 204
   teamwork and, 402–403
Outcomes, first- and second-level, expectancy theory
      and, 247, 249, 250
Outliers, as exceptions, 196
Outpatient ABC analysis of procedures,
      gastroenterology practice, 47, 48–49*e*
Outpatient services, 332, 332*f*
Outside relationships, in point system of job
      evaluation, 223, 223*t*
Outstanding balances, caps on, 94
Overdue accounts
   auditing, 105
   time standards for collection activities and,
      102–103
Overdue patient balances, collecting, 92–96
Overextension, 262

Overtime, 383
  equity and, 185
  unauthorized, preventing, 384
Overwork, 262
Owner's equity, 22, 23e
  negative, 23

**P**

Paid advertisements, 274–278, 279f, 280
Paige, Satchel, 269
Pareto, Vilfredo, 395
Pareto chart, receivables sources in 90+ days, 395,
    395f
Parking, 258
"Parole" evidence, 369
Participation, overcoming resistance and, 241e, 250
Partners
  "divorcing" from, 413
  mutual expectations and, 412–413
Patience, effective selection strategies and, 168
Patient characteristics, electronic media ads and, 277
Patient demand, marketing considerations and, 263
Patient education
  about financial obligations, 87, 89–90
  collection plan (partial) sample, 107
  physician and, 76
Patient intake process, 86–87
  collection plan (partial) sample, 107
Patient payment-file insurance strategy, 90
Patient payment problems, preventing, 92
Patient prepayment strategy, 92
Patients
  collecting from, 83–86
  e-mail correspondence with, 293, 293e
  Internet portal and, 292–293
  market segment development and, 287–289
  physician performance and, 133
  proper termination of, 363
  as referral sources, 285
  self-paying, 74
Payback analysis, 11–12, 14
  MRI facility, 12e
Pay levels, establishing, 187
Payment deals, for patients, 83–84
Pay raises, job performance improvement and, 132
Pay ranges, 199–202, 200t
  for jobs, 186–187
PDSA cycle, for creating short-term wins, 242f
Peer-review process, physician evaluation and, 133
Peers
  employee's perception of equity and, 186
  negotiating with, 303
Pension plans, 207–208

Perfection, examining need for, 414
Performance
  benefits and, 206–208
  general mental ability and, 147
  improving, 132
  incentive plans and, 203–206
  pay range and, 200
  physician compensation and, 210
Performance and skills tests, 158–160
Performance-appraisal interview, personal goals
    based on, 127e
Performance appraisals, 249
  accurate job descriptions and, 111–115
  annual reviews and, 116–117
  collection and, 80
  context of, 109–111
  control and, 50
  costs related to, 110–111
  employee responsibility and, 120–121
  fear and, 398
  feedback and, 115–116
    employees' equity judgments and, 186
  goal setting and, 117–119
  incentive plans and, 204
  job performance level and, 119–120
  pay range and, 200
  process of, 109
  proficiency in, 111
  realistic expectations and, 121
  reasons for development of, 110–111
  revenue collection and, 76
  salary matrix, 201t
  summary, 136
  terminating at-will employees and, 375
  360-degree process for, 123
  typical rating scales in, 131e
Performance evaluation
  data, 128–129
  excerpts, 124–125e
  physician compensation and, 211, 212t, 213
  report, writing of, 123
Performance indexes, variations in, 204
Performance planning, physician compensation and,
    211, 213
Performance standards, 129–130
  functional designs and, 335–336
  typical, 130e
Periodic reviews, 116–117
Persistence, negotiation and, 317
Personal Characteristics Inventory, 170
  section from, 171e
Personal contact, promotion through, 273–274
Personal digital assistants, 343

Personal goals, 250
    internal marketing and, 264–265
    performance-appraisal interview and, 127*e*
Personality disorders, collection and patients with,
    85, 86
Personality factors
    Big 5, 151*e*, 161, 169, 170
    conscientiousness, 148
    job success and, 149
Personal references, 165
Personal responsibility, assuming for, problem
    accounts, 105
Personnel actions, performance appraisals as basis
    for, 110
Personnel decisions, documentation and defending
    legal challenges to, 123
Personnel management process, 114*f*
Personnel management responsibility, 221, 222*t*
Personnel manuals, 375
Perspective, about running a business, 414
Petty cash account, establishing, 71
Phencyclidine, 162
Physical impairments, Americans with Disabilities
    Act and, 381, 382
Physical size and distance, integration and, 343
Physician appraisal process, introduction of, 134–135
Physician compensation, 209–215
    business strategy and performance goals related
        to, 211
    developing plan for, 213–214
    evaluating performance, setting goals, and
        performance planning, 211, 213
    rethinking, 206
    salary + incentive bonus, 214
    salary + market-based incentive, 214–215
    straight salary, 214
Physician evaluation, generic factors, 134*e*
Physician leaders
    aging history database reviewed by, 80
    balancing needs of various constituencies and, 401
    collection plan developed by, 104
    compensation plans and, 183
    continuous quality improvement and, 406–407
    effective, 121
    effective collection and, 74
    financial advisors and, 47, 50
    hiring physicians and, 168
    interviewing job applicants and, 156
    job performance evaluated by, 110–111
    negotiation skills required by, 326
    organizational quality and role of, 408–409
    performance appraisals and immediate feedback
        by, 115

quality improvement and role of, 396
    sound perspectives provided by, 57
    unique position of, in healthcare system, 1–2
    Web site designer and, 298
Physician leadership programs, 226
Physician managers
    collection and role of, 82
    effective communication between office manager
        and, 347*f*, 347–348
    integrating management skills of, 411
    personal challenge faced by, 411
Physician performance
    evaluating, 132–135
    360-degree evaluation form, 135*e*
Physician performance goals, critical, practice
        business strategy and, 211, 212*t*
Physicians
    business expectations and, 414–415
    collection and role of, 76–77, 80–82
    collection roles, problem areas and, 75*e*
    CQI algorithms and, 405, 407
    e-mail guidelines for, 293, 293*e*
    expectations of others and self, 411–414
    goal-setting discussion between business manager
        and, 118–119
    integrating roles of office manager and, 332
    leadership and management of organizations by,
        227
    local, news story with, 283*f*
    malpractice litigation and, 355
    motivation for, 246
    perfectionism and, 414
    retirement plans for, 207
    selecting, 168–170
    selection process directed by, 179
    Web site design and involvement by, 295
Piedmont Hospital (Atlanta), 5
Place, 257, 258, 271
    Internet and, 292–293
Place plans, 259
Point chart, 197
Point evaluation, of two benchmark jobs, 198*t*
Point plans, 191
Point-salary graph, 199*t*
Point system of job evaluation, 217–223
    base pay determined with, 198*t*
    description of, 197–199
    ingenuity, 217, 221*t*
    knowledge, 217, 218*t*
    nonsupervisory responsibility, 217, 219–220*t*
    outside relationships, 223, 223*t*
    personnel management responsibility, 221, 222*t*,
        223

Polygraph tests, 161, 162, 374
Portals, Internet, 292–293
Portfolio of services, analysis of, 7
Positioning organization, 290–291
Positions
    application exercise, 308*f*
    compensating, 187
    interests *vs.*, 307–309
    physician compensation plans and interests *vs.*,
        210–211
    of two adversaries, 309*f*
Positive leniency bias, 127
Postacquisition analysis
    achieving control and, 36, 38–39
    MRI facility after year 1, 37–38*e*
PPOs. *See* Preferred provider organizations
Practice-based cases, leadership ideas in, 226
Practice managers, coded wage and salary survey for
        (direct wages only), 195*e*
Preauthorizations, collection plan (partial) sample,
        107
Precedent, 314
Preferred provider organizations, 82, 258, 332
Pregnancy, discrimination on basis of, 379
Prenumbered checks, cash disbursements for
        practice expenses paid with, 71
Prepaid expenses, 28
Prepayment of fees, 27
Prepayment strategies, 92
Present value, 12–13, 13*t*
    annuities, 14*t*
    lease *vs.* purchase decisions and, 21–22, 21*e*
Press releases
    distribution of, 281
    sample, 281*e*
    writing, 280
Preventive law, 355
Price, 271
Price efficiency, 42
Price relative to quality, 257, 258
Pricing plans, 259
    for a psychiatrist, 272*e*
Principled negotiation, 314
Print layout, Ogilvy's formula for, 278, *279*
Print media, Web site advertising and, 299
Prisoners' dilemma
    as metaphor for negotiation issues, 318–321
    payoff matrix, 319*f*
Privacy, invasion of, 359
Privacy law, integrity tests and, 162
Private practice
    balance sheet for, 22, 23*e*
    cash flow statement for, 26*e*

cash management and collection in, 61–106
    income statement for, 25*e*
Proactive use of financial skills, 1–2
Problem accounts
    detection and timing, 102–103
    detection of, collection plan (partial) sample,
        108
    managing, 104–106
Procedural defense, 366
Processes, total quality management and, 395
Procurement, 5
Product, 257, 258, 271
    Internet and, 293–294
Product development, customer needs and, 401
Production quotas, quality and, 399
Productivity problems, pay dissatisfaction and, 183
Product plans, 259
    for a psychiatrist, 271*e*
Professional associations, wage-and-salary data
        through, 192
Professional employees
    Fair Labor Standards Act and definition of, 384*e*
    selecting, 168–170
Professional positions, filling, 148
Professional skills, internal marketing and,
        263–264
Professional standards, 314
Profit, quality and, 397
Profitability ratios, 34–36
Profit goals, reaching, 11
Profit margin, 35–36
Profit-sharing plans, 208
Pro forma budgets, developing, 264
Projected volume, 42
Projection calculation worksheet, for Oregon Sports
        Medicine, 56–57*e*
Promotion, 257, 258, 271, 273–286
    Internet and, 292
    local ethical standards and, 261
    paid advertisements, 274–278, 279*f*, 280
    performance appraisals as basis for, 110
    personal contact, 273–274
    to referring physicians, 285–286
    selection and development systems and, 346
    successful, 284–285
    unpaid advertisements, 280–284
    validity of, 379
Promotion plans, 259
    for a psychiatrist, 271–272*e*
Proprietary compensation plans, 184
Proximate cause
    malpractice and, 363, 364–365
    negligence and, 361

Psychiatric practice, case example: collection report data, 100–102
Psychiatrists
marketing plan for, 271*e*
price plan for, 272*e*
product plan for, 271*e*
promotion plan for, 271–272*e*
Psychographic segmentation, market segments and, 288*e*, 289
Psychological tests, 160
business manager applicant, 172
physician selection and, 169, 170
Public policy, contracts and violation of, 368–369
PV. *See* Present value

**Q**

QA. *See* Quality assurance
QC1, 401
QC2, 402
QC3, 402
QC4, 402
QI. *See* Quality improvement
Qualitative data, performance evaluations and, 129
Quality
of employees, 143
leadership and, 230
leading meetings and, 243
paramount concern about, 393
price relative to, 257
profit and, 397
Quality assurance, 340
Quality buyers, 289, 291
Quality control, 400
Quality improvement, 393–409, 400
higher quality and lower costs in dialysis case analysis, 405–408
break down barriers, 408
drive out fear, 407–408
physician leadership, 406–407
scientific method, 405–406
as ongoing process, 398
Six Sigma and, 404–405
teamwork: core of TQM and organization integration, 402–403
total quality management concepts and, 394–402
Quality management, 411
Quality planning, 400
meeting customer needs and, 400–401
Quality problems, 395
Quantitative data, performance evaluations and, 128–129
Question Mark phase, in Boston Consulting Group strategies, 268*e*, 269

Quick assets, 34
Quick ratio, 33
*Quid pro quo* sexual harassment, 380

**R**

Race
equal employment opportunity and, 170
prohibiting discrimination on basis of, 376
Radio
advertising, 274, 275*e*, 276–278, 283
Web site advertising and, 299
Radioimmunoassay tests, 162, 163
Radio programs
appearing on, 280
pointers for personal appearances on, 282
"Railroading," preventing, 346
Raises
for employees at top of pay range, 201
performance appraisals as basis for, 110
Ranking job evaluation method, 190
limitations with, 197–199
Rapid cycle improvement, 242, 350, 401
Rating forms, 130–132
Rating scales, typical, performance appraisal, 131*e*
Ratio analysis, 33
Ratios
analysis of, 33
current, 33
liquidity, 33–34
profitability, 34–36
quick, 33
solvency, 34
uses for, 33, 36
Readability, of Web sites, 295
Reading evaluations, 136
Realistic job previews, 167
Rebates, 386
Receipts, cash flow statement, 26*e*
Receptionist, order in waiting room and, 362
Reciprocity, 314
Recognition, performance appraisals and, 110
Record-keeping functions, keeping physical handling of cash separate from phases of, 70–71
Record-keeping requirements, Fair Labor Standards Act, 385*e*
Recruiting, job applicants, 138, 141–143
Recruitment, high applicant scores and, 147
Recurrent treatment patients, patient education and, 89
Red circling, of jobs, 196
References and recommendations, 165, 166–167, 168–169, 180*e*
business manager applicant, 172, 175

References and recommendations (*continued*)
    providing, guidelines for, 360–361
    for Web site designer, 295
Referrals, 273, 369, 391
    database maintenance for, 286
    Stark Law and, 386–387
Referring physicians, promoting to, 285–286
Registering domain name, 299
Regression analysis, point evaluation and, 198–199
Rehabilitation Act of 1973, 382
Rejected claims, examining, 100
Relative market share, Boston Consulting Group
    strategies and, 268, 268*e*
Relative Value Units, 213
Relevant ranges
    of fixed costs, 3
    imaging, 4*f*
Religion
    equal employment opportunity and, 170
    prohibiting discrimination on basis of, 376
Renal Physicians Association, 405
Rent, 40
    mixed costs and, 6
Reporters, responding quickly to, 282
Reporting, five Ws of, 280
Reports, financial statements, accounting statements
    and, 22–36
Reservation, adversary and, 305
Reservation prices, 306*f*
    interests *vs.* positions and, 307
    negotiating, 304
    negotiation dance and, 307
Residency, national uniform standards of, 363
Resignations, 209
*res ipsa loquitur,* 365
Resistance, 247, 249, 250
    to change, 237–238
        overcoming, 240, 241*e*
Resistors, change process and engagement of, 240,
    241*e*
Respect, decision making with, 350
Restructuring jobs, job performance improvement
    and, 132
Résumés, 138, 147, 158, 166, 180*e*
    of business manager applicant, 172
        disguised, 173*e*
    classifying, 166
    evaluating, 156–157
    screening, newspaper advertising and, 141
Retained earnings, 22, 31
Retaliation, negotiating situations and, 320–321
Retirement plans, 206, 207

equity and, 185
    judgments and, 367
Return on investment, 34–35
Return on total investment, 35
Revenue analysis, for Oregon Sports Medicine,
    52–53*e*
Revenue and procedure database report, 65–66, 66*e*
Revenue collection, as evaluation factor, 76
Revenue-generated figures, 65
Revenue-generating employees, dealing with those
    serving against their will, 372–373
Revenue projections, for general hospital MRI
    system case, 8
Revenues
    accrued, 27
    cost of long-term assets and generation of, 28
    deferred, 27
    increasing, turnaround strategy and, 270
    net income and, 24
    wage and salary survey data used to relate salary
        to, 214, 215*f*
Revocation of offers, 368
Reward component, in equity equations, 185
RIA tests. *See* Radioimmunoassay tests
Rich media, 299, 301*n*
ROI. *See* Return on investment
ROI-T. *See* Return on total investment
Run charts, 395, 396
    of receivables in 90+ days, *397*
Rutherford, Ernie, 405, 406, 407, 408, 409
RVUs. *See* Relative Value Units

**S**

Safari, 295
Safe harbor provision, 386
Safety equipment, properly located and maintained,
    362
Salami slicing tactic, 311
Salaries, 6, 31. *See also* Compensation plans; Equity
    benefit points based on, 207
    equal, for physician compensation, 214
    equitable, 184
        and issues other than, 185–186
    equity and, 185
    general hospital MRI system case, 8
    group practice budget, 40
    incentive bonus plus, for physician compensation,
        214
    market-based incentive plus, for physician
        compensation, 214–215
    net income and, 35
    physician, 206

Salary and benefits, business manager applicant, 173, 174, 179

Salary calculation, for Oregon Sports Medicine, 52–53*e*

Salary costs
   fixed costs and, 4
   imaging, 4*f*

Salary matrix, 200
   performance appraisal, 201*t*

Salary ranges, informing job applicant about, 167

Sashkin, M., 395

Satellite locations, 258

Scatter diagrams, 395

Schein, Edgar, 349

Schmidt, Frank, 147, 148, 149, 161, 163, 165

Scientific judgment, 314

Scientific method
   continuous quality improvement and, 405
   TQM method and, 403

Scott, J., 262

Scurvy, 237

Search engines, 295, 299

Second-level outcomes, expectancy theory and, 247, 249, 250

Selection and development systems, integration and, 346

Selection design services, 155

Selection failure, case application, 179

Selection methods
   hiring a business manager, 172–179
   research on validity of, 147–148

Selection procedures, 147–149, 151, 153–155

Selection process, steps in, 138

Selection rates, disparate impact and, 377

Selection ratios, 143, 144, 146

Selection sequencing, example of, 166, 167*e*

Selection strategy
   design of, 168
   implementing, 165–168

Self-evaluations, 121, 122*e*
   physician appraisal process and, 134

Self-improvement, encouraging, 399

Self-interest, 316, 317, 333, 413
   interests *vs.* positions and, 307
   negotiation and protection of, 304
   organizational integration and, 331

Self-knowledge, negotiation and, 304–305, 326

Self-paying patients, 74

Selling, marketing *vs.,* 257

Seniority, 202
   merit and, 201
   pay range and, 200

Sensitivity analysis, 10–11

Service buyers, 289

Services portfolio, analysis of, 7

Set term, 370

Sexual discrimination, 379

Sexual harassment, 359, 379–381

Sexual jokes, 380

Sharf, J. C., 378

Shewart, Walter A., 394, 396

Short-term financial and cash control, 2

Short-term projects, integrating around, 350

Short-term wins, obtaining, 242

Sick leave, 206, 207

Simpson, O. J., 357

Situational analysis, 259, 259*e*, 260, 300

Situational approach to leadership, 228

Six Sigma, 393, 394, 399, 404, 409

Size
   of market segment, 290
   Web site, 298

Skill, taking pride in, 399

Slander, 360

Slogans, eliminating, 398

Small claims court, process in, 96–97

Small practice structures, 347–350
   integrating acquisitions, 349–350

Social class, medical treatment and, 289

Social environment, marketing plan and, 260

Socialization standards, integrity tests and, 161

Socioeconomic status, chronicity of health problems and, 289

Solvency, 33

Solvency ratio, 34

Sorted aging report, 78

Sorting aging analysis (abridged), 78–79*e*

Source suppliers, best, identifying, 397–398

Specialty practices, growth of, 333

Special variance, 400

Speeches, 258

Sponsored Web site links, 299–300

Spreadsheet analysis, for private practice, 30*e*

SRs. *See* Selection ratios

Staffing, part-time, 6

Standard deviation, of value of performance for managerial and professional jobs, 144

Standards of care
   breach of, 362
   national uniform standards of, 363

Standards of practice, 414

Stark Law, 386–388, 391
   coverage under, 387*e*

Stars phase, in Boston Consulting Group strategies, 268*e*, 269

State employment commissions, wage-and-salary
    data through, 192
Statements, reports, and systems, 2
Static budgets, 42
Status, equity and, 185
Statutory law, 356
Stealing, 161
Strengths, examples of, 265–266
Strengths, weaknesses, opportunities, and threats
    analysis. *See* SWOT analysis
Structure, 333–342
    divisional, 333
    functional, 333
    matrix, 333, 338*f*, 338–342
    office manager, 347, 347*f*
Structured interviews, 149, 153
    business manager applicant, questions and
        responses to, 175, 176–178*e*
    characteristics of, 151
    elements measured in, 153–155
    physician selection and, 169
    questions and response categories, 154*e*
    training for, 156
    value system and, 154–155
Suboptimization, 331, 346, 401, 402
Subordinate performance, downgrading, 128
Subordinates
    annual review of, 116–117
    effective leaders and developing skills and abilities
        of, 229
    negotiating with, 303
    performance appraisal of, 136
Substantive defenses, against malpractice, 365
Success, changing probabilities of, 249
Successful leaders, characteristics of, 227
Superiors, negotiating with, 303
Supervisors, job-analysis performed by, 139
Suspending patients, 94
Sutter Health (California), 5
SWOT analysis, 259, 259*e*, 265–266, 271, 292, 300

**T**

Tardiness, pay dissatisfaction and, 183
Target analysis, 7, 10
Target marketing, 289
    adoption of, 286–287
Team building, 399
Team Competence factor, 233*t*, 234*t*, 235
Team effort, effective collection and, 74, 76
Teams, change-implementation, 239
Technical jobs, filling, 148
Technical schools, recruiting at, 143

Technical systems, integration of, within
    organizational cultures, 350
Telephone
    as collection tool, 94
    expenses, 40
    steps for collection administrator to follow on,
        95–96
Telephone interviews
    business manager applicant, 172, 174
        format and evaluation, 174*e*
Telephone skills, assessing, 164
Television
    advertising, 262, 274, 275*e*, 276–278, 283, 291,
        292
    infomercials, 258
    Web site advertising and, 299
Television programs
    appearing on, 280
    pointers for personal appearances on, 282
Television stations, press releases sent to, 281–282
Termination
    of at-will employees, 374
    of offers, 368
    of patients, 94
    preserving at-will options and, 375
    proper, 363
    of staff, problem accounts and, 105
    of treatments, 85
Termination clauses in employment contracts,
    wording of, 371
Termination decisions, performance appraisals as
    basis for, 110
Termination provisions, 372
Tertiary hospital services, 332, *332*
Testing, 180*e*
    design and conducting of, 155–156
    drug, 162–163
Testing companies, 155
Test publishers, selected, and potentially useful tests
    for practical selection, 160*e*
Tests, 147
    honesty/integrity, 161–162
    lie detector, 161
    performance and skills, 158–160
    psychological, 160, 169, 170, 172
    word-processing, 163–164
Texas Heart Institute, 266
Thanking referral physicians, 286
Theft
    daily activity by provider and deterrence of, 62
    deterring and identifying, 61
    gross receipts report and deterrence of, 63

integrity testing and reduction in, 161
lower revenues and, 66
Thin-layer chromatography, 162
Thirteenth Amendment, 376
Threats, examples of, 265
Time-driven model, leader participation model and, 234*t*
Timeliness
leadership and, 229, 230
leading meetings and, 243
Timeouts, 317
Time standards, for collection activities, 102–103
Time value of money, 12–15
Timing, media coverage and, 282
Tit for Tat, 319–320
TLC. *See* Thin-layer chromatography
Tone of voice, negotiation and, 321
Tortfeasors, 357
fear and actions of, 358
Tort law, seeking recovery under, 356
Torts, 355
classification of, 358
defined, 357
employment, 378
intentional, 358–361
negligence, 361–362
Total quality management, 352, 393, 394–402
collection process and, 77, 80
teamwork and, 402–430
*Toussaint v. Blue Cross and Blue Shield of Michigan,* 374
TQM. *See* Total quality management
Trade associations, wage-and-salary data through, 192
Trade libel, 359
Tradition, 314
Training
in filing procedures, 99
job performance improvement and, 132
performance appraisals and, 110
total quality management and, 398, 403
Transferred patients, fees on collections for, 369
Transportation problems, marketing plan and, 261
Tray fee, 58*n*
Treatment protocols, developing, 401
Triaging accounts, 105
"Triangling," collection, personality disordered patients and, 85, 86
Trust, 249
integrative situations and, 320
Tunnel information architecture, 297, 298*f*
Turnaround marketing strategy, 270–271
Turnover, pay dissatisfaction and, 183

**U**

UCL (upper control limit) line, in control chart, 394, 394*f*
Uniform Resource Locators, 299
United Family Practices, Ltd., 226, 228, 229, 230, 235, 236, 238, 239, 240, 242, 243, 245, 349
board-level issues, 255
finances of, 253
hiring of administrator for, 253
implementing changes at, 254–255
physician-staff reporting relationships at, 253–254
reservations about structure of, 254
United States system of laws, *356*
Unpaid advertisements, 280–284
Urgency, change process, and creation of, 239
Urine testing, 162
URLs. *See* Uniform Resource Locators
Ury, W., 313, 314, 317
Utility formula, application of, for employment method, 144

**V**

Vacations, 206
equity and, 185
mandatory, deterring cash diversion schemes and, 72
Valence, expectancy theory and, 247
Validity, 143–144
incremental, 147, 161, 165
of work samples, 163
Value buyers, 289
Variability, total quality management and, 394
Variable costs, 3, 5–6, 11
controlling, 5–6
examples of, 5
Verbal contracts, enforceability of, 369
Verbal language, negotiating and, 310
Verbal skills, evaluating job applicants on, 148–149
Verifications, collection plan (partial) sample, 107
Video, 292, 299
Web sites and, 295
"Virtual" groups, 388
"Virtual rounds" on patients, 262
Vision, 225, 247, 249, 250
change process and development of, 239–240
leadership and, 226
Vision correction surgery, 266
*Vogue,* 288
Volume, 7
actual, 42
equipment acquisition analysis and, 18

Volume (*continued*)
   fixed costs and, 4–5
   low costs and, 266
   MRI facility postacquisition analysis and, 39
   projected, 42
Voluntary action, of tortfeasor, 357
Volunteering, to write columns for local
      newspapers/newsletters, 280
Vroom, Victor, 229, 230, 231

**W**

Wage-and-hour law, 383
Wage-and-salary surveys, 214, 215
   benchmark information through, 192
   data from, used as starting point, 195
   data from, used to relate salary to revenue, 214,
     *215*
   Medical Group Management Association, 213
Wages payable, 33
Waiting room, toys eliminated from, 362
Walk-ins, patient education and, 89
*Wall Street Journal,* 393
Wal-Mart, 263, 267
"War on drugs," 260
Warrant by mail, 96
Warrant in debt, obtaining, 96
Washington Hospital Center, segment directed
      display ad using modified Ogilvy format,
      278, 279*f*
*Washingtonian Magazine,* 278
Weaknesses, examples of, 265
Web crawlers, 299
Web host, 299
   finding, 299
WebMD, 294
Web site designer, identifying, 295
Web sites, 258
   architecture level of design for, 295–298
   designing, 294–298

   developing, 291
   flexibility and, 297
   place and, 292
   promotion via, 292
   size and bandwidth issues for, 298
Weisner, W. H., 153
Welch, Jack, 228
WiFi access, 292
Wins, short-term, obtaining, 242, 242*f*
Wireless reception, 292
Wonderlic, E. F., 155
Wonderlic Personnel Test, 148
   cover page, 150*e*
   description of, 149*e*
Woodall, John, 237
Word-of-mouth recruiting, 141
   business manager applicant, 172
Word-processing tests, 163
Working conditions, equity and, 185
Work samples, 148, 153, 163–165, 180*e*
   business manager applicant, 172, 175
   constructing, 163–164
   physician selection and, 169
   résumés as, 156–157
Work smart, problem accounts and, 105
Write-off reports, physician manager and
      examination of, 73
Written contracts, 369
Wrongful discharge, 380

**Y**

Yahoo!, 295, 299
Yellow Pages advertising, 276

**Z**

Zero-sum-game, 309, 310
ZIP codes, market segments and, 286
Zone of agreement, 306*f*, 306–307